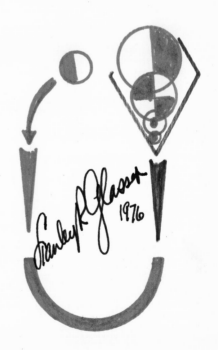

Ovum Transport
and
Fertility Regulation

Ovum Transport
and
Fertility Regulation

Proceedings of a Meeting of the
Task Force on Methods for the Regulation of Ovum Transport
organized by
the World Health Organization
and held at the Lutcher Conference Center of the
University of Texas, San Antonio
on 23–27 June 1975

EDITED BY

M. J. K. Harper
WHO, Geneva, Switzerland

C. J. Pauerstein
San Antonio, USA

C. E. Adams
Cambridge, UK

E. M. Coutinho
Bahia, Brazil

H. B. Croxatto
Santiago, Chile

D. M. Paton
Edmonton, Canada

PUBLISHED BY

Scriptor

Copenhagen

1976

Authors alone are responsible for the views
expressed in the Proceedings.
The mention of specific companies or of
certain manufacturers' products does not imply
that they are endorsed or recommended by the
World Health Organization
in preference to others of a similar nature
that are not mentioned.

A limited number of copies of this publication
are available for distribution from
The Human Reproduction Unit,
World Health Organization,
1211 Geneva 27, Switzerland.

Printed in Denmark
by Bogtrykkeriet Forum
Copenhagen

ISBN 87-87473-07-0

Contents

List of Participants

Dr. C. E. Adams
Agricultural Research Council
Unit of Reproductive Physiology
and Biochemistry
Cambridge, England

Dr. I. Aref
Department of Obstetrics & Gynecology
and Human Reproduction Research Unit
Al-Azhar University School of Medicine
Darrasa-Cairo, Egypt

Dr. J. P. Bennett
Syntex (US), Inc.
Palo Alto, California, USA

Dr. K. J. Betteridge
Physiology Section
Health of Animals Branch
Animal Diseases Research Institute
Ottawa, Ontario, Canada

Dr. G. Bialy
Contraceptive Development Branch
Center for Population Research
National Institute of Child Health
and Human Development
Bethesda, Maryland, USA

Dr. D. L. Black
Department of Animal Physiology
Laboratory for Reproductive Physiology
Paige Laboratory
Amherst, Massachusetts, USA

Dr. W. D. Blair
Department of Obstetrics & Gynecology
The University of Alabama in Birmingham
Birmingham, Alabama, USA

Dr. R. J. Blandau
Department of Biological Structure
University of Washington
School of Medicine
Seattle, Washington, USA

Dr. J. Brundin
Department of Obstetrics & Gynecology
Karolinska Institute
Danderyds Hospital
Danderyd, Sweden

Dr. M. C. Chang
The Worcester Foundation
for Experimental Biology
Shrewsbury, Massachusetts, USA

Dr. M. L. Chatkoff
Department of Obstetrics & Gynecology
and Biochemistry
Center for Research and Training in
Reproductive Biology
The University of Texas Health
Science Center
San Antonio, Texas, USA

Dr. S. Cheviakoff
Centro de Estudios en Biologia
de la Reproduccion
Universidad de Chile
Santiago, Chile

11

Dr. E. M. Coutinho
Department of Maternal Health
and Child Care
Maternidade Climerio de Oliveira
Universidade Federal da Bahia
Salvador, Bahia, Brazil

Mr. R. Crosby
Department of Obstetrics & Gynecology
Center for Research and Training in
Reproductive Biology
The University of Texas Health
Science Center
San Antonio, Texas, USA

Dr. H. B. Croxatto
Departmento de Fisologia y Embriologia
Instituto de Ciencias Biologias
Universidad Catolica de Chile
Santiago, Chile

Dr. E. E. Daniel
Department of Pharmacology
The University of Alberta
Edmonton, Alberta, Canada

Dr. J. Diaz
Departmento de Fisologia y Embriologia
Instituto de Ciencias Biologias
Universidad Catolica de Chile
Santiago, Chile

Dr. M. Doteuchi
Shionogi Research Laboratory
Shionogi & Company, Ltd.
Osaka, Japan

Dr. C. A. Eddy
Department of Obstetrics & Gynecology
and Physiology
Center for Research and Training in
Reproductive Biology
The University of Texas Health
Science Center
San Antonio, Texas, USA

Dr. E. Fromm
Department of Biological Sciences
Drexel University
Philadelphia, Pennsylvania, USA

Dr. B. Fuentealba
Departmento de Fisologia y Embriologia
Instituto de Ciencias Biologias
Universidad Catolica de Chile
Santiago, Chile

Dr. G. S. Greenwald
Department of Obstetrics & Gynecology
and Anatomy
University of Kansas Medical Center
Kansas City, Kansas, USA

Dr. E. Guiloff
Department of Obstetrics & Gynecology
Jose-Joaquin Aguirre Hospital
University of Chile
Santiago, Chile

Dr. E. S. E. Hafez
Department of Gynecology-Obstetrics
and Physiology
Wayne State University
School of Medicine
Detroit, Michigan, USA

Dr. B. J. Hodgson
Department of Obstetrics & Gynecology
and Pharmacology
Center for Research and Training in
Reproductive Biology
The University of Texas Health
Science Center
San Antonio, Texas, USA

Dr. G. R. Howe
Laboratory for Reproductive Physiology
Paige Laboratory
University of Massachusetts
Amherst, Massachusetts, USA

Dr. K. Humphrey
18 Lennox Street
Gordon, Sydney, Australia

Dr. A. Ibarra-Polo
Department of Obstetrics & Gynecology
Jose-Joaquin Aguirre Hospital
University of Chile
Santiago, Chile

Dr. J. N. Karkun
Division of Endocrinology
Central Drug Research Institute
Lucknow, India

Dr. D. Kennedy
Department of Medical Science
Neurosciences Section
Brown University
Providence, Rhode Island, USA

Dr. H. Koester
Department of Obstetrics & Gynecology
Staedtische Frauenklinik
Dortmund, Federal Republic of Germany

Dr. D. Kraemer
Department of Veterinary Physiology
and Pharmacology
Texas A & M University
College of Veterinary Medicine
College Station, Texas, USA

Dr. H. Maia
Department of Obstetrics & Gynecology
Maternidade Climerio de Oliveira
Universidade Federal da Bahia
Salvador, Bahia, Brazil

Dr. H. Maia, Jr.
Department of Obstetrics & Gynecology
Maternidade Climerio de Oliveira
Universidade Federal da Bahia
Salvador, Bahia, Brazil

Dr. J. M. Marshall
Department of Medical Science
Neurosciences Section
Brown University
Providence, Rhode Island, USA

Dr. A. H. Moawad
Department of Physiology
Karolinska Institutet
Stockholm, Sweden

Dr. T. S. Nelsen
Department of Surgery
Stanford University School of Medicine
Stanford, California, USA

Dr. C. Owman
Department of Histology
University of Lund
Lund, Sweden

Dr. D. M. Paton
Department of Pharmacology
University of Alberta
Edmonton, Alberta, Canada

Dr. C. J. Pauerstein
Department of Obstetrics & Gynecology
and Physiology
Center for Research and Training in
Reproductive Biology
The University of Texas Health
Science Center
San Antonio, Texas, USA

Dr. J. P. Polidoro
Division of Pharmacology
Ortho Research Foundation
Raritan, New Jersey, USA

Dr. C. H. Spilman
Fertility Research
The Upjohn Company
Kalamazoo, Michigan, USA

Dr. A. Talo
Department of Zoology
University of Turku
Turku, Finland

Dr. C. H. Van Nierkerk
Department of Human and
Animal Physiology
University of Stellenbosch
Stellenbosch, South Africa

Dr. M. I. Vargas
Department of Obstetrics & Gynecology
Center for Research and Training in
Reproductive Biology
The University of Texas Health
Science Center
San Antonio, Texas, USA

Dr. P. Verdugo
Department of Bioengineering
University of Washington
School of Medicine
Seattle, Washington, USA

WHO SECRETARIAT

Dr. M. J. K. Harper
Human Reproduction Unit
World Health Organization
Geneva, Switzerland

THE QUEST FOR A CONTRACEPTIVE METHOD FOR THE REGULATION OF OVUM TRANSPORT

In 1972, the World Health Organization launched a major research programme directed toward development of safe, acceptable, and effective methods for the regulation of human fertility.

Although presently available methods are considerably advanced over past methods, they remain relatively crude, and fail to meet the varied requirements of consumers and services in different countries, particularly developing ones. For these reasons, what has become known as the WHO Expanded Programme of Research, Development, and Research Training in Human Reproduction aims at improvement of existing methods of fertility regulation, assessment of their suitability in different populations, and development of new technology.

A major portion of the research effort is conducted by multidisciplinary, multinational collaborative Task Forces working in priority areas identified by the Advisory Group to the Expanded Programme. Initially, a review of the state of knowledge current in the particular field is made, and various approaches to the development of new methods of fertility control are discussed: a strategic plan is then developed that includes definition of short-term, intermediate, and long-term objectives. The steps by which the objectives can be achieved and initial estimates of the time and costs involved are identified. After approval by WHO, scientists who can make contributions to the research are invited to participate. All research projects are assessed on technical and ethical grounds by the Task Force and by an independent Review Group; those that are approved are supported by WHO.

The Advisory Group made the following statement at a meeting in January, 1972:

"It has been repeatedly shown, mainly in animal studies, that post-ovulatory fertility control can be achieved by interference with ovum transport in the Fallopian tube, and by altering implantation mechanisms in the uterus by non-steroidal and steroidal compounds. Accordingly a Task Force which included research on the reproductive processes involved, on pharmacological models, on contraceptive screening, and on clinical work where feasible in this area, could accelerate the development of post-ovulatory anti-fertility agents for human use. More specifically, such a Task Force would concern itself with components such as: (a) tubal events, e. g. ovum transport and development, and the hormonal, metabolic and pharmacodynamic milieu in which these events occur; (b) the uterine events, particularly around the time following implantation; e. g. development and differentiation of the blastocyst and the hormonal, metabolic (enzymatic, osmotic and ionic) and haemodynamic changes in the endometrium related to the implantation of the blastocyst; (c) compound synthesis based on research on tubal and uterine events and systematic "structure" activity relationship studies, for animal screening of potential post-ovulatory fertility regulating agents; and (d) clinical pharmacological studies where possible."

As a result the first meeting of a Task Force on Methods to Regulate Ovum Transport and Implantation was held in March, 1972, in Geneva. At this meeting, 11 scientists from 7 countries, and 4 members of WHO secretariat met to prepare a plan of action for the Task Force.

The group emphasized goal-oriented clinical problems, and recognized that chances of obtaining applicable results from existing animal models were remote. However, pertinent animal studies, especially in cases where human experimentation was not possible, were considered profitable.

Priority research areas were identified under three broad headings: (1) regulation of implantation, (2) regulation of events in the oviduct, and (3) intravaginal delivery systems for release of microdose progestins and other agents. This last area was considered a priority area by the participants in this meeting, although it was recognized that the mode of action of such a system could be not only on ovum transport and implantation, but also on sperm transport in the female reproductive tract.

With specific respect to the regulation of events in the oviduct, the following recommendations were made:

"The objective of this Task Force group is to develop a variety of fertility regulating agents and methods which interfere with fertilization and/or transport of the fertilized ovum.

Fertility regulation may be achieved by interference with the transport and metabolism of the fertilized ovum in the oviduct. However, there is insufficient knowledge concerning the factors that control normal oviductal motility and ovum transport. It is proposed to obtain information on such factors in untreated women and in women using various drugs for post-coital contraception. It is also proposed to recover the fertilized human ovum from the uterine cavity and to estimate the time required for this transport under normal cir-

16

cumstances as well as under the influence of steroidal contraceptives. These studies should be viewed together with others, in which the biochemical characteristics of the human oviductal fluid will be studied.

It has been suggested that post-coital drugs may interfere with ovum transport and/or implantation and clinical studies are proposed to replace the presently used emergency treatment which consists of the administration of rather toxic doses of estrogens with another method consisting of the administration of various progestins. There is a special need for the development of a new method of fertility regulation in women who are only infrequently exposed to the danger of unwanted pregnancy and the studies proposed would center on the needs of a group of women with low and irregular frequency of intercourse (say 4 or 5 per month). It is undesirable that such women should be exposed to contraceptive steroids on a continuous day to day basis."

These proposals were presented to the Advisory Group in June, 1972. After due consideration the Advisory Group recommended splitting this Task Force into two new Task Forces: (a) Methods for the Regulation of Ovum Transport and (b) Methods for the Regulation of Implantation. The proposed plan of action outlined above for studies concerning the regulation of ovum transport was also approved. As a consequence proposals to initiate the required research were solicited from appropriate experts and a second meeting of the newly constituted Task Force was held in September, 1972 to review these proposals. Eight scientists from 6 countries participated. Although it was felt that "Methods for the Regulation of Ovum Transport" was a less than perfect name for this Task Force, since such processes as ovum pickup, ovum transport, ovum retention at the uterotubal junction, ovum release from the oviduct, and ovum survival ought to be taken into account the name was retained for administrative purposes.

Following an extensive discussion of methods and compounds which could affect these processes, five areas of research were identified and rated for priorities. These areas and their ratings in descending order of importance were: occlusion of the oviduct (chemical/electrocoagulation), post-coital progestins, human ovum transport model, basic studies on human oviductal fluid, and basic studies on human oviductal motility. A strategic diagram showing the relationships of the research to be undertaken by the Task Force was then constructed (A, B, and C represent short term applied and D long term basic studies) (See page 18).

It was recognized that the proposals solicited up to this point heavily emphasized short term applied research and development; therefore the group recommended that another planning meeting should be held inviting representatives of disciplines not so far represented in this Task Force, e. g. bioengineer, biophysicist, steroid chemist, anatomist, ovum nutritionist, to develop new proposals in the area of human oviductal physiology and biochemistry.

17

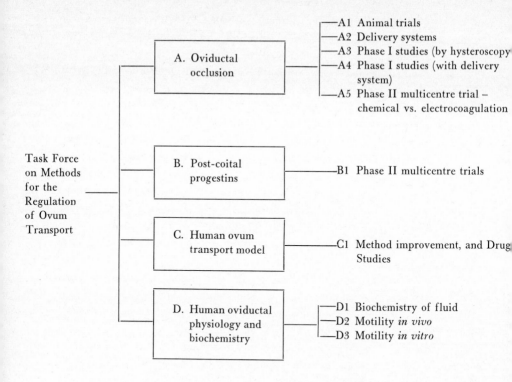

This proposal led to the Third Meeting of the Task Force (the first concerned solely with "Control of Human Oviduct Function") in Geneva in March, 1973. Eleven scientists from six countries attended this meeting. They agreed that if a contraceptive agent which acted by interfering with oviductal function could be found, alternate schedules of dosage or methods of delivery could be devised. Thus it was not necessary to envisage the objectives of this Task Force as limited to the development of a post-coital contraceptive. This view point was reinforced by a discussion which followed the presentation of a background paper on "Post-coital Contraception" which was pessimistic about this possibility. This paper has since been published (Shearman R. P., 1973, Post-coital contraception. A Review. *Contraception 1*, 459–476).

The objective of the Task Force was re-defined as follows: to develop a contraceptive method that acts through interference with ovum transport and/or development. Each major area of intervention was considered and a list of questions that needed to be answered before the objective could be reached were defined. Experiments were then outlined to seek answers to these questions. In most cases sequential steps of investigation were involved.

A. OVUM TRANSPORT IN THE HUMAN: METHOD IMPROVEMENT AND DRUG STUDIES/MOTILITY

Objective:

To interfere with ovum transport so that normal ovum development is prevented.

Questions:

The questions that require answers were defined as follows:

A1. What is the normal rate of ovum transport in women?

A2. Does interference with ovum transport in women reduce fertility?

A3. If A2 is true, how can we influence the rate?

A4. Do changes in motility affect transport rate and if so, how?

A5. What are the limitations of telemetry, as a tool for tracking ovum transport?

A6. Are all the smooth muscle fibres of the oviduct innervated, and how are contractions propagated?

A7. Is there any correlation between presence of the ovum and contraction or relaxation of the local oviductal segment?

A8. Do the number and/or activity of cilia in the oviduct change throughout the menstrual cycle? If so, are these changes hormonally controlled?

Plan of action

A1. *Determination of normal rate of ovum transport.*

This will be examined in human subjects and in sub-human primates. The time of ovulation will be determined by basal body temperature and LH assays. The ova will be localized in the genital tract by flushing or freeze-clearing.

A2. *Pharmacological modification of ovum transport.*

Can we influence rate of transport?

Using the information gained in A1., studies will be carried out in sub-human primates and in women with agents known to interfere with oviductal transport in laboratory animals, e. g. estrogens, progesterone, adrenergic agents (reversible α-blockade with phentolamine), and other compounds to be identified.

19

2*

A3. *Does altered rate of ovum transport interfere with fertility?*

This step is dependent upon being able to (1) measure ovum transport and (2) alter the rate of transport, and therefore would only follow steps A1. and A2. This question should be examined initially in sub-human primates using menstrual bleeding and assays of chorionic gonadotrophin as criteria for failure of conception.

A4. *Correlation of rate of ovum transport and motility.*

(a) Using knowledge obtained in A1. and A2. measurements of oviductal motility will be made in sub-human primates and women with agents known to influence transport (A2.) and those known to affect motility, e. g. ergot derivatives, ethanol, adrenergic agonists and β-stimulating agents. Experiments will also be performed to test the possibility of altering motility (and thus transport, provided initial experiments are favourable) with alternating electrical fields.

(b) The methods to be used for measuring motility should be compared with each other and the results evaluated in the light of the previous body of knowledge. Since studies of many of these agents have been done already in rabbits, experiments involving transducer evaluation and also radiotelemetric techniques could initially be done in this species more cheaply than in sub-human primates.

A5. *Factors influencing motility.*

This step is needed in order to develop in a rational manner further agents that affect motility. Questions that arise are:

1. What is the effect of the sympathetic innervation and how is this influenced by the menstrual cycle?

2. What are the characteristics of the α- and β-adrenergic receptors?

3. What is the relationship of electrical to mechanical events and how can this be modified?

Methods to be used would include: for electrical events, extracellular recording methods; and for mechanical events, catheters and strain gauges. There should also, at this stage, be studies of nerve-muscle relationships using electron-microscopy and histochemistry.

A6. *Determination of role of cilia in ovum transport.*

Assessment of the role of cilia is dependent upon considerable information about the mechanism of ciliary action(i. e. how do cilia beat, etc.). If ciliary action can be specifically interrupted (e. g. by nicotine), then their role could be assessed by studying ovum transport rates using methodology developed in A1.

A7. and A8. These questions were felt to have lower priority and therefore no research was planned until the more important questions had been addressed.

B. BIOCHEMISTRY OF FLUID AND TISSUE

There was some interest in the idea of collection of human oviductal fluid and its circulation to various collaborating biochemists for intensive analysis. However, until the group obtained good evidence that altered oviductal transport would influence fertility and that oviductal fluid provided essential substances for ovum development, they felt that such a project should not be initiated because of the low prospects of early success.

C. OVUM DEVELOPMENT

Objective

The viability of the ovum in the oviduct may be altered by changing essential processes required for its maintenance. The aim is to determine whether these processes are under hormonal control and then to develop means of altering this by pharmacological methods.

Questions

that require answers were defined as follows:

C1. a. Is there any specific component of oviductal fluid that is important for development of the ovum?

b. Is the oviductal environment necessary for ovum development (presence of or absence of component)?

c. Does the oviductal environment become noxious at a later stage (after the end of normal transport period)?

C2. How easy is it to fertilize and culture human ova *in vitro*?

C3. Can oviductal fluid be changed in composition so as to kill ova, e. g. by interference with circulation or secretion so that secretion stops?

C4. Does ectopic pregnancy occur in a discernible percentage of cases in sub-human primates? Can any such species be used as a model for the human?

Plan of action

To determine whether eggs will develop in non-synchronous oviducts and uteri. It is proposed to:

C1. Place fertilized ova in oviducts and uteri of castrate females; place fertilized ova in oviducts and uteri of castrate females stimulated with estrogen or progesterone or both in combination; place fertilized ova in oviducts and uteri in abnormal positions in normal cycling animals. These experiments will be performed in mice and rabbits. Some ova will be left in the test situation and others removed after various periods of time (12, 24 and 48 h) in the unnatural environment and retransferred to normal synchronous pseudopregnant recipients. The survival and cleavage rate of the ova will be determined.

C2. and C3. Research to answer these questions was left in abeyance until the answers to question C1. were obtained.

C4. It is also proposed to survey zoos and primate breeding laboratories to obtain more exact information on the incidence of extrauterine pregnancies in sub-human primates. It is also proposed to initiate experiments to attempt to induce oviductal pregnancies in sub-human primates.

Justification and future plans

If the ova develop in these abnormal or neutral environments or after exposure to such environments it will considerably decrease the urgency of further studies related to the definition of oviductal contents and secretions, because the importance of the oviduct for ovum development will obviously be minimal.

If the ova do not develop or development is retarded, additional studies will then be justified including:

(a) repeating the above experiments in a sub-human primate.

(b) cultivation of ova in fluid from the reproductive tract at different stages of development.

(c) mechanism of active secretion in the human oviduct.

(d) ultrastructure of the human oviduct as related to secretory function.

(e) characterization of human oviductal secretion, and relevant changes induced by hormones and pharmacological agents.

(f) characterization of steroid receptors in human oviductal tissue.

Following this Third and then the Fourth (San Antonio, September, 1973) Task Force meetings and Review group approval, a major portion of the Task Force supported research necessary to answer these questions began during 1973. Subsequent Task Force meetings have been held in Geneva, March, 1974; Bahia, September, 1974; and Geneva, February, 1975; the present one in San Antonio constitutes the Eighth in the series.

During informal discussion at the Fifth meeting in Geneva in March, 1974, one of us (CJP) suggested that it was an appropriate time to review the progress of work in the field. As a result, he solicited review papers from selected authorities in the field. Ten papers were submitted for publication in December, 1974, and appeared in print in June, 1975 (Pauerstein C. J. (ed.), 1975, Seminar on tubal physiology and biochemistry, *Gynecol. Invest. 6*, 101–264). The enthusiastic response of investigators and Task Force members to this initiative, and the quality of the manuscripts received encouraged the Task Force to plan a symposium on a broader scale and with the opportunity for personal interaction between the participants. In addition, scientists who had participated in the development of the Task Force plans outlined above, were obviously only a portion of those active in the field. Consequently at the Bahia meeting, September, 1974, it was decided to organize this Symposium in order to review as comprehensively as possible present knowledge concerning oviductal physiology and biochemistry and to determine whether Task Force supported research had answered any of the questions originally posed in 1973. To this end, 46 scientists from 15 countries gathered at the Lutcher Conference Center of the University of Texas in San Antonio on June 23–27, 1975. Many of these scientists had not previously participated in Task Force meetings, and therefore could provide fresh objective views on the regulation of ovum transport. Formal reports were presented on each of the five mornings of the meeting, and are printed in full. The morning sessions were moderated by recognized authorities in the designated areas. With the exception of the first session, each topic was discussed by two moderators. Although some overlap was inevitable, we hoped that different perspectives of the same subject might prove stimulating.

Afternoon sessions, except for one formal paper each on Thursday and Friday afternoons, were devoted to informal discussion. The participants were divided into 6 groups for this purpose. Each group was led by a member of the Steering Committee and after full discussion of the morning sessions, each group prepared a concensus report of their views concentrating on the following points: A. Summary of current knowledge; B. What needs to be established to achieve methods of contraception interfering with ovum transport; C. Experiments necessary to achieve this objective; and where applicable, D. Assessment of the feasibility and cost of such approaches.

A member of the Steering Committee was responsible for amalgamating the six documents prepared in each afternoon session into one composite statement. The purpose of this exercise was to establish different views on the same problem which would lead to fresh insights and approaches. These assignments were: Session 1 – "Biophysical and Bioengineering Considerations in Studies of Oviductal Physiology", Dr. Pauerstein; Session 2 – "Oviductal Contractility", Dr. Coutinho; Session 3 – "Autonomic Mechanisms in Ovum Transport", Dr. Paton; Session 4 – "Control of Ovum Transport in the Oviduct", Dr. Adams; and Session 5 – "Effects of Estrogen and Progesterone on Contractility and Ovum Transport", Dr. Croxatto.

Each member of the Steering Committee also did the initial editing of the formal papers presented on his assigned day. The final editing was done by us. We believe that the information contained in this volume supports our conclusion that many of the queries posed in March of 1973 have now been answered. We hope that the reader will concur. In the final paper we have attempted to indicate the directions for future research considered in the light of present knowledge and the objectives of the Task Force.

San Antonio, Texas, June, 1975.

M. J. K. Harper, Ph. D.   *C. J. Pauerstein,* M. D.

SECTION I

Biophysical and
Bioengineering Considerations
in Studies of
Oviductal Physiology

MODERATOR

R. J. BLANDAU

The Center for Research and Training in Reproductive Biology
and Voluntary Regulation of Fertility
and the Department of Obstetrics and Gynecology,
The University of Texas Health Science Center at San Antonio,
7703 Floyd Curl Drive, San Antonio, Texas, 78284

A BIOPHYSICAL MODEL OF THE MECHANISMS REGULATING OVUM TRANSPORT RATES

By

Marvin L. Chatkoff

ABSTRACT

A mathematical hydrodynamic model which partially simulates fluid bolus formation in the lumen of the oviductal isthmus was investigated. Using pressure-strain relationships measured in the rabbit isthmus, bolus length was found to be a sensitive function of luminal pressure developed by the musculature. For pressures exceeding 15 mgHg the lumen was found to be forced open throughout its length, however short closed boluses with diameter approximating natural ova could be formed. Differing segments of oviduct yield different boluses because of variability in wall compliance. Lighthill's theory of pressure forcing of pellets suggests particle velocities substantially less than Poiseuille models. Lighthill's principal velocity clearance and resistance parameters for a steady state pressure differential were evaluated as 0.6×10^{-5}, -0.4, and 400 respectively. These values are consistent with a slow propulsion and high resistance model. Relative isthmic traversal time as a function of ovum or particle diameter was estimated and compared to the available experimental evidence. Factors which limit the velocity for very small and very large spheres were also investigated.

A number of mechanisms have been suggested as determinants of ovum transport rates including ciliary stream formation, secretion flow effects, and contractile effects with or without hydrodynamic forces. It appears that the relative contributions from each of these force mechanisms depends on the location of the ova within the duct. A clear distinction can be made between mechanisms

27

of propulsion in the ampulla and the isthmus. Several factors lead to this conclusion. First the lumen of the ampulla is large relative to the ovum diameter and therefore wall effects except as transmitted through the oviductal fluids should be less important than in the isthmus. In the isthmus on the other hand, the ovum diameter is greater than the resting or non pressurized lumen diameter and the ovum must be forced forward against the resistance of the luminal walls. Secondly the gate at the ampullary-isthmic junction, and a possible second gate near the uterine junction, has profound effects on transport through the isthmus. In a recent publication (Chatkoff 1975), experimental evidence concerning ovum transport was reviewed and contrasted with the motions predicted by several theoretical models. It is clear that simplistic models cannot account for the complex dynamics exhibited by ova in their journey through the oviduct. Any realistic model must consider properties of the oviduct, its fluid contents and the ovum. In particular it was suggested that the elastic properties of the isthmic walls were a significant controlling element of ovum velocity (the time of transport). In artificial but revealing experiments with surrogates this property limits the maximum particle size capable of being transported (Pauerstein et al. 1975). It was also suggested that the oviductal junctions, in addition to functioning as time delaying gates, may influence the motion of ova during their course through the isthmus by placing boundary conditions on fluid motion.

An attempt was made to accommodate the commonly held concept that oviductal peristalsis is the predominant mechanism of isthmic transport (Brundin 1964). It was shown, however, that simple peristaltic pumping alone could not account for the observed motions partly because of the low pressure gradients generated. However, there is little evidence for continuous elastic waves with multiple and periodic pressure amplitudes. Extensions of the theory of simple peristaltic behaviour to a single bolus of fluid created by and propagated through muscular contractile activity appears to be capable of partly accounting for transport properties. Fluid motion of this type was first analyzed by Fung (1971). The analysis was based on the concept of a contractile wave, but unlike simple peristaltic motion the active region was limited to a single small segment of the tube. In this way a single bolus of fluid was propagated. The bolus could either be open or closed depending on conditions within the tube. Reflux flow, defined as sucking in fluid at the leading edge of the bolus and expelling it at the trailing edge, is also possible in this model. Although the model was constructed for the ureter, it also appears applicable to isthmus provided that the oviduct is free of obstruction. In the case of a closed bolus in which reflux does not occur, the analysis remains valid for obstructions in the lumen by ova provided they are not in the region of the bolus. When an ovum is introduced into the lumen, additional complications result. It is known that the resting luminal diameter in the rabbit is less than that of an ovum (mucin coated or not) and therefore the ovum acts as a localized plug. This suggests a controlling role for the ovum dependent on its physical properties especially its compliance and diameter. In a qualitative sense the theory may be described as the forcing of ova through a narrow lumen by localized pressure forces. The beginnings of such a theory have been explored for steady state differences between the upstream and downstream pressures in ideal tubes (Lighthill 1968; Fitz-Gerald 1969, 1972). In this theory the fit between the particle, or in our case the ovum, and the oviduct determines the dynamics. As the luminal pressure rises, pressure gradients develop across the ovum and at the same time, the lumen distends and the ovum distorts by amounts depending on their elastic properties. If the local pressure is high the ovum is transported and leak back flow develops providing a lubricating effect. Therefore the ovum is not viewed as a passive object carried along by a stream of fluid. This complex theory involves stress-strain relationships in the mucosa, the musculature and the ova; the contractile behaviour of the musculature including the contractile amplitude, the propagation velocity, and the propagation direction and frequency; the spatial distribution of contractile pulses; fluid properties especially the viscosity; and surface properties of the ova and walls. At present, sufficient experimental data is not available to warrant a complete simulation of the proposed mechanism. However, recent measurements of static stress-strain relationships in the inactive isthmic walls allow a limited application of the theoretical methods (Talo 1975). Fluid bolus formation can be analysed and interpreted in terms of the oviductal geometry. Preliminary evaluation of this model system is presented in this paper.

ANALYSIS

Evaluation of distensions of the isthmic lumen due to pressure gradients created by a moving contractile wave

Bolus formation theory which totally ignores contributions from particles in the luminal fluid, relates the strain induced in the walls of non-contracting segments to the tension (pressure) generated in adjacent active contracting regions (Fung 1971). In the actively contracting region the relationship between stress developed and muscular geometry is determined from Hill's equation (Hill 1938) and a sliding element model for the smooth muscles in the wall. Force-velocity measurements have yet to be accomplished for oviductal smooth muscle and therefore the portion of the theory dealing with active muscle presently cannot be evaluated without arbitrary assignment of constants. On the other hand, preliminary stress-strain relationships have been measured for 8 segments of rabbit oviduct by Talo (1975). Because the dynamic behaviour of the so called passive segment is uninfluenced by assumptions about the

29

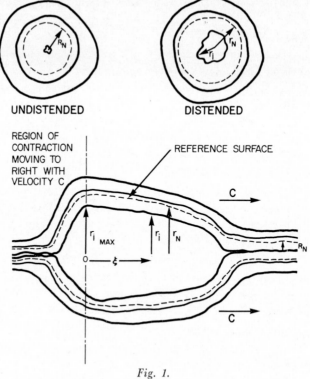

UNDISTENDED   DISTENDED

REGION OF
CONTRACTION
MOVING TO
RIGHT WITH
VELOCITY C

REFERENCE SURFACE

Fig. 1.

Coordinate definitions and bolus geometry in the isthmus of the oviduct.
The reference surface is arbitrarily located.

behaviour of the active musculature, except through boundary conditions imposed on the pressure at the active-passive interface, the solution in the passive region may be evaluated separately. The geometrical definitions of isthmic coordinates are presented in Fig. 1. For mathematical convenience but with some loss in accuracy, the elastic material is considered to be concentrated in a neutral surface. This concept, borrowed from the theory of beam bending, assumes that there is a transition neutral surface between regions of tension and compression. The location of the neutral surface need not be explicitly defined at the moment. The coordinate ξ measured downstream from the instantaneous position of maximum luminal diameter, moves with the bolus at velocity c. The fluid velocity within the bolus is a function of position within the bolus and is different from the bolus propagation velocity c. From Stoke's equation the fluid velocity can be shown to be parabolically distributed across the lumen with a maximum velocity on the axis. This distribution is independent of bolus formation and is a consequence of the no slip condition at the wall imposed by the viscosity. If reflux flow is prevented by conditions within

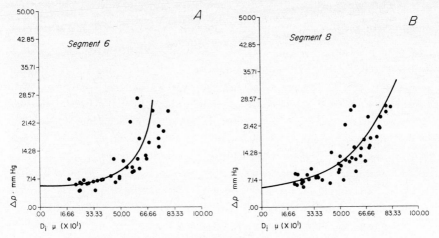

Fig. 2.
Luminal pressure-strain relationships in the rabbit isthmus (from Talo 1975).
Exponential curves were fitted to the data. The curves are defined in the text
and the parameter values given in Table 1.
A. Segment 6 of the isthmus.
B. Segment 8 of the isthmus.

the oviduct, then the maximum fluid velocity is equal to 2c at the maximum
radius $r_{i\ max}$.

In the oviduct the stress-strain relationship is complicated by the presence
of two distinct tissue types with differing rheological properties. The thick
mucosal layer has a different compliance than the thinner walled muscular layer.
Anatomical studies have shown that the ratio of outer mucosal radius to the
thickness of the muscular layer varies from approximately 2.5 at the ampullary junction to 1.5 proximal to the uterus (Talo 1975). This change in elastic
properties along the isthmus (Fig. 2) implies that the bolus of fluid will change
its diameter and shape as it travels.

Fung (1967, 1970) has shown that the stress-strain relationship in soft tissues
can often be approximated by a differential expression for the tension T of
the form

$$\frac{dT}{dr_N} = \frac{\alpha_1}{R_N} (T + \beta_1) \tag{1}$$

in which α_1 and β_1 are empirically fitted constants. This expression suggests
that the rate at which stress is developed with respect to strain is a linear
function of the stress. Equation (1) yields an exponential relationship between
stress and strain:

$$T = (T^* + \beta_1)e^{\alpha_1 \left(\frac{r_N}{R_N} - \lambda^*_1\right)} - \beta_1 \tag{2}$$

31

The integration constants T^* and λ^*_1 are evaluated as follows. T^* is the value of the stress T when $\dfrac{r_N}{R_N} = \lambda^*_1$. In the reference state $r_N/R_N = 1$ and the tension essentially vanishes defining λ^*_1. α_1 can be evaluated from the slope of Equation (1) and β_1 is the vertical intercept of dT/dr_N. Using the relationship of Equation (2), Stoke's equations and the equation of fluid continuity, equations were derived expressing the luminal pressure as a function of the displacement of the reference surface (4). In addition the reference surface was related to the longitudinal displacement ξ defined in Fig. 1. In the original derivation of bolus formation the wall was assumed to be composed of homogeneous muscular tissue for which it was natural to take a cylindrical sheet at half the maximum radius as the reference surface. In the oviductal isthmus non-homogeneity makes a rational choice of neutral surface difficult because the soft mucosa is approximately twice the thickness of the musculature. Thus an arbitrary assumption that the reference surface is at half maximum radius would put the reference surface in the mucosa. To circumvent this difficulty the equations were recast in terms of the luminal radius r_i rather than r_N. This may be accomplished as follows. The relationship between fluid pressure and stress is given by the Laplace relationship

$$\Delta p = T/r_U \tag{3}$$

in which Δp is the pressure difference across the neutral surface and is approximately the difference in pressure between the lumen and the peritoneal cavity. If the tension is describable by an exponential function of the reference radius r_N then the first derivative of pressure with respect to r_N is given by Fung (1971) as

$$\frac{d\Delta p}{dr_N} = \left(\frac{\alpha_1}{R_N} - \frac{1}{r_N}\right)\Delta p + \frac{\alpha_1 \beta_1}{R_N r_N} \tag{4}$$

The change in the longitudinal coordinate $\xi = x - ct$ with respect to the radial coordinate r_N in a passive or non-contracting segment of the oviduct is

$$\frac{d\xi}{dr_N} = \frac{1}{N}\left[\left(\frac{\alpha_1}{R_N} - \frac{1}{r_N}\right)T + \frac{\alpha_1}{R_N}\beta_1\right] \tag{5}$$

where

$$N = \frac{-16c\mu}{k^2 r_N}\ln\frac{k r_N}{A} \text{ and } k = (1 - R^2_N/r^2_N)^{1/2}.$$

The quantity in square brackets in Equation (5) is therefore expressible in terms of the rate of change of pressure and the radius of the neutral surface

$$\frac{d\xi}{dr_N} = \frac{r_N}{N}\frac{d\Delta p}{dr_N}$$

or in terms of r_i

32

$$\frac{d\xi}{dr_i} = \frac{r_N}{N} \frac{d\Delta p}{dr_i} \tag{6}$$

where

$$\frac{r_N}{N} = \frac{-k^2 r^2_N}{16c\mu \ln\left(\dfrac{kr_N}{A}\right)} \tag{7}$$

But because $kr_N = r_i$ and if reflux is prevented, the integration constant A is given by

$$A = r_{i\,max}\, e^{-1/2} \tag{8}$$

then

$$\frac{r_N}{N} = \frac{-r^2_i}{16c\mu\left[\ln\left(\dfrac{r_i}{r_{i\,max}}\right)+1/2\right]} \tag{9}$$

Thus $d\xi/dr_i$ may be expressed solely in terms of r_i and the choice of reference surface need not explicitly be made. Experimentally r_i is determined as a function of Δp, and the derivative on the right of Equation (6) can be evaluated directly from the data without recourse to explicit evaluation of the constants in Equation (2). Therefore for any radial deformation $r_{i\,max}$ caused by contractile activity in an adjacent segment of the oviduct, the deformation of the oviduct ahead of the contraction can be determined from (6) using (9) and the experimentally determined values for $\dfrac{d\Delta p}{dr_i}$. Once r_i is determined for each value of ξ the pressure at each ξ value can be determined from the experimental Δp versus r_i curve. In this way bolus behaviour may be calculated for any initial value of $r_{i\,max}$ and the luminal pressure at that radius. These initial values are proportional to the strength of the contractile activity.

Pressure-forcing of compliant particles through narrow elastic tubes

In the study of red cell motion through narrow capillaries, a theory of pressure-forcing of tightly fitting pellets has been proposed (5). This theory is applicable whenever the clearance between the pellet and the walls is small whether positive or negative. Negative clearance is defined for particles larger in diameter than the lumen at the downstream value of the pressure and is particularly applicable to ova in the isthmus. The theory is derived from the axisymmetric Navier-Stokes equation and the equation of fluid continuity; these are the same equations that determine bolus formation except that particle plugging effects are specifically accounted for. Flow past the pellet is assumed to take place and this flow acts as a lubricant. The analysis for mathematical simplicity is confined to a thin cylindrical film between the pellet and the wall and is a linearized theory. As the film thickness becomes large, *i. e.* the lumen distension increases, the theory extrapolates to Poiseuille flow, a theory which describes flow velocity profiles of a viscous fluid in a cylindrical tube. Therefore this theory appears capable of combination with bolus theory by replacing the steady state upstream and downstream pressures in pressure-forcing theory with the time variable pressures calculated for a moving bolus. The theoretical extension however, is very complex. In the interim the present pressure-forcing theory solutions are revealing. The solutions as described in terms of a non-dimensional parameter (L) (Lighthill 1968) given by

$$L = \frac{6\mu U \, (\alpha + \beta)}{(2Q/U)^{5/2} \, K^{1/2}} \tag{10}$$

where α and β are the compliances of the tube and pellet respectively, μ is the fluid viscosity, U is the pellet viscosity, K is the curvature of the deformed pellet and $2\pi r_0 Q$ is the rate of leakback of fluid past the pellet at the maximum radius r_0. For $L < 3.2$ the pellet clearance is positive. For ova in the isthmus the clearance is negative except for very large luminal pressures. Three principal parameters defined by Lighthill (1968) which describe the complex solutions are: the velocity parameter

$$A = \mu U \, (\alpha + \beta)/r^2_0 \, (Kr_0)^{1/2} \tag{11}$$

which measures velocity on a scale dependent on the fluid viscosity, the geometry and the elastic constants; the clearance parameter

$$B = (\alpha + \beta) \, [p(\infty) - p(O)] \, /r_0; \tag{12}$$

and the resistance parameter

$$D = [p_i(-\infty) - p(\infty)] \, r_0(Kr_0)^{1/2} \tag{13}$$

These quantities were evaluated for estimated values of isthmic geometry and pressures.

RESULTS

In the computed and plotted solutions, for definitiveness an arbitrary assumption was made that the bolus moves along the oviduct in either direction with a velocity of 1 cm/sec. This represents no loss in generality because the longitudinal coordinate ξ is inversely proportional to the velocity, that is the bolus will be elongated for smaller propagation velocities and compacted for the faster ones. At the limit when the velocity becomes very small, the lumen is distended throughout its length in both directions from the contracted segment.

By not explicitly modeling the dynamic properties of the musculature, complete solutions of the equations of motion cannot be obtained but are limited to the passive segment. As pointed out by Fung (1971) however, the active

34

region is only a small percentage of the total bolus length (on the order of 1 %). The active segment varies in length as a function of the maximum contractile velocity defined by Hill's equation. However, it is not the radial distension in the active region which is troublesome, but the computational observation that muscular activity forces the luminal pressure to be out of phase with the radial displacement, that is the peak pressure occurs at values of ξ upstream of the peak radial displacement. Calculations were made using peak pressure values corresponding to an in-phase relationship between pressure and radial displacement and also for an arbitrarily reduced pressure at half the value predicted from static pressure versus strain measurements. Also for concreteness, luminal pressure versus luminal diameter values measured by Talo corresponding to isthmic segment six in the rabbit were used in the calculation. This segment is the second segment from the ampullary-isthmic junction of 4 equal isthmic segments. Thus the calculations correspond to a region close to, but not at the ampullary-isthmic junction. In this segment the musculature is thinner than at the uterine end of the oviduct. The luminal pressure versus strain relationships for segment 6 and also for segment 8 are given in Fig. 2. An exponential curve of the form

$$\Delta p = \lambda_1 e^{kr_i} + \lambda_2 \tag{14}$$

was fitted to each data set. In Equation (14) r_i is the luminal radius, Δp is the luminal pressure and the constants λ_1, λ_2, and k are evaluated for the experimental data (Table 1). From Equation (14) the derivative $d\Delta p/dr$ was derived (Fig. 3) and used in the computations. The stress-strain curves indicate that the rabbit isthmic lumen is incapable of being expanded beyond 800–1000 μ in diameter by pressures in the physiological range. Thus particles greater in diameter than approximately 1000 μ (allowing for variations between animals) cannot be transported regardless of the conceptual model.

A contraction which results in 50 μ radial displacement of the oviductal lumen creates a bolus of fluid whose longitudinal extension is on the order of 125 μ for a velocity of 1 cm/sec or 1250 μ for a 0.1 cm/sec velocity (Fig. 4 A). Since reflux is prevented by blunt closure of the front end of the bolus at the

Table 1.
Best mathematical fits of the parameters λ_1, λ_2 and k to experimental pressure measurements in segments 6 and 8 of the rabbit oviduct.

Segment	λ_1	λ_2	k
6	0.04	4.96	0.01746
8	1.30	3.70	0.00722

35

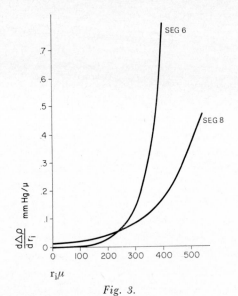

Fig. 3.

First derivates of the fitted curves in Fig. 2 as a function of the luminal radius.

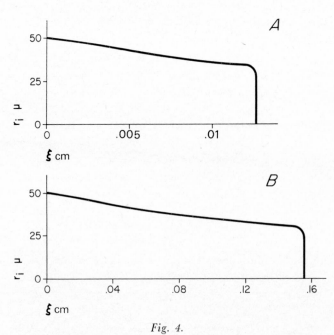

Fig. 4.

Geometric shape of a fluid bolus of maximum radius of 50 μ.
A. Calculated with the pressure-strain curve for segment 6.
B. Calculated with the pressure-strain curve for segment 8.

36

radius A, the presence of a low pressure bolus is not felt by an ovum until it is quite close. Because in the rabbit the diameter of an ovum exceeds 100 μ even prior to the accumulation of mucin coating, a bolus of 50 μ radius will not distend the oviduct sufficiently to free the ovum from contact with the walls. Profiles of boluses with larger radial displacement corresponding to larger pressures are shown in Fig. 5. The larger diameter boluses are elongated and a bolus with a 200 μ radial distention will open the oviductal lumen to its end. A 100 μ bolus at its forward end will just free an uncoated ovum. On the other hand a bolus of approximately 300 μ is needed to free a mucin coated ovum. A luminal radius of 300 μ corresponds to a steady state pressure of 12.5 mmHg for segment 6 of the oviduct. The ovum therefore acts like a luminal plug for all but very large pressure waves. At ratios of bolus diameter to ovum diameter slightly larger than 1, a nozzle effect is created with a corresponding pressure drop across the ovum. As the diameter ratio approaches 1, and the plugging becomes complete, the pressure drop approaches the difference in pressure between the bolus pressure and the downstream pressure. In this region recourse must be made to the theory of propulsion of tightly fitting spheres in narrow cylindrical compliant tubes. Under these conditions, the ovum has profound dynamic effects on the solutions.

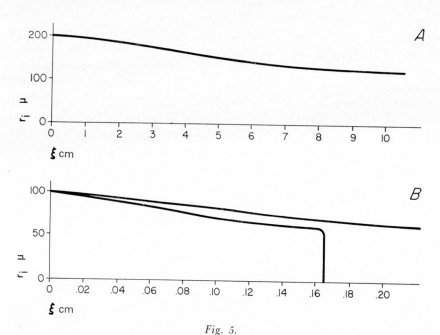

Fig. 5.
Shapes of fluid boluses of (A) 100 μ and (B) 200 μ radius. The shortened curve in B was calculated with half the maximum pressure for 100 μ radial displacement.

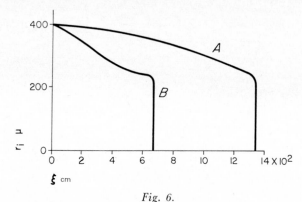

Fig. 6.
Shapes of fluid boluses of 400 μ radius.
A. Calculated with the pressure-strain curve for segment 6.
B. Calculated with the pressure-strain curve for segment 8.

The effect of the dynamic behaviour of the musculature on the luminal pressure and hence the radial displacement is demonstrated in Fig. 5 B. For a 100 μ bolus the reduced pressure at the interface between the active and passive regions causes the bolus to shorten. Of course, the reduced pressure also reduces the ovum velocity.

All of the above solutions were calculated using the elastic properties of segment 6 of the rabbit oviduct. For contrast calculations were also performed with the stress-strain data for segment 8 (Fig. 4 B). The 50 μ bolus is lengthened considerably for segment 8 data. This result is a consequence of the greater $d\Delta p/dr_i$ at the lower values of r_i (Fig. 3) and may reflect nothing more than inaccuracy in the measurement. On the other hand, there clearly is a significant difference in $d\Delta p/dr_i$ between segments 6 and 8 at a large luminal radius. For example at a 400 μ radius, segment 8 data yields a much shorter bolus (Fig. 6).

Lighthill's constants A, B and D (Lighthill 1968) were evaluated for rabbit oviductal geometry. Because the present form of the theory is limited to a linear stress-strain relationship, a drastic linearization of the exponential-like stress-strain curves had to be made. Nevertheless the calculated estimates for $A = 0.6 \times 10^{-5}$, $B = -0.4$ and $D = 400$ for a 1 cm/sec propagation velocity indicates how dramatically the plugging effect alters the solution. In particular, the resistance parameter which has a value of 16 for Poiseuille flow (viscosity of 0.01 poise) increases to 400 for the pressure-forcing- condition. The inverse relationship between resistance and velocity implies higher resistances for the lower velocities of larger diameter particles. Because for spherical particles Kr_0 is 1 the resistance increases linearly with the radius of the pellet, whereas the velocity parameter decreases with the square of the particle radius. Thus

38

large particles should travel considerably more slowly than smaller ones. Experiments in our laboratories indicate a definitely decreasing velocity for ovum surrogates of increasing size. In estimating the average isthmic velocity for surrogates of various sizes from position-time data, the ampullary delay time must be subtracted. In the small number of experiments run to date, the data suggests that the velocity may be more nearly inverse with the radius than inverse square. Because of the large dispersions in the data and the severe assumptions made in the analysis, especially in linearizing the stress-strain relationship, the discrepancies especially for large values are not surprising.

DISCUSSION

Let us consider an ideal pressure measuring instrument placed at some arbitrary location in the lumen of the isthmus: the detector is assumed to affect materially neither the dynamic stress-strain response of the walls nor the contractility of the musculature, and not to change the effective geometry of the lumen by partial obstruction. If a small diameter bolus is formed downstream it will be undetected, or if upstream it may not reach the detector before the active contractile pulse terminates. Therefore the detector may not indicate all contractions. A contraction of large amplitude as we have seen extends for a considerable distance and therefore if upstream of the detector the presence of the bolus will probably be registered. However, as has been demonstrated, the radial displacement downstream is less and the corresponding pressure is lower than at positions close to the active segment and the detector registers a reduced pressure. If a large amplitude contraction travels towards the detector the radial displacement and pressure will rise only modestly for short time intervals. Therefore it can be seen that the detector will exhibit a variable response to contractile activity, recording only those small pulses which are quite near and attenuating large pulses which are remote. Isolated pressure measurements give a distorted picture of true activity. For an ovum within the lumen, if the fit is close a large pressure drop develops across the ovum. Under these circumstances a downstream detector will not record the high upstream pressures.

The methods of calculation presented in this paper are very approximate in that muscle dynamic properties are not included. Fung's model of muscle activity (Fung 1971) is incomplete in that the contractile wave does not incorporate wave initiation dynamics nor does it simulate the finite active period and subsequent relaxation phase. The finite time character of the contractile pulse limits the travel of the bolus and therefore the displacement of ova on which it impinges.

Despite these limitations, the theory appears to have features consistent with experimental observations. Extension of the model may be appropriate after the contractile apparatus of the oviduct is better defined.

REFERENCES

Brundin J. (1964) An occlusive mechanism in the Fallopian tube of the rabbit. *Acta physiol. scand. 61*, 219–227.

Chatkoff M. L. (1975) A biophysicist's view of ovum transport. *Gynecol. Invest. 6*, 105–122.

Fitz-Gerald J. M. (1969) Mechanics of red-cell motion through very narrow capillaries. *Proc. roy. Soc. B 174*, 193–227.

Fitz-Gerald J. M. (1972) The mechanics of capillary blood flow. In: Bergel D. H., ed. *Cardiovascular fluid dynamics*, Vol. 2, pp. 205–239. Academic Press, New York.

Fung Y. C. (1967) Elasticity of soft tissues in simple elongation. *Amer. J. Physiol. 213*, 1532–1544.

Fung Y. C. (1970) Mathematical representation of the mechanical properties of the heart muscle. *J. Biomech. 3*, 381–404.

Fung Y. C. (1971) Peristaltic pumping: A bioengineering model. In: Boyarsky S., Gottschalk C. W., Tanagho E. A. and Zimskin P. D., eds. *Urodynamics*, pp. 177–198. Academic Press, New York.

Hill A. V. (1938) The heat of shortening and the dynamic constants of muscle. *Proc. roy. Soc. B 126*, 136–195.

Lighthill J. L. J. (1968) Pressure-forcing of tightly fitting pellets along fluid-filled elastic tubes. *J. Fluid Mech. 34*, 113–143.

Pauerstein C. J., Hodgson B. J., Young R. J., Chatkoff M. L. and Eddy C. A. (1975) Use of radioactive microspheres for studies of tubal ovum transport. *Amer. J. Obstet. Gynec. 122*, 655–662.

Talo A. (1975) *Functional properties of the oviduct with reference to the transport of ovum in the rabbit*. Reports from the Department of Zoology, Univ. of Turku, No. 5.

Laboratory of Reproductive Biology and Endocrinology,
Department of Obstetrics and Gynecology,
University Station,
University of Alabama in Birmingham,
Birmingham, Alabama 35294, USA

A SYSTEM FOR MEASUREMENT
OF OVIDUCTAL MOTILITY AND CONTRACTILITY AND
CHRONIC CHANGES IN LUMINAL DIAMETER

By

William D. Blair and Lee R. Beck

ABSTRACT

A technique has been developed that permits acute as well as chronic changes in luminal diameter of the oviduct to be measured in unrestrained animals. The fabrication and calibration of small doughnut-shaped intra-luminal Silastic transducers, sensitive to changes in their diameter, is described. A custom developed dual-channel telemetry system permits recordings to be made from unrestrained animals. Data is presented on the application of this system for measuring the effects of various endogenous hormonal changes and exogenous pharmacological agents on oviductal motility. Results are also presented that provide evidence that the isthmus of the rabbit oviduct exhibits a hormonally-induced constriction following HCG-induced ovulation. This constriction is temporal and coincides with the period when ova are known to be retained in the oviduct.

This work was supported by contracts from WHO Expanded Programme and Grant (RF 70097) from Rockefeller Foundation.
Several of the figures and tables have been reprinted from *Fertility and Sterility* with permission of the editor.

41

Contemporary emphasis on applied and basic research to develop new and better methods of contraception has resulted in the emergence of the oviduct as a reproductive organ of primary importance. There is growing evidence that mechanisms controlling gamete transport may be vulnerable to pharmacologic control. The development of new contraceptives that act at the oviductal level to disrupt normal transport is a distinct possibility. New techniques are needed for characterizing parameters of oviductal action that influence ova transport. A clear correlation between measurable parameters of oviductal activity and ova transport would provide a convenient means of screening compounds for potential contraceptive action.

During the last several years reproductive biologists, muscle physiologists, and clinicians have been intrigued with the idea of developing a system for quantitating changes in oviductal activity that could be correlated with gamete transport. Most early approaches relied on visual observation, pressure determination, and muscular electrical activity measurement. It is evident that the application of advanced engineering principles and techniques will be necessary to solve this biological problem. Such interdisciplinary emphasis has resulted in the development of custom-designed transducers to study oviductal motility. This paper concerns the fabrication, calibration, implantation and use of a newly developed transducer telemetric system. This system is unique in that the transducers permit not only the characterization of instantaneous oviductal motility, but also the determination of chronic changes in luminal diameter.

REVIEW OF PREVIOUS TECHNIQUES

A brief review of representative systems for determining oviductal activity will provide a perspective. Valuable information has been gained from several of these techniques and results obtained from them have been used to corroborate data from our newly developed system. Techniques previously employed may be classified in the following categories: (1) perfusion and flow studies; (2) visual observation; (3) measurement of intratubal pressure; (4) recording of muscular electrical activity; and (5) transducer measurement of muscular activity.

Perfusion and flow studies

To obtain an index of the state of contraction of the oviduct, Rubin (1947) recorded the pressure in a catheter inserted into different areas within the lumen of the oviduct. The catheter was perfused with 0.9 % NaCl solution at slow rate from a constant volume pump. Contraction of the oviduct was

42

measured as a resistance to fluid flow. Using the technique developed by Rubin, Davids and Bender (1940) inserted a glass cannula into the uterus. Oviducts were then insufflated with CO_2 delivered under a constant pressure and flow rate. Horton et al. (1965) and Brundin (1965) studied oviductal activity by inserting a polyethylene cannula into the oviduct, using a slow infusion system and a pressure transducer. Longley et al. (1968) made a small incision in the oviduct and inserted a polyethylene cannula. Using a perfusion apparatus muscular activity was measured as a change in resistance to fluid flow.

Visual techniques

Doyle (1954) used a pelviscope to study ovulation and oviductal contractions in the human; Black and Asdell (1958) introduced oil at the ovarian end of the oviduct and watched its movement; whereas Boling and Blandau (1971) used a double-walled chamber placed in the anterior abdominal wall to characterize oviductal motility in rabbits visually.

Measurement of intratubal pressure

The most widely used technique in recent years has been recording of intratubal pressure. Greenwald (1963) inserted a polyethylene catheter filled with physiological saline via the fimbriated end of the rabbit oviduct approximately 2 cm into the ampulla. The ampulla was ligated proximal and distal to the catheter creating a closed cavity within the oviduct. Another catheter was inserted into the contralateral isthmus through an incision in the uterus adjacent to the oviduct. Ligatures were applied to either side of the catheter. The saline filled catheters were connected to strain gauge transducers. Maia and Coutinho (1968) placed fenestrated polyvinyl catheter into the human oviductal lumen during laparotomy. The tip of the catheter was sealed and the fenestrated segment covered by a cylindrical natural rubber tube which was bound to the catheter. The free end of the catheter was taken through the abdominal wall, then filled with water and connected to a pressure transducer. In a follow-up study, Maia and Coutinho (1970) used a fenestrated catheter sheathed by a thin rubber diaphragm 1 cm long. Two catheters approximately 1 cm apart were placed in the lumen of the ampulla. In two patients an additional catheter was placed in the isthmus. Salomy and Harper (1971) used a polyethylene but with a small silicone tubing balloon sealed to it to record oviductal activity in which bubbles accumulated in the catheters, a second catheter was connected to the recording one through a 27 gauge needle to form a closed flushing system which allowed removal of air bubbles from the system. Catheters were inserted through the uterotubal junction (UTJ) into each oviduct. The other end of the catheter was exteriorized in the neck region and connected to pressure transducers. DeMattos and Coutinho (1971) used soft polyvinyl catheters

43

sheathed by a thin natural rubber membrane to study motility in the rabbit oviduct.

Muscular electrical activity of the oviduct

Brundin and Talo (1972) used five small suction electrodes attached along the rabbit's oviduct and correlated their activity with the response measured with a perfusion catheter/pressure system. Larks et al. (1971) implanted platinum electrodes in plastic collars on goat oviducts. The leads were exteriorized and activity was monitored for several days.

Transducer measurement of muscular activity

Maistrello (1971) used medical grade Silastic tubing (0.30 × 0.64 cm) cut to a length of 16 mm and filled with mercury to record motility in the rabbit oviduct. The mercury strain gauge was mounted within a U-shaped apparatus placed around the oviduct and fixed to the abdominal muscles and to a Teflon "button" placed subcutaneously. Hodgson et al. (1973) used an ultrasonic transducer to record oviductal motility in the rabbit. The transducer sensed contractions by measuring the attenuation of phase shift of low level ultrasound transmitted through the muscle. In some cases leads were exteriorized in the neck region and in others the transducer was implanted with a telemetry system. Jeutter et al. (1973) used carbon-doped Silastic as an extraluminal sensing element to record motility. The transducer was constructed from a 0.78 mm diameter conductive Silastic rod with gold plated nickel bands, having copper wire leads attached, crimped snugly about the Silastic material. The resistive Silastic element was pulled into a Silastic or polyethylene tube and the tube sealed. Sutures were tied around the tubes just over the bands and were used to attach the transducer to the oviduct. Duff et al. (1972) described a technique using small inductance coils attached to opposite sides of the oviduct to record motility as a change in mutual conductance between the two coils, whereas Nelsen and Nunn (1972) used miniature solid state force transducers attached to the oviduct to monitor motility.

Most techniques used to characterize muscular activity of the oviduct have severe limitations. Perfusion studies are quite involved and the flow rate can alter the results. These studies may be useful as an indication of overall oviductal activity, but cannot discern localized muscular action. Visual techniques have provided insight into the oviduct's role in gamete transport, but provide qualitative rather than quantitative information.

Intratubal pressure measurements may not sense only localized activity since the recorded pressure could be caused by contractions at points distant from the sensor forcing fluids into the region near the sensor. Gross movement of the oviduct caused by longitudinal muscular activity or contractions of the mesosalpinx could also cause pressure changes in the oviduct.

Recording of electrical activity is an indirect indicator of muscular activity in the oviduct, but could provide useful information if evaluated with a system for detection of isolated muscular activity. With the exception of ultrasonic transducers and the plans for the conductive silicone rubber device, all techniques require that the animal be either restrained or anesthetized.

Carbon-doped Silastic transducers offer the potential to record localized oviductal activity. Attachment to the oviduct could present a problem, and the technique may be subject to artifact from lead movement caused by visceral motility. The mercury-in-Silastic transducers provide good contractile information, but short lifetime and complex implantation techniques limit their utility. The ultrasonic transducer and housing is very elaborate and bulky. Artifact poses a major problem. When data from a mechanical transducer was compared to that from an ultrasonic transducer in isolated tissue, there was ambiguity with regard to contraction direction. Low signal to noise ratio compromises the effectiveness of this device. It is difficult to evaluate the inductance coil technique since no data are available at this writing.

It is obvious that an advanced method is needed to study oviductal activity as it relates to ova transport. Measurement of intraluminal diameter is potentially the most useful parameter to evaluate. Thus, transducers were developed that could be implanted within the oviduct to measure instantaneous perturbation as well as chronic increases or decreases in luminal diameter. A telemetry system has been incorporated with the transducers so that studies can be performed using unrestrained animals.

TRANSDUCER FABRICATION AND CALIBRATION

The most critical link in any instrumentation system is the input transducer. A transducer represents the sense organ for the electrical processing equipment and by its very nature is a highly specialized device theoretically possessing sensitivity to but one form of energy. An input transducer almost always extracts some energy from the measured source. Thus the measured quantity is often disturbed by the act of measurement, making perfect measurement impossible. Good transducers are designed to minimize this effect by reducing interaction between transducer and source.

Unique requirements of an oviductal motility transducer

The oviduct and its environment impose stringent requirements on transducer design. The extremely small size of the oviduct and its structural frailty renders it difficult to subject to instrumentation. A transducer capable of responding to minute changes in luminal diameter during contraction or relaxation must, of necessity, be extremely sensitive and small so as to cause minimal interference with normal oviductal functions.

After investigating several commercially available devices, as well as many custom-made transducers, conductive silicone rubber was selected as the primary material for an oviductal motility transducer. The material used for this transducer is Silastic S-2086 silicone rubber developed by Dow Corning Corporation. Silastic S-2086 is silicone rubber impregnated with carbon to make it conductive. Because it is synthetic rubber, it is very flexible and deformation produces an effect similar to that for strain gauges, *i. e.* as cross-sectional area changes, electrical resistance changes.

The Silastic material is extruded into rods approximately 1.0 mm in diameter (Fig. 1). Rods are embedded in paraffin and sectioned on a microtome to form disc-shaped devices 0.4 mm thick. A 0.5 mm hole is punched through the center

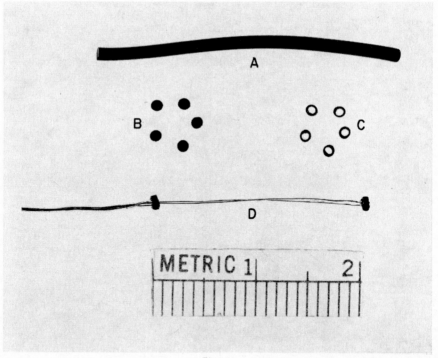

Fig. 1.

Silastic S-2086 extruded into a rod (A). Rods are embedded in paraffin and sectioned into discs (B). Holes are punched through the center to form doughnut-shaped devices (C). Dual transducers with stainless steel leads attached (D).

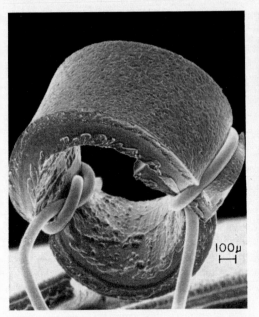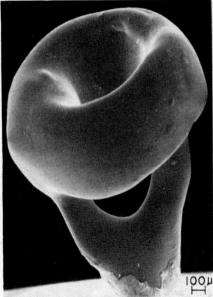

Fig. 2.
Scanning electron micrographs of uncoated and coated transducers with
0.076 mm diameter stainless steel leads.

of the disc to form a doughnut-shaped device. Electrical contact is made to the
conductive Silastic with 0.076 mm Teflon coated stainless steel wire (Fig. 2).
The transducer is then coated with 3 layers of medical grade Silastic. Dual
transducers are made by placing two transducers in tandem with the leads of
the distal transducer passing through the lumen of the proximal transducer.
All leads are placed in medical grade Silastic tubing (0.30 mm I. D. × 0.64 mm
O. D.). For long-term implants the leads are placed in 0.51 × 0.94 tubing filled
along its entire length with medical grade Silastic to prevent lead breakage
due to flexing. Conductive Silastic transducers made by this procedure are
extremely pliable, and the slightest deformation produces a change in electrical
resistance that is directly proportional to the change in diameter of the device.

Transducer calibration

The usefulness of any transducer is questionable unless it can be calibrated
and evaluated prior to actual use. Each transducer is calibrated to determine
static as well as dynamic characteristics. For the dynamic tests, the oviduct is
simulated with 1.02 mm × 2.16 mm Silastic tubing. Since the transducers are
developed to respond to changes in luminal diameter of the oviduct, it is necessary to control the diameter of the tubing to approximate a constriction, or

47

dilation, of the oviduct. The simulator constricts or dilates by applying negative or positive pressure to the tube. Changes in diameter of the tube are monitored by a displacement transducer housed in a test stand and positioned over the tubing at the site of the intraluminal transducer. The device used as a "standard" was a Hewlett-Packard 7DCDT-250 linear variable differential transformer (LVDT) displacement transducer. The low mass transformer core, sensitive to changes in diameter of this tubing, was positioned over the transducer being tested (Fig. 3) and movement produced a voltage output from the LVDT. Comparison of the response obtained by the commercial transducer to that obtained by the Silastic transducer provides a dynamic test for transducer hysteresis, linearity, and response to varying amplitude and frequency excitations (Fig. 4).

For static calibration, transducers are positioned at discrete locations along the inside of tapered glass calibration columns having known inside diameters (Fig. 5). The electrical resistance of the transducer is monitored at multiple stations along the length of the column to determine change in electrical resistance as a function of transducer diameter. This data establishes a calibra-

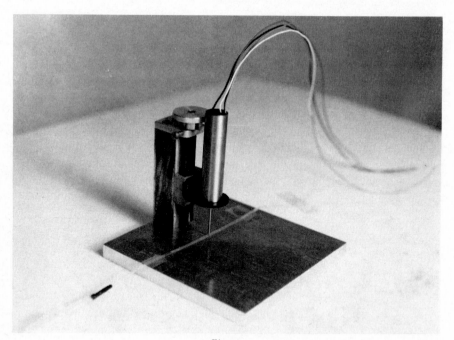

Fig. 3.
Hewlett-Packard 7CDT-250 LVDT transducer mounted on test stand. For dynamic calibration the oviduct is simulated with 1.02 mm × 2.16 mm Silastic tubing. Changes in the diameter of the tube are monitored by the displacement transducer positioned over the tubing at the site of the intraluminal transducer.

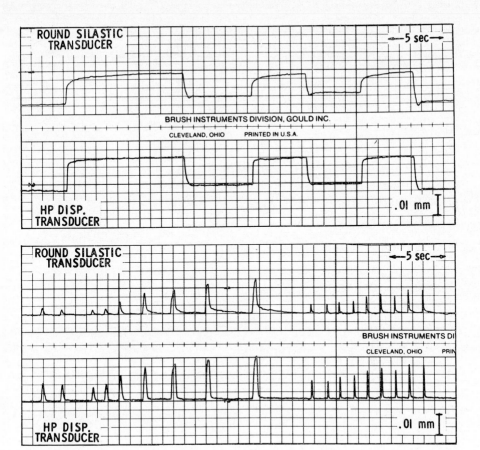

Fig. 4.

Comparison of response by commercial transducer to the intraluminal transducer. Dynamic testing characterizes hysteresis, linearity, and response to varying amplitude and frequency excitation.

tion curve for each transducer (Fig. 6). Only transducers that exhibit a linear response over the diameter range of the oviduct are selected for use. Identical calibration curves result when transducers are moved in either direction through the calibration column.

TELEMETRY SYSTEM

Requirements of an implantable telemetry system

An implantable telemetry system must be sufficiently small as to not disturb the animal physiologically. With the advent of integrated circuits, batteries are by far the largest single component. Low power consumption is therefore

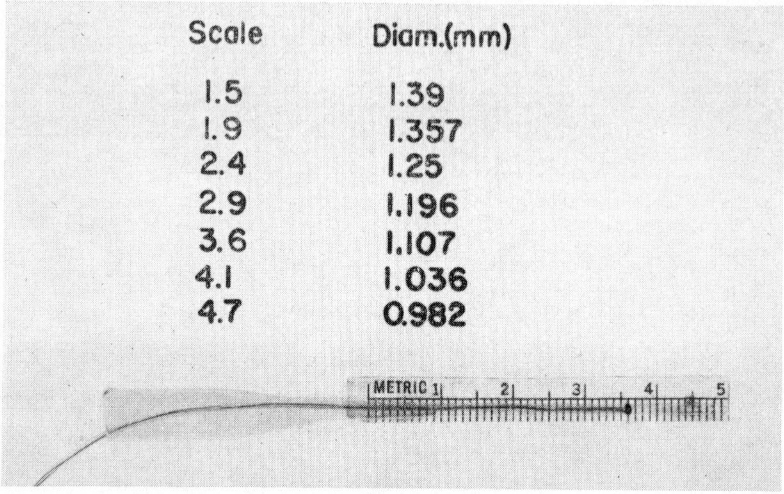

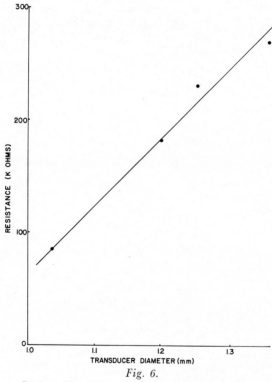

Scale
Diam.(mm)
1.5
1.39
1.9
1.357
2.4
1.25
2.9
1.196
3.6
1.107
4.1
1.036
4.7
0.982
METRIC 1
2
3
4
5

Fig. 5.
Transducer positioned inside tapered glass calibration column. For static calibration electrical resistance of the transducer is monitored at discrete locations within the column.

300
200
100
0
RESISTANCE (K OHMS)
1.0
1.1
1.2
1.3
TRANSDUCER DIAMETER (mm)

Fig. 6.
Static calibration curve for transducer in Fig. 5.

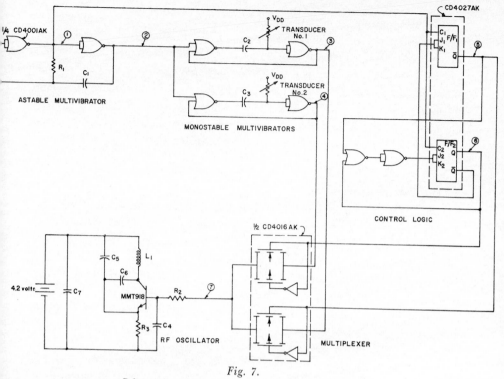

Fig. 7.
Schematic diagram for dual-channel transmitter.

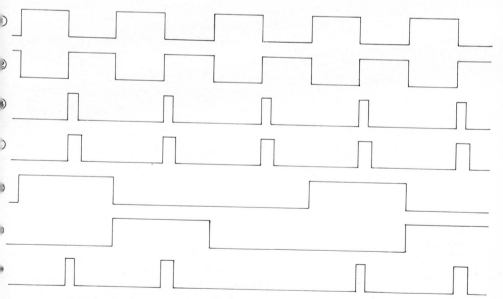

Fig. 8.
Timing diagram for transmitter circuit.

51

an important design requirement since long-term operation where batteries cannot be readily replaced is often essential. For implantation, proper sealing of electronic components is a stringent requirement. Body tissues and fluids present a hostile environment for electronic circuitry since small amounts of moisture can and do cause failure. The material used for sealing must provide adequate protection from moisture but must not react chemically or electro-chemically with the surrounding fluids and tissue. The implantable system must also be compatible for installation by standard surgical techniques.

Dual-channel transmitter

Fig. 7 is a schematic diagram of the dual-channel transmitter that is used for dual transducer studies. A timing diagram simplifies description of its operation (Fig. 8). This system is an outgrowth of an earlier successful single-channel transmitter. The astable in this configuration gates on a monostable for each channel, and also provides an output used as a clock pulse for the control logic. The control logic determines the manner in which the output of each monostable is gated through the bilateral switch multiplexer. From the timing diagram it can be seen that multiplexing produces a repeating series of two pulses followed by a blank. In each case the first pulse after the blank is the output of channel 1 monostable, while the second pulse is the output of channel 2 monostable. The blank pulse is necessary to provide a synchroniza-tion pulse for the demultiplexer. Output of the multiplexer turns the RF oscil-lator on and off. The RF stage used is a grounded-base Colpitts oscillator employing feedback from the collector tank circuit (Blair 1975).

Parameters controlling the frequency of the oscillator, and those controlling pulse duration of the two monostable multivibrators are selected to minimize power consumption of the transmitter. The oscillator is normally designed to operate at approximately 500 Hz. Pulse width of each monostable multivibrator is selected not to exceed 100 μ sec. Since the resistance of the transducer itself and its corresponding capacitor determines this pulse width, the transducer is selected before the capacitor. The proper selection of these components results in an overall low duty cycle. This minimizes on time of the RF oscillator and reduces average current drain. Operating at a supply voltage of 4.2 V, average average current drain of the entire system rarely exceeds 50 μ amps.

The dual-channel system is fabricated using COS/MOS integrated circuits plus necessary discrete components. Batteries are held in place between two pieces of 1/32" circuit board by means of a miniture screw and nut. The coil is constructed from three turns of number 30 wire placed in Silastic tubing. With $C5 = 47$pf, $C6 = 10$pf, the diameter of the coil was adjusted for trans-mitter operation at a frequency between 80 and 110 MHz. The stainless steel transducer leads are connected to the transmitter with conductive epoxy.

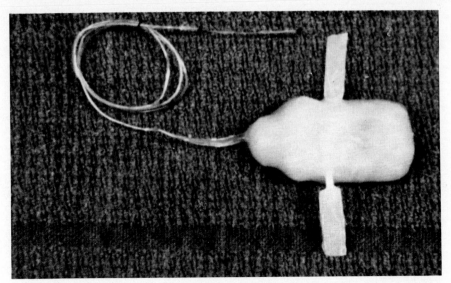

Fig. 9.
Dual-channel transmitter encapsulated with paraffin-beeswax and overcoated
with medical grade Silastic.

The dual-channel transmitter is encapsulated with a paraffin-beeswax mixture followed by an overcoating of medical grade Silastic (Fig. 9). Prior to Silastic outercoating, a narrow strip of 0.018 cm thick Dacron reinforced Silastic sheeting is attached to the transmitter. The strip is later used to suture the transmitter to the abdominal muscle. A thick coat of Silastic is built up around the transducer leads near the point where they leave the transmitter. This is done to reduce the possibility of lead breakage in this region due to flexing from animal respiration. The completed unit is approximately 4 cm × 1.8 cm, occupies a volume of 6 cubic centimeters, and weighs approximately 10 grams.

The transmitter is placed in a "pouch" beneath the skin and sutured to the abdominal muscle. Recordings are made from rabbits housed in a standard metal cage by a custom-designed antenna inside the cage.

Dual-channel demultiplexing

Demultiplexing and signal conditioning circuitry is used to extract data relating to contractile activity of the oviduct from dual-channel implants (Fig. 10). Prior to actual demultiplexing, the demodulated signal is buffered and pulse shaped. The heart of the demultiplexing process is the NE 555 timer used as a missing pulse detector. The output of this timer, after inversion, provides a synchronization pulse for the remainder of the control logic. A

timing diagram serves to explain the operation of the sequential logic that
controls the bilateral switch multiplexer (Fig. 11). Each output channel of the
multiplexer is filtered, level shifted, and amplified prior to recording. Data is
recorded on a strip chart recorder and on an FM tape recorder. The tape recorder provides a permanent record to permit further data reduction if required.

SURGICAL PROCEDURE

The reproductive organs are exposed by a mid-ventral abdominal incision
under halothane anesthesia (Fig. 12). A small incision is made in the uterine
horn within 1 cm of the uterotubal junction (UTJ). A 10 cm long 0.5 mm
diameter stainless steel wire is used to pull the transducers into the lumen of
the isthmus. A fine suture is passed through an eye at one end of the wire
and also through the lumen of the transducer. The free ends of the suture are
tied to form a loop. The wire is slipped through the incision at the uterine

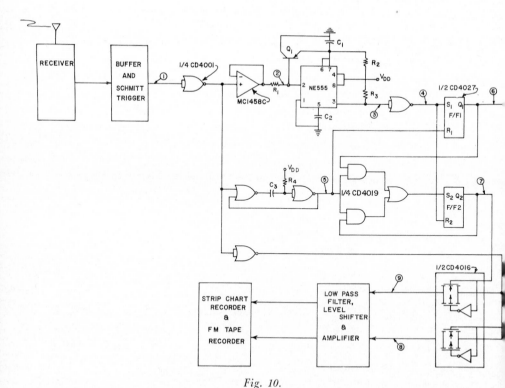

Fig. 10.
Schematic diagram of dual-channel demultiplexing and signal conditioning circuity.

horn and maneuvered through the uterotubal junction into the isthmus of the oviduct. It is then carefully worked through the oviduct to a position near the ampullary-isthmic junction, usually 6 to 8 cm from the UTJ. Here the tip of the needle is pushed through the oviductal wall and the transducers pulled into the isthmus by drawing the needle and the attached suture through the puncture wound. After retrieving the wire from the oviduct, the suture loop is used to maneuver the transducers into the desired positions within the oviduct. The suture loop is then cut and pulled free from the oviduct leaving the transducers in place. The tubing, with leads encased inside, is sutured to the horn of the uterus to hold the transducers in place. For hard-wired experiments the free end of the leads are passed through the abdominal incision and then subcutaneously to a position on the back of the animal between the front shoulders. Here the leads are exteriorized through a small stab wound. A plastic box is sutured over the wound to house the leads when not in use. For telemetry studies, the leads are passed through the abdominal incision and the transmitter is placed in a "skin pouch" and sutured to the abdominal muscular wall.

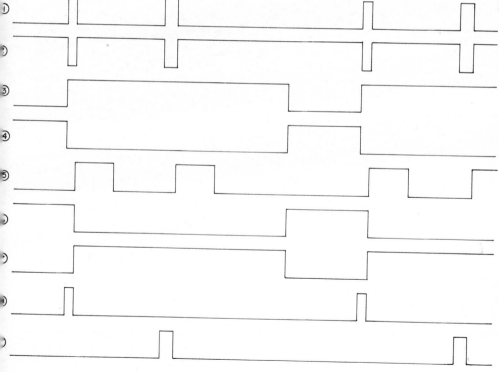

Fig. 11.
Timing diagram for dual-channel demultiplexer.

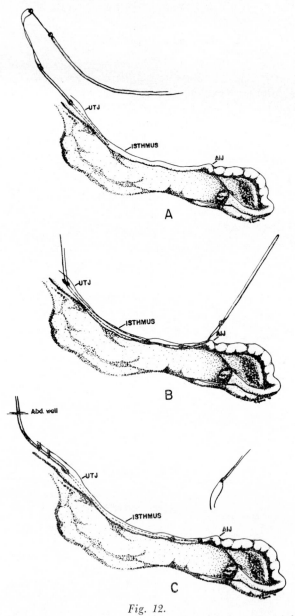

Fig. 12.

Surgical procedure. An incision is made in the uterine horn and stainless steel wire inserted into isthmus (A). Suture material attached to wire is used to pull the transducers into the lumen of the isthmus (B). After the transducers are positioned in the oviduct, the leads are sutured to the uterine horn (C).

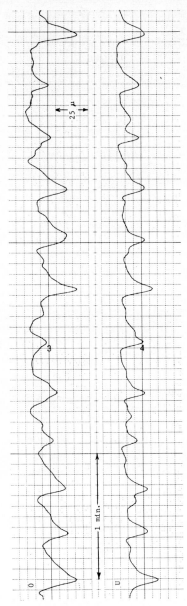

Fig. 13.

In vitro motility pattern. Transducer O and U are 2.5 cm and 2.0 cm respectively from the UTJ. Both transducers are responding in a similar fashion. An upward deflection from baseline represents a decrease in luminal diameter.

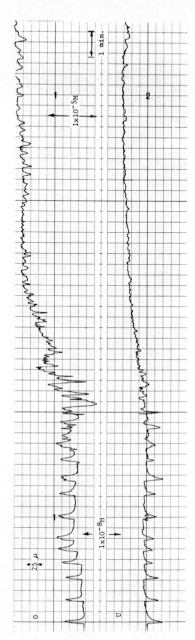

Fig. 14.

In vitro response to phenylephrine. Transducers O and U are 3.5 cm and 1.0 cm respectively from UTJ. Transducer O is experiencing decreases in luminal diameter while U is experiencing increases. As dose level is increased both approach a state of chronic constriction.

RESULTS

Once the transducers are calibrated it is necessary to demonstrate their sensitivity to changes in oviductal luminal diameter. Such determinations are made by *in vitro* evaluation. The instrumented oviduct is placed on hooks in a muscle bath containing Tyrode's solution at 37°C. Phenylephrine is added to the bath using a gradient mixer.

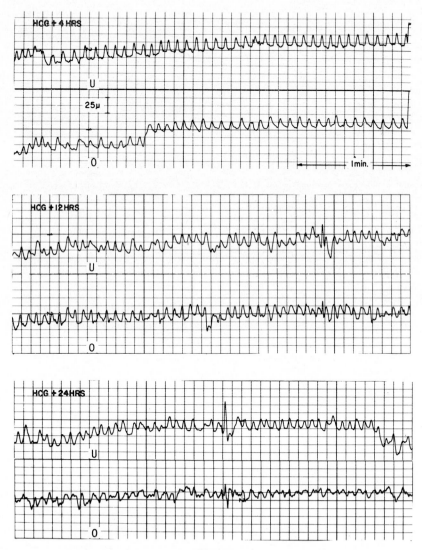

Fig. 15.
In vivo telemetry recordings after HCG-induced ovulation.

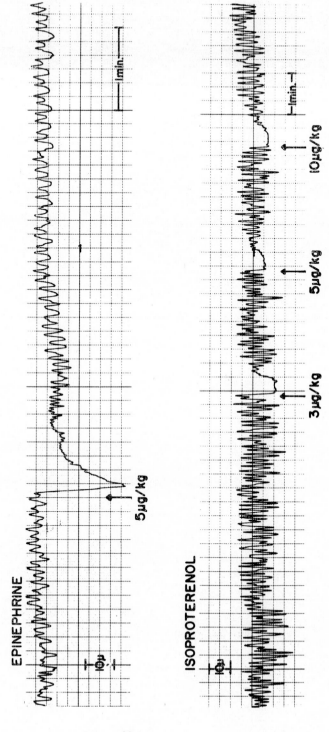

EPINEPHRINE

5 µg/kg

10 µ

1 min.

ISOPROTERENOL

3 µg/kg   5 µg/kg   10 µg/kg

1 min.

10 µ

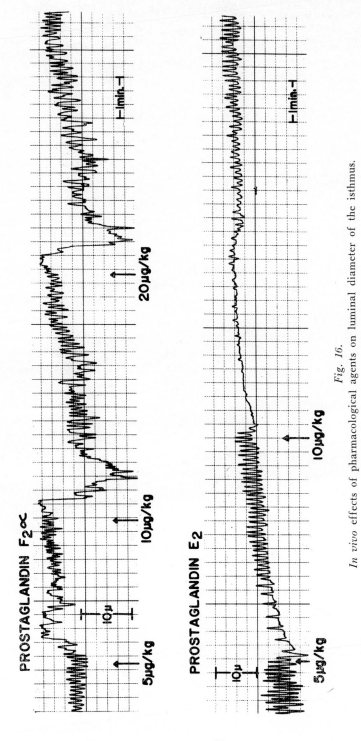

Fig. 16.

In vivo effects of pharmacological agents on luminal diameter of the isthmus.

The *in vitro* data of Fig. 13 clearly demonstrate that both transducers are responding to oviductal motility in a similar fashion. A downward displacement represents an increase in luminal diameter while an upward displacement represents a decrease in luminal diameter. The *in vitro* data in Fig. 14 are unique in that one transducer is sensing transitory decreases in luminal diameter while the other transducer is sensing transitory increases in luminal diameter. As the level of phenylephrine is increased, both portions of the isthmus approach a chronic constriction.

Once sufficient *in vitro* tests had been conducted, *in vivo* tests were commenced to evaluate transducer performance for extended periods of time. Initial testing measured the effects of HCG-induced ovulation on oviductal. motility (Fig. 15).

The effects of various pharmacological agents on luminal diameter have also been studied (Fig. 16). The administration of 5 μg/kg of epinephrine produces a transitory increase in luminal diameter followed by a gradual return to baseline and increase in rate of activity. Visual observation indicates that longitudinal muscles are stimulated by epinephrine causing a shortening of the oviduct and consequent increase in luminal diameter. Investigators using pressure transducers report an apparent increase in circular muscular activity. Our data suggest that the increase in intratubal pressure reported by these investigators may result from longitudinal contractions rather than increased circular muscular activity, especially since we measure a concomitant increase in luminal diameter.

Isoproterenol characteristically inhibits all muscular activity of the oviduct for several seconds followed by a return to normal baseline activity (Fig. 16). These results are consistent with other findings (Black 1974).

Preliminary experiments using prostaglandin (PG) $F_{2\alpha}$ resulted in changes in luminal diameter indicating variable bursts of dilatory activity (Fig. 16). Visual observations during PG $F_{2\alpha}$ administration indicate an increase in longitudinal activity. Spilman and Harper (1973) have reported that PG $F_{2\alpha}$ causes a spasmodic contraction followed by slight suppression of spontaneous activity.

Similar studies using prostaglandin E_2 produced a cessation of all activity for a variable length of time depending on dose levels (Fig. 16). Close observation shows a small chronic decrease in luminal diameter following treatment. These results are consistent with those reported earlier (Spilman and Harper 1973).

As mentioned previously, one of the important features of these intratubal transducers is that they are capable of responding to chronic changes in luminal diameter. Chronic changes in oviductal luminal diameter have been implicated in a post-ovulatory sphincter action of the rabbit isthmus (Blair and Beck 1975). Following recovery from surgery (5–7 days), determinations of transducer electrical resistance were made daily until fluctuations in the values became stable. A mean pretreatment control value for each transducer was established over a four day period following resistance stabilization. Rabbits were divided into four groups. Group 1 was an estrous control which received no treatment. Group 2 was injected with 100 IU of HCG (iv). Group 3 was treated with 100 IU of HCG (iv) and with 250 μg of 17 beta estradiol (im). Rabbits in group 4 were injected with 2.5 mg of progesterone (im) for three consecutive days and with 100 IU of HCG (iv) on the third day.

For the control group 1, time zero was designated as 24 h following last control determination of transducer resistance. For treatment groups 2–4, time zero was defined as the time of HCG injection. The experimental procedure was thereafter identical for all groups. All experiments were begun between 08.00 and 10.00 h and electrical resistance of each transducer was determined every 8 h for 104 h. Resistance of each transducer was monitored for a minimum of 10 min every 8 h. Continuous recordings were made to determine baseline resistance and to evaluate the frequency and amplitude of rapidly occurring shifts in resistance in response to oviductal contractions and/or relaxations. Baseline electrical resistance was converted to transducer diameter utilizing the calibration curve for the transducer being tested.

Changes in individual transducer diameter at 8 h intervals over the 104 h test period are shown in Tables 1–4. The control group comprises 12 transducers in four rabbits (Table 1). Experimental groups included eight transducers in five rabbits treated with HCG alone (Table 2); six transducers in four rabbits treated with HCG plus estrogen (Table 3); and 11 transducers in four rabbits treated with progesterone plus HCG (Table 4). The number of transducers varies since only those remaining functional throughout the study and confirmed to be within the lumen of the isthmus at autopsy were considered valid. The values expressed as change in transducer diameter in microns (μ) are calculated according to the formula $(R_2-\bar{x}R_1)$ TS $= \Delta$ diameter μ where

$\bar{x}R_1$ = mean pretreatment control electrical resistance;
R_2 = electrical resistance of the transducer at time of testing;
TS = sensitivity of the transducer determined from the slope of its calibration curve where transducer diameter = f (transducer resistance);
Δ dia. μ = change in transducer diameter in microns.

The mean change in transducer diameter from time 0 for the control is not significantly different from the mean value at any other time interval within this group (Table 1).

The mean change in transducer diameter at time 0 in HCG treated rabbits is significantly different ($P < 0.05$) from the mean values at 8, 16, 32, 40, 48,

Table 1.

The individual and mean change in transducer diameter (Δ dia.) at 8 h intervals for 104 h in control rabbits (N = 12 transducers in 4 rabbits).

Rabbit	#1		#2		#3				#4				Mean changes in trans. dia. (0–104 h)	
Trans.	R174S	R197S	R192S	R153S	R161S	R159S	R177S	R173S	R181S	R188S	R196S	R194S	$\bar{x}$ Δ dia. ± SD	h
$\bar{x}R_1(k)$(a)	149	521	174	301	188	118	230	614	235	191	306	521		
TS(μ/k)(b)	1.5	0.41	0.64	0.80	0.68	1.2	1.05	1.08	1.25	0.30	0.80	0.80		
	0.0	−4.5	−3.8	−16.8	−2.0	−2.5	+5.2	−15.1	0.0	−0.9	0.0	−2.4	−3.6 ± 6.3	0
	−13.5	−4.9	−2.6	−22.2	−8.8	−7.5	−1.0	−42.1	−11.2	−1.2	+7.2	+8.8	−8.3 ± 13.7	8
	−15.0	−8.6	−5.8	−0.8	−8.2	−6.2	−3.2	−36.7	+21.2	+12.0	+11.2	+27.2	−1.1 ± 17.2	16
	−15.0	−6.2	−4.5	−12.4	−8.8	−7.5	−3.2	−40.0	0.0	+6.3	+8.0	+30.4	−4.4 ± 16.5	24
	−10.5	−12.7	+3.2	−25.6	−8.2	−2.5	+3.2	−36.7	−2.5	+3.6	−4.8	+4.8	−7.4 ± 12.7	32
	−9.0	+0.4	−5.8	−24.8	−22.4	−6.2	+16.8	−43.2	+1.2	+0.9	−0.8	+1.6	−0.4 ± 17.6	40
	−12.0	−1.2	−4.5	−24.8	−19.0	−5.0	+10.5	−42.1	−1.2	+0.3	−4.8	+2.4	−8.4 ± 14.2	48
	−10.5	−9.0	−9.0	−4.8	−14.3	−5.0	+8.4	−36.7	+33.8	+7.2	−6.4	+0.8	−3.8 ± 16.5	56
	−18.0	−0.4	−2.6	−28.0	−20.4	−11.2	+9.4	−28.1	+13.8	−0.3	−0.8	+4.8	−6.8 ± 14.1	64
	−13.5	−2.9	−9.0	−12.8	−17.7	−10.0	+3.2	−38.9	+6.2	+1.2	−4.8	−0.8	−8.3 ± 12.1	72
	−16.5	+7.8	+6.4	−36.8	−19.0	−7.5	+5.2	−41.0	+21.2	+8.7	+12.8	+24.8	+0.3 ± 21.6	80
	−15.0	+1.2	−9.0	−16.8	−20.4	−8.8	+9.4	−47.5	+2.5	+3.9	−0.8	−2.4	−8.6 ± 15.2	88
	−10.5	+3.7	−7.7	−24.8	−21.8	−7.5	+6.3	−36.7	+3.8	+6.9	+6.4	−0.8	−6.9 ± 14.3	96
	−9.0	+27.1	−1.9	−20.8	−23.8	−16.2	+7.4	−57.2	÷5.0	+6.6	+4.8	−1.6	−6.6 ± 21.3	104

Individual changes in transducer diameter (μ)   Δ dia. = $(R_2 - \bar{x}R_1)$TS(c)

(a) $\bar{x}R_1(k)$ = mean pretreatment control transducer resistance in kilo-ohms.
(b) TS(μ/k) = transducer sensitivity in microns/kilo-ohms.
(c) R_2 = electrical resistance of transducer at time of testing.
* = mean change in transducer diameter is significantly different ($P < 0.05$) from the 0 h mean.

64

Table 2.

The individual and mean changes in transducer diameters (Δ dia.) in microns at 8 h intervals for a 104 h period. Rabbits treated with HCG (100 IU injected iv at time 0).

h	Rabbit #1 S38	R55S	#2 R51S	R58S	#3 R179S	#4 R160S	#5 R193S	R186S	Mean changes in trans. dia. (0–104 h) $\bar{x}\,\Delta$ dia. $\pm$ SD
$\bar{x}R_1(k)$(a)	24	365	190	85	118	328	192	264	
TS(μ/k)(b)	0.40	0.86	0.99	2.27	1.61	1.40	1.10	1.17	
0	−12.0	−10.3	−17.8	−15.9	−19.3	+11.2	+8.8	−1.2	−7.06 ± 12
8	−20.0	−19.0	−26.7	−56.8	−20.9	−39.2	−23.1	−4.7	−26.3 ± 15*
16	−0.20	−20.7	−50.5	−38.6	−30.6	−39.2	−24.2	−10.5	−29.3 ± 13*
24	−12.0	−21.6	−55.4	−32.2	−11.7	−4.4	+4.7	−30.5	−20.4 ± 19
32	−8.0	−23.3	−41.6	−38.6	−5.6	−23.1	−17.6	−36.3	−24.3 ± 14*
40	+4.0	−30.2	−61.4	−70.4	−38.6	−67.2	−22.0	−22.2	−38.5 ± 26*
48	−16.0	−16.4	−65.3	−77.2	−35.4	−46.2	−28.6	−12.9	−37.2 ± 24*
56	−20.0	−37.9	−74.2	−79.4	−37.0	−53.2	−11.0	−28.1	−42.6 ± 25*
64	−20.0	−30.2	−3.0	−13.6	−40.2	−4.2	−2.2	−21.1	−16.8 ± 14
72	−12.0	−10.3	−22.8	−13.6	−37.0	−39.2	−6.6	−28.1	−21.2 ± 12*
80	−20.0	−1.7	−57.4	−13.6	−41.9	−11.2	−2.2	−23.4	−21.4 ± 19
88	+20.0	+7.8	−55.4	−11.4	−32.2	−9.8	−18.7	−22.2	−17.7 ± 20
96	+12.0	+37.1	−66.3	−35.4	−7.0	−13.2	−28.1	−15.9	−14.6 ± 31
104	+12.0	+28.4	−28.7	—	−37.0	−16.8	−56.1	−4.7	−14.7 ± 29

Individual changes in transducer diameter (μ)

$$\Delta \text{ dia.} = (R_2 - \bar{x}R_1)\,TS\text{(c)}$$

(a) $\bar{x}R_1(k)$ = mean pretreatment control transducer resistance in kilo-ohms.
(b) TS(μ/k) = transducer sensitivity in microns/kilo-ohms.
(c) R_2 = electrical resistance of transducer at time of testing.
* = mean change in transducer diameter is significantly different ($P < 0.05$) from the 0 h mean.

65

5

Table 3.

The individual and mean changes in transducer diameter (Δ dia.) in microns at 8 h intervals for 104 h period in rabbits treated at time 0 with HCG (100 IU injected iv) and estrogen (250 μg injected im).

Rabbit	#1		#2	#3	#4		Mean changes in trans. dia. (0–104 h)	
Trans.	R37S	R82S	S32	R105S	R102S	R126S		
x̄R1(k)[a]	640	385	68	147	52	80	x̄ Δ dia. ± SD	h
TS(μ/k)[b]	0.42	0.64	4.0	2.11	5.0	3.08		
	+1.6	−19.9	0.0	−10.5	0.0	−9.3	−3.4 ± 15	0
	−137.0	−74.2	+8.0	−56.7	−55.1	−68.2	−63.9 ± 46*	8
	−140.7	−117.4	−16.0	−111.3	−95.6	−62.0	−90.5 ± 44*	16
	−138.6	−140.6	−72.0	−96.6	−84.8	−71.3	−100.6 ± 31*	24
	−131.1	−139.3	−72.0	−126.0	−84.8	−80.6	−105.6 ± 29*	32
	−141.5	−136.1	−48.0	−155.4	−110.0	−83.7	−113.5 ± 41*	40
	−144.4	−141.2	−32.0	−157.5	−75.4	−96.1	−107.8 ± 49*	48
	−146.9	−142.5	−32.0	−140.7	−100.5	−96.1	−109.8 ± 44*	56
	−146.1	−145.8	−88.0	−138.6	−100.5	−93.0	−118.7 ± 27*	64
	−149.8	−141.2	−100.0	−134.4	−105.2	−89.9	−120.1 ± 25*	72
	−146.9	−141.2	−64.0	−159.6	−110.0	−96.1	−119.6 ± 36*	80
	−146.9	−139.3	−52.0	−149.1	−84.8	−93.0	−110.8 ± 40*	88
	−149.8	−139.3	−108.0	−159.6	−110.0	−96.1	−127.1 ± 26*	96
	−147.7	−134.2	—	−159.6	−105.2	−93.0	−129.9 ± 28*	104

Individual changes in transducer diameter (μ)

$$\Delta\ \text{dia.} = (R_2 - \bar{x}R_1)\,TS^{(c)}$$

(a) $\bar{x}R_1(k)$ = mean pretreatment control transducer resistance in kilo-ohms.

(b) $TS(\mu/k)$ = transducer sensitivity in microns/kilo-ohms.

(c) R_2 = electrical resistance of transducer at time of testing.

* = mean change in transducer diameter is significantly different ($P < 0.05$) from the 0 h mean.

Table 4.

The individual and mean changes in transducer diameter (Δ dia.) in microns (μ) at 8 h in rabbits treated with progesterone (2.5 mg) for 3 days prior to injection with HCG at time 0 (100 IU iv).

Rabbit	#1			#2		#3		#4				Mean changes in trans. dia. (0–104 h)	
Trans.	S42	R53	R15	R35S	R71S	R137S	R146S	R100S	R93S	R104S	R120S	$\bar{x}\ \Delta$ dia. $\pm$ SD	h
$\bar{x}R_1(k)$[a]	119	116	91	450	111	117	57	200	70	65	56		
$TS(\mu/k)$[b]	0.41	0.58	0.82	0.77	0.80	2.25	1.67	2.38	2.50	1.50	1.63		
	−1.2	−12.8	−4.9	−22.3	+9.9	−11.0	−1.7	+4.8	−2.5	−3.0	−1.6	−4.2 ± 8.7	0
	+0.8	−10.5	+9.0	−26.0	+85.9	−11.0	+5.1	+79.2	−2.5	0.0	−3.2	+12.1 ± 36.4	8
	+1.2	−10.5	+0.8	+45.5	+29.9	−26.4	−8.5	+21.6	0.0	−4.5	−3.2	+4.1 ± 20.4	16
	+0.4	0.0	+2.5	+2.5	+89.1	−24.2	−10.2	+105.6	0.0	−4.5	−4.8	+14.2* ± 41.9	24
	+3.2	−0.6	−1.6	+11.7	+39.5	−24.2	−6.2	+43.2	−5.0	−6.0	−4.8	+4.47 ± 20.2	32
	+1.2	−3.5	+2.5	−9.1	+10.7	−19.8	−15.3	+38.2	−2.5	−6.0	−3.2	−0.6 ± 15.3	40
	+0.4	+1.2	−0.8	+12.5	+67.5	−26.4	−18.7	+31.2	−5.0	−4.5	−6.4	+4.6 ± 25.7	48
	+0.4	−7.0	−4.1	−5.2	+90.7	−33.0	−20.4	+12.0	−12.5	−7.5	−6.4	+0.6 ± 32.0	56
	+0.4	−8.8	−4.1	−16.0	+68.3	−35.2	−22.1	+2.4	−10.0	−7.5	−6.4	−3.5 ± 26.1	64
	+0.4	−14.6	−5.7	−52.9	+26.7	−37.4	−20.4	+14.4	−10.0	−4.5	−9.6	−10.3 ± 22.0	72
	−0.4	−8.8	−1.6	−29.8	+18.7	−37.4	−20.4	+21.6	−12.5	−7.5	−6.4	−7.7 ± 17.9	80
	+1.6	−9.3	−2.5	−22.1	+19.5	−37.4	−20.4	+7.2	−10.0	−4.5	−9.6	−8.0 ± 15.3	88
	+9.7	−10.5	−2.5	−37.5	+55.5	−41.8	−20.0	0.0	−12.5	−7.5	−9.6	−6.97 ± 26.0	96
	+2.8	−12.3	−7.4	−37.5	+25.1	−46.2	−20.4	+7.2	−5.0	−7.5	−9.6	−10.07 ± 19.7	104

Individual changes in transducer diameter (μ) Δ dia. $= (R_2 - \bar{x}R_1)/TS$[c]

(a) $\bar{x}R_1(k)$ = mean pretreatment control transducer resistance in kilo-ohms.
(b) $TS(\mu/k)$ = transducer sensitivity in microns/kilo-ohms.
(c) R_2 = electrical resistance of transducer at time of testing.
* = mean change in transducer diameter is significantly different ($P < 0.05$) from the 0 h mean.

56 and 72 h post-HCG injection (Table 2). However, no difference could be detected at 24, 64, 80, 88, 96 or 104 h post-HCG injection in this group. In each case where a difference occurred within this group, it was due to a decrease in mean transducer diameter.

In rabbits treated with HCG plus estrogen the mean change in transducer diameter from time 0 is significantly different ($P < 0.05$) from the mean values observed at all other time intervals tested (Table 3). The differences were due to decreases in transducer diameter following treatment.

In rabbits treated with progesterone plus HCG the mean change in transducer diameter from time 0 is not significantly different from the mean values observed at the other time intervals with one exception (Table 4). At 24 h post-HCG injection the difference was significant ($P < 0.05$), and was due to an increase in mean transducer diameter.

The mean changes in transducer diameter at each 8 h test period in the control and treatment groups are compared in Table 5 and Fig. 17. There is no significant difference between the mean change in transducer diameter observed at time 0 and the control and treatment groups. Comparison of the mean changes in transducer diameter between control rabbits (group 1) and the rabbits treated with HCG (group 2) appears in Table 5. Treatment with HCG resulted in significant decreases in luminal diameter when compared to mean

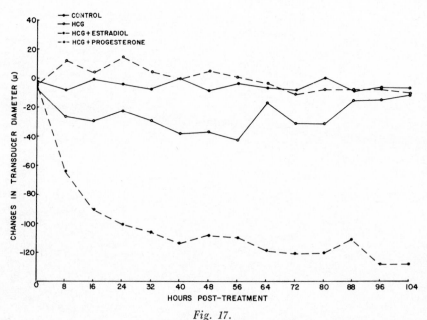

Fig. 17.

Mean changes in transducer diameter at 8 h intervals for control and treatment groups.

68

Table 5.

Statistical comparison of the mean changes in transducer diameters at 8 h intervals between the control (x̄ group 1) and treatment groups (x̄ group 2; x̄ group 3; and x̄ group 4).

Ex. group	1	2	3	4	Time	Student's t[a] value (P) Control group 1 (x̄ 1) vs. Treatment groups 2 (x̄ 2); 3 (x̄ 3); and 4 (x̄ 4):		
Treatment	Control	HCG	HCG + Estro.	Proges. + HCG		2	3	4
Rabbits/group	4	5	4	4				
Trans./group	12 (N)	8 (N)	6 (N)	11 (N)				
Mean changes in transducer diameter (Δ x̄ dia. ± SD)	-3.6 ± 6	-7.0 ± 12	-3.4 ± 15	-4.2 ± 9	0	0.7 ($P>0.05$)	0.1 ($P>0.05$)	0.2 ($P>0.05$)
	-8.3 ± 14	-26.3 ± 15	-63.9 ± 46	$+12.1 \pm 36$	8	1.66 ($P>0.05$)	2.3 ($P<0.025$)	0.9 ($P>0.05$)
	-1.1 ± 17	-29.3 ± 13	-90.0 ± 44	$+4.1 \pm 20$	16	2.18 ($P<0.025$)	2.8 ($P<0.01$)	0.6 ($P>0.05$)
	-4.4 ± 16	-20.4 ± 19	-100.6 ± 31	$+14.2 \pm 41$	24	2.32 ($P<0.025$)	2.9 ($P<0.005$)	1.3 ($P>0.05$)
	-7.4 ± 16	-24.3 ± 14	-105.6 ± 29	$+4.4 \pm 20$	32	1.7 ($P<0.05$)	2.9 ($P<0.005$)	1.6 ($P>0.05$)
	-0.4 ± 1	-38.5 ± 26	-113.5 ± 41	-0.6 ± 15	40	2.52 ($P<0.005$)	3.0 ($P<0.005$)	0.03 ($P>0.05$)
	-8.4 ± 14	-37.2 ± 24	-107.8 ± 49	$+4.6 \pm 26$	48	2.94 ($P<0.005$)	2.7 ($P<0.01$)	0.6 ($P>0.05$)
	-3.8 ± 16	-42.6 ± 25	-109.8 ± 44	$+0.6 \pm 32$	56	3.29 ($P<0.005$)	2.9 ($P<0.005$)	0.4 ($P>0.05$)
	-6.8 ± 14	-16.8 ± 14	-118.0 ± 27	-3.5 ± 26	64	1.14 ($P>0.05$)	3.0 ($P<0.005$)	0.4 ($P>0.05$)
	-8.3 ± 12	-21.2 ± 12	-120.1 ± 25	-10.3 ± 22	72	1.41 ($P>0.05$)	3.0 ($P<0.005$)	0.2 ($P>0.05$)
	$+0.3 \pm 22$	-21.4 ± 19	-119.6 ± 36	-7.7 ± 18	80	1.82 ($P<0.05$)	3.0 ($P<0.005$)	0.9 ($P>0.05$)
	-8.6 ± 15	-17.7 ± 20	-110.8 ± 40	-8.0 ± 15	88	0.89 ($P>0.05$)	2.8 ($P<0.01$)	0.1 ($P>0.05$)
	-6.9 ± 14	-14.6 ± 31	-127.1 ± 26	-6.9 ± 26	96	0.76 ($P>0.05$)	2.9 ($P<0.005$)	0.01 ($P>0.05$)
	-6.6 ± 21	-14.7 ± 29	-129.9 ± 28	-10.0 ± 20	104	0.85 ($P>0.05$)	3.3 ($P<0.005$)	0.4 ($P>0.05$)

(a) $t = \dfrac{\bar{x}_1 - \bar{x}_2}{S\bar{x}_1 - \bar{x}_2}$

69

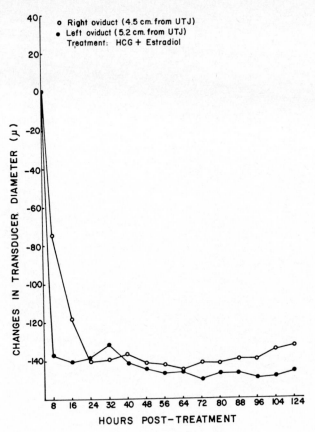

Fig. 18.

Response from two transducers in contralateral oviducts following administration
of HCG and estrogen.

control values at 16, 24, 32, 48 and 80 h post-HCG injection. There were no
differences between the mean control and treatment values at 0, 8, 64, 72, 96
and 104 h. Treatment with HCG at a dose level known to induce ovulation in
the rabbit resulted in a gradual decrease in mean transducer diameter, with
onset between 8 and 16 h post-HCG injection, and maximum by 56 h. After
56 h, mean transducer diameter increased and no significant difference could
be detected at 64, 72, 88, 96 and 104 h post-HCG treatment (Fig. 17). The
mean change in transducer diameter in HCG and estrogen-treated rabbits is
significantly different from the corresponding control values at all time intervals tested, with the exception of zero hour. As in rabbits treated with HCG
alone, the change is reflected as highly significant decreases in transducer
diameter (Table 5). Treatment with exogenous estrogen seems to enhance the

constriction induced by treatment with HCG as evidenced by an increase in both the magnitude and duration of constriction. The most noteworthy difference between these two treatment groups occurred between 56 and 104 h post-HCG injection. In HCG treated rabbits, the constriction relaxed during this interval as evidenced by a return to levels not significantly different from control values. In HCG and estrogen-treated rabbits, the mean change in transducer diameter remained significantly different from the corresponding control values during this period.

Comparison of the mean change in transducer diameter in control rabbits to those observed in rabbits with progesterone reveals no significant differences between the control and treatment means at any of the time intervals tested. Pretreatment with progesterone completely blocks the effect observed in both of the other HCG treatment groups.

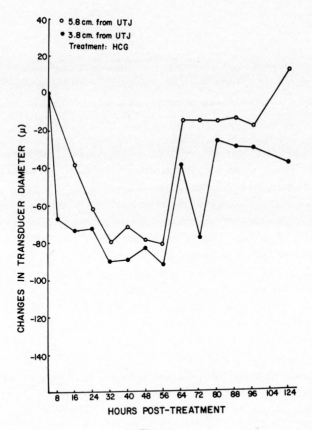

Fig. 19.
Response from two transducers in the same oviduct following administration of HCG.

Figs. 18 and 19 represent selected plots from individual transducers which illustrate two important findings made possible by use of multiple transducers in the same rabbit. Fig. 18 compares the response obtained from two transducers in the same rabbit. One transducer was 4.5 cm from the UTJ in the isthmus of the right oviduct. The second transducer was 5.2 cm from the UTJ in the isthmus of the left oviduct. The parallel response indicates that both oviducts respond in similar fashion to the same change in hormonal stimulation. Fig. 19 illustrates results obtained from two transducers in the isthmus of the same oviduct. One transducer was 3.8 cm from the UTJ with the second transducer 5.8 cm from the UTJ. This rabbit was from the HCG-treated group. The response from both transducers is typical of that observed in other rabbits treated with HCG. This provides evidence that constriction of the isthmus is not confined to a localized segment near the ampullary-isthmic junction as some have suggested.

DISCUSSION

Studies on the rate of ova transport in the rabbit have established a time frame of approximately 72 h from the time of ovulation until eggs reach the uterus (Harper 1961). However, egg transport through the ampulla occurs within minutes following ovulation (Harper 1961; Boling and Blandau 1971).

Others have shown that treatment with exogenous estrogen significantly extends the time that eggs are retained in the oviduct, and treatment with progesterone results in an accelerated rate of transport (Harper 1964; Chang 1966, 1969; Chang and Hunt 1970).

The theory that physiological constriction of the oviduct functions in the regulation of ovum passage from the ampulla to the uterus is not new. Brundin (1964) measured pressure changes in the isthmus of the rabbit oviduct following ovulation, and demonstrated changes in the resistance to oviductal insufflation suggestive of a functional oviductal occlusive mechanism. Blandau (1961) visually observed the transport of ova through the ampulla of the rabbit oviduct and reported the occurrence of a physiological constricture at the ampullary-isthmic junction, which retains ova in the ampulla. Histological and histochemical studies on the rabbit oviduct demonstrate a smooth muscular layer arrangement and neurological innervation characteristic of an adrenergic smooth muscular sphincter (Brundin and Wirsen 1964). Pharmacological studies on smooth muscular contractile activities demonstrate the occurrence of neurological control mechanisms representative of an adrenergic sphincter mechanism (Black 1974).

Although the evidence seems compelling, the occurrence of a functional estrogen-induced isthmic block to ovum transport resulting directly from smooth muscular constriction of the oviductal wall has not been previously established.

Our results provide direct evidence that the isthmus of the rabbit oviduct exhibits a hormonally-induced constriction following HCG-induced ovulation. We have shown that this constriction of the oviductal wall is temporal and coincides with the period when ova are known to be retained in the oviduct. The amplitude and duration of constriction is enhanced by treatment with exogenous estrogen and the post-ovulatory occurrence of the constriction can be effectively blocked by treatment with progesterone. These findings coincide with the observations by others that treatment of estrogen causes "tube-locking" of ova and treatment with progesterone accelerates the rate of ovum transport. Moreover, we have shown that constriction of the isthmus does not occur in the normal estrous rabbit in which transducers have been implanted. These findings considered in light of our observation that the isthmus of both oviducts responded in identical manner following HCG-induced ovulation provides evidence that the occurrence of the constriction is under direct ovarian hormonal control. The parallel response from transducers contained within the same isthmus indicates that the constriction is not confined to a localized segment of the oviduct, but occurs along the length of the isthmus.

Future studies utilizing this transducer and a newly developed telemetry system will be expanded to a primate model. Alteration of oviductal function may yield a novel approach to contraception.

REFERENCES

Black D. L. and Asdell S. A. (1958) Transport through the rabbit oviduct. *Amer. J. Physiol. 192*, 63–68.

Black D. L. (1974) Neural control of oviduct musculature. In: Johnson A. D. and Foley C. W., eds. *The Oviduct and its Function*, pp. 110–118. Academic Press, New York.

Blair W. D. (1975) *A dual-channel transducer/telemetry system for oviduct motility studies*. Dissertation Abstracts 35, N8, 3887B. (Order No. 75-4166, 131 pp).

Blair W. D. and Beck L. R. (1975) Demonstration of post-ovulatory sphincter action by the isthmus of the rabbit oviduct. *Fertil. and Steril.* (in press).

Blandau R. J. (1961) Biology of eggs and implantation. In: Young W. C., ed. *Sex and Internal Secretions 2*, 797–882. Williams and Wilkins, Baltimore.

Boling J. L. and Blandau R. J. (1971) Egg transport through the ampulla of the oviducts of rabbits under various experimental conditions. *Biol. Reprod. 4*, 174–184.

Brundin J. (1964) A functional block in the isthmus of the rabbit Fallopian tube. *Acta physiol. scand. 60*, 295–296.

Brundin J. (1965) Distribution and function of adrenergic nerves in the rabbit Fallopian tube. *Acta physiol. scand. 66*, Suppl. 259, 1–57.

Brundin J. and Talo A. (1972) The effects of estrogen and progesterone on the electric activity and intraluminal pressure of the castrated rabbit oviduct. *Biol. Reprod. 7*, 417–424.

Brundin J. and Wirsén C. (1964) The distribution of adrenergic nerve terminals in the rabbit oviduct. *Acta physiol. scand. 61*, 203–204.

Chang M. C. (1966) Transport of eggs from the Fallopian tube to the uterus as a function of oestrogen. *Nature (Lond.) 212*, 1048–1049.

Chang M. C. (1969) Fertilization, transportation and degeneration of eggs in pseudo-pregnant or progesterone-treated rabbits. *Endocrinology 84*, 356–361.

Chang M. C. and Hunt D. M. (1970) Effects of various progestins and estrogen on the gamete transport and fertilization in the rabbit. *Fertil. and Steril. 21*, 683–686.

Davids A. M. and Bender M. B. (1940) Effects of adrenalin on tubal contractions of the rabbit in relation to the sex hormones. *Amer. J. Physiol. 129*, 259–263.

DeMattos C. E. R. and Coutinho E. M. (1971) Effects of the ovarian hormones on tubal motility of the rabbit. *Endocrinology 89*, 912–917.

Doyle J. B. (1954) Ovulation and the effects of selective uterotubal denervation. *Fertil. and Steril. 51*, 105–130.

Duff G., Palm R., Boling J., Blandau R., Nelson C., Stegall F. (1972) *An implantable mutual inductance instrument for measuring oviduct diameter in mammals.* Proceedings Biomed. Eng. Soc., Baltimore, Md.

Greenwald G. S. (1963) *In vivo* recording of intraluminal pressure changes in the rabbit oviduct. *Fertil. and Steril. 14*, 666–674.

Harper M. J. K. (1961) The mechanisms involved in the movement of newly ovulated eggs through the ampulla of the rabbit Fallopian tube. *J. Reprod. Fertil. 2*, 522–524.

Harper M. J. K. (1964) The effects of constant doses of oestrogen and progesterone on the transport of artificial eggs through the reproductive tract of ovariectomized rabbits. *J. Endocr. 30*, 1–19.

Hodgson B. J., Ware R. W., Crosby R. J. and Pauerstein C. J. (1973) An ultrasonic transducer for recording oviductal motility. *J. appl. Physiol. 34*, 873–878.

Horton E. W., Main I. H. M. and Thompson C. J. (1965) Effects of prostaglandins on the oviduct studied in rabbits and ewes. *J. Physiol. (Lond.) 180*, 514–528.

Jeutter D. C., Fromm E. and Garcia C. R. (1973) *The study of reproductive tract motility by the use of implant telemetry.* Proceedings, 26, ACEMB *15*, 3.

Larks S. C., Larks G. G., Hoffer R. E. and Carlson E. J. (1971) Electrical activity of oviducts *in vivo. Nature (Lond.) 234*, 556–557.

Longley W. J., Black D. L. and Currie G. N. (1968) Oviduct circular muscle response to drugs related to the autonomic nervous system. *J. Reprod. Fert. 17*, 95–100.

Maia H. and Coutinho E. M. (1968) A new technique for recording human tubal activity *in vivo. Amer. J. Obstet. Gynec. 102*, 1043–1047.

Maia H. and Coutinho E. M. (1970) Peristalsis and antiperistalsis of the human Fallopian tube during the menstrual cycle. *Biol. Reprod. 2*, 305–314.

Maistrello I. (1971) Extraluminal recording of oviductal contractions in the un-anesthetized rabbit. *J. appl. Physiol. 31*, 768–776.

Nelsen T. and Nunn T. (1972) Personal Communication.

Rubin I. C. (1947) *Uterotubal Insufflation.* C. V. Mosby, St. Louis.

Salomy M. and Harper M. J. K. (1971) Cyclical changes of oviductal motility in rabbits. *Biol. Reprod. 4*, 185–194.

Spilman C. H. and Harper M. J. K. (1973) Effect of prostaglandins on oviduct motility in estrous rabbits. *Biol. Reprod. 9*, 36–45.

Departments of Surgery[1] and Electrical Engineering[2],
Stanford University, Stanford, California 94305, USA

MICROMINIATURE TRANSDUCERS FOR OVIDUCTAL MOTOR FUNCTION

By

Thomas S. Nelsen[1], Timothy A. Nunn[2]
and James B. Angell[2]

ABSTRACT

Using modern integrated circuit (IC) technology, a family of transducers has been developed which satisfy the stringent criteria of extremely small size, high sensitivity, and lack of functional interference. All devices measure 1 mm or less in their major dimension and sense linearly the electrical waves, mechanical contractions, and pressure waves of the rabbit (and human) oviduct. These are, respectively, etched platinum electrodes coated with flexible glass insulation, piezoresistive IC force transducers $1 \text{ mm} \times 50 \mu \times 20 \mu$ with integral silicon suture loops for attachment, and sensitive IC full-bridge piezoresistive pressure transducers 1 mm diameter $\times 200 \mu$ thick with an integral reference atmosphere. All devices are intended for prolonged *in vivo* use in unrestrained animals and should be particularly suitable for human use since their small size and rugged design will permit withdrawal of the transducers via the lead wires without reoperation.

A series of computer programs have been developed for the analysis of the data obtained from multiple transducer implants which provide estimation of frequency spectra and wave propagation characteristics of the oviduct.

The IC technology has the additional advantages of mass production capability with lowered cost and great uniformity from unit to unit; these transducers are also suitable for use on any other biological structure which bends, contracts, or generates an intraluminal pressure.

The devices described in this communication have been designed specifically for obtaining reliable recordings of electrical, force, and pressure information from the oviducts of awake, active, unrestrained, ostensibly normal rabbit does.

Such transducers must be physically scaled to the size of the rabbit oviduct (1 mm diameter) and sense the oviduct without altering the normal function of the thin muscle coats. Ideally, the devices should neither restrain free motion of the duct musculature, nor obstruct the lumen, nor surround the duct completely. They should not induce scarring, be easily attached, be electrically and mechanically stable, and be long-lived enough to permit chronic experiments (6–12 weeks). Each individual design should be compatible with all others, permitting multiple implants on a single oviduct of identical or different transducers without interference.

An additional desirable transducer characteristic is compatibility of the units with telemetry as well as hard-wired recording electronics. While not an important consideration for rabbits, the natural behaviour of many species precludes all recording techniques except telemetry if the experimenter wishes to obtain data from the animals in a condition approximating a normal or natural state. The behaviour of the reproductive system seems to be exquisitely sensitive to external influences and uncontrollable alterations in system be-

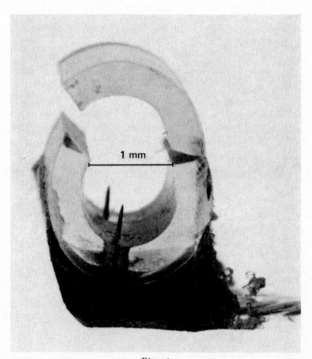

1 mm

Fig. 1.
The arrangement of two tapered Pt-Ir electrodes in a slotted cylindrical cuff of plastic for attachment to the oviduct.

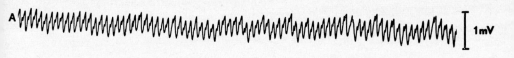

A ⊔ 1mV

B ⊔ 0.2 mV

C ⊔ 0.4 mV

D ⊔ 0.2 mV

|— 1 min —|

Fig. 2.

Example of recording from rabbit oviductal isthmus made with electrodes shown in Fig. 1 as a chronic *in vivo* implant. A and B from right oviduct on two different days (estrous doe). C and D from left oviduct of same animal on different days. Band pass of recording channel 0.05 to 7.5 Hz.

haviour can be minimized by maintenance of experimental animals in as natural a state as possible.

The final major influence on the transducer designs was the firm belief that the devices should be suitable for study of the human oviduct after surgical implantation (e. g., during an operation required for other reasons). If so used, they should be removable via the lead wires without reoperation or complications.

Accordingly, after consideration of all approaches it was decided that modern integrated circuit technology could produce transducers for force and pressure that were truly microminiature, sensitive, stable, easy to attach to the oviduct, removable without reoperation, non-reactive in tissue, long-lived, low-power, and most importantly, would not interfere with oviductal function.

77

The following describes separately the three transducers under development. The first design, largely complete, is an electrode assembly for the oviduct. The second design, in a useful but not final design phase, is the integrated circuit (IC) force transducer. The final and most complex device, an IC pressure transducer smaller than any other design heretofore available is in the prototype testing phase, *in vitro* and *in vivo*.

ELECTRODES

Satisfactory devices for chronic recording of electrical activity from oviductal smooth muscle have been constructed. The active portion of the electrodes is a length of tapered etched 90 % platinum – 10 % iridium wire. The tapered point is made by immersion of the Pt-Ir wire in a bath of 30 % NaOH solution saturated with NaCN and connecting the electrode and bath to an isolated 6 V alternating current supply. When microscopic inspection shows a tip diameter of desired size (about 10 microns), the voltage is reduced for polishing the wire.

Insulation of the Pt-Ir electrode is accomplished by immersion of the bare electrode in a bath of tert-amyl alcohol containing a suspension of Dow Corning 7575 glass. Passing the electrode through a heated wire loop bonds the glass to the wire, yielding a well insulated, strong, flexible electrode, particularly well suited for recording from moving muscular structures in acute experiments.

For chronic implantation, the Pt-Ir wires are made very short, soldered to flexible stranded # 40 lead wires and embedded in a cylindrical cuff or surround which is slotted for attachment to the rabbit oviduct (see Fig. 1). One or more electrodes are mounted in the cuff in a radial orientation with the tips pointing centripetally and the bases buried in the insulating cuff material. The cuff is stabilized on the oviduct by the penetration of the electrodes into the wall of the duct and a circumferential suture tied around the cuff which prevents slippage. Recordings obtained from chronic implants of these electrodes are of good quality and are shown in Fig. 2. Slow and fast electrical events are well demonstrated as well as pacemaker activity. The electrodes remain useful for weeks in chronic implants with a gradual increase in noise level. Because of the inherent problems of separating motion artefacts from local electrical events of muscle origin, we believe the greatest utility of these electrodes will be in conjunction with implants of force transducers and pressure transducers implanted on the same oviduct. The signals from the different transducers can be compared in time (frequency & phase) and amplitude; such correlations should aid in separation of artefact from the recorded electrical signals and may eventually provide enough insight to validate electrical recordings as a stand alone method from which physiologic conclusions can be drawn during *in vivo* chronic experiments.

FORCE TRANSDUCERS

1. *Development*

In the past four to five years, a major effort has been made to design, fabricate and test IC force transducers with dimensions and sensitivity commensurate with the size and power of the rabbit oviductal smooth muscle coats. This has dictated the use of modern integrated circuit technology. At the present time two viable designs are available, one, the so-called double-ended design, has been tested in chronic experiments and has been eminently successful (Nunn et al. 1973), the second, single-ended design, is beginning chronic testing.

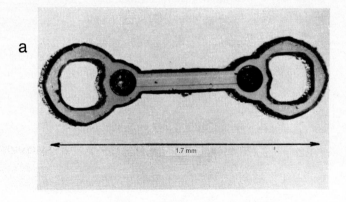

FORCE TRANSDUCER CROSS SECTION

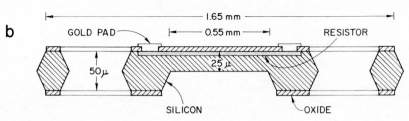

Fig. 3.

"Double-ended" IC force transducer showing integral suture loops of silicon and the bonding pads connected by the piezoresistive elements. Upper surface view (a) and cross-section diagram (b).

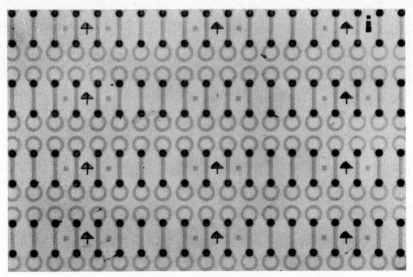

Fig. 4.
A portion of a silicon wafer during fabrication before separation
of individual elements.

The diffused resistor which serves as the strain gauge in the force transducer is clearly visible in Fig. 3, and extends along the entire length of the
thin portion of the transducers. Because low-resistance mechanically durable
contacts must be made to both ends of this resistor, considerable care and time
is required to form the ohmic contacts to the bonding pads at each end of the

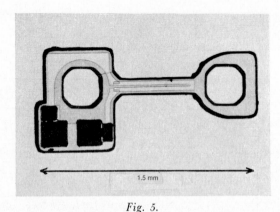

1.5 mm

Fig. 5.
"Single-ended" force transducer showing bonding pads at one end and
U-shaped piezoresistive element.

80

transducer. Fig. 4 shows a section of a silicon wafer of force transducers during processing and before separation. Each wafer contains 1200 individual elements.

Work on a related implantable transducer (a microminiature accelerometer, being developed with support from NASA) led to the suggestion of using a U-shaped diffused resistor, to which both ohmic connections could be made at one end of the transducer.

Fig. 5 shows a photograph of a transducer fabricated using this design. Because the two bonding pads are now close together, the leads which are attached to them can be part of a two-conductor cable. The cable can be considerably stronger and more durable than the single-conductor connections which are required for the double-ended transducer. At the same time, the cable to this single ended transducer does not have to be as pliant and flexible as the leads for the double-ended device.

2. Fabrication process

The batch fabrication process of force transducers using standard integrated circuit silicon technology consists mainly of six parts:

(1) Forming alignment marks for back side etching
(2) Forming the diffused resistor
(3) Forming the back side etch pattern
(4) Forming ohmic contacts and bonding pads
(5) Separation into individual transducers
(6) Lead attachments and testing

Each of the above six parts will be described briefly in the following. The detailed steps of the process are listed in Table 1.

(1) Forming alignment marks for back side etching

Since eventually we want to separate each individual transducer from the silicon wafer, it is essential that the etch pattern on the back side of the wafer be perfectly aligned to that of the front side. In order to achieve this, the alignment marks are anisotropically etched into the front side by using KOH solution. Due to its anisotropic nature, the etching of the alignment marks can be well controlled to stop at a pre-determined depth. Since the starting silicon wafer is much thicker than the final thickness of the transducer, the wafer has to be uniformly etched from the back side in a later thinning step as will be described in part (2) below. Once this etching to thin the wafer has proceeded to the bottom of the etched front-side alignment marks, we can see through the marks and the thinning is stopped so that we have both the needed alignment marks for back side etching and the right thickness for the final transducers.

81

Table 1.
Detailed steps of fabrication process.

(1) Forming alignment marks for back side etching

   1. Pre-oxidation cleaning
   2. Thermal oxidation
   3. Alignment mark (it also serves as the thickness indicator in the later thinning step) photolithography
   4. HF oxide etch
   5. Cleaning
   6. KOH anisotropic etch

(2) Forming the diffused resistor

   7. Pre-diffusion cleaning
   8. Thermal oxidation
   8.1. P+ diffusion photolithography ⎫
   8.2. HF oxide etch |
   8.3. Pre-diffusion cleaning   ⎬ For single-ended design only
   8.4. P+ diffusion |
   8.5. Remove boron glass   ⎭
   9. P-type resistor diffusion photolithography
   10. HF oxide etch
   11. Pre-diffusion cleaning
   12. P-type resistor predeposition
   13. Remove boron glass
   14. Chemical thinning of the wafer to 70 μ from the back side
   15. Pre-diffusion cleaning
   16. P-type resistor drive-in

(3) Forming the back side etch pattern

   17. Back side etch pattern photolithography

(4) Forming ohmic contacts and bonding pads

   18. Contact hole photolithography
   19. HF oxide etch
   20. Pre-diffusion cleaning
   21. Cr-Au evaporation
   22. Gold plating pattern photolithography
   23. Gold plating
   24. Remove unwanted field Cr and Au

(5) Separation into individual transducers

   25. Cleaning
   26. KOH etch to separate individual transducers
   27. Rinsing

(2) Forming the diffused resistor

The diffused resistor is the heart of the force transducer. The stress on this resistor induces a resistance change due to its piezoresistive properties. This resistor is formed by introducing p-type impurities (boron atoms) into the silicon at high temperature. After the predeposition step of the diffusion, the silicon wafer is thinned from the back side by using $HF-HNO_3$ solution so that SiO_2 can be grown on the back side during the drive-in step of the diffusion. This layer of SiO_2 on the back side will be used later as the back-side etching mask.

(3) Forming the back side etch pattern

This single photolithography step defines the back side etch pattern. The pattern is aligned with the front-side pattern through the alignment marks formed in part (1). This pattern also serves to make the diffused resistor region thinner than the rest of the area after the final separation etch.

(4) Forming ohmic contacts and bonding pads

The electrical contacts to the diffused resistor are formed by first evaporating Cr and then Au onto the silicon wafer. The choice of this two-layer metal structure gives both strong adhesion and good electrical contacts. After the evaporation, gold is selectively plated on the areas to which lead-bonding will be made. This plating procedure is done because we have found lead attachment is easier on a thicker layer of gold. The unwanted field Cr and Au is then etched away.

(5) Separation into individual transducers

The silicon wafer is then put into a warm KOH solution and silicon is etched away from both the top and the bottom in a way defined by the etch patterns on both sides. All the transducers will be separated from the silicon wafer when the etching from the two sides meets.

(6) Lead attachment and testing

Leads are then attached to the transducers by using the techniques described in section 3 below. The electrical characteristic of each transducer is also checked before the actual time-consuming implantation procedure.

In order to get some general idea about the degree of complexity of this fabrication process, the following table is prepared. In this table, the fabrication process of the force transducer is compared with the standard integrated circuit bipolar and MOS processes. The comparison has been made on the basis of the number of masks, the number of equivalent steps, and the number of diffusions involved in each of the three processes.

83

	Force transducer	MOS IC	Bipolar IC
Number of masks	5–6	4–6	6–8
Number of equivalent steps	30	25	40
Number of diffusions	1–2	1–2	5
			(Epitaxial growth included)

It is clear from the above comparison that the force transducer fabrication process is of about the same complexity as the standard MOS process and is definitely simpler than the standard bipolar process. The transducers are as amenable to mass production as the more common MOS and bipolar integrated circuit devices.

3. *Development of complete implantable assemblies*

Lead attachment failure, bonding pad adhesion, lead wire breakage, and insulation failures have been the major causes of the many problems encountered in developing a reliable, long-lasting force transducer assembly.

The first problem to be tackled was that of lead wire breakage. The choice of lead wire was based on three criteria: (1) the wires had to be strong enough to withstand the rigors of surgical implantation, (2) they had to be flexible so that movement of the leads transmitted a minimum of force to the transducers and (3) the wires had to be able to withstand considerable flexing without fatiguing. The original choice of 3 mil diameter copper wire proved to be acceptable with regard to the first two criteria but was found upon experimentation to fatigue quite readily when repeatedly flexed. Next 2-mil platinum-iridium (90 % Pt – 10 % Ir) was tried and was found to meet all the requirements. This wire was then chosen for our lead wires and has been in use for many months. Failures due to lead wire breakage have not been encountered since we switched to the 2-mil platinum-iridium wire.

The bonding pads presented a fairly formidable problem. On the one hand it was desirable to use a metal for the pads which readily oxidized thereby giving a strong pad to silicon bond; on the other hand, in order to make good electrical contact a non-oxidizing metal was called for. The technique for making the bonding pads, which we now use, utilizes a readily oxidizable metal, namely chromium, which is deposited in a vacuum at room temperature so that excellent electrical contact is also achieved. At the same time a thin layer of gold is evaporated on top of the chromium. Next a photolithography is performed and gold is then selectively electroplated to a thickness of approximately 5 microns over the bonding pad area. The photoresist is then removed and the excess evaporated gold and chromium is etched away. It is very important during this metallization procedure to avoid contamination. The bi-metal pads thus formed have excellent electrical and mechanical properties. Our experiments have shown that a force of 20 g is required to physically remove the bonding pad from the force transducer.

Various methods have been tried in the past for attaching the leads to the bonding pads. One of the first was thermocompression gold bonding which was simple to accomplish but was lacking in strength. Soldering was also tried, and in fact, used until near the end of this past year with varying results. Due to the fact that the bonding pads were gold it was necessary to use an indium doped solder in order to minimize the amount of gold leached by the solder. The indium doped solder however, would not adhere to the platinum wire necessitating an extra step of electroplating copper on the end of the platinum wire. This method of lead attachment proved to be strong enough quantitatively for our purposes but gave poor yields. The amount of flux, the amount of

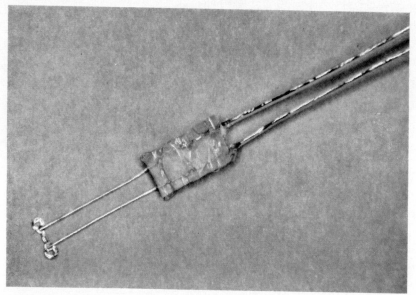

Fig. 6.
A complete force transducer assembly showing the sensitive element and the two individual 2-mil Pt-Ir wires soldered to two insulated stranded wires. The intermediate wire connections are insulated and stabilized by the rectangular patch of silicone rubber.

solder, the temperature of soldering, and the time had to be precisely controlled. Small variations in any of the above parameters often led to unacceptable bonds. However, this method of lead attachment, being the best available, was used for most of the force transducer assemblies this past twelve months.

A new method of lead attachment which uses a conductive silver epoxy has been under development for the past two months. Although this method is still undergoing final testing the preliminary results indicate that it will give much higher yields as well as a stronger bond in comparison to the solder method. The procedure for using the conductive silver epoxy is relatively simple. The silver epoxy, in paste form, is applied to the tips of the wire leads which are then brought in contact with the bonding pads on the force transducer. The epoxy is then cured by heating the force transducer assembly to 100°C for 30 min. Neither the temperature nor the time is critical for curing thereby making the quantity of epoxy applied to the lead wires the only step in the process which requires precise control. If no problems are encountered in the final tests this process will be used as our new method for lead attachment to the force transducers.

The last problem which still has to be solved concerns insulation failure The current method of insulation involves dissolving polyvinylchloride (PVC) in cyclohexanone and then painting this solution over the force transducer assembly being careful not to block the suture loop holes. Problems occur due to the tendency of the PVC solution to "ball up" leaving some areas with only a very thin layer of PVC insulation which has a tendency to crack.

A completed assembly is shown in Fig. 6, illustrating the sensitive element with bonding pads connected to the 2-mil Pt-Ir wires which are in turn soldered to insulated stranded # 40 wires. The pads are insulated with PVC, the intermediate solder joints with silicone rubber, the stranded wires with PVC and silicone rubber.

4. *Evaluation of completed transducers*

    A) Electrical characteristics
        The V-I characteristic of the force transducer is linear.

    B) Mechanical strength

    a) Lead attachment and bonding pad adhesion.
Transducers with lead wires attached have been subject to pulling test using a jig. The test results show that for transducers with leads properly attached, the breaking point is around 20 g. Observations of the transducers after the tests indicate that the bonding pads come off the silicon substrate.

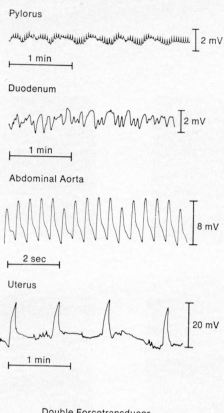

Single Forcetransducer Implant

Pylorus

2 mV

1 min

Duodenum

2 mV

1 min

Abdominal Aorta

8 mV

2 sec

Uterus

20 mV

1 min

Double Forcetransducer Implant

Oviduct

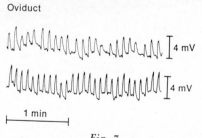

4 mV

4 mV

1 min

Fig. 7.

Examples of recordings obtained with the IC force transducer sutured to a variety of rabbit viscera showing the wide scope and utility of the devices.

Proximal 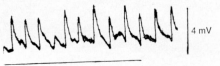 Distal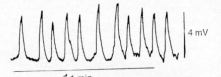

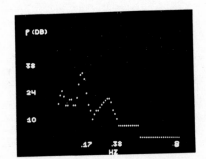

Cross Spectrum

Coherence Phase

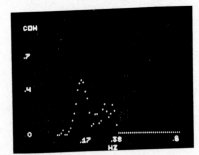

Fig. 8.

Tracings made 1 day post-implant from two force transducers chronically implanted on the right oviduct of an estrous rabbit doe. Distal refers to uterine end of oviduct. Upper two sections show simultaneously recorded raw tracings from the gauges spaced about 2 cm apart. Middle two sections of illustration show power spectra of the tracings immediately above. Bottom left section shows the frequency coherence of the cross-spectrum (COH), bottom right section shows the phase relationship (PHS) of the dominant coherent frequencies, if any (Jenkins and Watts 1968). The peak shown in all three spectra is a wave of 0.17 Hz which lags about 45° from proximal to distal gauge, permitting the conclusion that the recordings demonstrate a propagated wave toward the uterus at 0.17 Hz. Vertical scale on raw tracings indicate mV of bridge imbalance at the transducer with 1 V bridge energization. Power spectra are log scaled on the ordinate in relative power (P(DB)), linearly scaled in frequency on the abscissae (Hz). The cross-spectrum is linearly scaled in coherence (maximum of 1.0) on the ordinate, linear in frequency on abscissa. The phase of the cross-spectrum is scaled in degrees lead (up, +) or lag (down, –) of the right power-spectrum (distal) using the left power-spectrum (proximal) as a reference. The abscissa is linear with frequency.

88

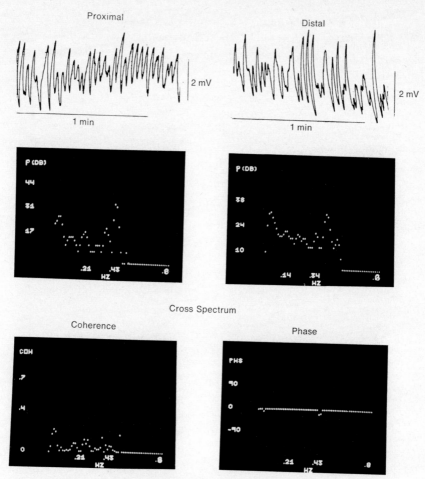

Fig. 9.

Tracings from same gauges on same rabbit oviduct made 6 days post-implant and 10 h post-injection of 100 IU of chorionic gonadotrophin. All scaling and diagram orientation unchanged from Fig. 8. Note significant high-frequency activity in all spectra at 0.43–0.46 Hz.

b) Mechanical strength of the silicon transducer body.

Between the two suture loops of the transducer is the diffused resistor region. Due to a compromise between mechanical strength and sensitivity of the transducer, the diffused region (~ 30 μM) has been made thinner than the rest of the transducer (~ 65 μM). As a consequence of this difference in thickness, the diffused resistor region is more vulnerable to breakage than the suture loops. When one end of the force transducer is fixed and the other free end is subject to some bending force by using a test, we find that the diffused resistor

89

region will break as the bending force is increased beyond 5 g. This force can by no means be considered small for such a small device, in fact, it is 1–2 orders of magnitude greater than the biological forces the transducer is intended to measure.

C) Sensitivity.

The resistance of the force transducer will change when there is stress present. The following graph is a resistance change versus bending force curve. As can be seen the response is rather linear up to a resistance change of 20 %. In biological use, ΔR is usually 1 % or less.

The force transducers have been used as single and double implants on rabbit oviducts with considerable success, the main difficulties encountered were in the leads and attachments, not the devices *per se*, limiting the utility of single devices to a life span from a few days to a few weeks. Fig. 7 illustrates the wave forms the devices are capable of recording from a variety of smooth muscle structures and from the rabbit aorta. The recordings are of high quality.

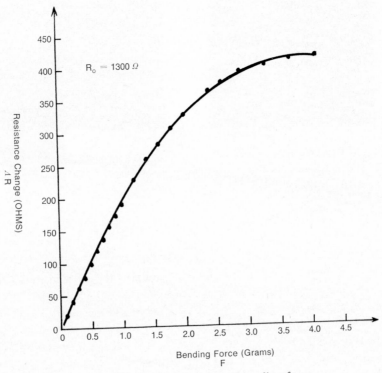

Ro = Resistance of transducer without bending force.

Spectral analysis of multiple gauge implant.

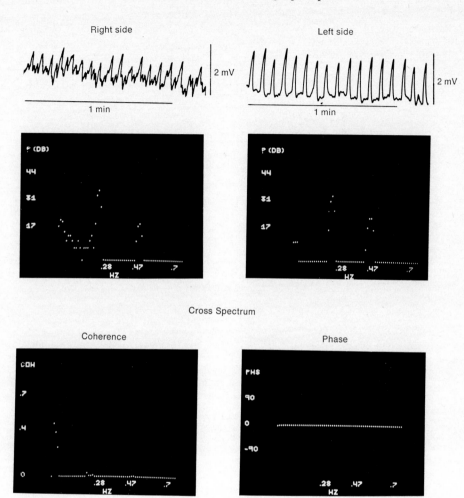

Fig. 10.

Tracings from two force gauges chronically implanted on the right and left oviducts of an estrous rabbit doe. Each is on the isthmus about 2 cm from the uterotubal junction. Recordings made 2 days post-implant and 8 h post-injection of 100 IU of chorionic gonadotrophin. Note peak of high frequency activity in both power spectra about 0.48–0.50 Hz. The COH and PHS show that the activity of right and left oviducts is similar but uncorrelated. See Fig. 8 for detailed explanation of legends.

Time series analysis.

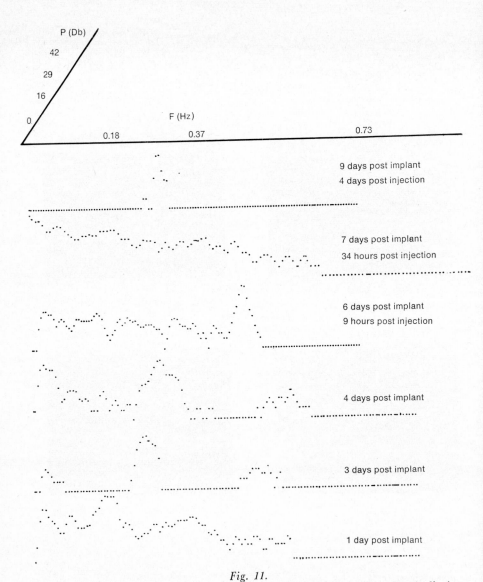

Fig. 11.

A series of power spectra made from recordings from a single gauge chronically implanted on the oviductal isthmus of an estrous rabbit doe. The scales at the top refer to all spectra. The raw traces are not shown. Note the wide variation in the spectra from day to day and the transient high frequency peak (0.45 Hz) in the 6 day post-implant spectrum made 9 h after injection of 100 IU of chorionic gonadotrophin.

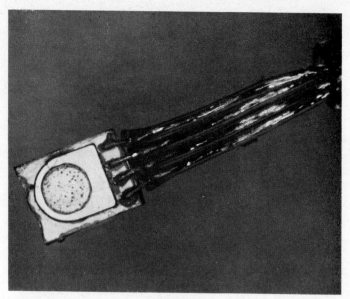

Fig. 12.

A completed pressure transducer showing the 1 mm diaphragm and the silicon block containing the reference atmosphere and bonding pads. The #40 stranded wires enter a silicone rubber tube at the right.

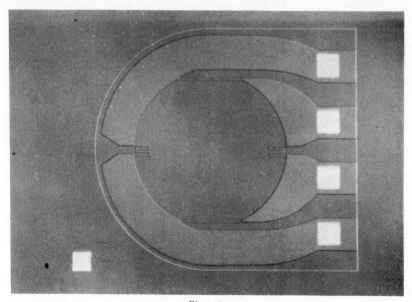

Fig. 13.

Close up of the sensitive diaphragm of the integrated circuit pressure transducer showing the bonding pads, integral conductive channels, and the four sensitive elements.

A number of implants were successful in rabbit does which were sub-sequently subjected to an induced ovulation by injection of 100 IU of chorionic gonadotrophin. Figs. 8 & 9 show recordings made from force transducers sutured to a rabbit oviduct (isthmus) before (Fig. 8) and 10 h after induced ovulation (Fig. 9). Spectral analysis of data has revealed a strong high frequency component in the oviductal contraction pattern which seems characteristic of the early ovulatory phase (Maistrello 1971; Talo 1974) (see Figs. 9 & 10). In rabbit does with a force transducer sutured to each oviductal isthmus and later subjected to induced ovulation, the fast frequency component appears bilateral-ly but the frequencies are not identical on cross-spectral analysis (see Fig. 10). The contraction frequency spectra from an individual gauge on the oviductal isthmus vary widely from day to day. A series of spectra from a single gauge over a 10-day span during which ovulation was induced are shown in Fig. 11. A strong high-frequency component (28 waves per min) is seen only in the spectrum from 9 h post-injection of chorionic gonadotrophin. More experi-ments need to be made before biological conclusions can be drawn but the illustrations indicate the power and scope of the multiple transducer implant as a research tool, particularly when modern data processing techniques are applied to the recordings.

MICROMINIATURE PRESSURE TRANSDUCERS

1. *Introduction*

These devices have also been scaled for use on the rabbit oviduct (1 mm diameter, 200 μ thickness) and are presently in the prototype testing phase. It is obvious that even this tiny device may obstruct the lumen of the rabbit oviduct isthmus but we hope it can be used on edge impaled through the ovi-

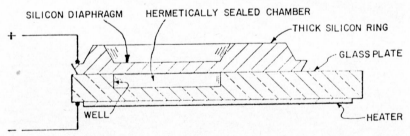

Fig. 14.

Cross-sectional diagram showing the details of construction of the pressure sensor. The heater and voltage supply are removed after bonding the glass plate to the silicon block, forming the integral reference atmosphere.

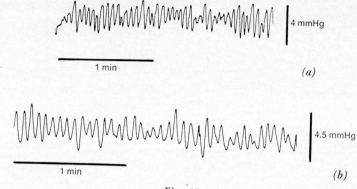

Fig. 15.
Two examples of recordings made with pressure transducer inserted in ampulla of rabbit oviduct *in situ* under pentobarbital anesthesia. The device produced partial occlusion. a, right, b, left.

ductal wall without producing obstruction. A photograph of the current version of the completed device is shown in Fig. 12 and a photograph of the sensitive diaphragm (Samaun et al. 1971) of the transducer is illustrated in Fig. 13.

The integrated circuit absolute pressure transducer (Fig. 12) consists of a glass cap that has a well etched in it and a silicon diaphragm containing four diffused piezoresistors connected to form a Wheatstone bridge. A cross-section of the transducer is shown in Fig. 14. The diaphragm is surrounded by a thick rim of silicon for support and protection. To construct the absolute pressure transducer, the glass with the well positioned directly over the diaphragm is anodically bonded to the silicon rim. The anodic bond is accomplished by heating the glass and silicon to 400°C and then applying a potential of 600 V to the silicon with the glass cap grounded (see Fig. 14). The bond is hermetic,

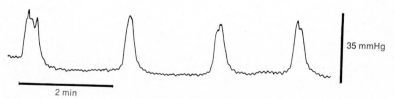

Fig. 16.
Example of recording made with pressure transducer inserted through rabbit uterine wall without luminal occlusion. Estrous doe under pentobarbital anesthesia, uterus *in situ*.

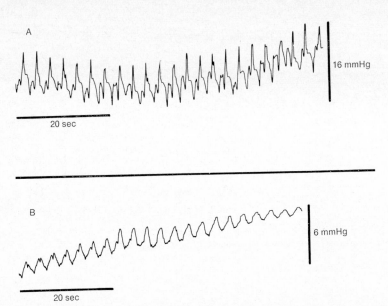

Fig. 17.

Two examples of recordings obtained from rabbit duodenum. The pressure transducer was inserted through the wall and was left free in the lumen. a. Made with duodenal occlusion 5 cm distal to the device. b. Made without occlusion. Duodenum *in situ*, pentobarbital anesthesia.

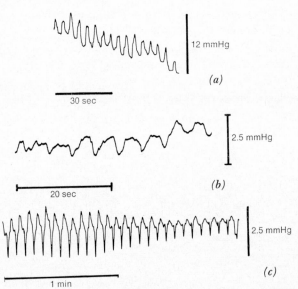

Fig. 18.

Three recordings made from rabbit ileum pressure transducer. a. With occlusion of lumen 8 cm distal. b and c. Without luminal occlusion.

and thus the well and diaphragm form a hermetically sealed chamber with a predetermined reference atmosphere trapped therein.

The diaphragm (Fig. 13) contains piezoresistive elements that form the four arms of a Wheatstone bridge. Their values change as the diaphragm flexes.

The overall dimensions of the absolute pressure transducer are $1.5 \times 2.0 \times 0.2$ mm. They have an intrinsic sensitivity of 30 μV/mmHg/V supply and a temperature drift equivalent to –2 mmHg/°C. The output voltage is linear with pressure for changes up to 300 mmHg. Experiments to date have revealed a long-term drift of less than 1 mm of Hg per month. This is much smaller than the long-term drift of commercially available pressure transducers. Initial biological testing of the prototype units has been satisfactory, demonstrating ability to resolve pressures of less than 1 mmHg over a range of 200 mmHg. The waveforms are clean and several examples of recordings made from rabbit hollow viscera with one of the devices are shown in Fig. 15 (oviduct), 16 (uterus), 17 (duodenum), 18 (ileum). Present efforts are aimed at improving the wire assembly for withdrawal without reoperation and producing versions for insertion through the walls of hollow organs (diaphragm on edge) as well as more conventional assemblies.

SUMMARY

Three different transducer assemblies have been specifically designed and fabricated for recording electrical waves, contractile activity, and pressure from the rabbit oviduct. All have met design performance criteria and are at various stages of refinement of design. The use of integrated circuit technology has yielded this great reduction in transducer size without loss of sensitivity or accuracy. We believe these devices will have use in many types of chronic and acute experiments on a variety of organs in many species and will be the first devices suitable for chronic implanted use in humans. The IC technology is inherently ideal for mass production with consequent lower unit cost for the devices.

ACKNOWLEDGMENTS

The authors are grateful to Walter Lau for construction of lead assemblies, to Holde Muller for the biological data collection, and to Alex Perel for computer programming. This work was supported by NICHD Contract NO1-HD 3-2774.

97

REFERENCES

Jenkins G. M. and Watts D. G. (1968) *Spectral Analysis and Its Applications*, pp. 363–420. Holden-Day, San Francisco.

Nunn T. A., Angell J. B. and Nelsen T. S. (1973) Force transducer for oviduct instrumentation. *Proc. Biomed. Eng. Soc.*, pp. 29–30, Los Angeles.

Maistrello I. (1971) Extraluminal recording of oviductal contractions in the unanesthetized rabbit. *J. appl. Physiol. 31*, 768–771.

Samaun F., Wise K. D., Nielsen E. D. and Angell J. B. (1971) An IC Piezo-resistive pressure sensor for biomedical instrumentation. *Proc. IEEE Solid State Circuits Conf.*, pp. 104–105.

Talo A. (1974) Electric and mechanical activity of the rabbit oviduct *in vitro* before and after ovulation. *Biol. Reprod. 11*, 335–345.

The Center for Research and Training
in Reproductive Biology and Voluntary Regulation of Fertility,
Department of Obstetrics and Gynecology,
The University of Texas Health Science Center at San Antonio,
7703 Floyd Curl Drive, San Antonio, Texas 78284

METHODS FOR STUDYING OVUM TRANSPORT RATES[1]

By

Robert J. Crosby, Marvin L. Chatkoff
and Carl J. Pauerstein[2]

ABSTRACT

A technique is described for producing plastic ovum surrogate microspheres (Dow cyclic sulfonium zwitterion XD8157L or XD8383) labelled
with radioactive isotope. Four microcuries of ^{125}I, sufficient for *in vivo*
detection within oviducts, were bound into microspheres of 180 to 200
micron diameter. Microspheres were placed in oviducts of rabbits using
a one microliter repetitive micropipetter. A collimated end window
Geiger-Muller tube located the position of the surrogates along the
lengths of oviducts to within ± 1 mm.

The ability to locate mammalian ova in the oviduct *in vivo* at various times
following ovulation would provide a means of assessing the capability of
various treatments to alter transport rates. Techniques presently used to determine the position of ova within the oviduct include *in situ* flushing of the
intact oviduct (Mastroianni and Rosseau 1965), surgical excision of the oviduct
followed by segmenting and flushing to recover ova (Greenwald 1959, 1961)
or clearing in benzyl benzoate to render ova visible within the excised oviduct

---

[1] Supported by World Health Organization Grant No. 3973 to Carl J. Pauerstein.
[2] Supported by a Research Career Development Award KO4-HD47279 from the
National Institute of Child Health and Human Development.

99

(Orsini 1962; Longley and Black 1968). No *in vivo* techniques exist for the isthmus.

The use of radioactive ovum models offers the possibility of defining the time course of ovum transport *in vivo* under normal, pathologic or pharmacologically modified conditions, both chronically and acutely.

Gamma rays penetrate the oviductal wall and high activity isotopes permit loading detectable but harmless levels of radiation (a few microcuries [μCi]) into either ova or plastic ovum-sized surrogates. To be suitable, surrogate ova must be transported with a time course similar to that of natural ova and possess sufficient radioactivity to be easily and accurately detected through the oviductal wall.

Commercially available vitreous carbon radioactive microspheres are labelled with relatively long half-life isotopes of low specific activity. They contain less than 0.48 μCi in each 200 micron diameter sphere making detection of these particular single microspheres difficult. Microspheres of size range 12 microns to 44 microns of human serum albumen labelled with ^{125}I have been described, but if these were enlarged to 200 microns with the same density of activity, each would have a theoretical activity of only 0.16 μCi (Zolle et al. 1970). Ion exchange resins labelled with radioactivity have been used as ovum surrogates (Harper et al. 1960; Harper 1961*a,b*; Bennett and Rowson 1961; Ishihama and Miyai 1969). The low specific activity of such microspheres necessitates excision of the oviduct and detection by scintigram or auto-radiogram. For these reasons a new technique was developed for producing large quantities of radioactive plastic ova simply and inexpensively.

The availability of monomer plastics which cure to hard, solvent-resistant hydrophobic polymers (Hatch et al. 1971) capable of binding significant amounts of radioactivity permits fabricating labelled spheres suitable for use as surrogate ova. At least 4 μCi of radioactivity may be incorporated in each 200 micron sphere, making chronic and acute detection of single surrogates possible.

METHODS

A. *Fabrication of microspheres*

[125]I radioisotope (10 mCi of specific activity ca. 400 mCi/ml) in aqueous solution with 0.1 N NaOH as a solubilizer was reduced in volume by evaporation from approximately 25 μl to less than one μl by directing a stream of dry nitrogen through a Pasteur pipette over the surface. The radioactive liquid in its V-vial container was retained in its lead shipping shield to reduce radiation exposure. A fume hood protected against accidental inhalation of radioactive vapours. 0.5 ml of monomer (cyclic sulfonium zwitterion) was blackened with one drop of India ink to provide visual contrast. Twenty μl of blackened

monomer was added to the concentrated isotope using an Eppendorf repetitive pipette and mixed thoroughly by repeated ejections and aspirations. Bubbles or foam formed by mixing were allowed to subside. An oil bath containing 1 ml of fluorosilicone fluid (130 cs viscosity; 1.26 specific gravity) in a 25 ml beaker was stirred with a 2.5 cm long smooth magnetic stirring bar (without spinning ring) at approximately 1 rps on a stirring hot plate at room temperature. The isotope-laden monomer was pipetted from the V-vial into the center of the slowly stirring oil bath. Because the monomer (1.04 specific gravity) floated on the heavy oil, the stirring velocity was increased momentarily to form a vortex and break up the few large drops into thousands of microspheres of various sizes. The stirring was stopped temporarily while the floating microspheres were visually examined to ensure that all of the excessively large drops had been broken up by the shearing forces produced during the period of rapid stirring.

The stirring plate was brought to a temperature of approximately 70°C, and the stirring speed maintained at 1 rps. Neither of these conditions was critical; however, an oil bath temperature of at least 60°C ensured curing of the plastic. The bath temperature was kept below 100°C to prevent water trapped within the monomer from boiling, causing possible formation of porous rather than solid microspheres. Slow stirring prevented the particles from sticking to the sides of the beaker or coalescing in the center, and also kept them from falling to the bottom and becoming flat. After approximately one-half hour at 70°C, the beaker was removed from the stirring plate and allowed to cool at room temperature.

The surrogates were poured into a Petri dish and sorted for size with the aid of a dissecting microscope using 100 x magnification. Surrogates were transferred using either a pipette with its tip pulled down to 250 microns diameter, or a repetitive one μl micropipette. Excessively large or small microspheres were removed by suction filtering through a 1 micron pore filter and the silicone fluid recycled for subsequent use. The film of silicone fluid adhering to the surrogate ova was removed by repeated washings with tetrahydrofuran, followed by rinsing in absolute ethanol, then 70 % ethanol for sterilization and storage. Prior to use, surrogates were rinsed and placed in sterile normal saline.

B. *In vivo testing*

Rabbits were used to determine the suitability of the microspheres as surrogate ova. New Zealand white virgin does were given 100 IU of human chorionic gonadotrophin (HCG) intravenously. Six hours later, they were anesthetized with intravenous sodium pentobarbital (30 mg/kg) and the oviducts exposed through a midline abdominal incision. Three or four radioactive plastic surrogates were placed within each ampulla, one to two cm from the fimbria, using a sterilized one μl pipette. The skin was moved to bring the incision over first the right and then the left oviduct so that the pipette could be inserted with minimum disturbance of the natural position of the oviduct.

The rabbits were sacrificed at 24 h intervals after HCG injection and the location of the microspheres was noted. The oviducts were excised and flushed with Tyrode's solution to recover natural and surrogate ova which were examined microscopically to evaluate their relative sizes and the thickness of mucin coatings.

Surrogates were located *in vivo* in oviducts of HCG-treated rabbits using a mica end window Geiger-Muller tube encapsulated in epoxy resin within a glass tube with a thin, flat bottom. For further resolution in locating the position of the surrogates, the glass tube was provided with a slip-on collimator made of 0.2 mm thick lead foil with a 1 mm by 10 mm slit. The collimator slit was aligned parallel to the longitudinal axis of the oviduct for gross location and turned perpendicular for fine location. A rate meter with audible count indication was used to drive the Geiger-Muller tubes.

Although the above technique is simple it was possible that anesthesia and unavoidable operative trauma interfered with ovum transport. Therefore an implanted system was developed for chronic monitoring, using a detector glued on the surface of the oviduct at a selected location, such as the ampullary-isthmic junction. Semiconductor radiation detectors including lithium-drifted silicone and chlorine doped cadmium telluride were considered for this application because they required a relatively low voltage power supply for direct conversion of the radiation into electrical impulses. However, they proved to be prohibitively expensive, fragile, too stiff, and difficult to shield from stray electromagnetic interference.

To avoid these difficulties, a system was designed using a cesium iodide scintillating crystal doped with thallium to detect the radiation. The resulting flashes of light were transmitted by a plastic fiber optic to a sensitive 13 stage photomultiplier tube. There the light was converted into electrical pulses, and amplified. The threshold was detected by a single channel analyzer, applied to a ratemeter, and recorded on a strip chart recorder through a low pass filter. The output was count rate versus time. This system emphasizes the desirable characteristics of the actual detector mounted on the oviduct (flexibility, small size, light weight, low cost, ruggedness) at the expense of a rather complicated electronic demodulation system and a large photomultiplier tube which requires a stable 940 V DC supply. It is suitable where the animal can be restrained, or on a cooperative subject.

Scintillator fibers were prepared by selecting plastic fiber optics of 0.3 mm diameter and 1 meter length that were free of optical and mechanical imperfections.

Crystals of scintillating material were cleaved with a scalpel under the microscope to approximately 0.5 mm diameter. They were attached to one square cut end of the plastic fiber with α-cyanoacrylate adhesive which held them in place while they were repeatedly dipped in cyclic sulfonium zwitterion monomer, air dried, and baked at 70°C for 15 min. This cycle was repeated approximately 15 times to produce a pinhole-free encapsulation on the crystal and the last 2 cm of fiber. The last 3 coats were applied with monomer blackened with India ink to reduce sensitivity to ambient light.

The fiber was inserted in a 2.5 mm diameter black flexible vinyl plastic tube to shield it from light and to give it mechanical support. Under barbiturate anesthesia, the fiber and tube were inserted through the rabbit's vagina and exposed by an abdominal midline incision. The vinyl tube was sutured to the uterus and the scintillating crystal was glued to the oviduct with surgical cement. The exterior end of the vinyl sheath was connected to an adapter tube where the inner fiber was cemented with quick setting epoxy resin. The end of the fiber was cut smooth and square, and coupled to the photomultiplier faceplate with silicone fluid.

RESULTS

The above technique produced plastic microspheres in a wide range of diameters containing relatively high levels of radioactivity firmly bound throughout their volume. The 180 micron plastic surrogates contained at least 4 μCi each, and less than 0.01 % of their activity leached out into sterile Tyrode's solution after a two week period of incubation at 37°C.

The surrogates accumulated less radial thickness of mucin (164 ± 3 microns SEM, n = 14) than did the natural ova (68.2 ±7 microns SEM, n = 11) at 60 h after HCG administration ($P < 0.001$). Thus 200 micron surrogates acquired a final diameter of approximately 220 microns compared to the approximately 300 microns overall diameter of natural ova including the mucin coat. Plastic ovum surrogates of 600 micrometers were found to track the natural ova reasonably well, with some tendency for smaller surrogates to travel too rapidly, while larger sizes were too slow. The ovum surrogates could be located to within ± 1 mm using the Geiger-Muller tube. Their position in the oviduct corresponded to that of natural ova as confirmed in benzyl benzoate cleared preparations.

Preliminary bench tests on implantable detector systems demonstrate that the system is capable of locating radioactive surrogates of 200 μ diameter or larger to within ± 1 mm. The tests were performed by placing surrogates within the excised isthmic lumens of rabbits. Surrogates separated by a few millimeters could be identified individually. In vivo measurements in restrained rabbits have proved the system capable of detecting surrogates passing single crystals. Further evaluation is in progress.

DISCUSSION

Cyclic sulfonium zwitterion monomers cure to hard, solvent-resistant, hydrophobic polymers with no organic by-products. The aqueous monomers mix readily with aqueous solutions of isotopes and are immiscible with the silicone oil in the bath allowing the surface tension to form the droplets into microspheres as they cure. Attempts to use a cottonseed oil bath were unsuccessful because its density was not sufficient to keep the microspheres from sedimenting when the stirring rate was slow enough to prevent breakup into excessively small particles. A density gradient made of cottonseed oil and tetrachloroethylene also failed because the chlorinated hydrocarbon prevented the monomer from polymerizing properly.

The first step in the curing process is the loss of water from the monomer as the oil bath temperature is gradually raised, with consequent shrinkage and increase in density. Polymerization proceeds with opening of the cyclic sulfonium ring to yield a long-chain, highly cross-linked polymer which binds the radioisotope firmly within the microspheres (Hatch et al. 1971). The polymer droplets shrink 70 % in volume and 34 % in diameter during the first part of the cure when the water is being driven off. The droplets are not initially spherical because the specific gravity of the monomer is only 1.04 while that of the silicone oil is 1.27. Therefore, the droplets float on the oil and assume a shape approximating a prolate spheroid which makes their final cured diameter difficult to estimate in the uncured state.

The scintillating crystal is the key element in the implanted system, and as yet a perfect one has not been found. Cesium iodide doped with thallium is the best compromise material, having high sensitivity and emitting a yellow light which is conducted well by the fiber. However, it deteriorates rapidly from moisture and was often unusable after three days of implantation, depending on the quality of the coatings.

Calcium fluoride doped with europium is much more resistant to moisture, but has only about half the sensitivity of cesium iodide and emits a blue-violet light that is severely attenuated by the plastic fiber.

Gadolinium oxysulfide doped with terbium has the highest conversion efficiency, resists moisture, and the wavelengths of its emissions are well matched to the fiber optics. Unfortunately it is available only as fine particles less than 20 microns in diameter. It might be suitable as the outer component of a composite scintillator with a crystal of calcium fluoride inside. The white gadolinium oxysulfide powder would serve as both a scintillator and a reflector of the light generated in the calcium fluoride.

For use in unrestrained primates, a system was designed using the same scintillator and fiber optic, but with a subminiature channel electron multiplier replacing the photomultiplier tube. This system together with its subminiature high voltage power supply and high energy lithium batteries, made it possible to consolidate the electronics into a back pack suitable for baboons or large rhesus monkeys, using an RF telemetry link to a remote receiver and pulse discrimination circuits.

Finally, a commercial personal radiation monitor (Baird Atomic Co.) about the size of a pack of cigarettes, was modified by removing its internal side window GM and mounting it on the end of a 30 cm flexible coaxial cable with appropriate potting materials to protect it from moisture. This probe was passed through the vagina and the uterine cervix to detect the arrival of the radioactive surrogate in the uterus. The monitor emitted audible signals when the surrogate approached to within approximately 3 cm of the detector. In conclusion, it has been demonstrated that radioactive ovum surrogates can be used to measure ovum transport rates directly *in vivo*.

ACKNOWLEDGMENTS

We wish to thank Dr. Horacio Croxatto, Catholic University, Santiago, Chile, for calling to our attention the paper of Dr. I. Zolle et al. explaining the technique for making human serum albumen microspheres. We also thank the Dow Chemical Company of Midland, Michigan, for providing samples of their monomers.

REFERENCES

Bennett J. P. and Rowson L. E. A. (1961) The use of radioactive artificial eggs in studies of egg transfer and transport in the female reproductive tract. *Proc. Fourth Int. Cong. Anim. Reprod.*, The Hague, p. 360–366.
Greenwald G. S. (1959) Tubal transport of ova in the rabbit. *Anat. Rec. 133,* 386.
Greenwald G. S. (1961) A study of the transport of ova through the rabbit oviduct. *Fertil. and Steril. 12,* 80–95.
Harper M. J. K., Bennett J. P., Boursnell J. C. and Rowson L. E. A. (1960) An autoradiographic method for the study of egg transport in the rabbit Fallopian tube. *J. Reprod. Fertil. 1,* 249–267.
Harper M. J. K. (1961a) Egg movement through the ampullar region of the Fallopian tube of the rabbit. *Proc. Fourth Int. Cong. Anim. Reprod.*, The Hague, p. 375–380.
Harper M. J. K. (1961b) The mechanisms involved in the movement of newly ovulated eggs through the ampulla of the rabbit Fallopian tube. *J. Reprod. Fertil. 2,* 522–524.
Hatch M. J., Yoshimine M., Schmidt D. L. and Smith H. B. (1971) Novel aryl cyclic sulfonium zwitterion that polymerizes when heated. *J. Amer. chem. Soc. 93,* 4617–4618.
Ishihama A. and Miyai T. (1969) Transport and cleavage of ova in rat and rabbit oviducts with the IUD. *Amer. J. Obstet. Gynec. 105,* 169–174.

Longley W. J. and Black D. L. (1968) Comparisons of methods for locating ova in the oviduct of the rabbit. *J. Reprod. Fertil.* 16, 69–72.

Mastroianni Jr. L. and Rosseau C. H. (1965) Influence of the intrauterine coil on ovum transport and sperm distribution in the monkey. *Amer. J. Obstet. Gynec.* 93, 416–420.

Orsini Margaret W. (1962) Technique of preparation, study and photography of benzyl-benzoate cleared material for embryological studies. *J. Reprod. Fertil.* 3, 283–287.

Zolle I., Rhodes B. A. and Wagner Jr. H. N. (1970) Preparation of metabolizable radioactive human serum albumen microspheres for studies of the circulation. *Int. J. appl. Radiat. Isotop.* 21, 155–167.

Drexel University*, Department of Biological Sciences,
Biomedical Engineering and Science Program,
Philadelphia, Pennsylvania, USA
and University of Pennsylvania(Department of Obstetrics
and Gynecology, School of Medicine, Philadelphia,
Pennsylvania, USA

PHYSIOLOGIC ASSESSMENT OF OVIDUCTAL MOTILITY – EXTRALUMINAL TELEMETRIC SUBJECT EVALUATION

By

E. Fromm, C-R. Garcia and D. C. Jeutter*

ABSTRACT

Characterization of oviductal contractility as it relates to ovarian cycle
status and alterations thereof is of widespread interest. The role such
activity plays, measures of its quantitative magnitude, timing relationships
and muscular effort expended are significant with respect to potential
contraceptive means. The program described offers such a characterization
with the use of specially developed transduction, data transmission,
acquisition and processing techniques. Subsequent to definition of pertinent parameters sensitive isotonic extraluminal transducers for chronic
implantation were developed. The associated chronically implantable bio-
telemetry system allowed multiple input force transmission and data
acquisition. Systems are statically and dynamically characterized prior to
implantation and subsequent experimentation in the unrestrained female
Macaca mulatta.

The Extraluminal Contractile Force Transducers (ECFT) make use of
conductive silicone rubber or piezoresistive silicon. The minimally loading
units allow chronic *in vivo* segmental contractility monitoring with demonstrated lack of interference with normal reproductive function. The
devices, which may be utilized in either the direct wire restrained subject
or the unrestrained subject with implanted biotelemeter, are calibrated to
forces of 15 g force providing average sensitivities of 1.5 % per g force
at frequencies to 3 Hz. These transducers are used in conjunction with
the chronically implantable telemetry system. The multichannel system is
of the PPM/FM type having an implanted operating life of 5 months and
range of 15 ft. with present power source configuration.

Physiologic experimentation has proceeded with implantation of these systems in four experimental groups of *Macaca mulatta*. In addition to continuous contractility measurements, correlative indices of plasma estrogen and progesterone, vaginal cytology and menstrual history are obtained for ovarian cycle timing. The continuous data is computer processed to retrieve quantitative information of magnitude, timing and expended contractile effort on a contraction by contraction basis. Analysis of this data proceeds in short (1, 8 and 24 h), medium (3 days) and long (entire cycle length) time frames for each of the quantitative measures. Short term analysis reveals variations within the day, while medium and long time frame analysis reveal timing and hormone related variations within and between experimental groups. While short term analysis reveals greater extremes, the range of cycle averages of contractile magnitudes is observed to be 0.8 to 3.3 g, contractile durations of 8.1 to 15.7 sec, contractile effort of 3.8 to 21.0 g-sec, intercontraction interval of 0.6 to 0.8 min and contractile frequency of 0.3 to 0.7 events per min. These values vary with treatment group and stage of cycle.

Contractile activity of the oviduct and its relationship to cyclic hormonal status is of interest owing to its suspected association with gamete transport, and with the pharmacologic modification thereof. Such activity is best studied at different levels of the oviduct in a chronic non-invasive manner having high resolution capabilities while monitoring small segmented contractions. Integration of such data with indices of ovarian status such as plasma steroid levels and vaginal cytology permit definition of quantitative parameters for motility measurement. Once defined in the normal cycle, variation from the norm in pharmacologically modified cycles may elucidate the physiologic mechanisms of oviductal motility.

Previously reported methods of monitoring contractile phenomena of the oviduct and uterus include experiments on excised strips of muscle tissue *in vitro,* the use of gas or fluid filled intraluminal catheters, and *in vivo* use of extraluminal contractile transducers. The *in vitro* investigations were quite different from the normal physiologic situation affording only relative qualitative inferences. Subsequent *in vivo* techniques more closely approach the reasonably normal environment yet seem to interfere or alter it in some manner. Catheter methods for recording intraluminal pressures reflect changes in oviductal radius arising from contractile activity along the organ's length. Extensive use has been made of the catheter-manometer method. Some investigators report average contractions of 6/min with increases during the periovulatory period (Seckinger and Snyder 1923). Others report low activity during menses (Sica-Blanco et al. 1971; Coutinho 1971) with increasing frequency of 3 to 4 and 4 to 5 contractions per min during the proliferative phase (Davids 1948; Sica-Blanco et al. 1971; Coutinho 1971). Coutinho also reports intermittent higher frequency bursts during this time with regular activity of

1 to 4 contractions per min during the secretory phase. Among the problems associated with the use of open-ended catheters are accumulation of potentially occlusive oviductal luminal contents, formation of air bubbles, and catheter or subject movement. Attempts to overcome these shortcomings have included fenestration of the catheter tip (Coutinho 1971; Neri et al. 1972), flushing mechanisms (Salomy and Harper 1971; Aref and Hafez 1973) and the fitting of microballoons to the catheter tips (Caldeyro-Barcia 1954; Maia and Coutinho 1968; Aref and Hafez 1973). While these modifications have increased the longevity of the technique to allow short term acute *in vivo* experimentation, the distension of the balloon or the presence of an intraluminally placed device may itself induce activity, interfere with the reproductive function of the organ, and generally respond as a temporal and spatial summation of total contractile activity as contrasted to activity at a more localized site.

Extraluminal contractile force transducers reported by others have been used to measure activity of the gut (Jacoby, Bennett and Bass 1962; Bass and Wiley 1965), common bile duct (Ludwick 1966) and uterus (Dominic and Reinke 1968). Their mass, dimensions and stiffness have made application to the oviduct unfeasible. In one study (Feit et al. 1968) it was necessary to support the weight of a miniaturized version of the device with an auxillary suture to the back muscles of the animal, while another (Dominic and Reinke 1968) noted interference with reproductive function.

Interest in obtaining quantitative measures of segmental contractile activity for multiple ovarian cycles, as well as the need for a chronic *in vivo* experiment having neither physical nor pharmacologic interference with subject mobility, activity or reproductive function led to the present investigation.

MATERIALS AND METHODS

To achieve the stated objectives has required definition of pertinent parameters, development of novel transduction techniques, development of chronically implantable transmission systems and their associated receivers, as well as the evolution of data acquisition and analysis techniques. The methods and procedures described have evolved over a number of years with the final versions in continuous use for the past two years.

Early work with the isotonic silicone rubber extraluminal contractile force transducer (ECFT) was described by Fromm (1967) and now has subsequent improvements (Jeutter and Fromm 1971a,b). The device is constructed by crimping previously formed gold plated nickel bands 0.5 mm wide × 0.08 mm thick about the 0.8 mm diameter cylinder of carbon-doped silicone rubber heat cured to a resistivity of 21 ohm-cm. Teflon-coated braided stainless steel wires (25 strands AWG50) are soldered to these bands prior to crimping. The nominal resistance of the unit is obtained by selecting the spacing between the nickel bands. For an approximate 1000 ohm device the spacing is consistently 2 mm. Assembly proceeds with insertion of the sensing element within a 1 cm length of silicone rubber sheath 0.8 mm i. d. by 1.3 mm o. d. along with an adjacent 0.13 mm × 0.5 mm mylar strip. After a single suture is tied snugly about the lead wires at the proximal end to prevent shearing motion the unit is injected with silicone rubber adhesive to ensure mechanical continuity and is allowed to cure. Theoretical mechanical operation of the device has been reported (Gallant and Fromm 1973) and may be likened to a strain gauge (silicone rubber element) mounted on a beam (mylar). As an applied force deflects the beam and gauge a change in electrical resistance results owing to the asymmetry of the cross-section. Prior to calibration and subsequent use the devices are saturated in 37°C saline for 10 days and monitored for stability. The hydrophobic nature of silicone rubber allows its electrical characteristics to change with environmental moisture. Stabilization occurs within this 10 day period and the units are kept in sterile saline until time of implantation.

The devices are subsequently dynamically and statically calibrated. A special test fixture holds the transducer in cantilever fashion and allows deflection by a knife edge while monitoring the applied force, resulting resistance change, and deflection. A servo-controlled driving mechanism is employed to develop forces of desired magnitude, frequency and waveshape on the transducer under test. The general characteristics of the silicone rubber ECFT are sensitivities of 1 to 2 % per gram force at the typical test deflection frequency of 0.5 Hz with a frequency response of 0.005 Hz to 1.5 Hz (–3db). Nominal resistances of completed devices may range from 500 to 1500 ohms. The silicone rubber ECFT maintains its high sensitivity to contractile forces while being able to withstand severe overstress which might result from extenuating intra-abdominal conditions. Thus, for example, the device may experience strong forces from an unusually strong uterine contraction without breakage and still allow collection of the normal contractile activity. Observation of the implanted device over the site of a developing rabbit embryo shows the ability to withstand *in vivo* 180° curvature without breakage. Experiments performed to evaluate the effect on reproductive function show no interference with blastocyst implantation, embryonic development, gestation or parturition (Epstein 1972). The minimal mechanical loading of the isotonically contracting musculature of the reproductive tract has made this silicone rubber ECFT a realistic choice for either oviductal or uterine measurements.

The ECFT used in oviduct contractility monitoring for the past several years employs a 2.5 mm × 0.25 mm × 0.025 mm thick piezoresistive silicon sensor mounted on a beam strip of heat-treated 0.2 mm thick beryllium copper (Jeutter 1974). Electrical connection is made with teflon coated stranded stainless steel wire soldered to an electrodeposited copper foil terminal pad along with a single strand of fine gold wire from the silicon sensor element. The use of conventional chemical etching techniques for beam strips and semiconductor fabrication allows repeatability of performance. These units are inserted into a silicone rubber sheath 0.64 mm i. d. by 0.81 mm o. d. followed by the injection of silicone rubber adhesive. After assembly, devices are calibrated in similar fashion to that described previously for the silicone gauge. Characteristics of this unit include 1.5 to 1.7 % resistance change from the nominal 1000 ohm initial gauge resistance per g force applied. Deflections of 0.5 mm per 10 g force are found while frequency response extends from 0 to 3 Hz (–3db).

The 1000 ohm nominal resistance for both transducers shown in Fig. 1, their high sensitivity to bending forces, and compatibility with the implanted environment make them useful for either short or long term experiments. Furthermore, their utility exists in either direct wire mode coupled to external circuitry and recorders or, as in this work, as the input devices to the chronically implantable biotelemeter developed for multi-site monitoring of contractility by PPM/FM telemetry.

The telemeters employed in this investigation were developed within this laboratory specifically for chronic *in vivo* utilization. Each system in this

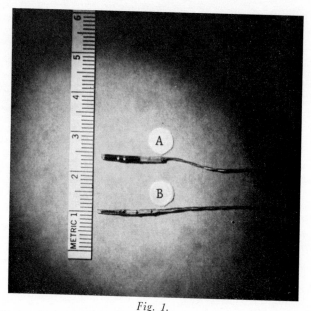

Fig. 1.
Assembled silicone rubber (A) and silicon gauge (B) transducers prior to organ attachment.

111

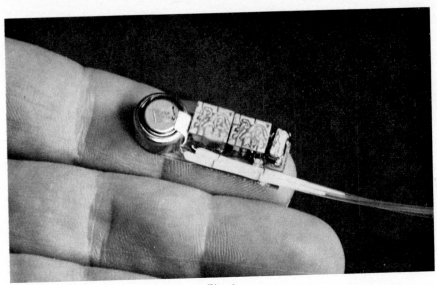

Fig. 2.
Two channel force measurement telemetry system prior to final encapsulation
and implantation.

study transmits two channels of contractile data. System design is of modular
form such that each channel of each variable is represented by a "plug-in"
block no larger than 6.5 mm × 6.5 mm × 3.5 mm (force module), though for
other variables they are half this size. The modules are interconnected through
the main circuit board to which they attached. Thus while this study utilizes
two force channels, the capability and flexibility of the system allows additional channels for the variables of temperature, biopotential, and pressure
measurement. The two channel system is designed for standard IRIG frequencies of 1.7 KHz and 3.9 KHz for each of the subcarrier oscillators
and 115 MHz for the carrier. The units are energized with two special biomedical mercury cells permitting up to 6 months of continuous operation. One
force transducer leadwire pair of each type is secured to the main circuit
board. An unsealed two channel force telemeter of this type is shown in Fig. 2.
Each system block is tested and calibrated individually as well as in a complete assembly. Characteristics of per cent input change (*i. e.* resistance) vs.
output frequency are obtained and related to force vs. frequency output change
via the transducer calibrations. Thus each channel of each system has a quantitative calibration of g force exerted by the muscle vs. system output change
prior to implantation. The systems are sealed and prepared for implantation
by encapsulating in a high dielectric imbedding paraffin followed by flexible
paraffin-polyethylene. This provides a moisture barrier as well as a flexible

sealed interface between the telemeter and the transducer leads. A final thin coating of silicone rubber is applied prior to cleansing and ethylene oxide sterilization in preparation for surgical implantation.

The surgical implantation technique has been developed to allow ease of implantation and to minimize intra-abdominal connective tissue growth due to foreign body response. Female Rhesus monkeys *(Macaca mulatta)* of approximately 3.5 kg body weight are used. Following the administration of 10 mg Sernylan® (Phencyclidine Hydrochloride) the telemeter is placed in a pouch created between the rectus muscles and the peritoneum just below the ribs. The lead wires are brought through a subcutaneous tunnel and the incision closed. A curved suture ligature carrier is inserted at the attachment of the round ligament with the uterus and carefully directed retroperitoneally to the point where the lead wires are brought through the abdominal wall. The wires are attached to the suture ligature carrier which is then withdrawn pulling the wires through with it. The technique provides a minimal foreign body within the peritoneal cavity and eliminates adhesions. Following attachment of the force transducers to the ampullary-isthmic junction of the oviduct (Fig. 3) and the uterine fundus, the abdomen is closed. Generally four telemetrically implanted monkeys are housed at one time in fiberglass cages located in a room containing the receiving, decoding, graphic chart and magnetic tape recording equipment. The FM receivers were commercially obtained whereas

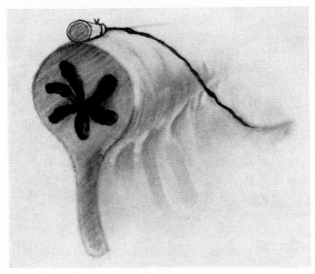

Fig. 3.
Schematic representation of transducer as attached to the oviduct.

113

subcarrier channel separation and decoding equipment was specially designed to fit the need for compatibility with the biotelemeter. The circuity designed for this purpose consists of unique Phase Locked Loop tracking filters for separating and enhancing the subcarrier channel S/N. The remainder of the circuitry restores the PPM information to analog contractile information for recording.

These systems have been employed in the study of oviductal motility as related to ovarian cycle status and its exogenous alteration. Each animal is the subject of four cycles of experimentation grouped into categories of control, estrogen or progesterone treatment, sequential therapy, and induction of ovulation with several combinations per animal. In each cycle, monitoring includes continuous motility information from the ampullary-isthmic junction (AIJ) as well as daily vaginal cytology and plasma estrogen and progesterone. Choice of the AIJ as the site of investigation has been predicted by its suggested importance in gamete transport and regulation by exogenous hormones.

Each channel of contractile data is recorded as a directly visualized analog record, as well as on magnetic tape with subsequent computer processing for specified parameters, statistics and their interpretation with respect to cycle timing. A series of user interactive computer operations has been developed for this type of data and begins with high speed "play back" of the magnetically recorded data into the A/D converters of the PDP-12 computer.

The sampling routine searches for specifically designated characteristics such as maximal and minimal values of a contraction, duration of contraction, and quiescent time between successive contractile events (Inter-Contraction Interval). Other pertinent information such as the detection threshold level and experimental identification information of monkey number, data and time, transducer/telemeter/receiving system calibration factors and playback speed are fed to the computer for subsequent calculations and output format. These allow retrieval of the information in g force with respect to contraction amplitude and real time restoration from the time-compressed playback data sampled. This resultant data is stored on computer tape or disk memory so that it may be later batch processed with additional operations or calculations and presented in several possible output formats.

The next phase combines the pre-processed data on tape or disk memory with the appropriate amplitude and time conversion factors and carries out several arithmetic operations prior to presenting a tabulated output. The result is a contraction by contraction line printer listing (Fig. 4) of contractile amplitude in g force, duration in min and sec, inter-contraction interval in min and sec, area enclosed within a force-time curve of a contractile event, and the number of contractions from the beginning of the particular record. The area enclosed within the force-time curve (g-sec) is a measure of the effort expended by the muscle segment. In this study the parameter is referred to

```
FIRST BLOCK = 076          ANIMAL NO. 390 ov    TIME START  1745
LAST BLOCK  = 107          DATE START 10-1-73   CHART PAGE 45165
SAMPLE PERIOD = 0.200 MSEC.
TAPE SPEED MULTIPLIER = 640
DC OFFSET = +      0 MV
THRESHOLD LEVEL = +   78 MV
FORCE FACTOR = 0.0164
```

CONT. AMPL. GRAMS	INTER-CONT. INTERVAL H M S	CONTRACT DURATION M S	TOTAL TIME H M S	PHILA. UNITS GM-SEC	CONT. NO.
.321	: : 3.58	: 8.70	: :12.28	14.44	1
4.772	: :26.36	1: .41	: 1:39.07	232.67	2
3.587	: :32.38	:45.05	: 2:56.51	126.57	3
2.114	: :16.76	: 6.14	: 3:19.42	11.62	4
4.772	: :54.91	1: 9.24	: 5:23.58	204.53	5
3.139	: : 8.70	:31.87	: 6: 4.15	64.35	6
5.317	: :41.21	:43.39	: 7:28.76	96.63	7
5.733	: :18.81	:48.25	: 8:35.83	115.60	8
4.612	: :56.44	: 7.42	: 9:39.71	14.68	9
4.996	: :52.35	:13.05	:10:45.11	20.78	10
4.324	: :10.49	: 6.65	:11: 2.27	13.18	11
5.092	: :17.92	: 5.88	:11:26.07	9.68	12
6.790	: 8:46.33	:38.01	:20:50.43	97.19	13
3.075	: 9:42.52	: 7.16	:30:40.12	11.48	14
2.017	: :32.25	: 9.08	:31:21.47	15.92	15
.608	: :11.64	: 3.71	:31:36.83	5.19	16
3.843	: 5:43.16	: 9.08	:37:29.08	16.78	17
4.804	: 3:48.09	:59.52	:42:16.70	107.24	18
.512	: : 2.56	:10.62	:42:29.88	16.62	19
.192	: : 5.50	: 1.15	:42:36.54	1.52	20
3.331	: :55.93	: 7.68	:43:40.15	14.55	21
1.537	: : 7.29	: 6.65	:43:54.19	11.24	22
3.715	:32:21.63	: 1.02	1:16:16.76	1.36	23
2.498	: 2:17.85	: 8.32	1:18:42.93	13.82	24
.416	: : 3.07	: 8.57	1:18:54.58	12.86	25
.192	: : 4.60	: 4.99	1:19: 4.18	6.82	26
3.203	: 5:23.58	:48.76	1:25:16.53	81.82	27
.192	: : 4.35	: 4.86	1:25:25.74	6.69	28
4.868	:34:42.56	: 9.72	2: :18.03	15.82	29
.096	: : 3.84	: 3.07	2: :24.94	4.07	30
.288	: :23.03	: .51	2: :48.49	.67	31
3.010	: 2:12.22	: 4.35	2: 3: 5.07	6.54	32
3.459	: 2:10.81	: 1.66	2: 5:17.55	2.22	33
4.804	:13:52.76	1: 7.71	2:20:18.02	107.13	34
.384	: : 9.08	:15.36	2:20:42.47	21.30	35
3.875	:10:23.48	: 2.94	2:31: 8.90	4.24	36
4.676	:48:54.65	: 3.96	3:20: 7.52	6.19	37
1.121	: :13.05	: 1.66	3:20:22.24	2.18	38
3.587	:15:25.69	: 2.68	3:35:50.62	3.81	39
1.601	: :44.28	: 2.94	3:36:37.85	4.35	40
2.242	: :33.02	: 4.99	3:37:15.87	7.53	41
2.946	: :35.32	: 7.93	3:37:59.13	16.18	42
2.402	: :27.13	: 6.27	3:38:32.54	10.06	43
3.107	: 8:13.31	:21.24	3:47: 7.09	32.25	44
3.651	:11:30.68	: 5.75	3:58:43.54	9.68	45
3.203	: :29.05	:31.10	3:59:43.70	47.58	46
.288	: : 5.88	: 5.88	3:59:55.47	8.33	47

Fig. 4.
Portion of oviductal contraction by contraction listing from the computer.

as a "Philadelphia Unit" while some versed in mechanics may recognize g-sec as the units for "impulse". This tabulated printing, which may be 20 or more such pages for a full day's record per contractile channel, becomes the basis for selection for further processing and analysis, being stored on digital tape or disk memory. It is subsequently addressed with processing routines for analysis of any desired time increment or set of identified contractions from those spanning time blocks of min to h, days or months. Inspection of the raw continuous 24 h recorded information suggests that changes may be noted in comparison of intervals of time within and between monkey cycles of as short as 10 min and as long as a month. Although investigation of the very short time segments by spectrum or frequency analysis through a sliding window or successive increment approach is contemplated in the future, the more immediate interests of full cycle and cycle segment analysis has led to the choice of time interval histograms of each of the parameters for 1 h and 8 h time blocks continuous for each ovarian cycle. This is followed with subsequent statistical evaluation and their combination for multiple day, cycle phase and full cycle comparisons.

The computerized generating and plotting routine provides histograms of these parameters on a single page for contractile records from min to days in length as the investigator may desire; in this case one and eight h. This is accomplished by specifying the first and last contraction numbers corresponding to the time segment length desired through reference to the "total time" column in the line printer listings. The shape and distribution of these histograms of the multiple contractile parameters allow not only an overall quantitative view for specified varying time intervals but shape and distribution give insight to the manner in which the contractions occurred and their physiologic interpretation.

The vertical axis represents the number of events within this time period which have the particular value of the parameter indicated on the horizontal axis. Such plots as this are used in the day-to-day, cycle-to-cycle, or cycle-to-phase comparisons for a given animal or between animals with varying treatments.

The computer stored histograms serve as the input to a further step in data reduction with the calculation of mean and mode for each histogram time block, plotted chronologically as to date and time, and presenting thereby a composite single graphic overview of the complete cycle for each of the parameters plus frequency. In addition, the mean values of each of the contractile parameters, including contractile frequency, and the standard deviations from the means are computed for three day segments. Added to the contiguous tabulating per cycle of these statistics are the plasma estrogen, progesterone, pyknotic index and medication information affording the comparison among cycle phases for each of the parameters of study.

Thus the small segment motility information is transmitted from the un-encumbered subject and quantitatively evaluated in short, intermediate and long time blocks with respect to the ovarian cycle.

RESULTS

The methodology and resulting long term continuous data from the un-restrained subject are believed to be the first such available information of oviductal activity. The instrumental aspects of this study have proved them-selves to be reliable methods by which chronically to study the oviduct quan-titatively in the unrestrained and reproductively functioning subject. Veri-fying transducer physiologic efficacy, a study (Epstein 1972) with more than 80 white New Zealand rabbbits indicated no interference with reproductive function as measured by blastocyst implantation, embryo development, gesta-tion or parturition. Split-image cinematography has verified the validity of retrieved contractile information illustrating contracting muscle beneath the transducer coincident with simultaneous system output changes.

Continuous motility data as well as plasma steroid and cytology information have been collected and processed in the manner described from 40 monkey ovarian cycles. These span control and experimental cycles of estrogen, pro-gesterone, Pergonal® and combination treatments, some of which are ovula-tory while others are anovulatory. All employ the described extraluminal force transducers and telemetry systems.

Evaluation of the information and assessment of its physiologic significance covers several levels or degrees of data reduction. Observation of the con-tinuous hard copy recorded information reveals various forms and patterns of contractions. Fig. 5 (A and B) shows representative tracings which illustrate some of the varied patterns one may observe and the rapidity with which these patterns may change. Each set (5 A and 5 B) represents 50 min from the con-tinuous record seen at the uterine fundus and AIJ of the oviduct. Note from the oviductal tracing of 5 A the burst pattern seen frequently during the peri-ovulatory period. These bursts range up to 5 min in duration and while those of this tracing are 16 min apart, they have been observed as close as 6 min apart. Within these periods of bursts we note contractions ranging between 0.1 and 0.3 g with a rather consistent frequency of 6 per min. Often these bursts are also associated with increases in oviductal muscular tone. At other times there may be less organized activity of the oviduct as seen in the same figure, with random amplitudes and frequency though the duration of contractions remains fairly constant. This less organized activity may proceed for very long periods. The changing forms of oviductal motility may be noted from Fig. 5 B. This figures demonstrates larger amplitude, regular rhythmic con-

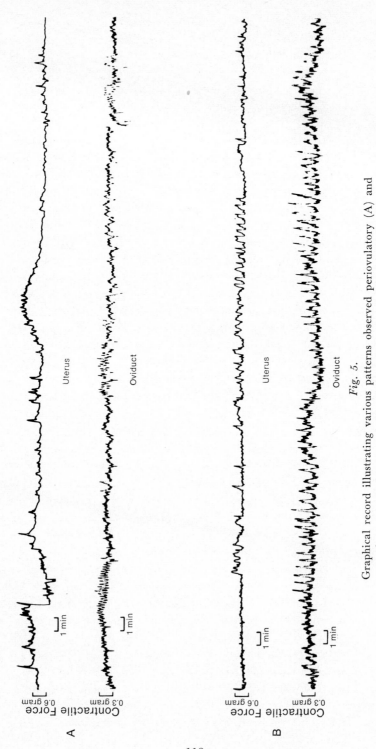

Fig. 5.

Graphical record illustrating various patterns observed periovulatory (A) and under estrogen dominance (B) as the result of exogenous administration.

Table 1.

Statistical measures of mean (x̄), mode (M), and standard deviation (σ) for the histogram set of Fig. 6.

Phase / Parameter	Early follicular freq. = 0.44 contraction/min	Estrogen domination freq. = 1.22 contraction/min	Progesterone domination freq. = 0.25 contraction/min	Pre-menstrual freq. = 0.04 contraction/min
Amplitude (g)	x̄ = 0.2 M = 0.1 σ = 0.1	x̄ = 0.5 M = 0.5 σ = 0.2	x̄ = 0.5 M = 0.1 σ = 0.3	x̄ = 0.4 M = 0.1 σ = 0.3
Duration (sec)	x̄ = 8.1 M = 5.0 σ = 8.8	x̄ = 14.5 M = 9.0 σ = 12.8	x̄ = 13.0 M = 5.0 σ = 11.4	x̄ = 6.9 M = 5.0 σ = 3.0
Phila. units (g-sec)	x̄ = 1.0 M = 0.6 σ = 1.0	x̄ = 3.7 M = 0.6 σ = 3.9	x̄ = 3.7 M = 1.4 σ = 3.2	x̄ = 2.0 M = 0.6 σ = 1.4
I.-C. I. (0–5 min)	x̄ = 0.7 M = 0.2 σ = 0.8	x̄ = 0.6 M = 0.2 σ = 0.8	x̄ = 0.6 M = 0.2 σ = 0.7	x̄ = 0.9 M = 0.2 σ = 1.0
I.-C. I. (0–30 min)	x̄ = 2.0 M = 0.2 σ = 3.9	x̄ = 0.7 M = 0.2 σ = 1.0	x̄ = 3.0 M = 0.2 σ = 5.1	x̄ = 3.2 M = 0.2 σ = 6.3

tractions of 0.2 to 0.6 g at frequencies of approximately 2 per min and contractile duration of 12 to 15 sec, approximately double that seen during the bursting pattern. This form of activity is more generally associated with high plasma estrogen levels.

While the primary effort of this work has been directed at oviductal contractility studies, uterine contraction data has been gathered coincident with that of the oviduct and is observed in Figs. 5 A and 5 B as well. Variations in activity with periods of uncoordinated random contractions, strong periodic and co-ordinated contractions, and tonus changes are also noted at various times in the uterus although not coincident with the oviductal activity.

As noted previously the contraction by contraction tabulation seen in Fig. 4 is used as a basis by which to select time increments for the generation of histograms pertaining to each of the contractile parameters. Figs. 6 (A), (B), (C) and (D) illustrate a sequence of such histograms at various cycle phases of an experimental animal. These each portray a single representative 8 h selection from the many contiguous histograms of each cycle phase. Table 1 includes the statistical measures for this set.

Observation of the shapes, distribution and position of the contractile parameter histograms and their statistics gives further insight about the type of oviductal contractility. A histogram with little dispersion or a low percentage of events in the tails is indicative of low variability and general regularity. One skewed right or left suggests a tendency for the values of that parameter towards higher or lower values respectively, while an associated dispersion indicates less regularity. Such a situation is evidenced by higher percentage of events in the tail of the distribution and separation of the mean and modal values. Further, a shifting of the overall distribution indicates that the average value of that parameter has shifted in that direction. Fig. 6 (A) is from the early follicular phase following menses when plasma estrogen and progesterone levels are low. Contractions at this early state of the cycle display some variability though all contractions are less than 0.6 g and the mean and modal

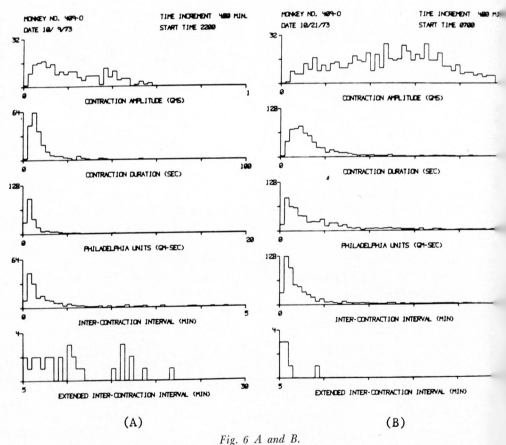

(A)   (B)

Fig. 6 A and B.

Histogram sequence of 8 h increments from each of the proliferative (A), estrogen dominant (B), progesterone dominant (C) and luteal phases (D).

120

values are somewhat separated. Contraction durations are rather short, most less than 20 sec while inter-contraction intervals show multiple large time spans sporadically interspersed between contractions. Thus, as typically seen under the hormonal conditions of the early proliferative phase, there appears to be moderate activity, non-uniform in duration with variable and random intervals between contractions.

Fig. 6 (B) illustrates the effect of very high levels of plasma estrogen on oviductal contractile activity. Very noticeable dispersion of the amplitude and duration distributions are noted as the estrogenic effects become substantial. Frequency of contractions has greatly increased with concomitant increase in contractile duration. Average contractile magnitude has greatly increased with a symmetrical distribution about the mean. Also noted is the spread of distribution of Philadelphia Units indicative of a greater number of contractions

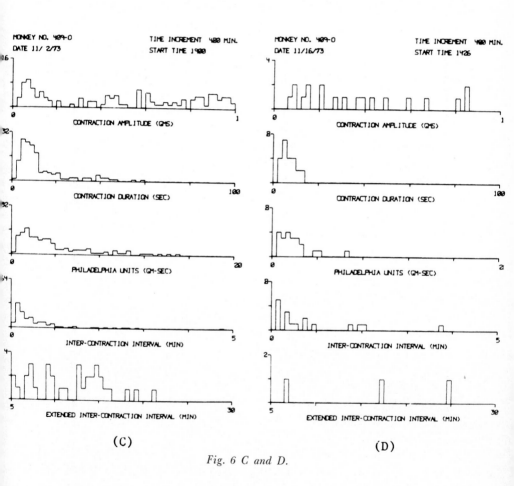

Fig. 6 C and D.

121

expending greater effort. The inter-contraction interval has decreased indicating greater tendency to rhythmicity and less randomness.

The effects of high progesterone and very diminished estrogen levels observed in this animal are exhibited by the low frequency of events with much greater variability in contractile amplitudes, durations and inter-contraction intervals as seen in Fig. 6 (C). These point to less rhythmicity and more irregularity in the events while the appearance of the contractile effort histogram indicates that even though contractions are much fewer in number, the distribution of effort by the existing contractions is similar to that during estrogenic dominance.

During the premenstrual phase, following the high estrogen and progesterone levels during the earlier phases of the cycle, the very low overall levels of activity are illustrated in Fig. 6 (D). The low number of contractile events have a very random dispersion of their amplitude and timing. The few events appear to be occurring sporadically. The histogram illustration and its physiologic interpretation depict that which is observed in the immediate pre-menstrual and menstrual phases.

As a further means of analysis and observation the mean values ($\bar{x}$) of each of the contractile parameters of the histograms, including contraction frequency, and the standard deviations from the means σ are computed for three day segments. These, tabulated for a complete ovarian cycle with the additional incorporation of plasma steroid, vaginal cytology and medication information as illustrated in Table 2, permit direct comparisons between the various contractile data parameters with cycle status. Note the trend of increasing average contraction magnitude during estrogenic dominance of the proliferative phase with a precipitous decline at ovulation and subsequent rise. The frequency of contractions increased and inter-contraction interval decreased just prior to the periovulatory period. Again indicative of greater organization and rhythmicity. Note that while frequency and amplitude of contractions increase prior to ovulation and then fall, the effort expended by the muscular segment per contraction does not rise and fall. To allow an overview of the contractile parameters of the complete cycle, a composite computer graphic presentation is also utilized wherein the means and modes derived from each stored histogram are plotted according to time and date.

As one averages the contractile parameters within greater time spans the specificity for hormonally influenced phase changes is lost. When one groups the cycles together this becomes even more the case but does permit the observations of average ranges. Thus while the short and medium time frame analysis reveals greater extremes, the ranges of multiple cycle contraction averages indicate average amplitudes of 0.9 to 3.3 g, durations of 8.1 to 15.7 sec, contractile effort of 3.8 to 21.0 g-sec, I.-C. I. of 0.6 to 0.8 min and frequency of contractions of 0.3 to 0.7 per min.

Cycle and cycle phase contractility statistics comparison in 3 day time segments.

Monkey 470   Cycle 1   Control ovulatory

Parameter		I	II	III	IV	V	VI	VII	VIII	IX	X	XI	XII	XIII	XIV
Amplitude (g)	x̄	0.97	0.94	0.94	1.52	1.11	1.04	1.23	0.67	0.65	1.00	0.98	0.87	1.09	1.03
	σ	0.08	0.10	0.07	0.50	0.05	0.14	0.27	0.10	0.07	0.15	0.12	0.15	0.28	0.18
Duration (sec)	x̄	6.12	7.16	8.28	12.55	8.45	7.44	9.04	11.43	11.85	15.49	14.13	16.53	16.53	15.15
	σ	0.54	0.74	1.32	1.94	1.40	0.88	1.13	0.95	0.78	1.36	2.00	1.87	2.36	1.69
Phila. U. (g-sec)	x̄	3.16	3.75	4.61	8.39	4.67	3.95	5.14	5.75	5.86	7.56	7.43	7.18	8.19	7.56
	σ	0.41	0.56	0.89	2.41	0.85	0.52	0.98	0.55	0.46	0.72	0.97	0.73	1.21	0.86
I.-C.I. (min)	x̄	1.23	1.15	0.92	0.69	0.84	0.78	0.56	0.79	0.82	0.72	0.73	0.93	0.77	0.65
	σ	0.24	0.21	0.08	0.22	0.20	0.22	0.22	0.11	0.08	0.12	0.08	0.13	0.07	0.09
Frequency (per min)	x̄	0.34	0.39	0.54	0.56	0.51	0.61	1.15	0.61	0.65	0.75	0.71	0.60	0.70	0.79
	σ	0.10	0.15	0.12	0.21	0.14	0.36	0.42	0.13	0.16	0.06	0.14	0.16	0.14	0.12
Plasma estrogen (pg/ml)		20	50	120	50	130	200	525	423	350	50	40	50	20	20
Plasma progesterone (ng/ml)		n. d.	n. d.	n. d.	n. d.	0.1	n. d.	n. d.	n. d.	0.4	5	6	5	n. d.	n. d.
Pyknotic index (0–100 %)			16	20	45	27	15	50	32		25	38	25	18	15
Phase code		M1	M1	Very EP	EP	MP	MP to LP	LP	O	PTO & EL	EL to ML	ML	LL	Very LL to PM2	M2
Medication day/dose													36 / 50 mg progesterone		

123

DISCUSSION

Oviductal motility patterns (*i. e.* frequency) have been reported by others to vary with cycle phase and our reported results agree with this generalization. What we have noted, however, is that agreement or disagreement with specifics of these changes (*i. e.* quantitative parameters of force and timing) may depend upon whether one makes the assessment for short time periods (*i. e.* 15 min to 1 h), whether the short term fluctuations are smoothed through intermediate time or long time averaging of the pertinent parameters and the association of the quantitative measures with accurate timing. During menses we also note the low frequency of activity reported by Sica-Blanco et al. (1971) and Coutinho (1971) but find that the amplitude of these contractions are quite varied and include a rather wide distribution of lower and higher contraction forces. Depending upon the particular animal, these may be in the range of 2 to 3 g of force exerted by the 2.5 mm length of muscle segment. During late proliferative and early periovulatory phases we sometimes note bursts as Coutinho reported. We find these at intervals of 6 to 16 min often superimposed on muscle tonus changes and with higher frequency (6 per min) than other contractile periods, with lower amplitudes (0.1 to 0.3 g) of contractile force as contrasted to that generally observed during other portions of the cycle. The influence of high estrogen effects are greater magnitudes of contraction with loss of the randomness associated with the menses or very early proliferative phases. The extent of this periodicity and increased force effect is seen to be dependent on the plasma steroid levels. The alterations at and prior to ovulation of peaking followed by dipping of the contractile force with an associated change of frequency, appears whether ovulation is spontaneous or exogenously induced. The changes, however, are often more dramatic with exogenous medication whereas the muscular effort expended per contraction remains high. The use of two or more transducers placed serially will allow propagational studies while 2 placed orthogonally allow longitudinal and circular muscle measurements.

The extraluminal contractile force transducers and implantable telemetry system described offer significant advantages for the monitoring of smooth muscle organs. The system and techniques afford the opportunity to evaluate the absolute quantitative measures of oviductal motility force and timing in both the long term chronic as well as the short term acute experiment. It enables the measure of segmental contractile activity in both force and timing relationships with neither physical nor pharmacologic intervention allowing subject mobility and non-interference with reproductive function.

ACKNOWLEDGMENTS

Supported by Contraceptive Development Branch of the Center for Population Research, NICHD.

REFERENCES

Aref I. and Hafez E. S. E. (1973) Oviduct contractility and egg transport in the rabbit. *Amer. J. Obstet. Gynec.* 42, 165–171.

Bass P. and Wiley J. (1965) Electrical and extraluminal contractile force activity of the duodenum of the dog. *Amer. J. Dig. Dis.* 10, 183–200.

Caldeyro-Barcia R. and Alvarez H. (1954). Effect of presacral nerve stimulation of the non-pregnant human uterus. *J. appl. Physiol.* 6, 556.

Coutinho E. M. (1971) Physiologic and pharmacologic studies of the human oviduct. *Fertil. and Steril.* 22, 807–815.

Davids A. M. (1948) Fallopian tube motility in relation to the menstrual cycle. *Amer. J. Obstet. Gynec.* 56, 655–663.

Dominic J. and Reinke D. (1968) Extraluminal force transducer for *in vivo* measurement of rabbit uterine contractile activity. *Fertil. and Steril.* 19, 945–952.

Epstein S .G. (1972) The physiologic effects of an extraluminal transducer on the utero-tubal junction. Drexel University M. S. Thesis.

Feit A., Freund M. and Ventura W. (1968) Effect of stage of the estrous cycle on the motility of the uterus in the guinea pig *in vivo*. *Amer. J. Obstet. Gynec.* 102, 202–211.

Fromm E. (1967) Myometrial contractile force telemetry from the unrestrained rabbit. Jefferson Medical College Ph. D. Thesis.

Gallant S. L. and Fromm E. (1973) The electromechanical analysis of a smooth muscle force transducer. *Proc. 26th Annual Conference on Engineering in Medicine and Biology* 15, 129.

Jacoby N., Bennett D. and Bass P. (1962) *In vivo* strain gage method for measurement of contractions and tone of gastrointestinal longitudinal and circular muscle. *Fed Proc.* 21, 261.

Jeutter D. C. (1974) A system for the study and the study of mammalian oviductal contractile activity, Drexel University Ph. D. Thesis.

Jeutter D. C. and Fromm E. (1971a) An implantable biologic force transducer. *Proc. 24th Annual Conference on Engineering in Medicine and Biology* 13, 201.

Jeutter D. C. and Fromm E. (1971b) Implantable telemetry from low impedance biologic transducers. *Fed. Proc.* 30, 699.

Ludwick J. (1966) Observations on the smooth muscle and contractile activity of the common bile duct. *Ann. Surg.* 164, 1041–1050.

Maia H. and Coutinho E. M. (1968) A new technique for recording human tubal activity *in vivo*. *Amer. J. Obstet. Gynec.* 102, 1043–1047.

Neri A., Marcus S. and Fuchs F. (1972) Motility of the oviduct in the Rhesus monkey. *Amer. J. Obstet. Gynec.* 39, 205–212.

Salomy M. and Harper M. J. K. (1971) Cyclical changes of oviduct motility in rabbits. *Biol. Reprod.* 4, 185–194.

Seckinger D. C. and Snyder F. F. (1923) Cyclic variations in the spontaneous contractions of the human Fallopian tube. *Proc. Soc. exp. Biol. Med.* 21, 519–521.

Sica-Blanco Y., Cibils L. A., Remedio M. R., Rozada H. and Gil B. E. (1971) Isthmic and ampullary contractility of the human oviduct *in vivo*. *Amer. J. Obstet. Gynec.* 111, 91–97.

125

Center for Bioengineering[1] and
Department of Biological Structure[2],
University of Washington,
School of Medicine, RK-15 Seattle,
Washington 98195

STOCHASTIC ELEMENTS
IN THE DEVELOPMENT OF DETERMINISTIC
MODELS OF EGG TRANSPORT

By

*Pedro Verdugo[1], Richard J. Blandau[2], Patrick Y. Tam[2]
and Sheridan A. Halbert[2]*

ABSTRACT

Elements of stochastic analysis have been applied to the study of egg transport in rabbit ampullae. Computer plots of egg position along the ampulla as a function of time were generated from data obtained by digitizing cinematographic records of transport in the exposed oviduct. Transport as observed in the ampulla of the rabbit is a discrete phenomenon composed of small "to and fro" movements of the cumulas mass. The *histographic representation* of these movements, according to their magnitude and direction, as well as the *cumulative distribution function* and the *probability density function* of egg velocities, were used to characterize the statistical structure of egg transport. Results show that under different patterns of egg transport and also different transport rates, the statistical structure of the process remains remarkably similar, suggesting that there must be some common factor in the intimate nature of ampullary egg transport that does not seem to be related to the absolute magnitude and frequency of the forward and backward movements but to the relative differences between these movements of the egg in the oviduct.

This work was supported by USPHS Grant Number HDO 3752, Contract Number HD 2788 and by NIGMS Grant GM-16436.

This may be the result of either some organized time-space programming of the muscular activity of the oviduct or of an interaction between muscle contraction and ciliary activity in which contractions of the oviduct may be randomly distributed in time and space, inducing random movements of the egg with the role of the ciliary activity being the production of an asymmetric frictional effect which would as a consequence, account for the net transport of the egg.

One of the most critical phases of reproduction is transport of gametes through the oviduct, and much interest has been focused on this process. Although tubal transport has been studied for over a century, we do not have at this writing, a complete understanding of the intimate nature of this phenomenon. Several mechanisms may act individually or in combination to facilitate tubal transport by controlling the movement of the gametes through the oviduct.

It seems widely accepted that the rate of egg transport is mainly controlled by the muscular activity of the oviduct, yet this relationship has not been unequivocally established. Until such time as a cause and effect relationship between the various mechanisms affecting tubal transport can be established, we cannot predict the egg transport process and reliably utilize the results of our study for fertility control.

This paper discusses a bioengineering approach to quantify the egg transport process.

Two different, although complementary, conceptual frameworks have been followed by our interdisciplinary research team to investigate gamete transport. One is an attempt to make a quantitative overall description of the transport process as a separate isolated and clearly defined phenomenon. Making no assumptions whatsoever as to what mechanisms are involved, we are introducing stochastic methods to quantitatively assess the statistical structure of certain elements of ampullary egg transport as observed in the "open dish" preparations (Blandau et al. 1971). The other is an analytical deterministic approach that seeks to evaluate the role of the various driving forces provided by the smooth muscle contractions, ciliary activity, and the hydrodynamic and rheological forces associated with the luminal fluids of the oviduct. The two approaches are complementary in the sense that, in order to evaluate the role of the various mechanisms involved in egg transport, we must first have an accurate quantitative assessment of the process of egg transport itself.

We realize that our research is limited, mainly because the preliminary evidence presented here has been obtained exclusively from the rabbit ampulla. The results of our study may not apply to other species and may not be valid for the entire oviduct. However, our goal is to assess the basic mechanisms underlying the gamete transport process itself, and in this sense ampullary transport represents a suitable model for the study of this phenomenon.

Stochastic vs. deterministic models in egg transport process

In studying egg transport, as in other biological phenomenon, both stochastic and deterministic models may be used. A deterministic model is one in which no randomness is assumed. The time behavior of the parameter that characterizes the phenomenon is determined by a well defined function. Even if this function is complex the time course of the characteristic parameter can be *predicted* for any particular moment. A rather simple example of this type of function is the cardiac output, which is equal to the product of the stroke volume and the heart rate.

Stochastic models describe those systems in which elements of randomness seem to exist, *i. e.*, elements for which we have no logical explanation. Obviously, we may imply randomness in a system both because some random elements may exist in the system and/or because of our lack of relevant information regarding the system. However, there are certain non-random elements in stochastic variables that allow us to give quantitative treatment to these types of phenomena. In fact, the relative frequency (probability) of occurrence of random events follows the "law of change". This "law" is expressed by the form and the parameters of the probability density function, elements which in fact are non-random. Therefore, a probabilistic approach can be used to *predict* when a phenomenon in which random elements are present, is characterized by a reproducible and consistent statistical structure. Whereas a purely deterministic approach excludes variations, the stochastic approach provides a descriptive tool for both the random and the non-random elements within random events. This feature gives to the probabilistic method a high noise immunity which makes it of practical interest, since the appearance of random fluctuations in a given phenomenon sometimes inhibits the ability to assess information that may characterize important aspects of the phenomenon. In reality, however, model development is an iterative process and these two approaches may be mixed; the information gathered by the probabilistic approach is used to adjust further a deterministic model.

Application of stochastic methods to describe egg transport

Since Harper first directly observed ampullary egg transport in rabbits in 1961 (Harper 1961), several laboratories have devoted much effort to evaluating surrogate egg transport in a variety of mammalian species at different periods of the reproductive cycle and under the influence of various hormonal or pharmacological interventions. Descriptions of the egg transport in the rabbit have been limited to the establishment that ampullary transport is a "to and fro" phenomenon and to the effects of hormones on the time it takes to move the egg from the infundibular ostium to the ampullary-isthmic junction. From direct observations of ampullary egg transport we know that many different patterns

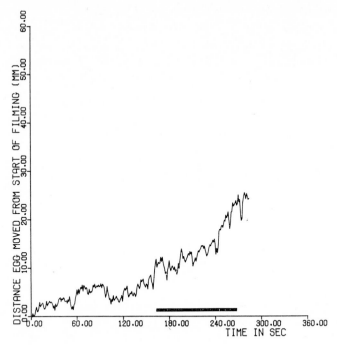

Fig. 1.

Graphic illustration of ampullary egg transport in a rabbit under estrogen withdrawal. Computer plots of egg position along the ampullary lumen as a function of time were generated from data obtained from cinematographic records of transport in the exposed ampulla, using the "open dish" technique. Ampullary egg transport in this animal is characterized by a pattern of rather small discrete "to and fro" movements. Data for these studies were obtained from the second 15 mm of ampullary egg transport. The solid line at the bottom of the figure shows the sampling time that corresponds to this segment of transport in the ampulla. Net forward transport rate in this sample was 9.8 mm/min.

of egg movement result in the same transport rate. A more sensitive and objective quantification of the egg transport phenomenon is mandatory if we are to arrive at a better understanding of the nature of this process. Since random elements seem to be apparent in egg transport phenomenon, our efforts have been oriented toward a quantitative stochastic description of ampullary egg transport as observed in the "open dish" preparation under various hormonal and pharmacological influences. Nine experiments were performed and two are presented in which, although the raw data and the rate of transport appear to be very different, the statistical structure actually shows remarkable similarities.

129

Definitions, data collection and data processing

Motion picture films of egg transport as observed in the "open dish" preparation were digitized to determine the position of the egg cumulus mass in the
ampulla of the rabbit as a function of time. Fig. 1 is a plot of egg position vs.
time in a rabbit under estrogen withdrawal induced by CI628, a nonsteroidal
estrogen antagonist. Transport as observed in the exposed ampulla may be described as a "to and fro", or better, as a discrete phenomenon. This discrete
movement that we label "spurt" may have different frequencies, magnitudes and
velocities, and its direction can be backward (pro-ovarian) or forward (anti-
ovarian). The magnitude of a "spurt" can be defined as the distance the egg
moves from the beginning of the "spurt" when the velocity of the egg is zero to
the end of the "spurt" when the egg velocity is again zero. For *net transport* to
occur, the summation of all the positive "spurt" magnitudes must be larger than
the summation of all the negative "spurt" magnitudes. Accordingly, the *transport
rate* is the ratio of net transport over time.

In a stochastic description, transport may be characterized by the probability
of occurrence of "spurts" of different magnitudes and velocities in both the
forward (anti-ovarian), and backward (pro-ovarian) directions. If under given
experimental conditions, ampullary egg transport shows reproducible statistical
patterns the method may be useful in characterizing this phenomenon.

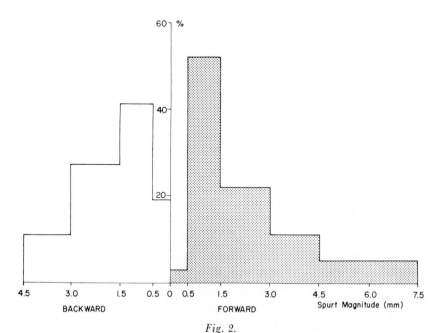

Fig. 2.

Histogram of frequency of occurrence (incidence) of spurts according to their magnitude
and direction from the sample marked by solid line in Fig. 1.

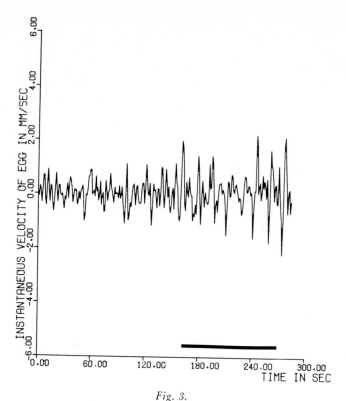

Fig. 3.

Plot of egg velocity vs. time corresponding to the transport illustrated in Fig. 1. The solid line at the bottom of this figure shows the sampling period of data used for the stochastic analysis.

One of the forms of stochastic analysis is the histographic representation of the frequency of occurrence of events. Fig. 2 is a histogram of the frequency of occurrence or incidence of "spurts" according to their magnitude and direction during the second 15 mm of ampullary transport in the same rabbit under estrogen-withdrawal. We observe first that the range of "spurt" magnitudes covers from 4.5 mm in the backward (pro-ovarian) direction, to 6.0 mm in the forward (anti-ovarian) direction, *i. e.*, the range of forward "spurts" is larger. Second, the highest incidence of occurrence is in the range below 3.0 mm in both forward and backward collections, *i. e.*, transport is predominantly characterized by small "spurts". Third, the *relative difference* between the forward and backward collections shows that in the small magnitude range (less than 0.5 mm) the backward "spurts" are dominant whereas in the larger magnitude range (more than 4.5 mm) the forward "spurts" are dominant. Fourth, the cumulative summation of backward "spurts" is smaller than the cumulative sum of forward "spurts",

131

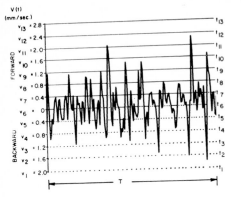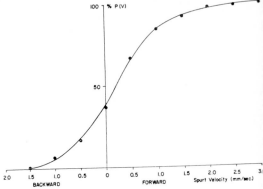

Fig. 4.

Graphical representation of the cumulative distribution function (CD) of egg velocities (right block). The velocity data (left block) are the same as illustrated in Fig. 3. CD is obtained by setting a collection of velocity levels, V_1, V_2, V_3, ... V_m. The cumulative time the egg velocity is at or below each velocity level (solid line) is represented by t_1, t_2, t_3, ... t_m. The probability P(V) of CD at each velocity level V_a is calculated at the ratio of the corresponding t_n to the total sampling time T, expressed in %. The probability P(V) of CD is zero below V_1, since the egg velocity is never less than V_1, *i. e.*, $t_1 = O$

and $\dfrac{t_1}{T} \times 100 = 0\ \%$. Similarly the probability of CD is 100 % at V_{13}, since the egg

velocity is always at or below V_{13}, *i. e.* $t_{13} = T$ and $\dfrac{t_{13}}{T} \times 100 = 100\ \%$. If the egg velo-

cities were completely randomly distributed, their average would be zero and P(V) of CD at V = O would be 50 %. Note that the probability of CD at V = O in this experiment is about 35 % which means that the forward velocities have a higher probability of occurrence than the backward egg velocities.

which implies that net forward egg transport was indeed observed in this experiment.

The statistical structure of transport may also be expressed with the *cumulative distribution function* and the *probability density function* of egg velocities. Fig. 3 shows a plot of egg velocities versus time as obtained from the same sample of egg transport data described above. Note that the range of velocities extend from 1.5 mm/sec in the backward to 2.8 mm/sec in the forward movements of the egg. Fig. 4 illustrates the cumulative distribution function (CD) of this sample. In its general form, the cumulative distribution function (CD) of velocity is defined as the probability or fraction of the sampling time the egg velocity is at or below a magnitude threshold level. (See Fig. 4 for a more detailed description of CD). Fig. 4 shows that CD is not symmetrical about V = O, which implies that, in this particular case, the forward velocities (anti-ovarian) have a higher probability of occurrence than the backward velocities (pro-ovarian). This is also evident when the probability density function (PD) of the velocity is calculated (see Fig. 5). PD is the first derivative of CD and it represents the probability of finding in the sample a velocity of any particular magnitude. Note in Fig. 5 that the velocities show an asymmetric distribution about V = O with the curve shifted to the positive side. This means, again, that the probability of occurrence of higher velocities is larger in the forward (anti-ovarian) movements than in the backward (pro-ovarian) movements of the egg.

The plot of egg position vs. time in a rabbit under estrogen dominance, is in Fig. 6. The corresponding velocity plot is shown in Fig. 7. The descriptive value of the stochastic methods may be appreciated by comparing the egg transport data of the estrous animal with those from the rabbit under estrogen withdrawal. The egg transport in the estrous rabbit is dominated by a pattern of large slow "spurts". Transport in the animal under estrogen withdrawal, on the other hand, consists primarily of a pattern of small fast "spurts". Fig. 8 shows an histogram of "spurt" magnitudes, and in Fig. 5 the probability density function of velocities

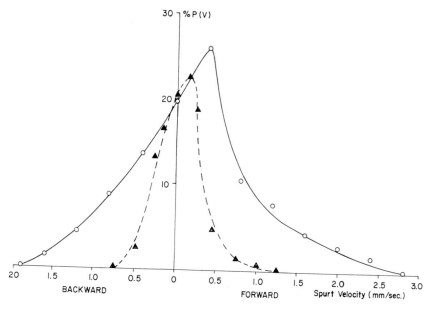

Fig. 5.
Probability density function (PD) of ampullary egg transport velocities in a rabbit under estrogen withdrawal (solid curve) and in a rabbit under estrogen dominance (dotted curve). Note that in both animals the egg transport velocities show an asymmetric distribution about V = O with the curve shifted to the forward side, *i. e.*, the probability of occurrence of higher velocities is larger in the forward movements than in the backward movements of the egg.

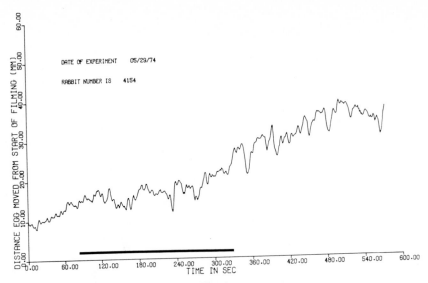

Fig. 6.

Computer plot of egg position along the ampulla as a function of time in a rabbit under estrogen dominance. Ampullary egg transport in this animal is characterized by the presence of rather large and slow "to and fro" movements. The solid line at the bottom of this figure corresponds to the data sampling of the second 15 mm of ampullary egg transport. Net forward transport rate in this sample was 3.39 mm/min.

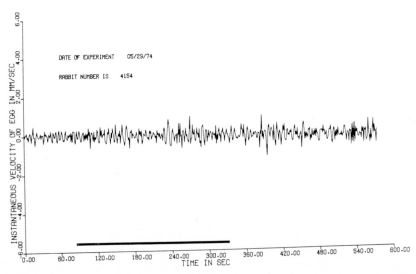

Fig. 7.

Computer plot of ampullary egg velocities from a rabbit under estrogen dominance. Instantaneous velocities were calculated from the transport data in Fig. 6. The solid line at the bottom of this figure represents the sampling period of data used for the stochastic analysis.

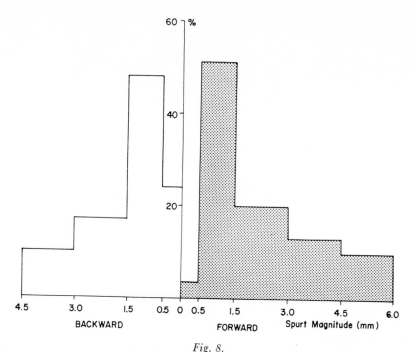

Fig. 8.

Histogram of frequency of occurrence of "spurts" according to their magnitude and direction. These data were obtained from the second 15 mm of ampullary transport in a rabbit under estrogen-dominance.

of the rabbit under estrogen dominance is illustrated in dotted lines. The *relative difference* in the backward versus the forward "spurt" collections as illustrated in Fig. 8 present remarkable similarities to the histogram of the rabbit under estrogen withdrawal in Fig. 2, although the *absolute range* of "spurt" magnitude is larger in the rabbit under estrogen dominance, extending from 4.5 mm in the backward (pro-ovarian) direction to 7.5 mm in the forward (anti-ovarian) direction. In both Fig. 8 and Fig. 2, the incidence of occurrence is highest in the range of small magnitudes. The *relative differences* between the two "spurt" collections show that in the small range the backward "spurts" are dominant, and in the larger magnitude range the forward collection of "spurts" is dominant. Finally, in both experiments the cumulative sum of forward is larger than the backward "spurts", therefore a net forward egg transport was indeed observed. The probability density function of velocities in this rabbit under estrogen dominance illustrated in Fig. 5 (dotted line curve), shows an asymmetric distribution about V = O, although it encompasses a smaller range of velocities than in the rabbit under estrogen withdrawal. Both curves show a

135

similar shift toward forward velocities thus demonstrating that the relative difference of the probabilities of occurrence between forward versus backward egg transport velocities is remarkably similar in these two animals.

DISCUSSION

These experiments provide some preliminary evidence that under very different absolute patterns of egg transport, the statistical structure of the process remains very similar, suggesting that there must be some common factor in the intimate nature of ampullary egg transport that does not seem to be related to the *absolute magnitude* and frequency of the forward and backward movement but to the *relative differences* between these movements of the egg within the ampulla. This rectifying effect that makes the forward conductivity higher than the backward conductivity in the ampulla may be interpreted either as a consequence of some rather organized programming on the activity of the muscle component of the wall of the oviduct or as the result of some asymmetric frictional factor due to a ratcheting effect produced by the ciliary activity within the ampulla.

A transporting program of the contractile activity of the oviductal wall could take the form of a bolus-driving peristaltic wave acting over limited distance along the oviduct. According to our results it would not necessarily be related to the magnitude and frequency of the contractions but rather to the time-space sequence of activation of the smooth muscle. On the basis of the evidence presented here, such a program should make the propagating contractile waves faster in the forward (anti-ovarian) direction than in the backward (pro-ovarian) direction. However, it may be important to emphasize at this point that there is no firm evidence that organized peristalsis does or does not exist in the oviduct.

An alternative interpretation that could account for this evidence is that the ciliary activity may be providing an asymmetric frictional (ratcheting) effect. This is especially appealing both because of its significance and because indirect evidence exists in support of it. In fact, Halbert et al., (1975) have shown recently that when the muscular activity of the oviduct is pharmacologically blocked with isoproterenol, ampullary egg transport changes its typical discrete ("to and fro") character and becomes continuous and *unidirectional*. This implies that the driving forces provided by the ciliary action are indeed asymmetric. Moreover, the suggested mechanism of a ratcheting frictional effect of the cilia can be supported further by work in Blandau's laboratory. Film studies have shown that the ciliary transport of the cumulus mass over the fimbria of the rabbit is unidirectional and that the ciliated epithelium of the fimbria not only functions as a transporting agent, but also firmly holds the cumulus mass in place, as evidenced by the unsuccessful attempts to remove the cumulus mass

136

from its surface with fine forceps. If this asymmetric frictional factor exists, there is then no need to postulate coordination of the contractile activity to account for the statistically dominant forward transport. In fact, under this premise, even a random pattern of contractions would lead to a net forward transport of the egg in the oviduct, the main characteristic being a pattern of statistically dominant higher forward velocities as found in the data presented here.

The evaluation of these preliminary data illustrates how the stochastic methods can be applied to study egg transport. It is obviously not conclusive; but it does give an interesting clue to the possible interactions of ciliary and smooth muscular functions on the mechanism of egg transport. It emphasizes also the unique role of stochastic analysis in evaluating the intimate statistical characteristics of the egg transport phenomenon.

REFERENCES

Blandau R. J. (1971) Observing ovulation and egg transport. In: Daniel J. C., ed. *Methods in Mammalian Embryology*, pp. 1–14. W. H. Freeman & Co., San Francisco.
Harper M. J. K. (1961) The mechanism involved in the movement of newly ovulated eggs through the ampulla of the rabbit Fallopian tube. *J. Reprod. Fertil.* 2, 522–524.
Halbert S. A., Tam P. Y. and Blandau R. J. (1975) The role of muscle and cilia in egg transport in the rabbit oviduct. Submitted for publication to Science.

Department of Biological Structure
and Division of Bioengineering,
University of Washington School of Medicine,
Seattle, Washington

Discussion Paper

AN OVERVIEW OF GAMETE TRANSPORT – COMPARATIVE ASPECTS

By

Richard J. Blandau and Pedro Verdugo

During the past decades, many investigators have explored the morphological, physiological, pharmacological, biochemical, biophysical and neurological factors involved in transporting gametes to the site of fertilization in the oviducts. Even though much information is available on this absorbing complexity, the fact remains that we cannot yet fully explain the mechanisms involved in gamete transport for any single mammal.

Transport of both eggs and spermatozoa within the oviducts involves at least four primary factors; (1) The frequency, force and programming of contractions in the various smooth muscle layers; (2) The rate of beat and direction of beat of cilia lining the mucosal folds; (3) The hydrodynamics and rheology associated with the luminal fluids at the critical times that sperm and eggs are being transported; and (4) The innate ability of sperm to flagellate and to move through the luminal fluids by their own power. In this brief summary we cannot elaborate on all the experimental methods which have and are being used to study the complex physiology of the oviducts as related to gamete transport. Nor can we pretend to establish any consistant theory regarding the physiology of the oviduct. We would prefer to describe and illustrate the problems involved in

Unpublished observations referred to in this chapter were supported by Grant HD-3752 and Contract HD-2788 from the National Institutes of Health.

searching out the complex mechanisms inherent to the transport of gametes within the oviducts. We wish to emphasize that even though the various techniques applied may give us some insight into the physiology of the oviduct, the mechanism of gamete transport will be clarified only when the respective roles of these primary factors and the intrinsic activities of the gametes, particularly the spermatozoa, can be fully ascertained and their integration clarified. Obviously we have not as yet attained this state of knowledge for any mammal. In reviewing the literature related to the various techniques used to study the physiology of the oviducts during the past decades, one is impressed with the overriding concept that gamete transport is accomplished primarily by variations in the contractile activity of the innate musculature of the oviduct (Blandau et al. 1975). There is, however, no hard evidence in any animal that gametes are transported primarily by muscle contractions. Furthermore, there appears to be significant species differences in the primary roles of muscles and cilia in accomplishing gamete transport. The frequent assumption that there exists a simple one-to-one functional relationship between oviductal contractions and gamete transport, has resulted in conclusions that may be misleading and it is perhaps not unfair to state that much of the data collected on oviductal motility may be irrelevant to gamete transport, particularly when one critically observes the phenomenon directly in the anesthetized animal. Before a quantitative analytical study can be made of the mechanism of oviductal transport, an accurate description of the normal transport process itself should be made upon which the assumptions for analytical studies may be used. We re-emphasize that although oviductal transport has been studied for over a century, we do not have a complete quantitative description of this process. Even the best qualitative descriptions are full of speculations since a large part of the process of both egg and sperm transport has not as yet been observed directly or completely in any animal. This emphasizes a very important fact, i. e., that not only are techniques needed to study the electrical, mechanical, biochemical and other aspects of oviductal physiology, but we require methods also to study accurately and describe quantitatively the gamete transport phenomena themselves and especially be certain that all parameters have been taken into consideration. In 1961 Harper described a technique in which he withdrew the oviducts through an incision in the lateral body wall of anesthetized rabbits, bedded them on moist cotton squares and observed the ampullary transport of eggs in cumulus. Harper's qualitative description of the transport of the egg to the ampullary-isthmic junction indicated roles for both the cilia and smooth muscles of the ampulla. These observations stimulated us to develop an experimental preparation which has provided a means for more precise and complete description of egg transport under what we would consider somewhat better physiologic conditions (Blandau 1970). The oviduct is maintained in an environment as nearly normal as possible with the nervous and blood supply intact. Yet it is sufficiently isolated from the abdominal cavity so that an unobstructed view of the entire oviduct is provided and high quality cinematographic records of oviductal activity are permitted. This preparation has been very useful in determining not only the time of transport of ovulated eggs through the ampulla of rabbits under a variety of endocrine conditions, but has impressed us greatly with the variety of phenomena that must be analyzed and considered if the full story of gamete transport is to be realized.

The role of the mesenteries

In observing the behaviour of the oviduct *in vivo* in the rabbit, cat, and rat, at the time of ovulation, one is impressed with the rigorous contractile activity of the mesovarium, the various ovarian ligaments, the mesosalpinx and the mesotubarium superius if such exists. The concentractions of the various mesenteries continuously change the position of the ovaries relative to the fimbria as well as the relation of the various subdivisions of the oviduct one to another. The patterns of contractions vary significantly in different animals and at various times in the cycle. The role of the mesenterial contractions in gamete transport is unknown for any mammal nor have they been described sufficiently, on a comparative basis, to even warn those of us who are placing various transducers in or on the oviducts that at least some of the contractile responses may be due to mesenterial influences and that we may not be recording purely oviductal muscular contraction. Very little is known concerning the hormonal interrelationships which effect mesenterial contractile activity and even less concerning the relationship of their contractile activity to gamete transport.

The anatomy of the fimbriae and gamete transport

The mechanism by which freshly ovulated eggs are transported into the oviducts depends on; (1) The anatomical configuration of the fimbria of the infundibulum and its relationship to the surface of the ovary at the time of ovulation; (2) The manner in which the cumulus oophorus and its contained egg is shed from the follicle at the time of ovulation; and (3) The physical characteristics of the antral fluids and the fluids that comprise the matrix of the cumulus oophorus. In some animals such as a rabbit, guinea pig, and cat, the fringed, fluted, and lansiform fimbriae surround the ovaries and form what is almost a complete *bursae ovarii*. Normally the ovulating eggs in these animals come into intimate contact with the ciliated cells lining the fimbriae immediately upon ovulation (Clewe et al. 1958). The intermittent contractions of the smooth muscles in the mesovaria and the various ligaments of the mesenteries attached to the ovaries and oviducts, act to change the surface relationship between the ovaries and the fimbriae. These rhythmic muscular contractions assure that the fimbriae remain in a constant position relative to the surface of the ovaries and that this position is altered frequently by the rhythmic contractions of the fimbriae. In contrast,

140

only a small portion of the diminutive fimbriae in the mouse, rat and hamster, come into direct contact with the ovaries. In these animals, the ovaries are enclosed completely by a thin membrane, the periovarial sac, into which the small, ciliated, anemone-like fimbria projects. Since the fimbriae in these rodents make only superficial contact with the ovaries, the question arises as to how the ovulated eggs are transported into the oviducts. At the time of ovulation, the periovarial sac is dilated with fluid, which causes its membrane to be lifted from the ovarian surface thus making possible the movement of eggs in cumuli within the periovarial space. In these animals, the eggs, embedded in the cumuli, are shed completely from the follicle into the fluids of the periovarial space. Intermittent contractions of the mesovarium displaces the ovary within the periovarial sac which in turn moves the eggs about at random within the fluids. of the periovarial space. The cilia on the cells covering the fimbria all beat in the direction of the ostium. When a cumulus mass comes into the sphere of influence of the fimbria, the currents in the fluid direct the egg toward the ostium. As soon as contact between the fimbria and the cumulus oophorus is established, the eggs are transported quickly over the fimbrial surface, through the ostium and into the ampulla of the oviduct. In contrast, the fimbriae of rabbits and cats form almost complete bursae about the ovaries at about the time of ovulation. Interestingly, in these animals, the cumulus masses adhere to the site of rupture. This is related to the viscoelastic properties of the matrix which form an integral part of the cumulus at about the time of ovulation. Thus, the highly polymerized matrix of the cumulus oophorus and the antral fluids are continuous one with another. The ovulated mass may be seen to be pulled into very long thin streamers as the cilia attempt to move them into the ampulla of the oviduct. This phenomenon is particularly striking in the cat where the matrix is highly polymerized and exceedingly sticky in contrast to that observed in the rat, mouse, or hamster. Thus, there seems to be a functional relationship between the anatomic configuration of the fimbria of the infundibulum and the manner in which the eggs are ovulated and transported into the ampulla. It should be emphasized that the decisive factors in egg transport appear to be whether or not the eggs are shed completely from the follicles at ovulation as well as the physical characteristics of the cumulus oophorus. There is a great need still to relate on a comparative basis, the anatomical configuration of the ampulla, the physical characteristics of the components of the cumulus mass and egg transport. We may conclude that despite a considerable anatomical variation of the fimbriae of the infundibulum, egg transport from the ovary and into the ampulla is an efficient biological phenomenon. Also irrespective of the anatomical configuration of the fimbria, the cilia covering its surface are programmed to beat in the direction of the ostium. In all animals studied to date, egg transport through the ostium itself and the first few millimeters of the ampulla is effected by the action of the cilia.

The role of cilia and muscle in gamete transport through the ampulla

Egg transport through the ampulla and to the ampullary-isthmic junction has now been observed in the living rat, rabbit and monkey (Blandau 1973). There are remarkable differences even in these three animals in the roles of the cilia and muscles in effecting transport of the ovulated cumulus mass. In all animals so far examined, including the rat, the rabbit, the cat, the cow, the sheep, the monkey and human, the cilia in the ampulla all beat in the direction of the ampullary-isthmic junction.

At the time of ovulation in the rat, the loops of the ampullae become greatly dilated. The size of the cumulus mass in relationship to the volume of the ampulla is relatively small. When the cumulus mass once passes into the ampulla, it is propelled to the ampullary-isthmic junction by vigorous peristaltic contractions. Normally it requires only a few seconds for the egg in cumulus to reach the ampullary-isthmic junction in this animal. In contrast egg transport in the rabbit is effected by 2 mechanisms; (1) by localized segmental, peristalic contractions that compress and elongate the cumulus mass and more or less "milk" it forward; and (2) the cilia, though capable of independently moving the egg forward, as readily demonstrated when isoproteronol is injected to inhibit muscular contractions, normally appear to play a role by holding the cumulus mass in position during the intermittent brief resting periods. In the rabbit, the egg in cumulus is carried to the ampullary-isthmic junction in about 6 minutes (Boling et al. 1971). At ovulation, the ampulla in the rabbit is slightly dilated with fluid. The role of this fluid in the transport process is completely unknown.

In the monkey, particularly *Macaca nemestrina*, the action of the cilia appear to play the dominant role in egg transport. The vigorous, segmental, peristaltic contractions seen in the rat and rabbit ampulla at ovulation are not visible in the anesthetized monkey. Egg transport through the monkey ampulla averages approximately 22 minutes (unpublished data) in contrast to the much more rapid rate described for the rat and rabbit. The complex arrangement of the numerous mucosal folds in the monkey ampulla almost completely fill the lumen so that there is only a potential space. Fluid is at a minimum; thus, the cumulus mass is in intimate contact with the ciliated mucosa.

We conclude that egg transport through the ampulla is accomplished variously in different animals but we must exercise care in not drawing broad conclusions from observations in only a few species.

Direction of ciliary beat in the isthmus and measurement of rate

With the exception of the work of Borell et al. (1957) and more recently Gaddum-Rosse et al. (1973), direct observations on the activity of oviductal cilia have rarely been reported in mammals. Parker (1928; 1930; 1931) was the first to show that in the turtle although most of the cilia in the isthmus beat towards the uterus, a narrow tract of cilia beat consistently towards the ovary. Similar observations were made on the isthmus of lizards, frogs and birds (Mimura 1937). It was concluded that the pro-ovarian ciliary currents served to transport spermatozoa to the site of fertilization. Yamada (1952) suggested that the dual currents served to rotate the eggs during the passage through the isthmus so that albumen and other egg membranes could be evenly deposited. There is considerable variation in the direction of ciliary beat in the isthmi of various animals. In those mammals in which ciliary beat has been evaluated, pro-ovarian ciliary pathways have been observed only in the isthmi of rabbits and pigs. All the cilia appear to beat in the direction of the uterus in the rat (Alden 1942), cat, cow, sheep, monkey and human (Gaddum-Rosse et al. 1973).

The role of cilia in the transport of eggs through the isthmus is still a mystery. This hiatus in our knowledge is related primarily to the technical difficulties in observing the behavior of the small gametes as they are transported through this thick-walled segment of the oviduct.

Borrell *et al.* (1957) were the first to suggest that there was a variation in the rate of ciliary beat depending upon the hormonal condition of the animal. His measurements, using high speed cinematography, revealed that the beat was significantly increased during the luteal phase of the cycle. Three methods are now available to study the rate of ciliary beat:

1. The high-speed cinematographic method though still used is cumbersome and has the disadvantage that a continuous measurement is not possible and minor effects of various substances tested would most likely be overlooked.

2. Photo-probe for the study of the ciliary beat is a system in which the rate of ciliary beat can be measured optically. A Rose chamber containing the ciliated specimen is placed on a stage of a phase-contrast microscope and transilluminated with an intense Zirconium arc lamp. The magnification (about 300 ×) is observed on the focal plane of a camera mounted on the microscope. The beating cilia are readily observed and the photo-probe placed at the desired site. The probe itself is a miniature phototransistor, Motorola MRD604, with a sensitive area about 0.55 mm in diameter. It is mounted in a piece of Lucite attached to a 6 × ocular. As the dark image of a cilium moves across the photo-probe, a varying electrical signal is generated. This signal is amplified and filtered, and then recorded directly.

The advantage of this method is that it yields a rapid and accurate determination of ciliary beat under well-controlled environmental conditions, and allows for the evaluation of the effects of hormones, anesthetic drugs, various pharmacological agents as well as of environment on the rate of cilia beat.

3. Recently we have introduced the use of Laser Photo Correlation Spectroscopy to study the kinetics of cilia beat, in cultured ciliated cells of the oviduct. This technique was first used by Bergé et al. (1967) to study motility of pro-

tozoa and later used by F. R. Hallett (personal communication) to evaluate motility in bull spermatozoa. The application of this method to study the activity of ciliated cells of the oviduct was first made at our Center for Bioengineering. The technique is based on the Doppler effect, i. e., the shift of frequency observed in the scattered light reflected by the ciliated cell culture illuminated with a Laser beam. The frequency shift being proportional to the average angular velocity and direction of the oscillating cilia. This method provides a unique tool to assess both the frequency of cilia beat, the amplitude of the ciliary oscillations, as well as the degree of coordination of beat within a group of ciliary units.

Gamete transport through the isthmus

The isthmus has the paradoxical facility to transport sperm to the site of fertilization before ovulation and to transport the egg in the opposite direction after fertilization.

Determining how sperm move through the isthmus has been thwarted by the complex technical problems involved in observing the behavior of the small, motile spermatozoa through the thick-walled isthmus. We have already pointed out the possible role of the pro-ovarian ciliary currents in the isthmi of pigs and rabbits in transporting sperm. Similar conditions do not exist in many other mammals. Therefore, the problem as to how sperm are transported rapidly to the site of fertilization needs to be explained.

Some insight into this problem has been obtained recently when a unique pattern of contraction that propels the luminal fluids upward toward the ovarian end has been observed in the pig, rabbit and human isthmi during the pre-ovulatory period (Blandau et al. 1974). If stained fluids are inserted into the junctura region of the isthmus, small amounts are pinched off and transported like boluses in a succession of constriction rings to the region just above the ampullary-isthmic junction. The physiologic constriction of the ampullary-isthmic junction normally retains the fluid within the ampulla. In the human isthmus, the pro-ovarian transport is somewhat less rigorous but nevertheless, obvious. Although we favor the theory that muscular contractions play the most important role in sperm transport through the isthmus and into the ampulla, we must evaluate in some way the significance of the pattern of ciliary beat in this process.

During the luteal phase, especially in the rabbit, the contractile activity of the isthmus changes dramatically from pro-ovarian contraction waves to a segmental, undulatory type that buffets the luminal contents backwards and forwards (unpublished observations). How the eggs finally reach the region of the junctura to be stored and finally moved into the uterus, is unknown for any mammal (Black et al. 1959).

Effects of environment

One of the principal reasons for developing various transducers which can be applied to the oviduct is to determine its behavior in an unanesthetized, free roaming animal. For years gynecologists have spoken about the so-called "spastic" oviducts observed during investigations of infertility problems. These conditions were observed particularly during insufflation procedures.

The effects of environmental conditions on the behavior of the oviduct is practically unknown. That investigators must pay attention to this parameter came to light recently when it was observed that painful stimuli, such as pinching the ear of the rabbit, could affect oviductal contractile activity especially of the ampulla, almost immediately and dramatically. There is also the possibility that visual, auditory and even pheromonal stimuli may play a part in the induction of changes in oviductal contractile activity.

CONCLUSIONS

From the limited observations mentioned here, we must conclude that the oviduct is indeed a most complex tubular system. Our understanding of the mechanism of gamete transport is in its inception. Until the respective roles of ciliary activity, oviductal muscular activity, rheology and hydrodynamics of the luminal fluids, contractions of the various mesenteries and ligaments and effects of sex hormones and catecholamines and environmental conditions, and even pheromones, can be ascertained and their integration clarified, the mechanism of gamete transport will remain a mystery.

REFERENCES

Alden R. H. (1942) The oviduct and egg transport in the albino rat. *Anat. Rec. 84*, 137–169.

Bergé Pierre (1967) Mise en évidence du mouvement propre de microorganismes vivants grâce à l'étude de la diffusion inélastique de la lumière. *C. R. Acad. Sci. (Paris) 265*, 889–892, Series D.

Black D. L. and Asdell S. A. (1959) Mechanism controlling entry of ova into rabbit uterus. *Amer. J. Physiol. 197*, 1275–1278.

Blandau R. J. (1973) Gamete transport in the female mammal. In: Greep R. and Astwood E. B., eds. *Handbook of Physiology and Endocrinology 2*, Part 2, Chapter 38, 153–163. American Physiologic Society, Washington D.C.

Blandau R. J. and Gaddum-Rosse P. (1974) Mechanism of sperm transport in pig oviducts. *Fertil. and Steril. 25*, 61–67.

Blandau R. J., Boling J. L., Halbert S. and Verdugo P. (1975) Methods for studying oviductal physiology. *Gynec. Invest. 6*, 123–145.

145

Blandau R. J. (1970) Methods of observing ovulation and egg transport. In: Daniel J. C., Jr., ed. *Methods in Mammalian Embryology,* Chapt. 1, pp. 1–14. Freeman, San Francisco, California.

Boling J. L. and Blandau R. J. (1971) Egg transport through the ampullae of the oviducts of rabbits under various experimental conditions. *Biol. Reprod. 4,* 174–184.

Borell U., Nilsson O. and Westman A. (1957) Ciliary activity in the rabbit Fallopian tube during oestrus and after copulation. *Acta obstet. gynec. scand. 36,* 22–28.

Clewe T. H. and Mastroianni L., Jr. (1958) Mechanisms of ovum pickup 1. Functional capacity of rabbit oviducts ligated near the fimbria. *Fertil. and Steril. 9,* 13–17.

Gaddum-Rosse P. and Blandau R. J. (1973) *In vitro* studies on ciliary activity within the oviducts of the rabbit and pig. *Amer. J. Anat. 136,* 91–104.

Gaddum-Rosse P., Blandau R. J. and Thiersch J. B. (1973) Ciliary activity in the human and *Macaca nemestrina* oviduct. *Amer. J. Anat. 138,* 269–275.

Harper M. J. K. (1961) The mechanisms involved in the movement of newly ovulated eggs through the ampulla of the rabbit Fallopian tube. *J. Reprod. Fertil. 2,* 522–524.

Mimura H. (1937) Studies on the ciliary movement of the oviduct in the domestic fowl. 1. The direction of the ciliary movement. *Okajimas Folia Anat. Japon. 15,* 287–295.

Parker G. H. (1928) The direction of the ciliary currents in the oviducts of vertebrates. *Amer. J. Physiol. 87,* 93–96.

Parker G. H. (1930) The ciliary systems in the oviduct of the pigeon. *Proc. Soc. exp. Biol. Med. 27,* 704–706.

Parker G. H. (1931) The passage of sperms and of eggs through the oviducts in terrestrial vertebrates. *Phil. Trans. Roy Soc. B 219,* 381–419.

Yamada F. (1952) Studies on the ciliary movements of the oviduct. *Jap. J. Physiol. 2,* 194–197.

146

SUMMARY OF DISCUSSIONS ON
BIOPHYSICAL AND BIOENGINEERING CONSIDERATIONS
IN STUDIES OF OVIDUCTAL PHYSIOLOGY

Reporter: *C. J. Pauerstein*

Some of the discussants of "Biophysical and Bioengineering Considerations in Studies of Oviductal Physiology" agreed to distinguish between oviductal "motility" and "contractility." The latter term was to be used in describing measurements such as force velocity curves and assessments of the active state. The designation "motility" was considered more descriptive of the measurements described in the papers presented in the morning session, such as intraluminal pressure, changes in transducer diameter and changes in wall tension.

The discussants then proceeded to a consideration of the papers presented in the morning session. The discussions focused upon three main issues: (1) the relative utility of various available sensors in measuring oviductal motility, (2) the correlation between oviductal motility and ovum transport rates, (3) the correlation in the human between ovum transport time and fertility.

SUMMARY OF CURRENT KNOWLEDGE

Three methods have been commonly used to measure oviductal motility *in vivo*. These are: (1) measurements of intraluminal pressure by open-ended or balloon-tipped catheters; (2) measurements of changes in luminal diameter by silastic rings; or (3) measurements of wall tension by extraluminal strain gauges of various designs. The discussion groups defined minimal criteria of an acceptable system for *in vivo* measurement of oviductal motility as non-interference with either fertility or fecundity, and non-disruption of the normal time-course of ovum transport.

147

Although many theoretical and some concrete objections to intraluminal recording were raised, it was generally agreed that the intraluminal methods have not been critically evaluated either by comparison to other methods, or by correlation with transport rates. Although such methods may not measure actual physiologic events, they seem to be useful for screening pharmacological agents. The balloon-tipped catheter appears quite useful for this purpose, and the silastic transducer may also prove useful. However, several observers voiced reservations about the use of the conductive carbon impregnanted silicone rubber device. Specific comments were that the system was pre-stressed when placed in the oviductal lumen, that the ring might buckle when intraluminal pressure rose, and that the amount of hysteresis in the system and the range over which the system is linear were undefined. One group suggested that these transducers may not actually record changes in the intraluminal diameter of the oviduct.

In more general terms, intraluminal devices were thought to provide less promise than extraluminal ones, because of the difficulty in correlating motility and ovum transport rates when intraluminal devices are used. In contrast, the consensus was that good data might be obtained by placing an array of external transducers along the isthmus, and by correlating the data so obtained with transport rates of ova or ovum models.

In the rabbit, the ampullary-isthmic junction, the uterotubal junction, and probably the isthmus, are involved in the regulation of ovum transport rates. With regard to the measurement of transport rates we now have developed radioactive ovum models that faithfully imitate the detailed time-course of normal ovum transport. Although it is possible that the transport of a surrogate might not be completely normal and if used to test pharmacologic agents, might thus not respond as a normal ovum would, two sets of data suggest that this is not a problem. First, treatments known to accelerate or delay ovum transport also accelerate or delay the ovum models. Further, in the case of estrogen-induced delay, the site of delay of the surrogate (ampullary-isthmic junction) is identical to that at which natural ova are delayed.

IDENTIFICATION OF NEEDED INFORMATION

The Task Force's impetus for the development of systems to measure oviductal motility depends upon the following chain of inference: 1) there is a reproducible correlation between oviductal motility and ovum transport rates; 2) it is possible pharmacologically to modify ovum transport rates in women; 3) pharmacologic agents that alter ovum transport rates would also alter motility and vice-versa; 4) pharmacologic modification of ovum transport rates would prevent pregnancy in women.

At this time, we lack definitive evidence for each of the items listed. It seems logical to begin by seeking immediate answers to the first and third items, because these premises can be tested by conducting relatively simple experiments in the rabbit.

In addition to seeking answers to these key questions, several participants thought that a need existed to develop techniques for recording tension and length in the longitudinal and circular axes of the oviduct, contraction of the mucosal folds within the oviduct, internal diameter, fluid currents, contraction of mesosalpinx and other ligaments, ciliary activity, and location of the ovum. However, the group did not consider the seeking of much of this information to be directly related to the goals of the Task Force. The consensus was that the rabbit experiments should be directed to the situation in the isthmus due to the brief sojourn of the ovum in the ampulla.

DEFINITION OF EXPERIMENTS NECESSARY TO ACHIEVE THIS OBJECTIVE

1) Experiments designed to correlate motility with ovum transport rates. This experiment would be done in rabbits during the immediate post-ovulatory period. Hormones or drugs known to accelerate or retard ovum transport will be used. A common experimental design specifying strain and weight of animals, dosage route and time of administration, will be prepared and sent to each participating laboratory. This experiment will clarify the relationship between ovum transport and parameters measured by each recording system. This information is considered essential in order to evaluate the relative performance of each recording technique under known conditions. 2) In subsequent experiments, those sensors judged to correlate most reliably with ovum transport rates in the first experiment will be utilized in experiments more directly correlating motility patterns with actual transport of ova or ovum surrogates. If the most reliable sensor proves to be one of the intraluminal group, motility in one oviduct would be correlated with transport rates in the contralateral oviduct. Although less than ideal, this approach appears to offer a workable compromise. 3) If a sensor yields information that consistently correlates with ovum transport rates, it can be used to screen agents for their effect on motility.

Finally, it was suggested that two separate approaches were needed to study the control of ovum transport. An *in vivo* system in which minimum interference was an objective and an *in vitro* system utilizing instrumentation which would allow definition of control mechanisms and their inter-relationships. It would then become mandatory to link these two methodologies.

ASSESSMENT OF FEASIBILITY AND COST
OF SUCH APPROACHES

The proposed crucial experiments (1 and 2) can be easily completed with current technology. A common protocol will be presented at the next meeting of the Task Force, and carried out in four or five laboratories currently engaged in measurement of motility and transport rates.

Further planning must await the results of these experiments.

SECTION II

Oviductal Contractility

MODERATORS

J. M. MARSHALL

and

E. E. DANIEL

Department of Neurosciences, Division of Biological and Medical Sciences, Brown University, Providence, R. I. 02912, USA

STUDIES OF OVIDUCTAL CONTRACTILITY
(Overview of in vitro approach)

By

J. M. Marshall

ABSTRACT

Studies on the contractile properties of the mammalian oviduct *in vitro* are discussed with respect to some anatomical considerations regarding the arrangement of the muscle layers and the methodology for recording mechanical and electrical activity of the muscle. Suggestions for future research are proposed. These include; further work on the anatomical arrangement of the muscle layers especially as related to the techniques for registration of contractile activity; quantitative approaches to the evaluation of the electrical characteristics of the muscle as it relates to the pattern and intensity of contractions and overall motility.

Over half a century of research has produced no definitive answer to the question: What is the role of oviductal contractions in the transport of ova in the mammalian oviduct? The task before us today is therefore a formidable one. My comments will be directed toward an overview of studies on the contractile behavior of the isolated oviduct since the *in vivo* approach will be considered by Dr. Daniel.

Studies of isolated organs circumvent, among other things, the effects of anesthetics, circulatory changes, and extrinsic nervous influences. In addition, they permit the composition of the extracellular medium to be manipulated more easily than *in situ*. Of course they are unphysiological in many respects, e. g. the

The author's research is supported by USPHE Grant HD-06963-10.

tissues are bathed in an artificial medium and are divorced from their normal neural and hormonal influences. Thus, as in most experimental situations, the investigator must compromise and choose the approach likely to give the most direct and reliable answers to the questions being asked. The present discussion on the *in vitro* approach focuses first on some anatomical considerations and then on selected experimental results obtained by various methods of recording contractions and electrical activity of the oviduct.

ANATOMICAL CONSIDERATIONS

From an anatomical viewpoint, studies on oviductal contractility present at least two difficulties. The first results from the heterogeneity of the cell types in the wall of the oviduct and the second from the arrangement of the muscle layers within the wall. In the oviduct, as elsewhere, smooth muscle cells coexist with a variety of other tissues including secretory, neural and connective tissue elements. Therefore, it is necessary to distinguish the effects of the experimental procedures on the muscle cells *per se* from those on the other tissue constituents. As in most hollow viscera, the smooth muscle layers in the wall of the oviduct can be oriented longitudinally, circularly or spirally. The specific orientation varies not only along the length of the oviduct, but also from species to species (Beck and Boots 1974; Nilsson and Reinius 1969). In all species so far examined, there is a transitional decrease in thickness of the muscular coat from the uterotubal junction to the infundibulum. In ungulates the muscle fibers are oriented spirally around the circumference of the oviduct, the individual muscle spirals traversing the muscularis from outside inward. In the mouse and the rat, the muscularis has a thin outer longitudinal layer and a thicker inner circular layer, while in the guinea-pig the orientation is reversed with the circular muscle on the outside. In rabbit and the human the circular layer lies between the inner and outer longitudinal layers which increase in thickness toward the uterus. These anatomical findings suggest that the nature of the contractions may vary from species to species and also within different regions of the oviduct. Thus, one factor which must be considered when isolating the oviduct for experimental purposes is whether a segment or the entire organ will be used and if the former, what anatomic portion is selected.

The patterns of innervation also vary in the different muscle layers and in different regions of the oviduct (Black 1974). Adrenergic innervation is especially prominent in the circular muscle layer of the isthmus and at the ampullary-isthmic junction. In these regions adrenergic nerve terminals come in close contact with individual smooth muscle cells (Hervonen and Kanerva 1972). In the ampulla and infundibulum the adrenergic nerves are limited primarily to the smooth muscle of the blood vessel walls. Our knowledge of the cholinergic

154

innervation is meagre, but hopefully this situation will be remedied later in this meeting.

The distribution of adrenergic nerves (and also perhaps cholinergic?), which varies from region to region and with the hormonal state of the animal in some species (see Brundin 1969) therefore should be considered in studies on the isolated oviduct since nerve terminals and ganglion cells may still be present and functional in the isolated organ. The effects of drugs, ions and other agents on these nervous elements must be distinguished from those on the muscle cells *per se*.

EXPERIMENTAL CONSIDERATIONS

A. *Mechanical properties*

In many studies on the mechanical properties of the oviduct, the isthmic portion is excised and suspended in a nutrient solution whose ionic constituents approximate those of the interstitial fluid. Although the nutrient solution usually contains glucose it rarely includes any of the essential amino acids or inter-mediates of the Krebs cycle. The temperature of the solution is sometimes re-duced to 20–25°C in order to minimize spontaneous motility. At this temperature the tissue sensitivity to various drugs and ions may be different than at normal body temperatures.

The longitudinal and circular muscle layers are especially prominent in the isthmus. Since muscle fibers usually contract in their plane of orientation an accurate quantitative registration of contractions depends, among other things, on the manner in which the tissue is arranged for recording. If the muscle is suspended along its longitudinal axis with one end fixed and the other tied to a force or linear motion transducer, the contractions of the longitudinal muscles will be predominantly registered. On the other hand, if circular rings are cut from the tube and suspended at right angles to the longitudinal axis contractions of the circular muscle will be predominantly registered (Hodgson et al. 1973; Higgs and Moawad 1974). Nevertheless, in both of these situations there is always some contribution of the circular or longitudinal muscle, respectively, to the contraction record. To my knowledge no one has ever tried to dissect the outer longitudinal muscle layer from the underlying circular muscle and study its mechanical properties separately.

Recently an attempt has been made to register the contractions of the longitu-dinal and circular muscle simultaneously in a segment of rabbit oviduct (Ueda et al. 1973). In this study, the isometric contraction of the longitudinal muscle was registered with a force transducer, while the circular muscle activity was monitored indirectly by an intraluminal microballoon. One of the unfortunate limitations of the intraluminal balloon technique for monitoring circular muscle

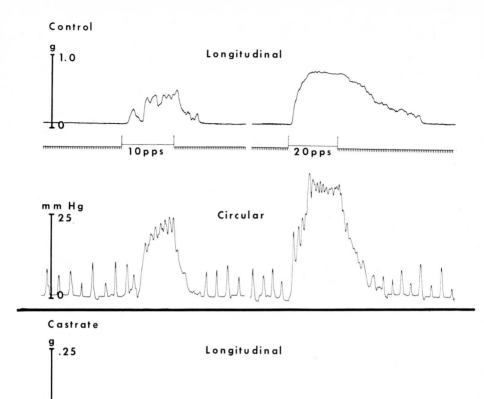

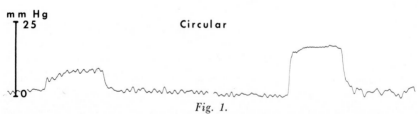

Fig. 1.

Effects of stimulation of the adrenergic, perivascular nerves on the contractions of the rabbit oviduct *in vitro*. Contractions of longitudinal muscle registered with a Statham force transducer, of the circular muscle indirectly by measurement of intra-luminal pressure changes with an open-ended polyethylene catheter (PE 10) connected to a Statham gauge (P 23 db). Nerve stimulation with rectangular pulses of 0.5 msec duration, 1.5 mA intensity at 10 and 20 pulses per second (PPS). Control animal = mature female Dutch rabbit; Castrate = mature female Dutch rabbit, 12 days post-ovariectomy (Kennedy and Marshall, unpublished).

156

activity is that it does not indicate whether the pressure changes are arising from local activity or are transmitted from distant sites. Thus, the extent and intensity of circular activity cannot be quantified with this technique. Despite these qualifications, the experiments are important because they represent one of the few attempts to register both longitudinal and circular muscle activity simultaneously in the same piece of tissue.

Using this technique we have studied the effects of perivascular stimulation of the adrenergic nerves on the contraction of the oviducts from rabbits under different hormonal conditions. The results from one of four experiments are shown in Fig. 1, where the activity in the predominantly longitudinally-oriented muscle and circularly-oriented muscle from a 12-day castrated rabbit is compared with that from a normal adult. Both layers of the muscle respond to nerve stimulation in the control animal, while in the castrate only the circular is activated. Whether this difference is due to a reduction in the content of the neurotransmitter (norepinephrine) in the castrate (as is known to occur – see Brundin 1969), to differing sensitivities of the 2 muscular layers to the transmitter (see Dr. Paton's paper in this volume) or to an interference with communication between the two layers are questions currently being investigated.

B. *Electrical activity*

Information about the electrical activity of the oviduct particularly its correlation with contraction, is much less extensive than for contractions alone since electrical activity is more difficult to record.

Two types of recording techniques are used in electrophysiology; intracellular and extracellular. An intracellular microelectrode gives precise, quantitative information about the membrane electrical characteristics of a single cell. Also, it can identify cells in pacemaker areas and in addition give a limited amount of information about the spread of excitation from cell to cell. If several microelectrodes are used together so that neighboring cells are impaled, then more precise information about cell-to-cell interaction can be obtained. Needless to say, the technical difficulties in such experiments are considerable.

An indirect, "quasi-intracellular" method for monitoring electrical activity, the sucrose-gap method (see Tomita 1970, for details), permits recording from small bundles of smooth muscle for prolonged periods of time, and together with the simultaneous monitoring of the muscle tension, provides a very useful approach to studies on electrical events and on excitation-contraction coupling. There is regrettably little quantitative information about the electrical characteristics of smooth muscle cells in the oviduct or their relation to contractility. One interesting observation, however, has recently been made on the guinea-pig oviduct using the sucrose-gap technique (Tomita and Watanabe 1973) Fig. 2. The spontaneous electrical activity of this muscle is composed of slow waves and spikes and resembles that from the small bowel (Prosser and Bortoff 1968). In the intestine the slow waves apparently originate in the longitudinal muscle and control the level of the membrane potential over many cell lengths. The spikes trigger contractions. Slow waves are thought to be induced in the circular muscle by activity in the overlying longitudinal muscle. Spikes also trigger contractions in the circular muscle. Whether this analogy applies to the guinea pig oviduct remains to be established as does evidence for electrical or mechanical coupling between the muscle layers.

The tracings in Fig. 2 also show that the amplitude of the slow wave can be altered by changing the level of the membrane potential, hyperpolarization (an increase in potential difference across the membrane) increasing and depolarization (a decrease in potential difference) diminishing the amplitude. The frequency of pacemaker discharge is, however, not altered by changes in membrane polarization. In these respects, the oviduct behaves like intestinal muscle.

Neither the intracellular microelectrode nor the sucrose-gap method lends itself to the mapping of electrical activity over the entire oviduct, the determination of direction and speed of propagation, or localization of pacemaker areas. The elegant studies with extracellular suction electrodes by Drs. Talo and Brundin, have provided valuable information about the spread of electrical

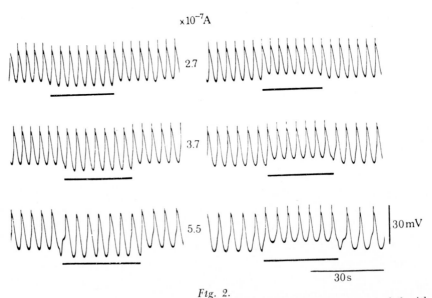

$\times 10^{-7} A$

2.7

3.7

5.5

30 mV

30 s

Fig. 2.

Spontaneous electrical activity in the isolated oviduct of the guinea pig recorded with the double sucrose gap method. Effects of hyperpolarizing (left) and depolarizing (right) current application (horizontal bars) with increasing intensities as indicated. (From Tomita and Watanabe 1973, by permission of the Royal Society).

activity, pacemaker areas, frequency gradients for activity along the oviduct. In some of their experiments, intraluminal pressure was measured by the microballoon technique, while in others changes in the diameter of the luminal radius were monitored by the constant perfusion method. Although we will hear more about this work today and later in this meeting, I should like to mention briefly one of the recent studies (Talo and Brundin 1973) because it bears on the relationship between longitudinal and circular muscle. In this work, they recorded the electrical activity in the longitudinal muscle (whereas most of their previous work had been done on the isolated rabbit oviduct whose longitudinal muscle had been removed) and registered the intraluminal pressure simultaneously with a miniature balloon. They found that the electrical activity of the longitudinal muscle layer was similar to that in the longitudinal layer of the myometrium, *i. e.*, a train discharge of action potentials. The electrical discharge in the circular muscles (as monitored in their previous studies) was of short, pulsatile bursts or single discharges. The longitudinal train discharge triggered a fused tetanus-type contraction, whereas the bursts triggered brief, phasic contractions. The longitudinal muscles appeared to function independently of the circular, in agreement with earlier findings (Hasama 1932). Thus, unlike the intestine, electrical activity in the longitudinal muscle layer may not influence that in the circular muscle. The functional consequence of this situation is that ovum transport may be independent of ovum retention; the former being related to contractions of the longitudinal muscle and the latter to the contraction of the circular layer. This important possibility deserves further experimental consideration.

FUTURE RESEARCH STRATEGY

On the bases of these somewhat biased and highly selected examples of studies on the oviduct *in vitro*, I submit the following suggestions for consideration by the Task Force for future research.

1. *Contraction*

a) Improve methods for simultaneous registration of longitudinal and circular muscle layers. What are the most feasible, relatively non-interruptive techniques?

b) Initiate a series of carefully controlled studies on the comparison between the different muscular layers with respect to humoral, hormonal, ionic and neural influences.

2. *Electrical activity*

a) Obtain precise quantitative information about the electrical characteristics of individual smooth muscle cells, including effects of drugs, ions, hormones and neural influences.

b) Encourage studies with extracellular electrodes along the lines of Drs. Talo and Brundin.

c) Attempt to devise techniques and experiments designed to study the electrical interaction (or lack thereof) between muscle bundles in the different muscular layers.

3. *Excitation – contraction coupling*

a) Utilize microelectrode or sucrose-gap recording techniques to study this relationship under various hormonal, humoral and ionic conditions.

b) Utilize a multiple extracellular electrode technique for similar studies.

REFERENCES

Beck L. R. and Boots L. R. (1974) The comparative anatomy, histology and morphology of the mammalian oviduct. In: Johnson A. D. and Foley C. W., eds. *The Oviduct and Its Functions*, pp. 1–52. Academic Press, New York City.

Black D. L. (1974) Neural control of oviduct musculature. In: Johnson A. D. and Foley C. W., eds. *The Oviduct and Its Functions*, pp. 65–118. Academic Press, New York City.

Brundin J. (1969) Pharmacology of the oviduct. In: Hafez E. S. E. and Blandau R. J., eds. *The Mammalian Oviduct*, pp. 251–269. Univ. of Chicago Press, Chicago.

Hasama B. (1932) Die elektrische Vorgänge am isolierten Eileiter bei der Ablauf der peristalishen Kontraktion. *Pflügers Arch. 231*, 311–331.

Hervonen A. and Kanerva L. (1972) Adrenergic and noradrenergic axons of the rabbit uterus and oviduct. *Acta physiol. scand. 85*, 139–148.

Higgs G. W. and Moawad A. H. (1974) The effect of ovarian hormones on the contractility of the rabbit oviductal isthmus. *Canad. J. Physiol. Pharmacol. 52*, 74–83.

Hodgson B. J., Sullivan K. G. and Pauerstein C. J. (1973) The role of sympathetic nerves in the response of the uterus and oviduct to field stimulation. *Europ. J. clin. Pharmacol. 23*, 107–110.

Nilsson O. and Reinius S. (1969) Light and electron microscope structure of the oviduct. In: Hafez E. S. E. and Blandau R. J., eds. *The Mammalian Oviduct*, pp. 57–83. Univ. of Chicago Press, Chicago.

Prosser C. L. and Bortoff A. (1968) Electrical activity of intestinal muscle under *in vitro* conditions. In: Code C. F., ed. *The Alimentary Canal*, Sect. 6, Vol. IV of Handbook of Physiology, pp. 2025–2050. Waverly Press, Baltimore.

Talo A. and Brundin J. (1973) The functional significance and contractile function of the upper reproductive tract in female rabbits. *Biol. Reprod. 9*, 142–148.

Tomita T. (1970) Electrical properties of mammalian smooth muscle. In: Bülbring E., Brading A. F., Jones A. W. and Tomita T., eds. *Smooth Muscle*, pp. 197–243. Williams and Wilkins, Baltimore.

Tomita T. and Watanabe H. (1973) Factors controlling myogenic activity in smooth muscle. *Phil. Trans. R. Soc. Lond. B. 265*, 73–85.

Ueda M., Mattos C. E. R. and Coutinho E. M. (1973) The influence of adrenergic activation and blockade on the motility of the circular and longitudinal muscle layers of rabbit oviduct *in vitro*. *Fertil. and Steril. 24*, 440–447.

Department of Zoology, University of Turku,
20500 Turku 50, Finland

ELECTROPHYSIOLOGY OF THE OVIDUCT

By

Antti Talo

ABSTRACT

Electrical activity of the oviduct has been very little studied. Intracellular or sucrose-gap measurements of resting and action potentials and other membrane properties have been studied hardly at all. Since there is wide variation between the electrical properties of different smooth muscles, no attempt has been made to extrapolate from studies in other organs. This review is restricted to those few studies which have been made on the oviduct.

When recorded by suction electrodes *in vitro,* the filtered electrical activity consists of a single spike or of a short burst of spikes, depending on the hormonal state. In unfiltered recordings, one or few spikes appear on a slower depolarization. A few such depolarizations with spikes correspond to the burst of filtered activity.

The electrical activity of the oviduct differs from the electrical activity of other structures of the upper reproductive tract at least in its duration. The duration of bursts is always short, being only a few seconds, while the other structures typically discharge longer trains of spikes. Corresponding to the short duration of the bursts, the contractions are of a short, phasic type.

The rabbit oviduct exhibits multipacemaker activity with shifting pacemaker location. Normally the highest pacemaker activity is at the distal isthmus or at the ampullary-isthmic junction. In postovulatory rabbits electrical activity is generated at some distance from the previous generation rather than at the same place. The frequency of generation may vary in a short segment.

Electrical activity often propagates in both directions, faster in the isthmus than in the ampulla. The speed of propagation is normally low, only a few mm/sec, but reaches nearly 20 mm/sec in the isthmus of castrated, estrogen-treated rabbits. The proportion of antiperistaltic propagation of the total number of propagating bursts depends on the hormonal and on the functional state. This is also the case for the distance of propagation. The frequency of electrical activity varies between the oviductal regions and with time in respect to mating. In most cases the highest frequency is found at the distal isthmus or at the ampullary-isthmic junction.

When wire electrodes are used to record electrical activity *in vivo* it is difficult to avoid recording the activity of nearby peritoneal structures.

The electrophysiology of the oviduct is inadequately known. There are no reliable measurements of resting and action potentials by microelectrodes or by the sucrose-gap technique. The values reported by Zastowt (1969), about 30 mV for resting potential and 20 mV for action potential, are lower than is generally accepted for smooth muscles (Kuriyama 1970).

Electrical activity has been characterized only by extracellular recording methods. It varies from a single spike (Talo and Brundin 1971; Paton 1974) to a short burst of spikes (Nishimura et al. 1969; Brundin and Talo 1972; Talo

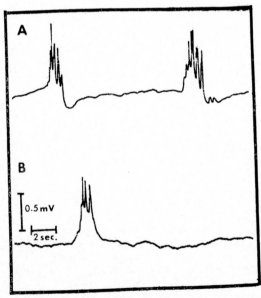

Fig. 1.

Electrical activity recorded from the ampullary-isthmic junction of the rabbit oviduct *in vitro* at 91 h after mating. Recording by suction electrodes using 1 sec time constant in A and DC recording in B.

1974). In the author's studies low frequency components were filtered. Unpublished recordings (Talo 1972) suggest that the spikes are superimposed on a slow depolarization (Fig. 1). Filtering off this component might thus at least partly explain the low amplitude of the spikes in the oviduct. A spike amplitude over 1 mV has been rare in the oviduct, particularly in the isthmus, while amplitudes of over 5 mV are commonly recorded at nearby peritoneal structures using suction electrodes. This difference in amplitude might partly be explained by asynchronous activity in the oviduct.

The duration of the bursts seems to be lower in the oviduct than in the nearby peritoneal structures (Talo and Brundin 1972). This difference should not however be overemphasized, since the activity of the peritoneal structures is controlled by ovarian hormones (Talo and Brundin 1973; Halbert and Conrad 1975), which may result in variation in burst duration. Burst durations of 0.7–2 sec have been reported in estrogen-treated rabbits (Nishimura et al. 1969; Talo and Brundin 1971). Unpublished measurements of the duration of bursts in postovulatory rabbits have provided mean values between 0.7 and 1.5 sec.

The speed of propagation of electrical activity is slow in the oviduct. Values from 2–17 mm/sec have been reported (Nishimura et al. 1969; Talo and Brundin 1971; Paton 1974).

The majority of electrophysiological studies have had the objective of analyzing contractile activity of the oviduct by measuring the site of generation, and the frequency, direction and distance of propagation of electrical activity. The site of generation has been studied by mapping out contractions by means of several electrodes rather than by measuring prepotentials. This technique is accurate only when short interelectrode distances are used or when the electrical activity propagates regularly and fast (Talo and Brundin 1971; Talo 1974). In estrogen-treated castrated rabbits electrical activity generated regularly at the distal isthmus (Talo and Brundin 1971). In other states the oviduct showed multipacemaker activity with changing pacemaker location, although the highest frequency of generation was in this same region (Brundin and Talo 1972; Talo 1974). In postovulatory rabbits, electrical activity began as frequently in the uterine as in the ovarian direction from the preceding generation (Talo 1974). Some evidence was also obtained that electrical activity had a tendency to generate at a given distance from the previous generation and that this distance was shorter in the distal isthmus than in the ampulla (Talo 1974).

The frequency of electrical activity in the rabbit oviduct is affected by the hormonal state of the animal. In estrogen-treated castrates the frequency was similar throughout the isthmus but lower in the ampulla (Talo and Brundin 1971). In nontreated castrates and estrogen- and progesterone-treated castrates the frequency was highest at the distal isthmus (Brundin and Talo 1972). This was also the case at 5 h and 91 h after mating or induction of ovulation by

163

injection of human chorionic gonadotrophin (Talo 1974). At 17 h, on the other hand, the frequency was low and similar in all segments of the oviduct. It increased in the ampulla and the ampullary-isthmic junction up to 43 h and remained high at 71 h. It has been suggested that changes of frequency of electrical activity affect ovum transport (Talo 1974).

The direction in which electrical activity spreads is probably the most significant variable of the contractile activity affecting ovum transport. When electrical activity initiates irregularly in many locations, e. g. after ovulation (Talo 1974), the prevailing direction should be down the frequency gradient. Although excitation spreads in both directions (Nishimura et al. 1969; Talo 1974; Paton 1974), a common phenomenon is that it spreads asymmetrically (Talo 1974). Often this was due to the fact that two bursts spread towards each other and canceled each other out. The direction of propagation can be most reliably studied by electrode pairs with short interelectrode distances (Talo 1974). Although the results of this study were based on a small number of experiments owing to technical difficulties, there are some interesting obser- vations. Bursts propagated with nearly identical frequency in the ovarian as in the uterine direction at 17, 43 and 71 h after mating except at the ampullary- isthmic junction at 17 h and at the proximal isthmus at 71 hours. At 17 h about 90 % of bursts spread in the ovarian direction in the ampullary-isthmic junction and about 80 % in the uterine direction at 71 h in the proximal isthmus. Although these findings cannot be taken as conclusive they are in agreement with earlier findings by Maia and Coutinho (1970) on the human oviduct *in vivo*, and suggest that the change in direction of propagation could play a decisive role in ovum transport.

The correlation between electrical activity and intraluminal pressure has

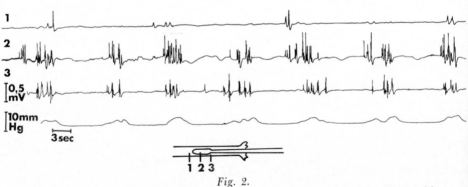

Fig. 2.
Electrical activity and intraluminal pressure in the ampulla of the rabbit oviduct recorded *in vitro* by suction electrodes and through a balloon-tipped catheter. The locations of electrodes and the catheter are illustrated schematically.

not been easy to demonstrate when intraluminal pressure is measured by the perfusion method. When electrical activity propagates regularly in one direction this task, however, is simpler (Talo and Brundin 1971). The main problem is that the contractile activity is normally complex and irregular, and the mapping of all contractions is difficult even when several electrodes are being used. It has been shown, however, that the amplitude of pressure cycles depends on the distance of contraction from the tip of the perfusion catheter, on the direction of propagation, and on the distance of the contracting segment (Talo 1975). It should also be recognized that the effects of these factors are modulated by the luminal volume and elasticity of the wall (Talo 1975). The correlation between electrical activity and intraluminal pressure is much simpler to establish when intraluminal pressure is recorded by the balloon technique (Fig. 2).

The *in vitro* studies have provided important information concerning the optimal placement of electrodes in order to obtain various types of information. The reliability of *in vitro* studies must, however, be questioned until their results have been confirmed *in vivo*, preferably in unanestethized, unrestrained animals. Such studies have been hampered by technical difficulties. It should be stressed that if the technical difficulties are overcome, recording of wall activity by chronically implanted electrodes would permit detailed analysis of contractile activity of the oviduct while permitting its normal function of gamete transport. Nishimura et al. (1969) recorded the electrical activity of the oviduct by three Ag-AgCl needle electrodes in anesthetized rabbits with opened abdomen. Larks et al. (1971) implanted platinum electrodes in a plastic collar in the infundibulum and isthmus of nonpregnant goats. They recorded trains of spikes with amplitudes up to 600 μV and reported changes in activity during the estrous cycle. Nishimura et al. (1969) recorded short bursts in the ampulla and isthmus but also long bursts in the isthmus. Such bursts have been recorded in the peritoneal smooth muscles covering the isthmus (Talo and Brundin 1973), but not in the oviduct when the peritoneal structures have been removed (Brundin and Talo 1972; Talo 1974). Due to intimate contact between the oviductal circular musculature and the peritoneal structures, the placement of electrodes *in vivo* is critical to avoid recording of electrical activity of the peritoneal muscles simultaneously with the oviductal activity.

I have been recently involved in a feasibility study of recording chronic electrical activity of the rabbit oviduct *in vivo* and wish to report here some of the preliminary data. Using the method described by Grivel and Ruckebush (1972), NiCr wire electrodes (62.5 μm thick) were implanted in the isthmic wall of ten rabbits and the wires exteriorized laterally. The plug in which the wires were attached was protected by a small aluminum box sewed to the skin. The wires were insulated except, in an area of about 0.5 mm long which was placed inside the oviduct wall. The results with estrous and postovulatory rabbits were variable and usually had only limited success. The main problem

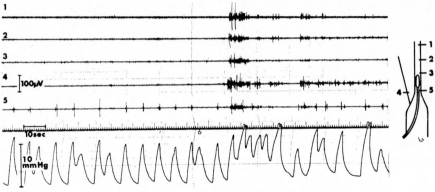

Fig. 3.

Chronically recorded intraluminal pressure and electrical activity in the rabbit oviduct and mesotubarium superius. The rabbit was ovariectomized 7 days previously and treated with 0.25 μg estradiol twice daily for three days, the last injection 11 h before recording. The locations of electrodes and the balloon-tipped catheter are illustrated schematically on the right. Electrode no. 4 was implanted in the mesotubarium superius. Electrical activity of variable amplitude was recorded in electrode no. 5 in nearly perfect synchrony with the intraluminal pressure cycles. When activity begins in electrode 4, it is recorded in all electrodes, while a typical "outburst" with elevated baseline is recorded intraluminally.

was how to be sure that the electrical activity was indeed from the oviduct. This was solved by using recordings of intraluminal pressure through a balloon inserted in the isthmic lumen through the uterine lumen, by recording the electrical activity of the mesotubarium superius with one electrode near the uterus, and by measuring the electrical activity with four electrodes implanted in the isthmic wall (Fig. 3). These rabbits were ovariectomized and treated with estrogen using the same schedule as in Talo and Brundin (1971). Although two nearby electrodes have not been implanted successfully so far the results are in close agreement with those made *in vitro* (Talo and Brundin 1971). The pressure cycles were regular and appeared in synchrony with the electrical activity, which consisted of spikes of variable amplitude. Interestingly, when electrical activity was recorded by means of the electrode placed in the meso-tubarium superius, the intraluminal pressure increased and a typical "outburst" was recorded as had occurred *in vitro* (Talo and Brundin 1973). At the same time electrical activity of a similar type was recorded in all the other electrodes, suggesting that the peritoneal activity was also recorded in the electrodes implanted in the isthmic wall. Although the results are still based on only a few successful recordings (3), the similarity between them and the *in vitro* studies increases their reliability. Although the method is still in need of further refinement, the results are promising.

166

REFERENCES

Brundin J. and Talo A. (1972) The effects of estrogen and progesterone on the electric activity and intraluminal pressure of the castrated rabbit oviduct. *Biol. Reprod. 7*, 417–424.

Grivel M-L. and Ruckebusch Y. (1972) The propagation of segmental contractions along the small intestine. *J. Physiol. (Lond.) 227*, 611–625.

Halbert S. A. and Conrad J. T. (1975) *In vitro* contractile activity of the mesotubarium superius from the rabbit oviduct in various endocrine states. *Fertil. and Steril. 26*, 248–256.

Kuriyama H. (1970) Effects of ions and drugs on the electrical activity of smooth muscle. In: Bulbring E., Brading A. F., Jones A. W. and Tomita T., eds. *Smooth Muscle*, pp. 366–395. Williams & Wilkins, Baltimore.

Larks S. D., Larks G. G., Hoffer R. E. and Charlson E. J. (1971) Electrical activity of oviducts *in vivo*. *Nature (Lond.) 234*, 556–557.

Maia H. and Coutinho E. M. (1970) Peristalsis and antiperistalsis of the human Fallopian tube during the menstrual cycle. *Biol. Reprod. 2*, 305–314.

Nishimura T., Nakajima A. and Hayashi T. (1969) The basic pattern of electrical activities in the rabbit Fallopian tube. *Acta Obst. Gynaec., Jap. 16*, 97–103.

Paton D. M. (1974) Personal communication.

Talo A. (1974) Electric and mechanical activity of the rabbit oviduct *in vitro* before and after ovulation. *Biol. Reprod. 11*, 335–345.

Talo A. (1975) Amplitude variation of the pressure cycles in and between segments of the rabbit oviduct *in vitro*. *Biol. Reprod. 13*, 249–254.

Talo A. and Brundin J. (1971) Muscular activity in the rabbit oviduct: A combination of electric and mechanic recordings. *Biol. Reprod. 5*, 67–77.

Talo A. and Brundin J. (1973) The functional connections and contractile function of the upper reproductive tract in female rabbits. *Biol. Reprod. 9*, 142–148.

Zastowt O. (1969) Badania nad zjawiskami bioelektrycznymi błony komórkowej mieśniówki jajowodów. Gin. Pol. *40*, 371–376.

W. H. O. Collaborating Center for Clinical Research
on Human Reproduction,
Maternidade Clímério De Oliveira, Federal University of Bahia,
Salvador – Bahia – Brazil

RELATIONSHIP BETWEEN CYCLIC AMP LEVELS AND OVIDUCTAL CONTRACTILITY

By

H. Maia Jr., I. Barbosa and E. M. Coutinho

ABSTRACT

Dibutyryl Cyclic AMP (7 mM) induced relaxation of the musculature of the isthmus and ampulla in rabbits, guinea pigs and humans. The response of the rabbit oviduct to norepinephrine (0.2–1 μg/ml) and prostaglandin $F_{2\alpha}$ (1–2 μg/ml) was decreased by dibutyryl cyclic AMP (1 mM) *in vitro*. Theophylline (10 mM) increased cyclic AMP levels in the rabbit oviduct and inhibited both spontaneous and prostaglandin $F_{2\alpha}$-induced contractility. The relaxing effect of beta adrenergic stimulatory compounds on human oviduct was enhanced by theophylline. Imidazole (10 mM), a phosphodiesterase activator, increased the contractility of the guinea pig, human and rabbit oviduct *in vitro*. The effect of imidazole was abolished by either removal of calcium ions from the medium or by theophylline.

Prostaglandin E_2 (2–5 μg/ml) inhibited the contractility of the rabbit isthmus *in vitro*. PGE_2 increased cyclic AMP levels in the isthmus, but not in the ampulla of pseudopregnant animals. Basal levels of cyclic AMP also decreased in the rabbit isthmus during the first three days after ovulation. Addition of PGE_2 (5 μg/ml) restored these levels to estrous values. These studies show that changes in cyclic AMP levels alter the contraction rate of the oviductal musculature.

The concept of cyclic AMP as a "second messenger" of hormonal action was first introduced in 1960 by Sutherland to explain the glycogenolytic effect of epinephrine (Sutherland and Rall 1960). Later this concept was extended to several other hormones, such as LH, FSH, MSH, ACTH, vasopressin and prostaglandins. Biochemical studies have further shown that cyclic AMP is formed from ATP by a direct reaction that is catalysed by a membrane-bound enzyme, adenylate cyclase. Activity of this enzyme is under hormonal control. Inactivation of cyclic AMP, on the other hand, is accomplished by several cyclic nucleotide phosphodiesterases which are present mainly in the cytoplasm. These enzymes are susceptible to inhibition by methylxanthines, such as theophylline, aminophylline and cafeine. Compounds like imidazole, on the other hand, are capable of stimulating phosphodiesterase activity *in vitro* (Sutherland et al. 1968). Thus an increase in cyclic AMP levels may come about in two ways, either by a stimulation of adenylate cyclase activity or by the inhibition of phosphodiesterase. Conversely, a decrease in the intracellular levels of cyclic AMP may result from either a reduction in adenylate cyclase or an increase in phosphodiesterase activity.

In the past few years, it has been shown that cyclic AMP plays an important role in several reproductive processes, such as gonadotrophin release (Labrie et al. 1975), ovarian and testicular steroidogenesis, luteinization (Channing 1974), ovarian contractility (Coutinho et al. 1974), and spermatozoal motility and metabolism (Gray et al. 1971). With respect to steroid action, on the other hand, it has been established that most of the features of steroid action cannot be ascribed to cyclic AMP (Baulieu 1974). However, it is possible that cyclic AMP does interfere with steroid action secondarily.

It has been established that in the intestine an increase in cyclic AMP is related to relaxation, in addition to possible roles for the nucleotide in regulating the metabolism of such muscle (Anderson and Nelson 1972). In this communication we will discuss the interaction of cyclic AMP, prostaglandins and catecholamines in the oviduct. The studies include *in vitro* experiments which were carried out in our laboratory during the last three years.

MATERIALS AND METHODS

All the experiments were carried out *in vitro* with segments of oviduct excised during laparotomy from women or obtained from various laboratory animals immediately after sacrifice. After careful dissection of adhering tissue, the chosen segment of the oviduct was suspended in an organ bath containing Krebs' solution. The temperature of the bath was maintained at $37°C$, and a gas mixture (95% $O^2 : 5 \%$ CO^2) was constantly bubbled into the solution. To record isometric contractions, one end of the segment of the oviduct was fixed to the bottom of the container, and the free end was attached to a force-displacement transducer (FT 100, Sanborn).

RESULTS

Interaction between cyclic AMP and catecholamines in the oviduct

Both alpha and beta adrenergic receptors were identified in the rabbit, human and guinea pig oviduct. The reactivity of the oviduct to catecholamines is modulated by ovarian steroid hormones (Coutinho et al. 1971). During estrogen dominance the adrenergic receptors in the oviduct are predominantly excitatory (alpha receptors) whereas under luteal dominance they are inhibitory (beta receptors). Based on these and other observations, it was suggested that ovum transport was under adrenergic control (Pauerstein et al. 1970; Coutinho et al. 1971). However, this model was criticized recently when it was shown that the chemical or surgical denervation of the oviduct could prevent the pharmacologic effects of steroid hormones on ovum transport, but did not interfere with normal transport (Pauerstein et al. 1974).

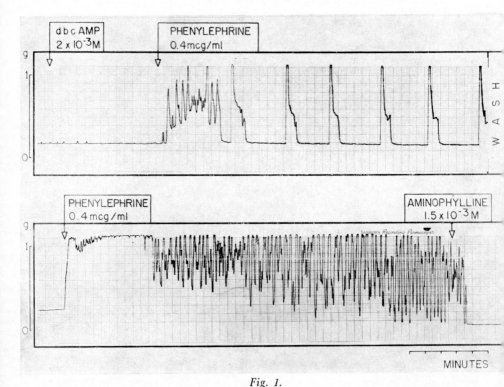

Fig. 1.
Effect of dibutyryl cyclic AMP on the response of the isthmus from an estrous rabbit to phenylephrine *in vitro*. Note that following dibutyryl cyclic AMP, the response to phenylephrine is greatly reduced.

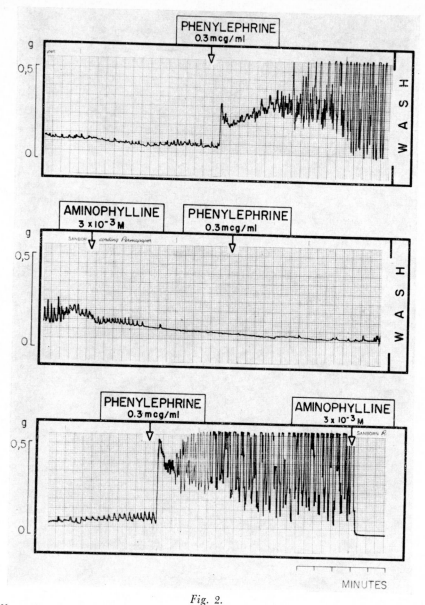

Fig. 2.
Effect of aminophylline on the response of the isthmus from an estrous rabbit to phenylephrine *in vitro*. Note that aminophylline pretreatment reduces the effect of phenylephrine.

Nevertheless, oviductal contractility seems to be greatly influenced by catecholamines and prostaglandins. In the rabbit oviduct, a mutual antagonism between E prostaglandins and catecholamines was recently reported *in vivo* (Spilman and Harper 1974). In view of these findings, it was suggested that prostaglandins could act as local regulators of the effects of catecholamines on the oviduct. In adipose tissue, a similar antagonism between catecholamines and prostaglandins was also found, and in this case it was at the level of adenyl cyclase (Butcher and Sutherland 1969). In the oviduct, the participation of cyclic AMP in this mechanism is not totally established. Experimental results have shown that dibutyryl cyclic AMP and phosphodiesterase inhibitors, such as aminophylline, can inhibit the response of the rabbit oviductal isthmus to alpha adrenergic compounds during estrus, mimicking therefore the effect of PGE_2 (Figs. 1 and 2). High doses of dibutyryl cyclic AMP and aminophylline cause complete oviductal relaxation *in vitro* in several mammalian species, including man (Maia, Jr. and Coutinho 1974a,c) (Fig. 3). This inhibitory effect is not antagonized by beta adrenergic blockers, such as propranolol (Maia, Jr. and Coutinho, in press).

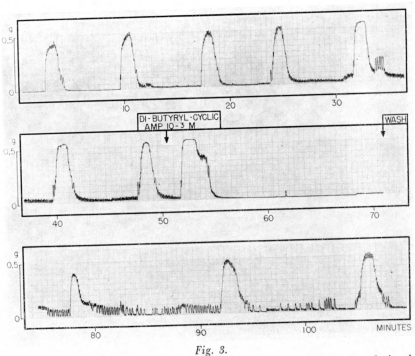

Fig. 3.

Response of the oviduct of a guinea pig to dibutyryl cyclic AMP *in vitro* during late pregnancy. Note the suppression of outbursts following dbc AMP.

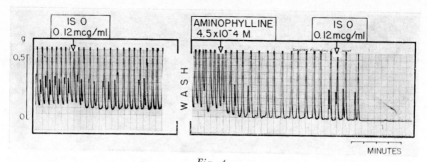

Fig. 4.

Potentiation of the effect of low doses of isoproterenol on the human oviduct *in vitro* by aminophylline. The oviduct was isolated during the luteal phase (day 22).

Beta adrenergic compounds, like isoproterenol, on the other hand, increased cyclic AMP levels and induced oviductal relaxation *in vitro* as well as *in vivo* (Brunton 1972). In humans, low doses of aminophylline do not markedly inhibit oviductal contractility, but they do enhance the inhibitory effects of sub-threshold doses of isoproterenol (Fig. 4). This indicates that the effects of beta adrenergic activation are mediated by cyclic AMP. This assumption is supported by the observation that isoproterenol causes an acute elevation of cyclic AMP levels in the oviduct (Brunton 1972) and that dibutyryl cyclic AMP can mimick the relaxing effects of beta activators (Maia, Jr. and Coutinho 1974a).

Effect of imidazole on the oviduct

Imidazole increased oviductal contractility in humans and guinea pigs under different hormonal conditions. In humans, the stimulatory effect was observed

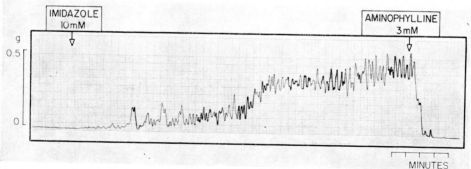

Fig. 5.

Response of the human oviductal isthmus during the late luteal phase to imidazole *in vitro* (day 22). Note the sustained increase in tonus following imidazole and the blockade by aminophylline.

173

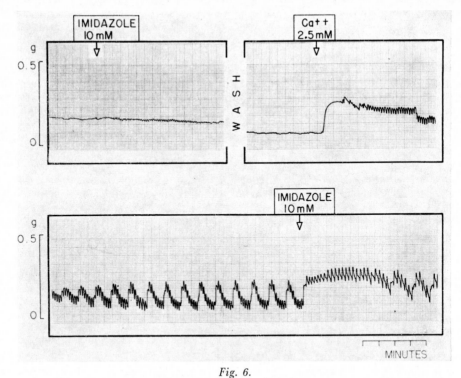

Fig. 6.

Effect of calcium on the response of the guinea pig oviduct during early pregnancy to imidazole *in vitro*. Note that the stimulatory effect of imidazole is absent in the calcium free-Krebs, but is restored after the addition of 2.5 mM Ca^{++}.

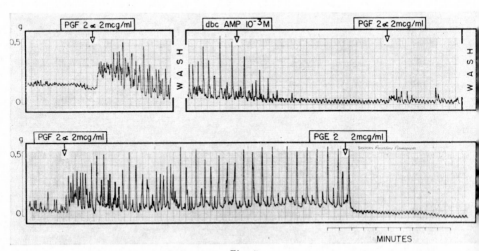

Fig. 7.

Inhibitory effect of dbc AMP on the response of the isthmus from an estrous rabbit to PGF$_{2\alpha}$ *in vitro*.

174

throughout the menstrual cycle, as well as during pregnancy (Fig. 5). The response to imidazole was characterized by an increase in the tonus of the oviduct with the appearance of rhythmic contractions in a quiescent preparation. Incubation of the human oviduct with aminophylline greatly reduces the response to imidazole (Maia, Jr. and Coutinho 1974b).

The effect of imidazole on the guinea pig oviduct is very similar to that recorded in humans. During both estrus and pregnancy, imidazole caused an increase of oviductal contractility which was suppressed by aminophylline. The response to imidazole was inhibited also in calcium free-Krebs (Fig. 6).

Effect of prostaglandins and cyclic AMP on oviductal contractility

Prostaglandins affect oviductal contractility in several species, both *in vivo* as well as *in vitro* (Spilman and Harper 1973). In rabbits and humans, prostaglandin $F_{2\alpha}$ activates oviductal contractility while PGE induces relaxation.

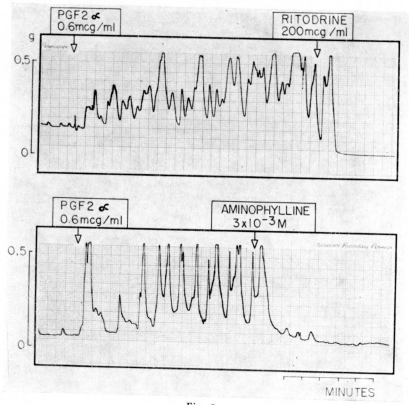

Fig. 8.

Inhibitory effect of ritodrine and aminophylline on the response of the human isthmus during the luteal phase to $PGF_{2\alpha}$ *in vitro*.

175

These effects are influenced by ovarian steroids. Progesterone increases the response to PGE_2, while at the same time decreases the effect of $PGF_{2\alpha}$ (Spilman 1974). In rabbits and hamsters, the response of the oviductal isthmus to $PGF_{2\alpha}$ is inhibited by dibutyryl cyclic AMP, aminophylline and PGE_2 *in vitro* (Maia, Jr. and Coutinho 1974a) (Fig. 7). *In vivo*, PGE^2 and $PGF_{2\alpha}$ are also mutually antagonist in man and in the rabbit (Coutinho and Maia 1971; Spilman and Harper 1973). In the human oviduct the response to $PGF_{2\alpha}$ is decreased by beta adrenergic activators and phosphodiesterase inhibitors (Fig. 8). It is thought that this inhibition may result from the accumulation of cyclic AMP in the oviduct.

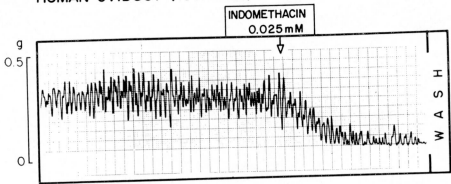

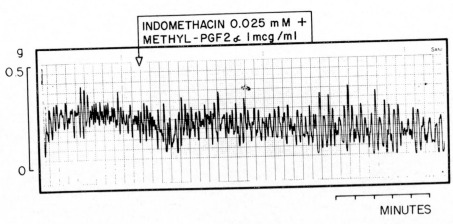

Fig. 9.
Inhibitory effect of indomethacin on the contractility of the human oviduct *in vitro* during the proliferative phase (day 12). Note that the effect of indomethacin is not observed in the presence of $PGF_{2\alpha}$.

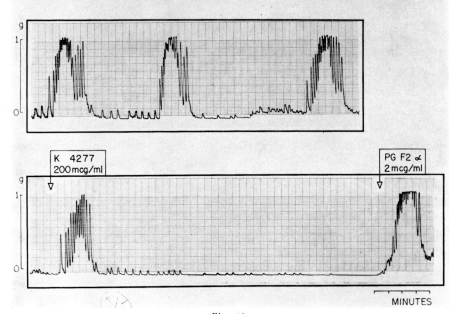

GUINEA PIG OVIDUCT (ESTRUS)

Fig. 10.
Effect of K4277 on the contractility of the guinea pig oviduct *in vitro*.

The fact that E and F series prostaglandins exert opposite effects on the oviductal isthmus suggest that they may be involved in the regulation of oviductal contractility and ovum transport (Spilman and Harper 1973). It was suggested that F prostaglandins may act to retain the eggs in the oviduct by virtue of their occlusive effect on the isthmus, while E Prostaglandins would abolish this effect, permitting therefore the entry of ova into the uterus. It is well established that itshmic occlusion is an important mechanism preventing the premature passage of the eggs to the uterus (Spilman and Harper 1975). This model is in agreement with our observation that indomethacin, a known inhibitor of prostaglandin synthesis, decreases the tone and the contractility of the oviduct in rats, guinea pigs, rabbits and humans *in vitro*, (Maia, Jr. and Coutinho 1974b). This effect is totally prevented by addition of prostaglandin $F_{2\alpha}$ (Fig. 9). Preliminary studies with other inhibitors of prostaglandin synthesis, such as propoxyphene, K4277, RU15167, have revealed that these compounds depress oviductal contractility *in vitro* in guinea pigs, humans, and rats. The occurrence of outbursts *in vitro* in guinea pigs is also suppressed by these compounds (Fig. 10).

177

Effect of oxytocin and aminophylline on the oviduct

Oxytocin does not have any effect on the rabbit oviduct, while it markedly increases the contractility of the guinea pig and hamster oviducts *in vitro*. In both species the response to this neurophypophyseal hormone *in vitro* is greatly reduced by aminophylline pretreatment (Maia, Jr. and Coutinho 1974c).

Effect of PGE₂ and theophylline on cyclic AMP levels in the oviduct

The effect of PGE_2 and theophylline on cyclic AMP production by the oviduct was recently studied by us in the rabbit during estrous and pseudo-pregnancy, (Maia, Jr. et al. 1975). Control levels of cyclic AMP were found to be significantly ($P < 0.05$) lower in the isthmus during the first three days of pseudopregnancy than in estrus, but were not different in the ampulla. Ampullary cyclic AMP levels were not increased by incubation with PGE_2 in either hormonal condition. Incubation with PGE_2 significantly increased cyclic AMP levels in the isthmus of pseudopregnant animals ($P < 0.001$), but

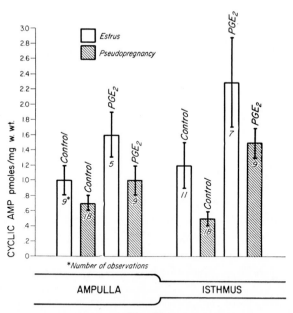

Fig. 11.
Effect of PGE_2 on cyclic AMP levels in the isthmus and in the ampulla during estrous and pseudopregnancy. The increase in isthmic cyclic AMP levels was significant during pseudopregnancy ($P < 0.001$) but not during estrus. The basal levels of cyclic AMP in the isthmus were also lower during pseudopregnancy ($P < 0.05$) than during estrus. The addition of PGE_2 restored cyclic AMP to estrus values.

178

not of estrous ones. In estrous animals, the response of the isthmus to PGE_2 was variable. The increased levels of cyclic AMP induced by PGE_2 in the isthmus of pseudopregnant rabbits were not statistically different from either control or post-PGE_2 incubation levels of estrous animals (Fig. 11). Exposure to theophylline significantly increased cyclic AMP above control levels of both isthmus and ampulla of pseudopregnant animals.

FINAL COMMENTS

The present report deals with the effects of cyclic AMP on oviductal contractility. The inhibitory effect of this nucleotide is probably due to inhibition of calcium release from the cell membranes. In other smooth muscle cells, cyclic AMP increases the binding of calcium to the microsomal fraction, reducing thereby the ionic concentration in the sarcoplasm (Anderson and Nelson 1972). Conversely, a decrease in cyclic AMP levels facilitates calcium release from the membranes, which in turn activates the contractile proteins. This is probably the mechanism by which imidazole increases oviductal contractility *in vitro*. A similar situation also occurs in the rabbit isthmus during the three post-ovulatory days, when the drop in basal cyclic AMP levels contributes to maintaining the musculature constantly activated (Maia, Jr. et al. 1975). In the narrow regions of the isthmus this should result in the closure of the lumen. It is interesting to remember that in the rabbit there is a considerable delay in the movement of surrogates through the oviduct during the first days of pseudopregnancy (Pauerstein et al. 1975). In other species, the occurrence of a barrier to this progression of the ovum through the isthmus after ovulation is widely recognized. It was recently suggested that prostaglandin E_2 acts to relax the isthmic sphincter after ovulation, thus permitting the entry of the ova into the uterine cavity (Spilman and Harper 1973). This model agrees with our observation that PGE_2 increases cyclic AMP levels in the isthmus, but not in the ampulla, during the first three post-ovulatory days in the rabbit (Maia, Jr. et al. 1975). $PGF_{2\alpha}$ on the other hand, seems to be necessary for the activation of oviductal musculature (Maia, Jr. and Coutinho 1974d). Compounds that block prostaglandin synthesis cause a decrease in the tonus, amplitude and frequency of oviductal contractions. This effect can be reversed by $PGF_{2\alpha}$ (Maia, Jr. and Coutinho 1974b). In the rabbit, it has also been shown that there is an increase in PGF levels in the contracting segments of the oviduct during the post-ovulatory phase (Saksena and Harper 1975). The response of the oviduct to $PGF_{2\alpha}$ is decreased by cyclic AMP derivatives, theophylline and prostaglandin E_2. The mechanism of action of these compounds is through the elevation of cyclic AMP, which renders the oviduct insensitive to the stimulatory effect of $PGF_{2\alpha}$ (Maia, Jr. and Coutinho 1974a).

179

ACKNOWLEDGMENTS

This work was supported by Ford Foundation and World Health Organization. Aminophylline was a gift of Byk-Procienx of Brazil.

REFERENCES

Anderson R. and Nelson K. (1972) Cyclic AMP and calcium in relaxation in intestinal smooth muscle. *Nature New Biology* 238, 119–120.
Baulieu E. E. (1973) A 1972 survey of the mode of action of steroid hormones. In *Proceeding of the Fourth International Congress of Endocrinology*, Excerpta medica, International Congress Series No. 273, 30–62.
Brunton W. J. (1972) Adenylcyclase activity in rabbit oviduct. Stimulation by iso-proterenol and prostaglandins. Proc. Fifth Ann. Meeting Soc. Study Reprod. *Biol. Reprod.* 7, 106 (Abstr. 20).
Butcher R. W. and Sutherland E. W. (1967) The effects of the catecholamines, adrenergic blocking agents, Prostaglandin E and insulin on cyclic AMP levels in the rat epididymal fat pad *in vitro*. *Ann. N.Y. Acad. Sci.* 139, 849–859.
Channing C. (1974) Temporal effects of LH, HCG, FSH and dibutyryl cyclic AMP upon luteinization of rhesus monkey granulosa cells in culture. *Endocrinology* 94, 1215–1223.
Coutinho E. M. and Maia H. (1971) The contractile response of the human uterus, Fallopian tubes and ovary to prostaglandins *in vivo*. *Fertil and Steril.* 22, 539–543.
Coutinho E. M. and Maia H., Jr. (1974) Regulation of ovarian contractility by cyclic AMP. *Proceedings from VIII World Congress of Fertility and Sterility*, Buenos Aires, Abstr. 312.
Coutinho E. M., Mattos C. E. R. and da Silva A. R. (1971) The effect of ovarian hormones on the adrenergic stimulation of the rabbit Fallopian tube. *Fertil. and Steril.* 22, 311–317.
Gray J. P., Hardman J. G., Hammer J. L., Hoos R. T. and Sutherland E. W. (1971) Adenylcyclase, phosphodiesterase and cyclic AMP of human sperm and seminal plasma. *Fed. Proc. 30* (II), 1267.
Labrie F., Pelletier G., Borgeat P., Drouin J., Savary H., Côté J. and Ferland L. (1974) Mechanism of action of luteinizing hormone – releasing hormone. In: Coutinho E. M. and Fuchs F., eds. *Physiology and Genetics of Reproduction*, Part A, pp. 289–303. Plenum Press N.Y.
Maia H., Jr. and Coutinho E. M. (1974a) Cyclic AMP and oviduct contractility. In: Coutinho E. M. and Fuchs F., eds. *Physiology and Genetics of Reproduction*, Part B, pp. 167–176. Plenum Press, N.Y.
Maia H., Jr. and Coutinho E. M. (1974b) Efeitos da Indometacina e imidazol sobre a contractilidade tubária *in vitro*. *Proceedings of the VI meeting of the Latin American Society for Investigation of Human (ALIR)*, Abstr. 311.
Maia H., Jr. and Coutinho E. M. (1974c) Effect of aminophylline, oxytocin and acetylcholine on the contractility of the hamster oviduct *in vitro*. *Cienc. Cult.* 26, 781–782.
Maia H., Jr. and Coutinho E. M. (1974d) Inhibition of oviduct motility by aminophylline and indomethacin. *Proceedings of the VIII World Congress of Fertility and Sterility, Buenos Aires*, Excerpta Medica, International Congress Series, Abstr. 163.

Maia H., Jr., Deal M., Hodgson B. and Pauerstein C. J. (1975) Effects of prostaglandin E_2 on oviductal cyclic AMP during estrus and pseudopregnancy. *Fertil.
and Steril.*, in press.

Pauerstein C. J., Fremming B. D. and Martin J. E. (1970) Estrogen-induced tubal
arrest of ovum. *Obstet. and Gynec. 35*, 671–675.

Pauerstein C. J., Hodgson B. J., Fremming B. D. and Martin J. E. (1974) Effects of
sympathetic denervation of the rabbit oviduct on normal ovum transport modified
by estrogen and progesterone. *Gynec. Invest. 5*, 121–132.

Pauerstein C. J., Hodgson B. J., Young R. T., Chatkoff M. L. and Eddy C. A. (1975)
Use of radioactive micropheres for studies of tubal ovum transport. *Amer. J. Obstet.
Gynec. 122*, 655–662.

Spilman C. H. (1974) Oviduct response to prostaglandins. Influence of estradiol and
progesterone. *Prostaglandins 7*, 465–472.

Spilman G. H. and Harper M. J. K. (1973) Effect of prostaglandins on oviduct
motility in estrous rabbits. *Biol. Reprod. 9*, 36–45.

Spilman G. H. and Harper M. J. K. (1974) Comparison of the effects of adrenergic
drugs and prostaglandins on rabbit oviduct motility. *Biol. Reprod. 10*, 549–554.

Spilman C. H. and Harper M. J. K. (1975) Effects of prostaglandins on oviductal
motility and egg transport. *Gynec. Invest. 6*, 186–205.

Sutherland E. W. and Rall T. W. (1960) The relationship of adenosine 3'5'-phosphate
and phosphorylase to the actions of catecholamines and other hormones. *Pharmacol.
Rev. 12*, 265–299.

Sutherland E. W., Robison G. A. and Butcher R. W. (1968) Some aspects of the biological role of adenosine 3'5'-monophosphate. *Circulation 37*, 279–306.

The Center for Research and Training in Reproductive Biology
and Voluntary Regulation of Fertility,
Departments of Obstetrics & Gynecology and Pharmacology,
The University of Texas Health Science Center at San Antonio,
7703 Floyd Curl Drive, San Antonio, Texas 78284

THE ROLE OF CALCIUM
IN CONTRACTION OF THE OVIDUCT

By

Barrie J. Hodgson and Susan Daly[1]

ABSTRACT

$^{45}Ca^{2+}$ movements have been studied in oviducts removed from rabbits 24 h after HCG (I), 72 h after HCG (II), 24 h after HCG with an ovum transport accelerating dose of progesterone (III), or 72 h after HCG with an ovum transport retarding dose of estrogen (IV). Total calcium content of 72 h isthmus was 3.32 ± 0.17 mmoles/kg wet weight, of which 66 % was exchangeable. $^{45}Ca^{2+}$ exchange was 72 % complete within 10 min. $^{45}Ca^{2+}$ uptake in different regions of the oviduct after 60 min was significantly greater in isthmus than in ampulla in all groups. $^{45}Ca^{2+}$ uptake into ampulla and isthmus was not different between Groups I–III but was significantly elevated in Group IV. In contrast, uptake into AIJ was not different for Groups II–IV but was significantly decreased in Group I. Efflux curves of $^{45}Ca^{2+}$ from isthmus into Ca^{2+}-free medium indicated a multicompartment system. Curves were resolved into three exponentials after subtraction of a small (< 0.1 mmoles/kg) slowly exchangeable fraction, in an attempt to delineate physiologically meaningful compartments. The fastest phase of efflux represents loss of extra-

This work was supported by N. I. H. Grant HD-09339-01.

[1] Present address: Department of Pharmacology, Chelsea College, University of London, London SW3 6LX, England.

cellular calcium and corresponds to loss of potassium-induced contractions (half-times < 3.0 min) in Ca^{2+}-free medium. Phenylephrine (PE)-induced contractions were lost with half-times which are similar to those of the 2nd phase of efflux. However, hormonal differences in amplitude of responses to agonists, in rate of loss of PE contraction and $t\frac{1}{2}$ for $^{45}Ca^{2+}$ efflux did not correlate with each other.

These data suggest that changes in calcium binding and exchange may represent an hormonal site of regulation of oviductal contractility but further experimentation is required to elucidate the mechanisms of hormone-Ca^{2+} interactions.

Under physiologic and pharmacologic conditions intracellular free calcium concentration mediates the effects of chemical, mechanical or electrical stimuli to cause activation or inactivation of contractile proteins and hence contraction or relaxation of smooth muscle cells. Contraction-related calcium may be either extracellular, gaining access to the interior by influx, or may be bound at some location within the cell membrane, or inside the cell, gaining access to the contractile proteins by release from binding sites. Calcium may be removed from the cell interior by energy-requiring pumping into cell organelles such as mitochondria or to the exterior or by rebinding.

Ova are likely to be transported through the mammalian oviduct by propulsive forces generated by contractions. Although there is little consistency in the literature concerning contractile patterns of the oviduct during ovum transport, the concept of hormonally-induced alterations of contractions is well established for both the oviduct and the uterus. Much emphasis has been placed on the control of ovum transport and oviductal contractions by factors derived from non-muscular sources. However, by altering calcium binding or exchange, hormones could readily alter amplitude of contractions or rate of contraction or relaxation and hence frequency of contractions. Hormonal action could alter the size of calcium pools, the affinity of binding sites for calcium or the permeability of membranes to divalent ions.

The present experiments were designed to study radiocalcium movements in isolated rabbit oviducts removed during the period of ovum transport. Tissues studied were from estrous animals, and pseudopregnant animals killed 24 h (when ova are entering the isthmus), or 72 h (when ova have entered the uterus) after Human Chorionic Gonadotrophin (HCG). Tissues were also studied from animals given a regimen of progesterone that accelerates ovum transport (killed 24 h after HCG, when ova are entering the uterus), and animals given a "tube-locking" dose of estradiol (killed 72 h after HCG, when ova are at the ampullary-isthmic junction).

MATERIALS AND METHODS

Experimental animals and tissue preparation

New Zealand white does were injected with 100 iu HCG and then isolated for 30 days under constant light and temperature environment. Estrous animals were killed with no further treatment. The remaining animals were injected with 100 iu HCG and were divided into four groups: Groups I were killed 24 h after HCG; Group II were killed 72 h after HCG; Group III received 2.5 mg progesterone i. m. on the two days preceding and on the day of HCG injection and were killed 24 h after HCG; Group IV received 250 μg estradiol cyclopentylpropionate i. m. at the time of HCG injection and were killed 72 h after HCG. Animals were killed by an overdose of barbiturate. Tissues were rapidly removed and were equilibrated with at least two washes of Tyrode's solution. Oviducts were trimmed free of fat and associated membranes. Ovaries were examined for ovulatory stigmata. Portions of ampulla, ampullary-isthmic junction (AIJ) and isthmus used in these studies were taken from the following regions, expressed as percentage of the length of the oviduct from the ovarian end: ampulla, 20–40; AIJ, 50–60; isthmus, 75–90.

For measurement of contractions, rings of oviductal isthmus 0.3 cm wide were mounted as described previously (Hodgson and Pauerstein 1974).

Measurement of $^{45}Ca^{2+}$ movements

For measurement of $^{45}Ca^{2+}$ uptake, segments of oviducts 0.5–1 cm in length were mounted on hooks, equilibrated for 30 min and then incubated in Tyrode's solution containing $^{45}Ca^{2+}$ (0.1 μC/ml), for 10, 30, or 60 min. They were then rapidly rinsed in Tyrode's solution to remove surface $^{45}Ca^{2+}$, blotted, weighed and digested in Protosol tissue solubilizer (New England Nuclear). $^{45}Ca^{2+}$ was counted using a Picker Scintillation Spectrometer (Model 3320) and counts per min (cpm) were corrected for quenching using the channels ratio method. At least 3 aliquots of medium were also counted. $^{45}Ca^{2+}$ exchanged was expressed as mmoles/kg tissue wet weight.

For measurement of uptake with lanthanum wash, Tris-buffered Tyrode's solution was used throughout. After 60 min incubation with labelled Tyrode's, tissues were transferred to Ca^{2+}-free solution containing 2 mM lanthanum chloride for 60 min and were blotted, weighed, digested and counted.

For measurement of $^{45}Ca^{2+}$ efflux, isthmic tissues were mounted on hooks, equilibrated and then incubated in Tyrode's solution containing 1 μC/ml $^{45}Ca^{2+}$ for 60 min. They were then transferred to successive tubes containing 5 ml of Ca^{2+}-free Tyrode's for specific time intervals for a total of 3 h. Tubes were bubbled with 95 % O_2/5 % CO_2 to ensure mixing and oxygenation. At the end of efflux, tissues were blotted, weighed, digested and counted, and

184

duplicate aliquots of efflux solutions and incubation medium were also counted. From the $^{45}Ca^{2+}$ content of the tissues at 180 min, and from the total $^{45}Ca^{2+}$ released during efflux, the $^{45}Ca^{2+}$ remaining in the tissue at each interval was calculated.

Analysis of efflux curves

Since it became necessary to describe efflux curves quantitatively for comparison between groups, efflux of $^{45}Ca^{2+}$ was tentatively considered to occur from a multicompartment system. Efflux could be described as the sum of a minimum of 3 exponential processes. However, for compartmental analysis, the final phase of efflux must be from a single homogenous compartment. Such a condition requires that the efflux curves (cpm) have the same rate constant as the curves for rate of loss of $^{45}Ca^{2+}$ (counts per min per min, cpm^2), i. e. the curves be parallel on a log plot. Parallelism was achieved by subtraction of a small slowly exchangeable, or bound, fraction (see inset to Fig. 4) (Dick and Lee 1964). The 'curve peeling' technique (Solomon 1960) was utilized to reveal the size and rate constants of 3 exponentials. Thus efflux curves were described by the equation:

$$Y_t = A_o e^{-k_1 t} + B_o e^{-k_2 t} + C_o e^{-k_3 t} + D$$

where Y_t is the amount of radioactivity remaining at the time t; A_o, B_o, C_o and D are the sizes of the three compartments and bound fraction at t_o and k_1, k_2 and k_3 are respective rate constants in min^{-1}.

Drugs and solutions

Tyrode's solution had the following composition (mM): NaCl, 154; KCl, 2.8; $MgSO_4$, 1.0; $CaCl_2$, 1.8; $NaHCO_3$, 11.9; and glucose, 5.1. It was maintained at 37°C in all experiments, was continuously gassed with 95 % O_2 and 5 % CO_2 and had a pH of 7.1. For Tris-buffered Tyrode's, sodium bicarbonate was replaced by 5 mM tris-(hydroxymethyl)-aminomethane, adjusted to pH 7.1. This solution was bubbled with 100 % O_2. For Ca^{2+}-free solution, calcium chloride was omitted; trace amounts of Ca^{2+} were probably present. Strontium-Tyrode's contained 1.8 mM $SrCl_2$ in place of calcium chloride. The following drugs and hormones were used: estradiol cypionate (Depot Estradiol, Upjohn), Human Chorionic Gonadotrophin (APL, Ayerst), lanthanum chloride (Fisher), 1-phenylephrine (Sigma) and progesterone (Proluton, Schering).

RESULTS

Calcium-45 uptake into isthmus with time was studied in Group II tissues. Sixty-six percent of the total calcium (3.32 mmoles/kg wet weight) was exchangeable, and exchange was 72 % complete after 10 min (Fig. 1). All subsequent measurements of $^{45}Ca^{2+}$ uptake were carried out after 60 min incubation.

In all groups, uptake of $^{45}Ca^{2+}$ into isthmus was significantly greater than uptake into ampulla (Table 1). Uptake into ampulla was significantly different from uptake into AIJ for Groups I, II and IV, whereas uptake into AIJ was significantly different from isthmus only for estrous and Group I tissues.

In the ampulla, $^{45}Ca^{2+}$ uptake was significantly elevated in Group IV tissues, compared to all other groups, which were not significantly different from each other. In contrast, uptake into AIJ was only significantly different for Group I tissues, where uptake was decreased (Table 1, Fig. 2). It is noticeable that uptake

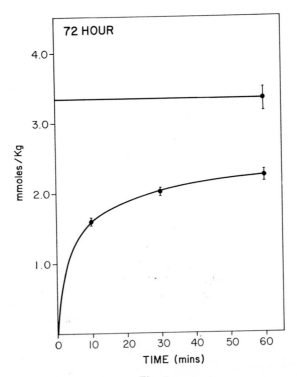

Fig. 1.

$^{45}Ca^{2+}$ uptake with time into isthmus 72 h after HCG (Group II). Upper line is the total calcium content. Each point represents the mean ± SE of at least 4 tissues. Ordinate: mmoles/kg $^{45}Ca^{2+}$ uptake obtained by dividing counts · min⁻¹ · kg⁻¹ by counts · min⁻¹ · mM⁻¹ of the medium. Abscissa: time of incubation in min.

Table 1.
Influence of hormonal treatments on $^{45}Ca^{2+}$ uptake of rabbit oviduct.

Treatment	Segment	Number of tissues	mmoles/kg $^{45}Ca^{2+}$ (mean ± SE)
Estrous (E)	Isthmus (I)	8	2.53 ± 0.20[bcd]
	A-I Junction (AIJ)	4	1.88 ± 0.14
	Ampulla (A)	8	1.67 ± 0.14[e]
24 h HCG	I	27	1.95 ± 0.08[ae]
(I)	AIJ	10	1.66 ± 0.05[cde]
	A	20	1.46 ± 0.06[e]
72 h HCG	I	12	2.12 ± 0.10[ae]
(II)	AIJ	6	2.23 ± 0.27[b]
	A	12	1.60 ± 0.07[e]
24 h HCG +	I	12	2.08 ± 0.06[ae]
progesterone	AIJ	6	1.91 ± 0.08[b]
(III)	A	12	1.66 ± 0.12[e]
72 h HCG +	I	12	2.46 ± 0.10[bcd]
estradiol	AIJ	6	2.34 ± 0.23[b]
(IV)	A	12	2.01 ± 0.08[abcd]

Superscripts indicate significant difference ($P < 0.05$) from corresponding region in:
[a] estrous group;
[b] 24 h HCG (I);
[c] 72 h HCG (II);
[d] 24 h HCG + progesterone (III); or
[e] 72 h HCG + estradiol (IV).

into AIJ tissues in Group III (progesterone 24 h) resembles that in 72 h groups. In the isthmus, uptake was significantly decreased in Groups I, II and III, compared to estrous and Group IV tissues.

Efflux curves for loss of $^{45}Ca^{2+}$ from isthmus were similar for Groups I and II, but efflux was increased and decreased for Groups III and IV respectively, during the early portion of efflux (Fig. 3). By extrapolating the slowest compartment back to zero and subtracting from the "cpm minus bound" curve, the efflux curve was peeled into three exponentials (Fig. 4). The sizes, as percentage of exchangeable $^{45}Ca^{2+}$, of these three hypothetical calcium compartments, their half-times and the size of the bound fraction (in mmoles/kg wet weight) are shown in Table 2. There were no differences in the size of the bound fraction of $^{45}Ca^{2+}$. Half-times for the three compartments were not different between groups. The sizes of compartments were identical for Groups I

187

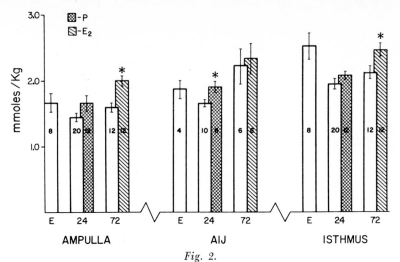

Fig. 2.

Uptake of $^{45}Ca^{2+}$ into different regions of oviducts removed from estrous animals and from animals killed 24 or 72 h after HCG. Cross-hatched bars are uptake into progesterone pre-treated tissues and shaded bars uptake into estrogen-treated tissues. Vertical lines represent $\pm$ SE. Asterisk indicates significant difference of hormonally treated group compared to tissues from corresponding time after HCG ($P < 0.05$). Ordinate: mmoles/kg $^{45}Ca^{2+}$ uptake. Abscissa: region of oviduct at times shown. E = tissues from estrous animals.

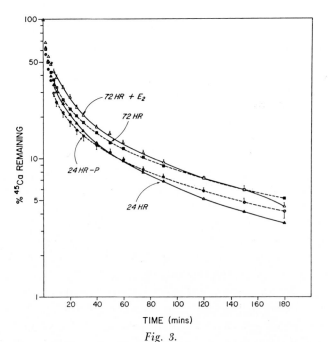

Fig. 3.

$^{45}Ca^{2+}$ efflux into Ca^{2+}-free medium, from isthmus for different groups as shown. Each point is the mean $\pm$ SE of at least 8 tissues. Ordinate: radioactivity remaining in oviduct as a percentage of the amount at zero time. Abscissa: time in min of efflux.

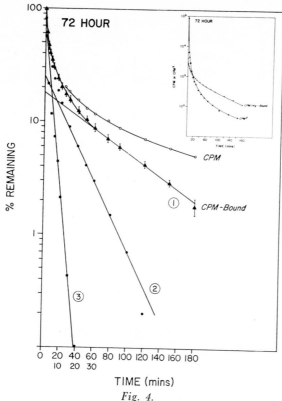

Fig. 4.

Resolution of $^{45}Ca^{2+}$ efflux into 3 compartments, curve shown is for 72 h (Group II) tissues. Original efflux curve is shown as open circles; efflux curve after subtraction of bound fraction shown as closed triangles. Curve-peeling is shown: extrapolation of the final phase to zero time and subtraction from cpm-bound curve yields curve 2 (●) and the same procedure yields curve 3 (■). Ordinate: counts per min remaining in tissue. Abscissa: time after removal from labelled medium in min. Inset shows parallelism of cpm and cpm² curves after subtraction of the bound fraction.

and II. Group III showed an increase in the size of the fastest compartment (A) and a corresponding decrease in size of the second compartment (B). However, only the increase was significant and then only when compared to Groups II and IV. Significant differences were observed for Group IV tissues, in which the fastest compartment was decreased in size and compartments B and C were elevated. The sizes of compartments in mmoles/kg are shown in Table 3, and the ratio of the size of each compartment relative to Group I is shown for each group. Sizes of compartments B and C are significantly greater in Group IV compared to all other groups. The sizes of the fastest compartment,

Table 2.

Compartmental analysis of $^{45}Ca^{2+}$ efflux from rabbit proximal oviductal isthmus.

Treatment	No. tissues	A %	A t½	B %	B t½	C %	C t½	D mmoles/kg
Group I (24 h HCG)	7	61.7 ± 4.0[d]	2.3 ± 0.6	20.8 ± 3.1[d]	11.3 ± 1.4	17.5 ± 2.1[d]	58.3 ± 7.8	0.07 ± 0.02
Group II (72 h HCG)	8	60.7 ± 2.5[cd]	2.6 ± 0.3	21.1 ± 1.8[d]	9.8 ± 1.0	18.2 ± 1.4[d]	54.9 ± 3.5	0.07 ± 0.003
Group III (24 h HCG+P)	7	68.9 ± 2.1[bd]	2.2 ± 0.2	15.6 ± 2.0[d]	11.2 ± 1.3	15.3 ± 1.3[d]	68.6 ± 11.5	0.05 ± 0.005
Group IV (72 h HCG+E)	8	43.5 ± 4.8[abc]	2.4 ± 0.4	31.9 ± 3.2[abc]	10.5 ± 1.5	24.6 ± 2.0[abc]	52.1 ± 4.6	0.05 ± 0.01

Superscripts indicate significant difference ($P < 0.05$) from tissues of other groups within the same compartment, i. e.:

[a] 24 h HCG (I);
[b] 72 h HCG (II)
[c] 24 h HCG + progesterone (III); or
[d] 72 h HCG + estradiol (IV).

190

Table 3.
⁴⁵Ca²⁺ compartmental sizes.

Treatment	A		B		C		After La^{+3} wash	
	mmoles/kg	Ratio[e]	mmoles/kg	Ratio	mmoles/kg	Ratio	mmoles/kg	Ratio
Group I (24 h HCG)	1.35 ± 0.09	1.0	0.45 ± 0.07d	1.0	0.38 ± 0.05d	1.0	0.114 ± 0.006	1.0
Group II (72 h HCG)	1.34 ± 0.06cd	0.99	0.47 ± 0.04d	1.01	0.40 ± 0.03d	1.04	0.132 ± 0.005c	1.16
Group III (24 h HCG + P)	1.55 ± 0.05bd	1.2	0.35 ± 0.04d	0.75	0.34 ± 0.03d	0.88	0.10 ± 0.004bd	0.88
Group IV (72 h HCG + E)	1.06 ± 0.12cb	0.79	0.78 ± 0.08abc	1.53	0.60 ± 0.05abc	1.41	0.142 ± 0.014c	1.26

a–d = As for Table 1.
e = Ratio of size of compartment for different groups, Group I = 1.0.

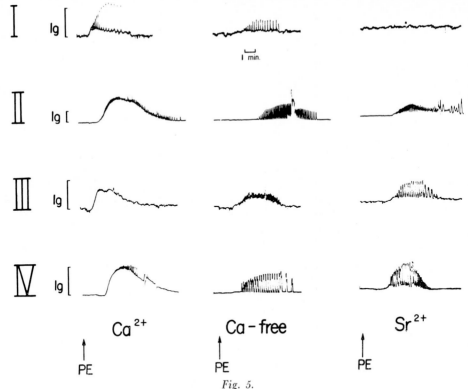

Fig. 5.

Effect of Ca^{2+}-free solution on response to phenylephrine (PE) for isthmic tissues from Groups I–IV. Traces at left are responses to PE (5×10^{-5} M) in normal Tyrode's solution for each group. Center traces are responses to the same dose 15–16 min after changing to Ca^{2+}-free solution. Right traces are 5 min after changing to Sr^{2+}-Tyrode's solution.

A, in Groups II, III, and IV are significantly different from each other, but Group I tissues were not different compared to other groups.

After lanthanum wash, the ratios for different groups are similar to those for compartments B and C. A statistical difference only occurred between Group II and Groups III and IV.

Changes in contractility *in vitro* between groups were evaluated by measuring the maximum isometric tension generated in response to maximal doses of phenylephrine (PE) (5×10^{-5}M), an alpha adrenergic agonist, and of potassium ions (K^+, 80 mM) which cause contraction through depolarization. Amplitude of contraction was not different between groups for K^+-induced contractions. However, Group II tissues were consistently able to generate greater tension to acetylcholine and phenylephrine: Group I tissues generated much less tension, with Groups II and IV intermediate (Table 4).

192

Table 4.

Effect of hormonal treatments on amplitude of contractions to agonists.

Treatment	Amplitude (g)[e]			Mean % recovery in strontium[ef]	
	ACh^g	PE	K^+	PE	K^+
Group I (24 h HCG)	0.56 ± 0.11[bc]	0.33 ± 0.07[bcd]	0.46 ± 0.10	12.0 ± 9.0[d]	32.0 ± 11.0
Group II (72 h HCG)	1.22 ± 0.12[ad]	1.44 ± 0.12[acd]	0.51 ± 0.10	22.0 ± 8.0	24.0 ± 10.0
Group III (24 h HCG+P)	0.94 ± 0.17[ad]	0.65 ± 0.09[abd]	0.59 ± 0.10	33.0 ± 4.0	37.0 ± 5.0
Group IV (72 h HCG+E)	0.58 ± 0.08[bc]	0.9 ± 0.04[abc]	0.57 ± 0.10	37.0 ± 4.0[a]	47.0 ± 11.0

[a–d] = As for Table 1.

[e] = Mean amplitude of first contraction to agonist for at least four tissues for each group.

[f] = Mean percentage of recovery in Strontium Tyrode's after loss of contraction in calcium-free medium. Because usually only phasic contractions in response to PE occurred in Sr^{2+}, contraction is mean half-amplitude of phasic contractions compared to contraction (tonic) in Ca^{2+}. Contractions to K^+ in Sr^{2+} were tonic and amplitude is expressed as percentage of contraction in Ca^{2+}.

[g] = Data from Hodgson and Pauerstein (1975).

ACh = acetylcholine;
PE = phenylephrine.

193

Table 5.
t½ for loss of phenylephrine contraction in calcium-free Tyrode's.

Treatment	t½ PE contraction[a]
Group I (24 h HCG)	9.6 ± 1.6
Group II (72 h HCG)	9.9 ± 1.1[b]
Group III (24 h HCG + P)	14.6 ± 1.8[b]
Group IV (72 h HCG + E)	13.4 ± 2.8

[a] = N > 4 tissues for each group.
[b] = Significantly different from each other at $P < 0.05$.

Half-times for loss of contractions to K^+ when tissues were placed in Ca^{2+}-free Tyrode's were less than 3 min for all groups. In contrast, PE was able to induce contractions for at least 20–30 min in Ca^{2+}-free Tyrode's (Fig. 5). Half-times for PE-contractions are shown in Table 5. Although half-times for loss of phenylephrine contractions and $^{45}Ca^{2+}$ efflux from the second compartment of isthmus are the same order of magnitude, no consistencies for half-times were observed in differences between groups. During exposure to Ca^{2+}-free Tyrode's, the tonic contraction to PE was consistently lost first. Regular phasic contractions were prominent. When tissues were placed in Sr^{2+}-Tyrode's after depletion of contraction-related calcium, PE-induced contractions returned although these were primarily only phasic. Contractions returned in Groups II, III, and IV, but little or no recovery was observed for Group I tissues (Fig. 5). Tonic contractions in response to K^+ partially returned in Sr^{2+} in all groups.

DISCUSSION

Calcium exchange in rabbit oviduct resembles that in other smooth muscle tissues, particularly myometrium. Exchange is rapid but not all calcium is exchangeable (Lullman 1970). Significant changes in $^{45}Ca^{2+}$ uptake occur in different regions of the oviduct. Uptake is decreased in the AIJ 24 h after HCG; a possible relationship therefore exists between delay of ova at the AIJ and decreased $^{45}Ca^{2+}$ uptake. However, estrogen "tube-locking" must be considered to act through separate mechanisms. Such a hypothesis is not unlikely (Pauerstein et al. 1974). Uptake in the isthmus is decreased at 24 and 72 h after

HCG and 24 h after HCG with progesterone. Estrogen treatment restores isthmic uptake to estrous levels. The relationship of such alterations in binding to changes in contractility is not clear. However, since estrous oviducts rapidly transport transferred ova (Chang 1966) whereas estradiol treatment "tube-locks" ova, any relationship cannot be a simple one.

Efflux of $^{45}Ca^{2+}$ from oviducts cannot be described by a simple two-compartment system. Curves have been tentatively analysed to yield three compartments. This has been attempted for other smooth muscles (see Lullman 1970 and Prosser 1974 for examples). Compartmental analysis can only be considered as an empirical quantitative method of describing efflux curves, unless other data indicate that compartments are physiologically meaningful. The fastest exchanging compartment in oviduct appears to comprise extracellular calcium and this correlates well with loss of contractions induced by K^+ depolarization. Thus, K^+-induced contractions are caused by influx of extracellular Ca^{2+}. In contrast, PE utilizes a less labile pool of Ca^{2+} for both tonic and phasic contractions. Strontium apparently cannot support tonic PE contractions but can support phasic contractions, even though strontium is not thought to be able to bind at sites which bind Ca^{2+} (Daniel 1963).

Loss of PE contractions has a half-time similar to that of the second compartment of Ca^{2+} efflux but this cannot be taken as evidence that this compartment is contraction-related calcium. In order to reveal the size of the contraction-related compartment with time, all or a proportion of it must be released to induce a response. The proportion of released Ca^{2+} which is rebound or lost is unknown. Thus the half-time for loss contraction is probably an underestimate of the true half-time in the absence of stimulation. Our data are not sufficient to determine whether compartments B and C represent physiological compartments. Collagen, which comprises a considerable portion of oviductal tissue, is able to bind Ca^{2+} (Villamil et al. 1973) but whether collagen binding is related to these compartments is not known.

Estrogen treatment consistently decreased the extracellular compartment, which could be related to changes in extracellular space. The slower compartments were significantly elevated. If compartment B and/or C is related to contraction, Group IV tissues might be expected to either show the largest contractions to agonists, or the longest $t\frac{1}{2}$ for PE-induced contractions, depending upon which model of contraction is used. In fact, Group II tissues consistently generated greatest tension to acetylcholine or PE, and $t\frac{1}{2}$ for PE was not greatly different for any group. Similarity of responses to K^+ suggest that differences in tension generated are not due to differences in tissue cross-sectional area. The poor responses of 24 h isthmic tissues to agonists, failure of strontium to restore responses and similarity of $^{45}Ca^{2+}$ exchange of these tissues to 72 h tissues suggest poor ability of 24 h tissues to utilize calcium for contraction.

13*

Lanthanum has high affinity for Ca^{2+}-binding sites and displaces Ca^{2+}. Although reports are contradictory concerning the degree to which lanthanum reveals contraction-related calcium, it has been used in these experiments to displace non-specifically bound calcium. The relative sizes of lanthanum-revealed calcium are similar to those derived from uptake and efflux experiments but do not correlate with agonist-induced contractions.

These data represent initial experiments to define calcium distribution and exchange in the oviduct and the source of calcium for contractions. The location of ova in oviducts from similarly treated animals has been established (Pauerstein et al. 1974). Some correlations between the ability of segments to transport ova and calcium exchange were observed. However, given the numerous unknowns concerning the possible relationships of these parameters, it is premature to speculate, particularly in the absence of consistent *in vivo* motility data. It is not surprising that the fraction of calcium related to concentraction is not readily quantified; a satisfactory description of calcium movements remains to be formulated. Thus, although Ca^{2+} binding and/or exchange might represent a site of hormonal control of contractile activity, such alterations are likely to be complex.

REFERENCES

Chang M. C. (1966) Effects of oral administration of medroxyprogesterone acetate and ethinyl estradiol in the transportation and development of rabbits eggs. *Endocrinology 79*, 939–948.

Daniel E. E. (1963) On roles of calcium, strontium and barium in contraction and excitability of rat uterine muscle. *Arch. int. Pharmacodyn. 146*, 298–349.

Dick D. A. and Lee E. J. (1964) Na fluxes in single toad oocytes with special references to the effect of external and internal Na concentration on Na efflux. *J. Physiol. 174*, 55–90.

Hodgson B. J. and Pauerstein C. J. (1974) Effect of ovulation on the response of rabbit oviduct to adrenergic agonists *in vitro. Biol. Reprod. 10*, 346–353.

Hodgson B. J. and Pauerstein C. J. (1975) Effects of hormonal treatments which alter ovum transport on Beta-adrenoceptors of the rabbit oviduct. *Fertil. Steril. 26*, 573–578.

Lullman H. (1970) Calcium fluxes and calcium distribution in smooth muscle. In: Bulbring E., ed. *Smooth muscle*, pp. 151–165. Arnold, London.

Pauerstein C. J., Anderson V., Chatkoff M. L. and Hodgson B. J. (1974) Effects of estrogen and progesterone on the time-course of tubal ovum transport in rabbits. *Amer. J. Obstet. Gynec. 120*, 299–308.

Prosser C. L. (1974) Smooth muscle. *Ann. Rev. Physiol. 36*, 503–535.

Solomon A. K. (1960) Compartmental methods of kinetic analysis. In: Comar C. and Brommer F., eds. *Mineral metabolism*, pp. 119–167. New York Academic Press.

Villamil M. F., Rettori V. and Yeyati N. (1973) Calcium exchange and distribution in the arterial wall. *Amer. J. Physiol. 224*, 1314–1319.

Fertility Research, The Upjohn Company,
Kalamazoo, Michigan 49001

PROSTAGLANDINS, OVIDUCTAL MOTILITY
AND EGG TRANSPORT

By

C. H. Spilman

ABSTRACT

Prostaglandin (PG)E_1 and PGE_2 relax, while $PGF_{1\alpha}$ and $PGF_{2\alpha}$ contract the oviductal muscle in humans, sub-human primates and rabbits. The effects of E- and F-series PGs on oviductal muscle activity are mutually antagonistic, and are dependent on the time interval between the administration of the PGs. Ovarian steroids influence the response of oviductal muscle to PGs; progesterone increases the response to PGE_1 and decreases the response to $PGF_{2\alpha}$, while estradiol decreases the response to $PGF_{2\alpha}$. Oviductal tissue concentrations of $PGF_{2\alpha}$ increase after human chorionic gonadotrophin administration, the peak values occurring at 10 h in the distal isthmus and at 30 h in the proximal isthmus. Proximal isthmus binding of PGE_1 tended to be greater in 72 h pregnant rabbits than in estrous rabbits, while binding of $PGF_{2\alpha}$ was greater in estrous than in pregnant animals. Based on available data, a mechanism by which PGs contribute to the physiological control of egg transport is described. Preovulatory increases in ovarian steroid secretion may stimulate PGF synthesis in the oviductal isthmus in a sequential fashion, the peak value occurring when the oviductal isthmus is most sensitive to stimulation by $PGF_{2\alpha}$. The postovulatory increase in progesterone secretion may then cause a decrease in tissue concentrations of PGF and a decrease in the response of the isthmus to $PGF_{2\alpha}$, thus allowing a progressive movement of eggs through the oviduct into the uterus. In view of the more rapid transport of eggs through the entire oviduct in estrous rabbits than in normally ovulated animals, it appears that the oviduct in estrous animals promotes rapid egg transport; and that some event associated with mating and/or ovulation changes the oviduct from an organ that promotes egg transport to an organ that actually prevents egg trans-

197

port into the uterus. PGs may play an important physiological role in causing these changes in muscular activity, and thus in the regulation of egg transport rate.

One of the primary functions of the mammalian oviduct is to regulate the time at which eggs enter the uterus. In a few experimental animals it has been demonstrated that the embryo and endometrium must be at nearly synchronous stages of development for the successful continuation of pregnancy (Chang and Pickworth 1969). Many investigators have suggested that an effective contraceptive method would be one that caused an accelerated transport of eggs through the oviduct, thus disrupting the normal developmental synchrony between the embryo and endometrium.

It is generally agreed that the isthmus is primarily responsible for preventing premature passage of eggs through the oviduct by virtue of an occlusive mechanism (Black and Asdell 1958; Brundin 1964; Greenwald 1967). The physiological control of this occlusion is not clearly defined. However, it has been through the oviduct, thus disrupting the normal developmental synchrony between the embryo and endometrium.

The present paper briefly reviews the investigations demonstrating the effects of PGs on oviductal motility and egg transport. A more complete review has recently been published (Spilman and Harper 1975). Based on these investigations and a review of the literature, a mechanism by which PGs are involved in the physiological control of egg transport is suggested.

MATERIALS AND METHODS

Oviductal motility

Mature, female New Zealand rabbits were caged individually and provided a standard rabbit diet and water *ad lib*. The method used to record oviductal motility has been reported in detail previously (Spilman and Harper 1973). Silicone balloon-tipped catheters were placed in the lumen of the oviductal isthmus. The recordings were made in conscious animals by attaching the distal end of the saline-filled catheters to Statham P-23Ac transducers. Oviductal motility changes were recorded on a Grass polygraph.

A similar balloon-tipped catheter has been used to record muscular activity of the oviductal ampulla in rhesus monkeys during the menstrual cycle (Spilman 1974a).

Oviductal binding of prostaglandins

PGE_1 and $PGF_{2\alpha}$ binding was determined in slices of oviductal tissue from estrous rabbits and rabbits mated 72 h previously. Tissue aliquots were distri-

198

buted to vials and incubated for 1 h at 37°C with continuous shaking. The incubation medium contained either ^{3}H-PGE$_1$ or ^{3}H-PGF$_{2\alpha}$, with or without a 100-fold excess of non-radioactive PGE$_1$ or PGF$_{2\alpha}$, respectively. Specific binding was assessed as the difference between ^{3}H-PG in tissue in the presence and absence of excess non-radioactive PG. Details of the methods have been published previously (Wakeling et al. 1973; Wakeling and Spilman 1973).

Egg transport

Ovulation was induced in Dutch-belted rabbits by injecting 100 IU human chorionic gonadotrophin (HCG) intravenously (iv). Phosphate buffer vehicle (0.2 M, pH 7.3), PGE$_1$ or PGF$_{2\alpha}$ were administered subcutaneously at either 14, 19 or 23 h after HCG. These times are approximately 4, 9 and 13 h, respectively, after ovulation (Harper 1963). Prostaglandins were administered at a dose of 2.5 mg/kg body weight. Animals were sacrificed 2 h after treatment and the reproductive tracts were examined by the freezing-clearing method described previously (Orsini 1962). The location of tubal ova was expressed as a percentage of the total oviductal length. The ovarian end of the oviduct was referred to as 0 %, and ova that were not found in the oviducts were considered to have been transported 100 %.

The effects on egg transport of vaginal suppositories containing 1.0 mg 15[S]15-methyl-PGF$_{2\alpha}$ have also been studied (Spilman and Roseman 1975). Vaginal suppositories were administered to New Zealand rabbits at 18 and 24 h after HCG, and the animals sacrificed at 48 h after HCG. The location of oviductal ova was determined as mentioned above.

RESULTS

Prostaglandin effects on motility

Rabbit. – PGF$_{1\alpha}$ and PGF$_{2\alpha}$, administered at doses of 10–40 μg/kg iv, caused a sustained, spasmodic contraction of the oviductal isthmus (Fig. 1). The spasmodic contraction was followed by either a short period of suppression or an increase in the amplitude and frequency of contraction.

PGE$_1$ and PGE$_2$ administered at doses of 5–20 μg/kg iv completely suppressed spontaneous activity of the oviduct (Fig. 1). When very large doses of PGEs were administered (greater than 30 μg/kg) the initial response was often a contraction of the oviduct which was followed by a suppression of activity.

The rabbit oviduct is apparently more sensitive to PGE$_1$ and PGE$_2$ than it is to PGF$_{1\alpha}$ and PGF$_{2\alpha}$; the dose of PGF required to cause a significant increase in activity was usually two times the dose of PGE required to suppress activity.

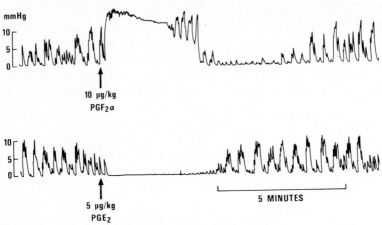

Fig. 1.

Effects of PGF$_{2\alpha}$ and PGE$_2$ on spontaneous activity of the
oviductal isthmus in estrous rabbits.

The effects of subcutaneously administering 3 mg/kg PGs were qualitatively
the same as they had been following intravenous administration PGEs caused
a complete suppression of activity, while PGFs caused a significant increase
in both the frequency and amplitude of contraction. An interesting observation
was that the mean duration of the effect of PGE$_2$ lasted only 1.4 ± 0.3 h
(mean $\pm$ SE, $n = 8$), while the duration of the PGE$_1$ effect lasted 5.4 ± 1.6 h

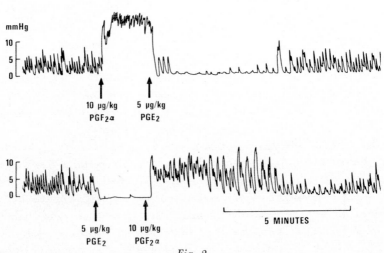

Fig. 2.

Mutually antagonistic effects of PGE$_2$ and PGF$_{2\alpha}$ on oviductal motility in the rabbit.

(mean ± SE, n = 7). There was no difference between the duration of the effects of $PGF_{1\alpha}$ and $PGF_{2\alpha}$, the mean length of effect being 3.0 ± 0.3 h (n = 7) and 3.4 ± 0.5 h (n = 6), respectively.

In view of the opposite effects of PGEs and PGFs on oviductal motility, it was of interest to determine if the effects of these PGs were antagonistic. The spasmodic contraction induced by $PGF_{2\alpha}$ could be suppressed by a subsequent injection of PGE_2 (Fig. 2). Similarly, the suppressed activity caused by PGE_2 could be overcome by $PGF_{2\alpha}$ administration (Fig. 2). This mutual antagonism could be demonstrated for all combinations of PGE_1 or E_2 and $PGF_{1\alpha}$ or $F_{2\alpha}$. However, the PGs were antagonistic only when the second PG was administered at least 2 min after the first PG.

Spontaneous spasmodic contractions were observed in many animals. These contractions could be abolished by administering either PGE_1 or E_2. Furthermore, the spontaneously occurring spasmodic contractions could be mimicked almost exactly by administering the proper dose of either $PGF_{1\alpha}$ or $F_{2\alpha}$ (Fig. 3).

Monkey. – PGE_1 and PGE_2 had little effect on the oviductal ampulla during all phases of the menstrual cycle in rhesus monkeys. Spontaneous bursts of activity, which occurred during the post-ovulatory phase of the cycle, could be suppressed by administering PGEs in some animals. Changes in the response of the primate oviduct during the menstrual cycle were more evident following $PGF_{2\alpha}$ administration. During the follicular phase of the cycle $PGF_{2\alpha}$ had no effect on spontaneous activity, but just prior to expected ovulation $PGF_{2\alpha}$

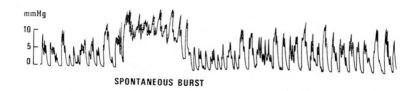

SPONTANEOUS BURST

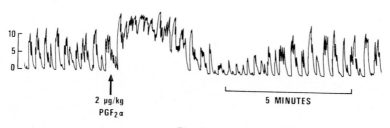

2 µg/kg
$PGF_{2\alpha}$

5 MINUTES

Fig. 3.
Spontaneous burst of activity in the oviductal isthmus of the rabbit, and a similar type of activity induced by $PGF_{2\alpha}$.

201

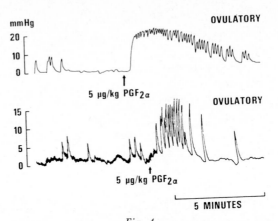

Fig. 4.

Effects of PGF$_{2\alpha}$ on the activity of the oviductal ampulla during the ovulatory phase of the rhesus monkey menstrual cycle.

caused an increase in the amplitude of contractions. At ovulation the oviduct became extremely sensitive to stimulation by PGF$^2_\alpha$, often responding to as little as 5 μg/kg iv (Fig. 4). The burst of activity which could be induced by PGF$_{2\alpha}$ (lower tracing, Fig. 4) was very similar to the spontaneous bursts of activity which were prevalent during the first few days following expected ovulation. During the luteal and pre-menstrual phases of the cycle the oviduct could still be stimulated by PGF$_{2\alpha}$, but a larger dose was required (Fig. 5).

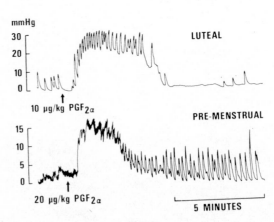

Fig. 5.

Effects of PGF$_{2\alpha}$ on the activity of the oviductal ampulla during the luteal phase of the rhesus monkey menstrual cycle.

202

Interaction of ovarian steroids and prostaglandins

Prostaglandin-induced changes in isthmic motility had been observed to vary considerably from day to day in some rabbits. It was suspected that these changes were due, at least in part, to changes in ovarian steroid production. In experiments using ovariectomized rabbits it has been demonstrated (Spilman 1974b) that the duration of PGE_1 (5 μg/kg iv)-induced suppressed activity was significantly longer ($P < 0.05$) in progesterone treated animals than in untreated or estradiol-treated animals (Fig. 6). The response to 10 μg/kg $PGF_{2\alpha}$ iv lasted significantly longer ($P < 0.01$) in untreated, ovariectomized rabbits than in animals treated with either estradiol or progesterone (Fig. 6). Progesterone was more effective than estradiol ($P < 0.05$) in decreasing the response to $PGF_{2\alpha}$. Although the duration of response to $PGF_{2\alpha}$ was decreased by both estradiol and progesterone treatment, estradiol apparently decreased the threshold dose of $PGF_{2\alpha}$ required to cause a spasmodic contraction. Progesterone had the opposite effect; the magnitude of response to $PGF_{2\alpha}$ tended to be less after progesterone treatment.

Tissue binding of prostaglandins

Significant specific binding of PGE_1 was detected in all sections (ampulla, distal and proximal isthmus) of the oviduct in both estrous and 72 h pregnant rabbits. There were no statistically significant differences in PGE_1 binding

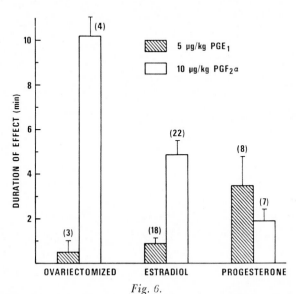

Fig. 6.
Duration of effects of PGE_1 and $PGF_{2\alpha}$ on the oviductal isthmus in ovariectomized rabbits and ovariectomized rabbits treated with either estradiol or progesterone.

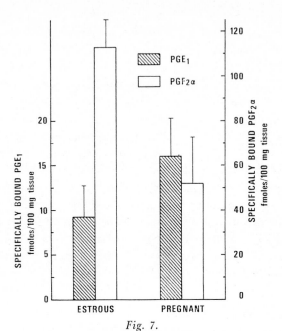

Fig. 7.

Binding of PGE$_1$ and PGF$_{2\alpha}$ by the proximal isthmus of estrous
and 72 h pregnant rabbits.

between estrous and pregnant animals, although the binding in the proximal
isthmus tended to be lower in estrous than in pregnant animals (Fig. 7). Significant specific binding of PGF$_{2\alpha}$ was detected in all cases except in the proximal
isthmus of pregnant animals. There were no statistically significant differences
in PGF$_{2\alpha}$ binding of the ampulla and distal isthmus between estrous and
pregnant rabbits, but there was significantly less ($P < 0.02$) binding of PGF$_{2\alpha}$
in the proximal isthmus of pregnant animals at 72 h after mating than in
estrous animals.

Prostaglandin effects on egg transport

The results of these experiments are presented in Table 1. The mean position
of oviductal eggs was similar in all three control groups, and all eggs were
located on the ovarian side of the ampullary-isthmic junction (AIJ). An average
of 85.4 % of the eggs were recovered from the oviducts in control animals.
The mean distance traveled, taking uterine and unrecovered eggs as 100 %,
was 56.5 % in the control group.

PGE$_1$ treatment altered the position of eggs when administered at 9 and
13 h after ovulation, but not when administered at 4 h after ovulation. When

animals were treated with PGE_1 at 4 h after ovulation 79 % of the eggs were recovered from the oviducts, but only 9.1 % and 27.8 % of the eggs were recovered when animals were treated at 9 and 13 h, respectively. The mean distance traveled in animals treated at 4 h was not different than in the control animals, but was greater in animals treated at 9 and 13 h than it was in controls.

$PGF_{2\alpha}$ treatment was effective in altering egg transport at all time periods. Only 11.8 % of the eggs were recovered from the oviducts in $PGF_{2\alpha}$ treated animals. All oviductal eggs were located on the ovarian side of the AIJ; their positions varied from half way between the ovarian end and AIJ to just slightly above the AIJ. In contrast to the PGE_1 group, treatment with $PGF_{2\alpha}$ as early as 4 h after ovulation caused a complete loss of eggs from the oviducts. The mean distance traveled for eggs in the $PGF_{2\alpha}$ treated groups was 93.0 %.

Vaginal suppositories were formulated to contain 1.0 mg 15[S]15-methyl-$PGF_{2\alpha}$ in a lipid base. The suppositories were placed deep in the rabbit's vaginae with the aid of blunt forceps. The oviductal motility tracings (Fig. 8) demonstrate the significant stimulatory effect of 15[S]15-methyl-$PGF_{2\alpha}$ suppositories in estrous rabbits. The amplitude of contractions began to increase within 30 min after treatment, and the increased activity persisted for an

Table 1.
Effect of prostaglandins on the distribution of eggs in the rabbit oviduct.

Treatment group	Treatment time[1]	Position of eggs[2]	Position of eggs relative to AIJ[3]	Per cent eggs in oviduct[4]	Mean distance traveled[5]
Control	4	52.0	− 2.3	66.7	68.0
	9	45.0	−10.4	89.5	50.8
	13	50.7	− 6.4	100	50.7
PGE_1	4	50.2	+ 1.0	79.0	60.7
	9	91.0	+29.0	9.1	99.2
	13	58.8	+ 8.0	27.8	88.6
$PGF_{2\alpha}$	4	None	None	0	100
	9	23.3	−21.7	14.3	89.0
	13	52.8	− 1.5	21.1	90.1

[1] Hours after ovulation.

[2] Percentage of total oviductal length. Animals sacrificed 2 h after treatment.

[3] Position on the ovarian (−) or uterine (+) side of the AIJ as a percentage of total oviduct length.

[4] Based on total number of ovulation points.

[5] Percentage of total oviductal length, missing eggs considered as 100 %.

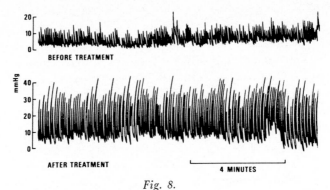

Fig. 8.

Activity of the rabbit oviductal isthmus before and after treatment with a vaginal suppository containing 15[S]15-methyl-PGF$_{2\alpha}$.

average of 2 h. Pretreatment and post-treatment amplitudes and frequencies of contractions were compared using the paired *t*-test (Snedecor and Cochran 1969). The maximal amplitude of contraction following suppository treatment (27.1 ± 7.9, mean ± SE, n = 11) was significantly ($P < 0.02$) greater than that before treatment (6.6 ± 1.3; mean ± SE, n = 11). In general, the amplitude of contractions following suppository treatment was 3-times greater than pre-treatment levels.

When animals were treated with one vaginal suppository at 18 and another at 24 h after an injection of HCG and sacrificed at 48 h after HCG, there was a statistically significant ($P < 0.05$) decrease in ovum recovery. All the ova were recovered from the control animals, while only 43.7 ± 18.9 % (mean ± SE) of the ova were found in the oviducts of treated animals. The mean distance traveled in the control group was 78.1 ± 3.3 % (mean ± SE), but in the treated group it was 90.2 ± 3.1 % (mean ± SE).

DISCUSSION

It has been sufficiently demonstrated that exogenous PGEs and PGFs have characteristic effects on oviductal motility *in vivo* (see Spilman and Harper 1975 for review). PGE$_1$ and PGE$_2$ administered intravenously or subcutaneously suppress spontaneous oviductal activity while PGF$_{1\alpha}$ and PGF$_{2\alpha}$ stimulate activity when administered by similar routes. PGE$_1$ when administered topically (Salomy and Halbrecht 1973) and PGE$_2$ when administered subcutaneously (Aref et al. 1973) reportedly caused a biphasic effect on motility, first a suppression of activity followed by an increase in activity. In view of the very rapid metabolism of PGs (Samuelsson et al. 1971), it seems unlikely that these

206

latent effects of PGE_1 and PGE_2 are due to direct effects of the PG on oviductal muscle.

The response of oviductal tissue to PGs in rabbits (Horton et al. 1965; Spilman and Harper 1973) and rhesus monkeys (Spilman 1974a) is influenced by the endocrine status of the animals. The monkey ampulla responds very little, or not at all, to PGE_1 and PGE_2 during the follicular phase of the menstrual cycle. During the luteal phase spontaneous oviductal activity could be suppressed, but the response was variable from animal to animal. $PGF_{2\alpha}$, which had no effect on the ampulla during the follicular phase, caused an increase in the amplitude of contractions when administered during the ovulatory and early post-ovulatory phases of the menstrual cycle. It is interesting that the effects of $PGF_{2\alpha}$ on the monkey oviduct were greatest at ovulation when eggs would be expected to be found in the oviducts. This increase in the sensitivity of the oviduct to $PGF_{2\alpha}$ stimulation just prior to expected ovulation suggests that PGs may be important in sperm and/or egg transport. The dramatic changes in blood hormone levels which occur prior to ovulation (Bosu et al. 1972; Hotchkiss et al. 1971) may be responsible for the change in oviductal sensitivity to PGs. Results in recently ovariectomized rabbits (Spilman 1974b) demonstrated that the oviductal isthmus is minimally responsive to PGE_1, but maximally responsive to $PGF_{2\alpha}$. Progesterone treatment significantly increased the response to PGE_1 and decreased the response to $PGF_{2\alpha}$. Estradiol treatment also decreased the response to $PGF_{2\alpha}$, but had no effect on the response to PGE_1. These effects of ovarian steroids on the response of the oviduct to PGs may play an important role in the physiological control of egg transport.

Recently, Saksena and Harper (1975) reported that the oviductal tissue concentrations of PGF changed after HCG administration. Of particular significance are the changes in PGF which occurred in the distal and proximal halves of the isthmus. The concentration of PGF in the distal isthmus increased to the highest level by 10 h after HCG injection, and then fell to its lowest level during the next 20 h. In the proximal isthmus there was first a fall in tissue PGF at 10 h after HCG, and then a 5-fold increase at 30 h. By 50 h after HCG the concentration of PGF in the proximal isthmus had fallen to levels less than those measured in estrous rabbits. Simultaneous determinations of oviductal egg location demonstrated that the majority of eggs were recovered from the distal and proximal sections of the oviduct only at those times when tissue levels of PGF had fallen to the lowest values.

The changes in specific binding of PGs by the oviduct (Wakeling and Spilman 1973) correlate well with functional changes during the time of egg transport and with observed changes in the response of the oviduct to PG administration (Spilman 1974b). A physiological function of the oviduct is to retain eggs for approximately $2\frac{1}{2}$ days, and then promote transporation of the eggs into the uterus. High binding of $PGF_{2\alpha}$ relative to PGE_1 as was measured in the isthmus of estrous rabbits may be important in the maintenance of oviductal tone and the retention of eggs in the oviduct. A reduction in oviductal occlusion, which then allows passage of eggs into the uterus, may be the result of a decrease in $PGF_{2\alpha}$ binding and an increase in PGE_1 binding as was measured at 72 h after mating. The decrease in the response of the isthmus to $PGF_{2\alpha}$ and increase in the response to PGE_1 following progesterone treatment agrees well with changes in PG binding observed in 72 h pregnant rabbits in which endogenous progesterone secretion is increasing (Hilliard and Eaton 1971).

Numerous investigators have demonstrated that PG administration alters the normal rate of egg transport (see Spilman and Harper 1975). In the rabbit both PGE_1 and $PGF_{2\alpha}$ cause a significant reduction in the recovery of eggs from the oviduct, but PGE_2 has no effect. This failure of PGE_2 to affect egg transport may be related to the relatively short duration (1.4 h) of effect on oviductal motility as compared to PGE_1 (5.4 h). Both PGE_1 and PGE_2 delay egg transport in rats. It has not been possible to affect egg transport with PGs in the hamster.

The freezing-clearing technique used in the experiments reported here has allowed several interesting observations to be made regarding the effects of PGs on egg transport. The difference in location of oviductal eggs following PGE_1 or $PGF_{2\alpha}$ treatment may be due to their different effects on muscular activity of the oviduct. PGE_1, by decreasing spontaneous activity and occlusion of the isthmus, would allow eggs to move in an abovarian direction beyond the AIJ. Eggs which were recovered from the oviducts in PGE_1 treated animals were on the uterine side of the AIJ (Table 1). By greatly increasing muscular activity, $PGF_{2\alpha}$ may cause the ova to be propelled in both directions. Thus, oviductal eggs were found on the ovarian side of the AIJ (Table 1), while those eggs that were propelled in the other direction were likely transported into the uterus. It is not known if eggs were lost from the fimbriated end of the oviduct following $PGF_{2\alpha}$ treatment, although this is possible.

Horton et al. (1965) reported that solutions of crude PGs administered vaginally decreased the activity of the rabbit oviduct, but there are no published reports of the effect of vaginally administered PGs on the rate of egg transport. The present data using vaginal suppositories containing 15[S]15-methyl-$PGF_{2\alpha}$ demonstrate that such treatment causes a significant increase in oviductal activity similar to that caused by the subcutaneous injection of $PGF_{2\alpha}$ (Spilman and Harper 1973). Furthermore, treatment with only two suppositories caused a partial expulsion of eggs from the oviducts. It is possible that the ability of PGs, administered vaginally, to accelerate egg transport will depend upon the time of administration relative to the time of ovulation. Such a temporal effect has been reported for the effects of PGs administered subcutaneously (Aref et al. 1973; Chang et al. 1974; Ellinger and Kirton 1974).

Spilman and Harper (1972, 1973) suggested that PGs might be involved in the physiological control of egg transport. This suggestion was based on the observed antagonistic effects of PGEs and PGFs. Although we had suggested that PGFs retained eggs in the oviduct by virtue of their occlusive action and PGEs allowed passage of eggs into the uterus by reducing tubal occlusion, it was not clear how this mechanism operated physiologically. Additional experiments have helped to elucidate this mechanism (Spilman and Harper 1975).

Ovarian venous estradiol and 20α-hydroxypregn-4-en-3-one concentrations increase within 4 h after mating in the rabbit (Hilliard and Eaton 1971). This endogenous increase in steroid production could stimulate PGF synthesis in the oviductal isthmus in a sequential fashion as was reported to occur following HCG injection (Saksena and Harper 1975). These investigators also reported that exogenous estradiol increased oviductal tissue concentrations of PGF; but the effect, if any, of 20α-hydroxypregn-4-en-3-one on PGF synthesis is not known. Following the preovulatory increase in steroid secretion there is a fall so that at ovulation and immediately thereafter steroid secretion is at nadir (Hilliard and Eaton 1971). The proximal isthmus of the rabbit oviduct is most sensitive to $PGF_{2\alpha}$ stimulation during the first few days after ovariectomy (Spilman 1974b), a time when endogenous levels of circulating steroids would be decreasing. The preovulatory increase in steroid secretion, perhaps primarily estradiol, may cause a delayed increase in oviductal tissue PGF concentration. The peak concentration of PGF occurs at a time when the oviductal isthmus is most sensitive to stimulation by $PGF_{2\alpha}$. The steroid-induced changes in oviductal tissue concentrations of PGF and changes in sensitivity to $PGF_{2\alpha}$ could cause tonic muscular contraction which would increase occlusion of the isthmus, and prevent premature passage of eggs into the uterus. A gradual increase in progesterone secretion following ovulation (Hilliard and Eaton 1971) could cause a decrease in tissue PGF (Saksena and Harper 1975), and at the same time a decrease in the response of the proximal isthmus to $PGF_{2\alpha}$ and an increase in the response to PGE_1 (Spilman 1974b). These changes would then allow a progressive movement of eggs through the isthmus into the uterus. It is not known if tissue concentrations of PGE change during the time of oviductal transport, nor if PGE levels are affected by steroid treatment.

It should be recognized that egg transport through the entire oviduct is more rapid in estrous, unmated rabbits than in normally ovulated animals. Unpublished observations in my laboratory have demonstrated that when eggs are transferred to the infundibulum of estrous rabbits, only $15.9 \pm 7.0\%$ (mean $\pm$ SE) of them can be recovered from the oviducts 48 h later. Chang (1966) also reported that within 40–41 h after transferring eggs to the oviducts of estrous rabbits only 34.1% could be recovered from the oviducts. Thus, there is evidence that the oviduct in estrous animals promotes rapid egg transport;

and that some event associated with mating and/or ovulation, presumably the preovulatory increase in steroid secretion, changes the oviduct from an organ that promotes egg transport to an organ that actually prevents egg transport into the uterus. An increase in oviductal muscle activity which causes an occlusion of the isthmus after ovulation may be responsible for preventing passage of eggs through the oviduct. Transport of eggs into the uterus might then occur only after tonic muscle contraction has decreased and oviductal occlusion is reduced. As discussed above, PGs may play an important physiological role in causing these changes in muscular activity, and thus in the regulation of egg transport rate.

ACKNOWLEDGMENTS

I sincerely appreciate the excellent assistance of M. E. Meissner in preparing this manuscript, and of D. C. Beuving, A. E. Finn, A. D. Forbes and J. F. Norland in various phases of the experimental work.

REFERENCES

Aref I., Hafez E. S. E. and Kamar G. A. R. (1973) Postcoital prostaglandins, *in vivo* oviductal motility, and egg transport in rabbits. *Fertil. and Steril. 24,* 671–676.

Black D. L. and Asdell S. A. (1958) Transport through the rabbit oviduct. *Amer. J. Physiol. 192,* 63–68.

Bosu W. T. K., Holmdahl T. H., Johansson E. D. B. and Gemzell C. (1972) Peripheral plasma levels of oestrogens, progesterone and 17α-hydroxyprogesterone during the menstrual cycle of the rhesus monkey. *Acta endocr. (Kbh.) 71,* 755–764.

Brundin J. (1964) A functional block in the isthmus of the rabbit Fallopian tube. *Acta physiol. scand. 60,* 295–296.

Chang M. C. (1966) Effects of oral administration of medroxyprogesterone acetate and ethinyl estradiol on the transportation and development of rabbits eggs. *Endocrinology 79,* 939–948.

Chang M. C. and Pickworth S. (1969) Egg transfer in the laboratory animal. In: Hafez E. S. E. and Blandau R. J., eds. *The Mammalian Oviduct*, pp. 389–405. Univ. of Chicago Press.

Chang M. C., Saksena S. K. and Hunt D. M. (1974) Effect of prostaglandin $F_{2\alpha}$ on ovulation and fertilization in rabbit. *Prostaglandins 5,* 341–347.

Ellinger J. V. and Kirton K. T. (1974) Ovum transport in rabbits injected with prostaglandin E_1 and $F_{2\alpha}$. *Biol. Reprod. 11,* 93–96.

Greenwald G. S. (1967) Species differences in egg transport in response to exogenous estrogen. *Anat. Rec. 157,* 163–172.

Harper M. J. K. (1963) Ovulation in the rabbit: the time of follicular rupture and expulsion of the eggs, in relation to injection of luteinizing hormone. *J. Endocrin. 26,* 307–316.

Hilliard J. and Eaton L. W., Jr. (1971) Estradiol-17β, progesterone and 20α-hydroxy-pregn-4-en-3-one in rabbit ovarian venous plasma. II. From mating through implantation. *Endocrinology 89*, 522–527.

Horton E. W., Main I. H. M. and Thompson C. J. (1965) Effects of prostaglandins on the oviduct, studied in rabbits and ewes. *J. Physiol. (Lond.) 180*, 514–528.

Hotchkiss J., Atkinson L. E. and Knobil E. (1971) Time course of serum estrogen and luteinizing hormone (LH) concentrations during the menstrual cycle of the rhesus monkey. *Endocrinology 89*, 177–183.

Orsini M. W. (1962) Technique of preparation, study and photography of benzyl-benzoate cleared material for embryological studies. *J. Reprod. Fertil. 3*, 283–287.

Saksena S. K. and Harper M. J. K. (1975) Relationship between concentration of prostaglandin F (PGF) in the oviduct and egg transport in rabbits. *Biol. Reprod. 13*, 68–76.

Salomy M. and Halbrecht I. (1973) Immediate and late effect of PGE$_1$ on the rabbit oviduct (*in vivo* studies). *Adv. Biosci. 9*, 795–803.

Samuelsson B., Granström E., Gréen K. and Hamberg M. (1971) Metabolism of prostaglandins. *Ann. N. Y. Acad. Sci. 180*, 138–161.

Snedecor G. W. and Cochran W. G. (1969) In *Statistical Methods*, 6th Edition, pp. 93–94. Iowa State Univ. Press, Ames.

Spilman C. H. (1974a) Oviduct motility in the rhesus monkey: Spontaneous activity and response to prostaglandins. *Fertil. and Steril. 25*, 935–939.

Spilman C. H. (1974b) Oviduct response to prostaglandins: Influence of estradiol and progesterone. *Prostaglandins 7*, 465–472.

Spilman C. H. and Harper M. J. K. (1972) Effect of prostaglandins on oviduct motility in conscious rabbits. *Biol. Reprod. 7*, 106.

Spilman C. H. and Harper M. J. K. (1973) Effect of prostaglandins on oviduct motility in estrous rabbits. *Biol. Reprod. 9*, 36–45.

Spilman C. H. and Harper M. J. K. (1975) Effects of prostaglandins on oviductal motility and egg transport. *Gynecol. Invest. 6*, 186–205.

Spilman C. H. and Roseman T. J. (1975) Effect of vaginally administered 15[S]15-methyl-PGF$_{2\alpha}$ on rabbit oviducts. *Abs. Book*, p. 147, Int. Conf. Prostaglandins, Florence, Italy.

Wakeling A. E., Kirton K. T. and Wyngarden L. J. (1973) Prostaglandin receptors in the hamster uterus during the estrous cycle. *Prostaglandins 4*, 1–8.

Wakeling A. E. and Spilman C. H. (1973) Prostaglandin specific binding in the rabbit oviduct. *Prostaglandins 4*, 405–414.

Fertility Research and Research Programming,
The Upjohn Co., Kalamazoo, MI. 49001

ACQUISITION AND COMPUTER ANALYSIS OF OVIDUCTAL MOTILITY DATA

By

C. H. Spilman and M. L. Sutter

ABSTRACT

A system has been developed which provides rapid, repeatable and un-biased analysis of oviductal motility data. Analog signals from a Grass polygraph are interfaced to an 8-channel scanner; from one to eight channels can be sampled at a rate of 7.5 times per sec. The analog input module uses an analog-to-digital converter which accepts voltages (V) from the polygraph between –5 V and +15 V DC. The data from each channel are recorded as 3 digit numbers on a 9-track incremental magnetic tape recorder in IBM compatible format. A manual data entry panel containing 35 decimal thumbwheel switches is included to record coded experiment identification and event marks. A computer program has been developed to process the recorded digital data and quantitate several motility parameters. The validity of the computer quantitation of oviductal motility has been tested by comparing data obtained by computer calculation with those obtained by manual measurement of the original chart paper tracings. This system has application not only in oviductal motility studies, but also in the measurement of other physiological parameters in which the usual output is a chart paper tracing.

Oviductal motility data has usually been analyzed by hand measuring such parameters as amplitude and frequency of contractions, duration and interval between contractions, area under the contraction curve and rate of rise of contractions. These measurements have been made from the original chart paper output. Because of the length of some experiments, one is faced with either a very long and tedious job of analyzing all the data or the task of objectively selecting a representative portion of the data for analysis. In both cases, the analysis is subject to human error and results can vary between replicate measurements made by the same person and between measurements made by different investigators.

Within the last decade attempts have been made to develop data acquisition systems which allow computer analysis of contractile data recorded on magnetic tape. These systems have been used to evaluate uterine activity during labor (Hon 1965; Hon and Paul 1973), non-pregnant uterine activity (Braaksma et al. 1971) and myocardial activity (Zieske and Levy 1968; Smith and Schwede 1969; Voland et al. 1972). While all of these systems have some common features, none is necessarily adaptable to one's own requirements. Individual investigators must develop a system that is compatible with existing facilities and within certain budgetary restrictions.

The present report describes the data acquisition system and computer program which have been developed for the analysis of oviductal motility data. The system permits rapid, unbiased analysis of data. For comparative purposes, data are presented which have been analyzed both by hand and by computer.

MATERIALS AND METHODS

Oviductal motility. – The balloon-tipped recording method used to monitor activity of the oviductal isthmus in New Zealand rabbits has been described in detail previously (Spilman and Harper 1973). Briefly, recording catheters were attached to Statham P-23 Dc pressure transducers. Oviductal motility was recorded on a Grass Model 7 polygraph using 7 DA driver amplifiers and 7 Pl preamplifiers. Motility tracings were obtained on Grass fan-fold curvilinear chart paper.

Data acquisition system.[1] – A schematic diagram of the system is shown in Fig. 1. The analog signals from the Grass driver amplifiers are connected to an 8-channel scanner. Two thumbwheel switches are provided to select the number and location of channels scanned. The operator can select from 1 to 8 channels, the only requirement being that the channels are in sequence. For example, channels 1, 2, 3 and 4, channels 3 and 4 or channels 6, 7 and 8 may be selected. The scanner's stepping rate is controlled by a line frequency-synchronized time base generator. Scanning is arranged so that the time between samples of any one channel is always the same and independent of the number of channels being scanned. The scanning rate is always 60 channels per sec,

---

[1] Manufactured by Adams-Smith, Inc., P. O. Box 363, Needham, Massachusetts 02192.

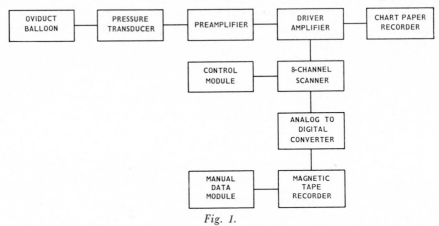

Fig. 1.

Schematic diagram of oviductal motility recording and data acquisition systems.

thus, each channel is sampled at a rate of 7.5 times per sec. When less than 8 channels are scanned, the scanner pauses at the end of each scan until the time slot has elapsed.

The analog input module uses an analog-to-digital converter which accepts voltages varying between –5 V and +15 V DC. For convenience, a special voltage supply is included which permits the input analog voltages to be offset; a zero voltage output from the polygraph (i. e. center scale on the chart paper) is recorded as +5 V. The polarity of the volt meter has been changed so that a decrease in voltage output from the polygraph, which causes an upward pen deflection, causes an increase in the meter reading.

The data from each channel are recorded as 3 digit numbers on a 9-track incremental magnetic tape recorder. The letter *S* is recorded at the start of each scan and the letter *E* is recorded after each channel reading. The data are recorded in IBM compatible format.

A manual data entry panel is included which has 35 decimal thumbwheel switches arranged in 7 groups. Four of these groups are labelled as follows: animal number, date, sensor location and preamplifier sensitivity. The remaining three groups are unlabelled and can be designated and coded by the operator. These manual data switches are used to record experiment identification and event marks indicating when a particular treatment was administered. Each thumbwheel group has a push button adjacent to it for initiating the recording of that group on tape. An additional push button is provided for recording all seven groups at once. The letter *C* and the group number are always recorded before each entry of manual data. When manual data are

214

entered during a recording, the scan in progress is completed, the manual data are recorded and then a new scan begins on the first channel. One complete scan, approximately 133.36 msec, is lost when manual data are recorded.

The number of scans between inter-record gaps may be selected by setting four thumbwheel switches. This may be selected from 0 to 9999 scans. Push buttons are provided for the manual generation of inter-record gaps and end-of-file marks.

The program is capable of analyzing from one to four channels of data recorded on magnetic tape. The data for each channel are gathered and analyzed independently, except for events affecting an animal which has been recorded on more than one channel.

The program first evaluates the thumbwheel parameters to determine the number of channels to be analyzed, the sensor locations, the sensitivity settings, and information about the animals recorded. The data are then gathered for each channel until either a predetermined amount of data has been gathered or some event affecting a channel or channels is encountered. Once the data have been gathered, the affected channel(s) is analyzed.

The remaining discussion refers to the analysis of the data gathered for some segment of time on one channel.

The basic assumption used in the calculations within the program is that the baseline of the data can be approximated by a straight line over some interval of time. Ten minutes has been assumed as a reasonable span of time.

The first step of the analysis is to compute an approximation of the baseline

CALCULATION OF BASELINE

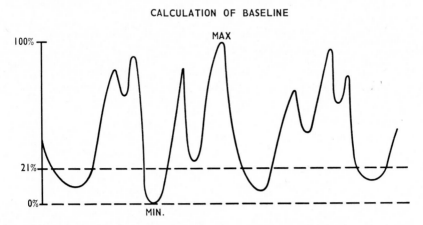

Fig. 2.

The mean baseline is approximated by first computing a band which is at least 21 % of the difference between the absolute maximum and minimum. All data points which are within this band are then averaged to obtain an approximation of the mean baseline.

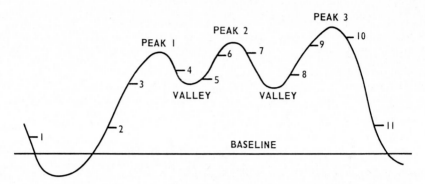

Fig. 3.
Calculation of peaks and slopes.

Test	Decision
1. X > Mean B +0.10 × Range	Lost to Setup
2. X > Mean B +0.15 × Range	First point of 1st slope
3. X > Mean B +0.20 × Range	Second point of 1st slope possible
4. X < Peak 1 −0.20 × (Peak 1 − Mean B)	At least a single peak
5. X > Valley +0.10 × (Valley − Mean B)	First point of 2nd slope
6. X > Valley +0.20 × (Valley − Mean B)	Second point of 2nd slope possible
7. X < Peak 2 −0.10 × (Peak 2 − Mean B)	At least a double peak
8. X > Valley +0.05 × (Valley − Mean B)	First point of 3rd slope
9. X > Valley +0.10 × (Valley − Mean B)	Second point of 3rd slope possible
10. X < Peak 3	Multiple peaks
11. X ≤ Mean B +0.20 × (Peak − Mean B)	Cut-off

(Fig. 2). The approach is to compute a band or interval based on the maximum and minimum meter readings, and then to compute the mean within the band as an approximation of the baseline. The band is computed from the minimum plus a percent of the *range* (difference between the maximum and minimum meter readings).

The width of the band depends on the linearity of the true baseline. The minimum bandwidth is 21 % of the *range*. The mean baseline (*mean B*) is then computed within the resultant band. If more than 90 data points are encountered before *mean B* plus 10 % of *range*, then the bandwidth is increased by 3 % increments until less than 90 data points are lost. If the bandwidth exceeds 45 % of *range*, then the analysis is terminated. A bandwidth greater than 45 % implies that the true baseline cannot be approximated by a straight line.

The term *pulse* is used to describe a portion of the data from a cut-in value (*mean* $B + 0.10 \times range$) to a cut-off value [*mean* $B + 0.20 \times (peak\text{-}mean\ B)$]. *Peak* refers to the last maximum encountered within a pulse.

Fig. 3 is a diagram with a list of the formulas used to determine the number of peaks within a given pulse. The tests for determining where and if slopes can be computed are also shown.

Each segment of the recorded data is analyzed independently. Therefore since the program does not know what has happened preceeding the segment under analysis, the data points preceeding test # 1 are tallied and referred to as "lost to setup".

A pulse which has no data points above *mean* $B + 0.15 \times range$ or a pulse which has data points greater than 220 units above the minimum meter reading, is disregarded. The last pulse in the segment is also ignored if the cut-off value is not encountered before the data are exhausted.

A pulse having data points greater than *mean* $B + 0.15 \times range$ is evaluated to determine the number of peaks it has. A maximum value will be detected as a first peak if it attains a height of at least $0.15 \times range$ above *mean B*, and if the data points following the maximum value drop at least 20 % of the distance between the maximum value and *mean B*. A second maximum value will be detected as a second peak if a first peak has been found, if the second peak attains a height of at least 10 % of the distance between the previous valley and *mean B*, and if the data points following the maximum value drop at least 10 % of the distance between the maximum and *mean B*. A third maximum value will be detected as a third peak if a second peak has been found, if the third peak attains a height of at least 5 % of the distance between the previous valley and *mean B* higher than the previous valley, and if the data points following it are smaller. Only the first three peaks are considered by this program.

The formulas used to compute the remaining variables are listed in the Appendix.

RESULTS AND DISCUSSION

The time base used for analysis, usually 10 min, can be changed depending on the requirements of the experiment. For example, the time base can be shortened for the analysis of experiments in which the pattern of oviductal motility is changing rapidly. In experiments in which a treatment has been administered, the manual entry of an event marker will cause the analysis to be interrupted. The program will compute the data parameters up to that point and then begin computations again.

A log book is kept to indicate the definition of code numbers for the three unlabelled thumbwheel groups. The definition of these can be changed as needed by changing a statement in the program.

The mean amplitude, frequency, area, slope and number of single, double and multiple peaked contractions are calculated according to the methods described above. Several "housekeeping" items are printed at the end of each printout to indicate the number of data points which were not used in the calculations.

During a typical experiment several data printouts are obtained at 10 min intervals. The data obtained can then be averaged for each parameter, thus giving a mean quantitation of each parameter for the entire experiment.

In order to establish the validity of the computer quantitation of oviductal motility data it was necessary to compare statistically the data obtained by computer calculation with those obtained by manual measurement of the original chart paper tracings. For this comparison only the amplitude and frequency of contractions have been determined manually. The area under the curves and the rate of rise of the contractions (slope) were not calculated manually because these are functions of the amplitude and a fixed variable, time. The assumption has been made that if the computer calculation of the amplitude is valid, the calculation of area and rate of rise will also be valid.

The comparison of manual and computer quantitation of oviductal motility data is shown in Table 1. The data calculated by computer program represent the mean ± se of 21 ten min intervals taken from recordings in five rabbits. The manually calculated data represent means of five min intervals; a five min interval on the chart paper tracing was selected from each of the ten min intervals used in the computer calculations. The data for both methods of quantitation were compared using Wilcoxon's signed-rank test (Snedecor and Cochran 1969). There was no statistically significant difference between the two methods of calculation for the amplitude of contractions, but the computer calculation resulted in a smaller frequency of contractions than did manual measurement ($P < 0.012$). Because of the specifications mentioned above and shown in Fig. 3, the computer program was biased to not include small peaks

Table 1.

Comparison of manual and computer calculation of oviductal motility data.

Parameter	Manual quantitation	Computer quantitation
Amplitude (mmHg)	6.2 ± 0.4*	6.3 ± 0.3
Frequency (cont./min)	9.0 ± 0.6	7.5 ± 0.7

* Tabular values are means ± se for 21 recording intervals taken from five rabbits.

218

as separate contractions. However, these might be counted if the frequency was manyally calculated from the original motility tracings. The precision of the computer calculations of motility parameters is likely to be better than that for manual calculations since the same specifications are always used by the program, while individual investigators may use different specifications when making manual calculations.

Experiments in which the basal tone fluctuates widely can result in computer calculations of mean amplitude which do not agree with manual computations. Because the amplitude of individual contractions is calculated using an average baseline for each time interval, a shifting baseline causes an underestimation of the true baseline and thus a calculation of amplitude greater than would be calculated by hand.

The data acquisition system and computer program described in this report permit rapid, reliable and repeatable quantitation of oviductal motility data. The use of a standard procedure for quantitation of these data removes all biases that the investigator may have formed from his initial interpretation of the chart paper tracings. Because the data are stored on magnetic tape they can be retrieved easily and analyzed by other programs at a later time. The system is very flexible and could be used for the acquisition and analysis of most types of data which use chart paper as the usual form of output.

REFERENCES

Braaksma J. T., Veth A. F. L., Jr., Janssens J., Stolte L. A. M., Eskes T. K. A. B., Hein P. R. and van der Weide H. (1971) A comparison of digital and nondigital analysis of contraction records obtained from the nonpregnant uterus *in vivo. Amer. J. Obstet. Gynec. 110,* 1075–1082.

Hon E. H. (1965) Computer aids in evaluating fetal distress. In: Stacy R. W. and Waxman B., eds. *Computers in Biomedical Research,* Vol. 1, pp. 409–437. Academic Press, New York.

Hon E. H. and Paul R. H. (1973) Quantitation of uterine activity. *Obstet. Gynec. 42,* 368–370.

Snedecor G. W. and Cochran W. G. (1969) In *Statistical Methods,* 6th Edition, pp. 128–129. Iowa State Univ. Press, Ames.

Smith N. T. and Schwede H. O. (1969) Rapid computation of myocardial contractility in intact animals. *J. appl. Physiol. 26,* 241–247.

Spilman C. H. and Harper M. J. K. (1973) Effect of prostaglandins on oviduct motility in estrous rabbits. *Biol. Reprod. 9,* 36–45.

Voland J., Souhrada J. F. and Smith J. W. (1972) Computer evaluation of peak isometric tension and resting tension of isolated myocardial muscle strip. *J. appl. Physiol. 32,* 724–727.

Zieske H. A. and Levy M. N. (1968) A cardiac contractility computer. *J. appl. Physiol. 24,* 419–423.

Conversion factors:

SVT = sensitivity conversion factor for a given channel

Sampling rate = 7.5 data points per sec or 450 per min

Formulas:

Mean amplitude of contraction $= \dfrac{\Sigma Ai}{N}$

where $A_i =$ (maximum peak − mean B) for pulse 1

N = number of pulses

Range = minimum A_i to maximum A_i

Total area (integrated using trapezoidal rule)

$$\text{Area} = \frac{\text{SVT}}{7.5} \times \Sigma \, \frac{(X_i + X_{i+1})}{2} \text{ where } X_i, \, X_{i+1} > \text{mean B}$$

Average area = area/N, N = number of pulses

Frequency of contractions $= \dfrac{450 \times (\text{NP1} + 2 \times \text{NP2} + 3 \times \text{NP3})}{M}$

where NP1 = number of single peaked pulses

NP2 = number of double peaked pulses

NP3 = number of multiple peaked pulses

M = number of data points gathered

Note: Multiple peaked pulses are considered to have 3 peaks.

Average rate of contraction $= \dfrac{\Sigma S_K}{N}$

where $S_K = 7.5 \times \text{SVT} \times \dfrac{(X_i - X_j)}{(i-j)}$

N = number of slopes computed

First slope = slope of first peak of single, double, and multiple peaked pulses.
Second slope = slope of second peak of double and multiple peaked pulses.
Third slope = slope of third peak of multiple peaked pulses.

WHO Collaborating Center on Clinical Research in Human Reproduction,
Maternidade Climério de Oliveira,
Federal University of Bahia, Salvador – Bahia, Brazil

MOTILITY OF THE HUMAN OVIDUCT IN VIVO

By

Hugo Maia and Elsimar M. Coutinho

ABSTRACT

The spontaneous motility of the human oviduct varies during the menstrual cycle. During menstruation the motility of the oviduct is exaggerated, with frequent outbursts of activity characterized by tonic contractions superimposed on contractions of high frequency. After ovulation oviductal activity changes markedly. During the luteal phase activity is depressed and outbursts of increased motility become less intense and of shorter duration.

The pharmacologic reactivity of the human oviduct also changes during the menstrual cycle. During menstruation and throughout the proliferative phase the oviduct is very sensitive to alpha adrenergic compounds and oxytocin. After ovulation and throughout the period of luteal domination the response to norepinephrine and oxytocin is depressed. The inhibitory effects of beta adrenergic compounds, on the other hand, are more pronounced during this phase.

The motility of the human oviduct is affected by prostaglandins. Prostaglandin $F_{2\alpha}$ increases oviductal motility while prostaglandin E_2 decreases it. The inhibitory effect of PGE_2 seems to be greater during the luteal phase.

The oviduct is a complex and dynamic organ involved in human reproduction whose main function is to transport ova from the ovary to the uterus, and to provide an appropriate environment for the gametes to meet and fertilization to occur. Because longitudinal muscle fibers, which cause shortening, and circular muscle fibers, which cause annular constriction, are constantly activated, the contractile pattern of the human oviduct is very complex. Additional complicating factors are the contractile activity of the mesosalpinx, the uterus and the supporting ligaments, and ciliary movement.

Changes in intratubal pressure have been recorded *in vivo* in different animals and in humans (Aref and Hafez 1973). These studies have shown a great similarity between oviductal contractility in humans and monkeys (Maia and Coutinho 1968; Neri et al. 1972).

Although the rabbit oviduct seems to respond to ovarian steroids in the same fashion as the primate oviduct, it does not respond, as does the human oviduct, to several other hormones and smooth muscle activators, such as oxytocin, vasopressin and ergot derivatives. Because of this difference, the findings obtained with the rabbit oviduct cannot be readily extrapolated to the human only studies done in primates, preferably in women, provide an adequate model for studying human oviductal pharmacology.

MATERIALS AND METHODS

Several techniques have been used to study oviductal motility *in vivo* and *in vitro*. All these techniques are still far from perfect, and several limitations have been observed with each of the methods currently used. In our department we have initially used an open end catheter inserted into the oviductal lumen in order to record variations in intratubal pressure. However, this technique was soon discarded due to the great number of technical artifacts produced, and the

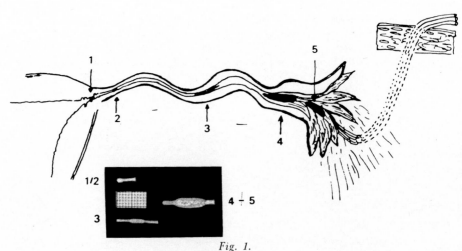

Fig. 1.
Schematic drawing of the different sizes of microballoons which are used to record human oviductal motility *in vivo*.

222

great risk of infection. The technique of using a closed system to record intratubal pressure was developed at the University of Bahia in 1967, and has been
used by us in more than 150 patients. This technique permits chronic recording
of intratubal pressure in ambulatory patients for as long as two complete menstrual cycles. The complete description of this method has been published
elsewhere (Maia and Coutinho 1968). Essentially it consists of the use of a
thin catheter (polyvinyl) which is fenestrated and occluded at one end by a
microballoon. The size of the microballoon varies according to the diameter
of the segment of the oviduct in which it is placed. The external end of the
catheter is connected to a pressure transducer which transmits a signal to a
Sanborn Recorder 321 (Fig. 1). One limitation of this technique is the fact
that the microballoon can act as a foreign body in the oviduct, possibly stimulating oviductal motility. However, the use of small balloons and the chronic recording over long periods of time, are certainly important factors in reducing this
source of mechanical interference to an acceptable degree.

RESULTS AND DISCUSSION

In most of the patients the microballoons were inserted in the oviduct during
the premenstrual phase of the cycle. Using this technique, it was possible to
detect changes in intratubal pressure during the menstrual cycle that were
reproducible from patient to patient.

In some patients four microballoons were inserted in different segments of
the oviduct in order to study the differences in contractile patterns during a
complete ovulatory cycle. Fig. 2 shows the contractility of four different regions
of the human oviduct on day 15. In the intramural portion oviductal motility was
characterized by strong contractions that had an amplitude of 30–40 mmHg
occurring at intervals of 3–5 min. In the isthmus small contractions of 5–10
mmHg, interspersed at regular intervals of 20–30 min, with outbursts of
increased activity when intratubal pressure reached values of 30–40 mmHg
were observed. In the ampulla, these outbursts are still recorded near the
ampullary-isthmic junction (AIJ), but not at the fimbriated end. These studies
show that the various segments of the oviduct display different contractile
patterns during the ovulatory phase of the menstrual cycle. The changes in
oviductal motility during the menstrual cycle are more pronounced in the intramural portion than in other segments. Fig. 3 shows that from day 8 to day 22
there is a progressive decrease in the amplitude and frequency of the contractions. In this respect the intramural portion behaves more like the uterus
than the other segments of the oviduct. In the isthmus, recordings of intrabubal
pressure also revealed cyclic changes during the menstrual cycle due to ovarian

steroids (Coutinho and Maia 1970). During menstruation the motility of the oviduct is exaggerated with frequent outbursts of increased activity. A progressive increase in overall oviductal motility takes place during the ovulatory phase. It is only after ovulation that oviductal motility changes markedly. During the luteal phase, activity is depressed in all segments of the oviduct and the outbursts become less intense and of shorter duration.

The response of the human oviduct to pharmacological agents also changes during the menstrual cycle. During menstruation and throughout the proliferative phase the response to oviductal activators, such as oxytocin and norepinephrine, is always greater than during the luteal phase (Coutinho et al. 1970). Ergot derivatives, on the other hand, are powerful activators of oviductal motility in all phases of the menstrual cycle. The motility of the oviduct is inhibited by

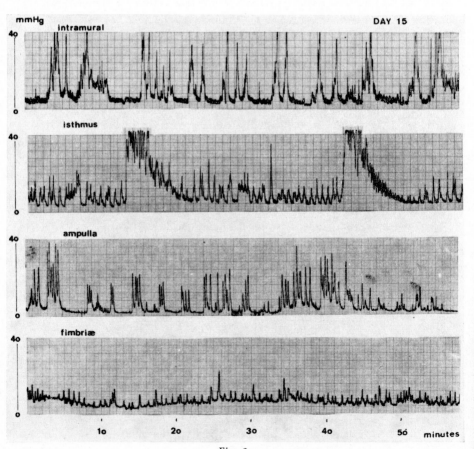

Fig. 2.

Motility patterns of different segments of the human oviduct on day 15
of the menstrual cycle.

224

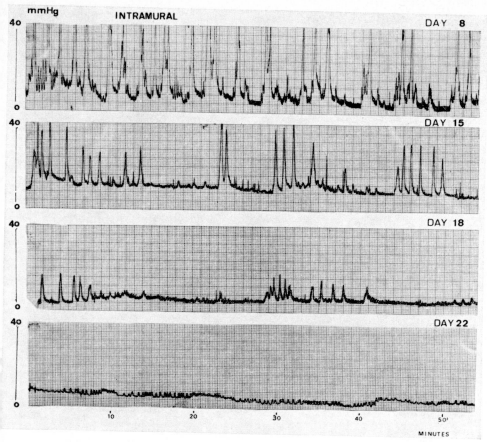

Fig. 3.
Changes in the motility of the intramural portion during the menstrual cycle.
Note that activity is markedly depressed during the late luteal phase.

several groups of compounds that include beta adrenergic activators, phospho-diesterase inhibitors, prostaglandin E_2, and prostaglandin synthetase inhibitors (Coutinho and Maia 1971; Spilman and Harper 1973; Fig. 4). These compounds act through different mechanisms and their effects are observed in all phases of the menstrual cycle.

Another aspect of oviductal physiology that can be studied using different pressure receptors is the direction of propagation of the contractions through-out the menstrual cycle. By recording intratubal pressure in different portions of the oviduct we have been able to study peristalsis and antiperistalsis during the menstrual cycle (Maia and Coutinho 1970). By recording at very high paper speed (100 mm/min) we have been able to record contractions beginning

225

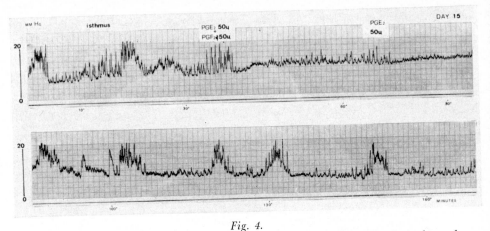

Fig. 4.

Response of the human isthmus to $PGF_{2\alpha}$ *in vivo* on day 15. Note that when administered simultaneously, PGE_2 inhibits the stimulatory effect of $PGF_{2\alpha}$.

in the infundibulum and going all the way down to the isthmus and vice-versa (peristalsis and antiperistalsis respectively). During menstruation antiperistaltic waves are not observed, but during the late proliferative and ovulatory phase they represent about 40 % of the contractions. This indicates that although peristalsis is still predominant at mid-cycle, the occurrence of antiperistalsis is increased during the ovulatory period. This is probably the result of the overall increase in frequency of oviductal contractions induced by estrogen dominance at this stage of the menstrual cycle. Progesterone seems to decrease both the frequency and amplitude of the contractions, but not to interfere with the occurrence of antiperistaltic waves. The speed of propagation in either direction is reduced under progesterone dominance. The simultaneous occurrence of both peristalsis and antiperistalsis, either before or after ovulation, indicates that the direction of the contractile wave in the oviduct appears to depend on the origin of the impulse. If the fimbriated end contracts first the contractions spread from the adovarian portion toward the isthmus. If, however, the isthmus or ampullary segment is stimulated, the contractile response originating in this area will spread toward the fimbria. The regulatory influence of the ovarian steroids seems to be exerted mainly on the excitability and conduction properties of oviductal smooth musculature. Under combined estrogen-progesterone domination the speed of propagation in either direction is considerably reduced. Under estrogen alone, the contractile wave propagates much faster, but it is during menstruation that the displacement of peristaltic waves along the oviduct is fastest.

226

REFERENCES

Aref I. and Hafez E. S. E. (1973) Utero-oviductal motility with emphasis on ova transport. *Obstet. Gynec. Surv. 28,* 679–703.

Coutinho E. M. and Maia H. (1970) The influence of the ovarian steroids on the response of the human Fallopian tubes to neurohypophyseal hormones *in vivo. Amer. J. Obstet. Gynec. 108,* 194–202.

Coutinho E. M. and Maia H. (1971) The contractile response of the human uterus, Fallopian tubes and ovary to prostaglandins *in vivo. Fertil. and Steril. 22,* 539–543.

Coutinho E. M., Maia H. and Filho J. A. (1970) Response of the human Fallopian tube to adrenergic stimulation. *Fertil. and Steril. 21,* 590–594.

Maia H. and Coutinho E. M. (1968) A new technique for recording human tubal activity *in vivo. Amer. J. Obstet. Gynec. 102,* 1043–1047.

Maia H. and Coutinho E. M. (1970) Peristalsis and antiperistalsis of the human Fallopian tube during the menstrual cycle. *Biol. Reprod. 2,* 305–314.

Neri A., Marcus S. L. and Fuchs F. (1972) Motility of the oviduct of the rhesus monkey. *In vivo* studies with and without intrauterine contraceptive devices. *Obstet. Gynec. 39,* 205–212.

Spilman C. H. and Harper M. J. K. (1973) Effects of prostaglandins on oviduct motility in estrous rabbits. *Biol. Reprod. 9,* 36–45.

227

Department of Physiology, Monash University,
Clayton, Vic. 3168, Australia

Discussion Paper

A CRITICAL INTRODUCTION TO ANALYSIS OF THE ROLE OF OVIDUCTAL MOTILITY IN OVUM TRANSPORT*

By

*E. E. Daniel***

ABSTRACT

The main problems for deciding the role of motility of the oviduct in determining ovum transport are considered. Some appear to be conceptual. Others, unfortunately, are methodological. The current methods for recording oviductal motility are considered critically and found wanting. Even if conceptual clarity is achieved methodological advances may be required before valid answers can be obtained.

Consideration of the role of motility of the oviduct in ovum transport requires conceptual and methodological analyses.

Conceptually we must define the questions to be answered and the approaches to such answers. Methodologically we must determine whether techniques which have been applied can yield meaningful answers.

* Supported by grants to D. M. Paton by W.H.O. and to E. E. Daniel by the Medical Research Council of Canada.

** Visiting Scientist of the Medical Research Council of Canada.
Permanent address: Department of Pharmacology, University of Alberta, Edmonton, Alberta, Canada.

CONCEPTUAL CONSIDERATIONS

There seems to be little disagreement that in mammals the timing of passage of the ovum down the oviduct is critical in relation of fertilization, development and ultimate implantation of the ovum in the uterus. There is considerable agreement too that the ovum with associated cumulus enters the infundibulum, passes rapidly through the ampulla and thereafter is delayed for many hours before it passes into the uterus. During this delay, fertilization by sperm which have entered the oviduct from the uterus and development of the ovum to a stage appropriate for implantation both occur; then the control of the oviduct changes and the blastocyst is allowed to enter the uterus. These changes are influenced by ovarian hormones. From this analysis onward there is no agreement as to mechanisms and, I contend, no critical evidence about them.

Many mechanisms have been proposed as to the oviductal locking and unlocking of ova described above: theoretically one could consider:

1) mechanical blocking, such as from edema;

2) blocking of myogenic origin, such as, a) from sustained contraction of circular muscle in the isthmus, b) from contractions organized by myogenic pacemakers which are somehow coupled in time and space such that they do not propel ova predominantly in a uterine direction, c) from local or general relaxation of muscle so that no motive force exists to propel the ova in an aduterine direction;

3) blocking from neurogenic changes which control one of the above myogenic mechanisms (instead of their resulting from direct changes in muscle, e. g. a mechanism such as sustained release of epinephrine onto circular muscle cells which respond by contracting, instead of one like an alteration in Ca^{2+} entry and release, leading to increased intracellular Ca^{2+});

4) blocking from hormonal changes which act on a myogenic or neurogenic mechanism (e. g., on the amount and function of intracellular organelles which control Ca^{2+} binding and release, or on the predominance of alpha (a) or beta (β) adrenergic receptors in oviductal muscle or alternately on the nerves, to alter their innervation of muscles or their release or reuptake of mediator).

Since the presence of "tube-*locking*" requires the occurrence of "tube-*unlocking*" at the appropriate time the same type of analysis would have to be applied to mechanisms for this change.

It is evident from the above type of analysis that the clues as to the mechanisms of "tube-locking" or "tube-unlocking" must first be found in an analysis during ovum transport of myogenic activity of the oviduct, particularly the isthmus. Whatever the initiating mechanism, there is a high probability that its final manifestation will be in altered myogenic activity. Later we will consider some of the evidence available concerning altered myogenic activity during "tube-locking" and "unlocking".

CONCEPTUAL PROBLEMS RELATED
TO TERMINOLOGY

First, however, it may be valuable to consider some terms loosely used in relation to control of oviductal motility, since they may have contributed obfuscation rather than clarity. Secondly we need to consider methodologies for recording oviductal motility. The terms I wish to consider are: sphincter, peristalsis and antiperistalsis, and segmental contraction.

Sphincters of smooth muscle exist in many organs, e. g. eye, bladder and throughout the gastro-intestinal tract. The broadest definition would have to imply a circular muscle system which could exert active tension over long periods producing closure of some orifice. In some organs such as the sphincter pupillae of the eye, this tension may originate from persistent release of mediator, in other organs such as the gut, and in particular the lower eso-phageal sphincter, it originates at least in part from myogenic mechanisms (since the tension is not relaxed by tetrodotoxin, an agent which inhibits action potentials in nerves); thus it does not originate chiefly from sympathetic nerve activity. In nearly all cases, a special neural mechanism for relaxation of this active tension has evolved; in the gut, non-adrenergic inhibitory neurones are directly involved in the relaxation. There is often no morphologically iden-tifiable sphincter. Thus to establish the existence of a functional sphincter, active tension in circular muscle of myogenic or neurogenic origin and a special relaxatory mechanism should be demonstrated. It is not sufficient to show that nervous mechanisms to initiate contractions exist; they must be shown to be contributing to continuing active tension of circular muscle. A mechanism to produce relaxation of this tension must also be present. No such demonstration has been made for isthmic circular muscle.

Unfortunately analysis of the papers of Brundin (1965) and Seitchik et al. (1968) on adrenergically-controlled sphincteric properties of the isthmus near its junction with the ampulla (AIJ) does not suggest that this evidence is complete. For example, aside from methodological problems discussed below, no one has shown that chronic sympathetic denervation *per se* relaxes this region or affects ovum transport.

Peristalsis is a term most widely used to describe the coordinated aboral movements of the mammalian small bowel in response to distension. It is also used in other regions of the bowel, and in other smooth muscle organs like the ureter to describe progressive annular contractions. In the guinea pig small intestine, usually ileum, distension produces a complex sequence of neurally mediated events with the following essential components: a distally (anally) progressing radial band of inhibition followed by a similar band of excitation, leading to distal-going propulsion of gut contents. The neuronal control systems are complex, involving primarily reflex arcs which are intramural (intrinsic to the gut itself) and contain sensory receptors, afferent neurones, and inhibitory and excitatory efferent neurones (Hirst and McKirdy 1974; Hirst et al. 1975). No such intramural neuronal system exists in the oviduct.

However, gradually there has been recognition that neuronally controlled peristalsis is only one means of providing a coordinated, directed movement of a tubal organ leading to propulsion. Indeed the peristalsis of the guinea pig ileum may be, in part, an artefact of the experimental situation and of lesser importance in most regions of most mammalian intestine than in guinea pig ileum. Peristaltic movements can also be of myogenic origin. Myogenic control systems which behave as coupled systems of relaxation oscillators have been documented for the distal stomach, small and large intestines of several species (see Nelsen and Becker 1968; Sarna et al. 1971; Sarna and Daniel 1973). In such systems, oscillators have an intrinsic frequency of pacemaking activity when isolated (i. e. uncoupled) but when electrically coupled (intact) the high frequency oscillators pull up the frequencies of lower frequency oscillators. These, too, provide for co-ordination and spread of activity by having the coupled oscillator with highest (uncoupled) intrinsic frequency proximal, thus providing either a higher frequency of contraction proximally or a proximal contraction with phase lead over a distal contraction; both lead to distal transit. A stimulus, such as distension, is required to bring about release of acetylcholine and couple the electrical oscillations to contractions. Since oscillators in the gut are mutually coupled and intrinsic oscillation frequency can be modulated by neuronal, hormonal or metabolic events, the system (e. g. during vomiting) can show direction reversal; something not readily possible with the neurally controlled type of peristalsis. In the latter, the connections (i. e. the wiring) determines directionality and these are complete in the gut wall. No doubt both types of systems operate in an integrated fashion in the living intestine. However, in the oviduct the structural basis does not seem to exist for a neuronal control of directionality and the possibility of coupled myogenic oscillators has not been explored. All we have are visual descriptions and photographs of progressive contractions.

Segmental and peristaltic contractions are easily related to activities of systems of coupled relaxation oscillators. If the oscillators are not sufficiently tightly coupled so that all share the same frequency, then proximal higher frequency oscillators will produce more segmental contractions than distal lower frequency ones, and lead to distal propulsion. If these oscillators are

231

sufficiently tightly coupled to show phase-locking and identical contraction frequencies, then the proximal contraction will show phase lead over the distal one. The only apparent difference from neuronally controlled peristalsis in the latter case would be the absence of a preceding distal-going wave of inhibition or relaxation. To my knowledge, such a wave of inhibition has never been demonstrated in the oviduct associated with so-called peristalsis.

METHODOLOGICAL CONSIDERATIONS

The recording of motor activity of the oviduct presents difficult problems. These arise from the narrow, variable caliber of the lumen and of the outer muscle coat, the small volume of the lumen, the lack of distinct, separable, well-oriented muscle layers, the presence of substantial amounts of fat, connective tissue and collagen around the outer coat, and the variable occurrence of secretions by the oviduct. There is the further difficulty that the ultimate trial of any recording technique is its non-interference with ovum transport, but observation of ovum transport is itself inherently difficult.

An ideal recording system would provide accurate records of the length or volume changes in muscles, or the resultant tension or pressure changes during active contractions and indicate when tension or pressure changes are not arising from local activity but are secondary to distant activity. Furthermore, it would provide such records without interference with the normal systems for initiation, coupling and termination of muscular activity and would not in itself provide a stimulus to initiate or terminate activity. Also it should be capable of distinguishing activity in various geometries: i. e., from longitudinal muscle or circular muscle contractions. Finally, it should be compatible with normal ovum transport.

No such methods are available in the oviduct, and furthermore, it appears probable that most methods fall short of this ideal in gross terms rather than in a few insignificant or quantifiable ways. Few critical evaluations have been made of recording techniques in the oviduct. These gross failings arise from attempts to apply methods worked out in other systems to the oviduct with its special problems.

METHODS USED IN VIVO

Essentially the *in vivo* methods involve one of 4 approaches: 1) to observe a) the accompanying propulsion of ovum or surrogate visually, often with photographic recording, and to infer the causality for b) from a); 2) to place one or more pressure-sensitive monitors in the lumen and infer the effect on ovum transport from the observed pressure changes; these pressure-sensitive monitors have varied from open-ended unperfused tubes to perfused tubes and closed, balloon systems; 3) forcing a fluid (gas or liquid) through the oviduct and inferring) something about resistance of the whole oviduct or some part of it from the back pressures generated in the process; 4) extraluminal strain gauge transducers sewed to the outer wall.

Visual observation of the oviduct and its contained ovum or ovum surrogate has many advantages. It need not interfere with ovum transport. With care, there need be minimal local interference with the oviduct and its control systems. However, the animal is usually anesthetized and the abdomen opened, this may effect some control systems and limits the duration of observations. The timing of events can, however, be checked by comparison with experiments in which ovulation is timed and ova localized by killing the animals at various times after ovulation. The first limitation with such techniques arises, I think, from the two dimensional nature of the recording. That this occurs is obvious when a camera is used; but even visual observations are limited by surrounding and supporting structures and become, I believe, essentially two dimensional. Thus part of the activity is not observed. The second limitation arises from the necessity to infer cause of ovum movement from previous or concomitant motor activity without additional information about intraluminal pressures, wall tension, isometric contraction or relaxation etc. The only connection between the two events is time and there is no way to exclude coincidence without causality or to include relevant events which are unnoticed or do not involve visible wall motion (e. g., isometric contraction). Nevertheless this mode of recording can provide valid observations of ovum motions in time and space for which oviductal motility changes must account.

The use of intraluminal monitors has a variety of serious limitations. Common to all techniques is the probability that the available probes are so large that they distend the oviduct and the certainty that their existence in the oviduct precludes normal ovum transport (so that the validity and relevance of the motor activity for normal function cannot be checked). It is not even clear that they accurately record the abnormal events to which they may contribute. Open-ended, fluid filled tubes are notoriously unreliable for recording from the much larger lumina of the gastro-intestinal tract because of partial or complete blockage of the tip (they are often pressed against the wall and record components of wall motion rather than intraluminal pressure and it may not be possible to distinguish the two), and because they often show considerable damping in practice and cannot accurately follow rapid pressure events.

Attempts to overcome the limitations of unperfused tubes have included the use of a steady perfusion or the covering of the tip with a rubber sheath to make it into a balloon. In the lower esophageal sphincter it has been shown

233

that perfused tubes probably record a yield pressure (the pressure required to force the fluid out of the fenestration past the occluding wall) and can provide accurate recordings when such pressure changes rapidly only if perfused at rates approaching 6 ml/min, or with high performance perfusion apparatus unaffected by back pressure. Such perfusion rates are not conceivable in the oviduct and no such high performance apparatus has been applied. It seems probable that any reasonable perfusion rate (say 0.6 ml/min) will both distort the normal control systems by causing distension and lead to inaccurate recording of rapid events. In any case, these problems have not been evaluated in any study known to me and the relation of published results to normal events is uncertain.

Covering the tip of an open-ended catheter with a balloon may prevent occlusion of the tip but creates other problems. It allows accumulation of air bubbles which may be unobserved and/or difficult to remove. Damping may be markedly increased. These distort recordings. It also creates an artificial closed system which may not have the same dimensions as the closed system of physiological relevance and which may have its own pressure-volume relations superimposed on or replacing those of the physiological system. Thus the relation between pressure events in the balloon and in the oviduct are obscure. The balloon is usually a distending stimulus; furthermore, unless rigid precautions are adopted the degree of distension varies from experiment to experiment (e. g., in chronic recordings) and this variation is exaggerated if oviductal dimensions vary with time. There are other limitations, but these suffice to show why I cannot accept the physiological relevance of balloon recordings reported in the literature.

All intraluminal techniques suffer two most serious further limitations. First they provide records from only one or a very few sites. There is reason to believe that the oviduct consists of many local systems, each with partial or complete independence, so that these recording techniques cannot provide adequate sampling in time or space to yield sufficient information about the whole oviduct. Second, they cannot provide insight into what muscular or other activity contributes to the observed pressure changes since the origin of these may be anywhere within the natural or artefactual closed system affecting the pressure transducer (i. e. proximal or distal). As a consequence of the limited number of sites sampled and the lack of insight into the origin of pressure changes at such sites, the significance of pressure changes at such sites, the significance of pressure changes for ovum transport (accelerated or slowed) cannot be determined.

Experiments with insufflation of gas or liquid into the oviduct also have serious limitations. They are often carried out without preliminary analysis of the pressure-volume relations of the delivery and recording system and hence inferences from the records about resistance in the oviduct may be meaning-

234

less. The site of resistance to flow cannot be determined without further experimentation and may not be the oviduct or the isthmus. As with other intraluminal techniques, and even more so, the measurement requires a distending stimulus. Mechanism of resistance (active muscular contraction, flap valve mechanism, mechanical obstruction) cannot be inferred from the results without further experimentation. Usually the fluid flow during insufflation is from isthmus to ampulla while the ovum moves from ampulla to isthmus.

The currently available extraluminal recorders have serious limitations as well. Most have dimensions too large to be applied to the oviduct without distorting and limiting wall motion. Further, they may produce injury reactions. The number which can be applied may, as with intraluminal transducers, be too small to provide sufficient information about the components of the total system. Furthermore, there may be no possibility of determining whether there is motion in all axes. As a consequence, the effect of wall motion on intraluminal pressure or transport is often obscure.

The above rather pessimistic analysis of the recordings to date of oviductal motility is only partly determined by the special problems of oviductal structure. In part, these problems exist for any system and the attempt to analyze wall motion, pressure changes and their consequences for transport. In my opinion, only a combination of techniques can possibly provide definitive answers. These might include a combination of observations of ovum or surrogate motion with measurement of wall motion. Such may be possible with photographic techniques and with sufficiently small extraluminal transducers.

METHODOLOGIES FOR IN VITRO STUDIES

Properly conceived, methodologies for *in vitro* studies are simpler, more valid and more reliable. Isotonic or isometric recordings have limitations which are probably widely appreciated. The main limitation of *in vitro* techniques is that such studies can only provide information about the potentialities of a fragment of the total system, isolated from the whole and hence missing many of the possible control systems. Nevertheless, in my opinion, such studies can provide important insights by determining operating limits for a control system supposed to operate *in vivo*. For example, a neurogenically controlled "spasm" of circular muscle is an unlikely mechanism for "tube-locking" if stimulation of the nerve in question causes relaxation *in vitro*. Coupled pacemakers of myogenic origin are not a likely mechanism in the absence of electrical pacemakers in the muscle *in vitro*. The possibility that *in vitro* preparations have lost a vital control system must always be considered, but it is certain that new ones will not be acquired.

In the reports that are included in this session I hope we will critically consider what we should accept as valid and reliable from current information about motility and what directions we should follow to provide such information in the future.

RESEARCH STRATEGIES

In light of the above analysis, I would suggest the following research strategy for consideration by the workshop.

Attack the problem on two fronts:

1) Define the operating limits for various control systems in the oviduct during different stages of the cycle using *in vitro* techniques. Either human oviduct or an appropriate animal model could be used.

2) Develop technology to allow recording of oviductal motility without interfering with ovum transport; test this technology by showing lack of such interference and utilize it to determine how the control systems defined in 1) are operating *in vivo*.

REFERENCES

Brundin J. (1965) Distribution and function of adrenergic nerves in the rabbit Fallopian tube. *Acta physiol. scand. 66*, 5–57.

Hirst G. D. S., Holman M. E. and McKirdy H. C. (1975) Two descending nerve pathways activated by distension of guinea-pig small intestine. *J. Physiol. (Lond.) 244*, 113–127.

Hirst G. D. S. and McKirdy H. C. (1974) A nervous mechanism for descending inhibition in guinea-pig small intestine. *J. Physiol. (Lond.) 238*, 129–144.

Nelsen J. S. and Becker J. C. (1968) Simulation of the electrical and mechanical gradient of the small intestine. *Amer. J. Physiol. 214*, 749–757.

Sarna S. K. and Daniel E. E. (1973) Electrical simulation of gastric electrical control activity. *Amer. J. Physiol. 225*, 125–131.

Sarna S. K., Daniel E. E. and Kingma Y. J. (1971) Simulation of slow wave electrical activity of small intestine. *Amer. J. Physiol. 221*, 166–175.

Seitchik J., Goldberg E., Goldsmith J. P. and Pauerstein C. J. (1968) Pharmacodynamic studies of the human Fallopian tube *in vitro*. *Amer. J. Obstet. Gynec. 102*, 727–735.

SUMMARY OF DISCUSSION
ON OVIDUCTAL CONTRACTILITY

Reporter: *E. M. Coutinho*

SUMMARY OF CURRENT KNOWLEDGE

In vivo studies of contractile and electrical activity of the smooth musculature of the genital tract have been carried out in several species with a variety of techniques. None of the available techniques appear to be completely satisfactory, since the devices used as sensors have to remain in prolonged contact with the oviduct, becoming themselves a source of mechanical stimulation. Moreover, intraluminal sensors interfere with ovum transport, prohibiting studies of correlations between ovum transport and oviductal motility.

In vitro studies of oviductal motility are intuitively difficult to accept as faithful models of normal contractility because the organ is far removed from its physiological conditions. The advantage of *in vitro* studies is that recording conditions and other variables can be more closely controlled.

Several individuals felt that little of the material presented in the morning session had any immediate application to contraception, nor had the reports revealed major leads that could be exploited for contraception. No absolute correlation between motility of the oviduct and ovum transport had been proved up to the present, and the available information was insufficient to determine the exact roles of prostaglandins, cAMP, cGMP and calcium ions in controlling oviductal function.

It was agreed that despite their shortcomings the studies performed *in vitro* and *in vivo* with available techniques had provided important information regarding some basic properties of oviductal muscular function. *In vivo* recordings of intratubal pressure with intraluminal catheters or balloons are very useful for screening and identifying compounds which may be used as activators or inhibitors of oviductal contractility. The question that has not been resolved is whether intraluminal balloons record activity of the mesosalpinx rather than motility of the oviductal wall.

237

IDENTIFICATION OF NEEDED INFORMATION

It is generally agreed that better techniques for studying oviductal contractility should be developed. Some of the sensors discussed at this meeting may apparently be used without interfering with ovum transport. They should be subjected to careful comparative studies with other available techniques and evaluated in several different species.

Although no correlation between the various patterns of oviductal contractility and ovum transport has been clearly established, it may be reasonably assumed that such a correlation exists. If this is so, some of the compounds stimulating oviductal contractility, such as prostaglandins, alpha adrenergic agonists and ergot alkaloids, may be used to accelerate ovum transport.

Another mechanism closely related to oviductal contractility and which may be the key to the control of ovum transport, is the sphincter-like action proposed for the isthmus. Although the mechanism of isthmic activation during "tube-locking" is unknown, it seems clear that at least in some laboratory animals it is under endocrine control. "Tube-locking" and "unlocking" of ova may be induced in some species by appropriate treatment with estrogens and progestins. Studies of the mechanism responsible for the sustained active tension of the circular muscle during "tube-locking" may provide clues which could lead to the development of methods of exogenous control.

EXPERIMENTS TO BE PERFORMED

Despite the general lack of enthusiasm for much of the work that had been done previously because of methodological criticisms, all participants agreed that such studies should be continued to help elucidate the physiology and pharmacology of the oviduct. It is clear that much remains to be done. The relationship of electrical events to changes in motility, and the relationship of both to ovum transport have to be established. Other studies should be concerned with the regulation of excitation-contraction coupling and with the roles of cAMP and prostaglandins in regulation of oviductal function. At least two groups felt very strongly that use of isolated oviducts *in vitro* permitted much useful information to be collected with only minimal problems of methodological artefact. It was also recognized that the absence of an intact nervous system from such preparations might introduce some difficulties of interpretation.

In vivo experiments especially in primates should be limited to the period of ovum transport, i. e. the first three days following ovulation. Of all methods presently in use, the use of multiple electrodes to measure electrical activity was felt to be most potentially valuable and should be improved to give better and more sensitive recordings *in vivo*. Great care must be taken to ensure that appropriate methodology is used for such determinations and that rigorous control experiments are done at the same time.

Studies with multiple extraluminal transducers combined with recordings of electrical activity from similar sites may be even more informative, especially if combined with use of ovum surrogates. In all such experiments ultimate human application should be borne in mind.

Additional experiments were suggested which would have fundamental interest but were unlikely to be of immediate profit for achievement of WHO's objectives. These included studies on investigation of follicular fluid effects on all components of ovum transport, contraction of fimbria, ciliary beat, transport from the ampulla and swimming ability of spermatozoa, and the extent of species differences and similarities between rabbits (no PGs in semen) and man and monkey (high levels of PGs in semen). It is recommended that wherever possible such studies should be done in humans, at least under *in vitro* conditions.

ASSESSMENT OF FEASIBILITY AND COST
OF SUCH APPROACHES

In view of the fact that many of the recommended studies were felt to be of lesser importance for the WHO program the question of costs of such research was not directly addressed. Feasibility of experiments varied and to a large extent depended upon the state of the methodology involved. For example, measurement of electrical activity *in vitro* is useful and feasible, but such experiments *in vivo* are still fraught with difficulties. At the moment it is therefore difficult to undertake studies *in vivo* measuring both electrical activity and pressure force changes. Although it would be useful to use arrays of extraluminal transducers, manufacture of the transducers still presents problems. Conversely studies of the role of PGs and cAMP are now feasible and should be actively pursued, first in rabbits (about which some information is already available) and then in primates. The methodology for pursuing such studies has been largely worked out and may well provide new leads to the control of ovum transport.

It was stressed that ultimate success in obtaining a contraceptive active on the oviduct depended not only on finding an effective compound but also on the ability to detect ovulation and to deliver the compound effectively.

SECTION III

Autonomic Mechanisms
in Ovum Transport

MODERATORS

D. L. BLACK

and

J. BRUNDIN

Department of Obstetrics & Gynecology, Karolinska Institute,
Danderyds Hospital, S-182 03 Danderyd, Sweden

ADRENERGIC MECHANISMS
IN OVUM TRANSPORT

By

J. Brundin

ABSTRACT

A review is presented of our knowledge of the noradrenergic mechanisms involved in oviductal functions. Emphasis has been laid upon the activities of the oviductal adrenergic receptors in view of the reported endocrine influences on ovum transport. The known effects of the appropriate stimulators and inhibitors of adrenergic receptor activities are presented as well as the pharmacological effects of certain adrenolytic drugs on muscular functions in the oviduct. A discussion is given on the possible role in oviductal physiology that a recently discovered and functionally specific set of receptors may possess. These are sensitive enough to respond to the circulating concentration of catecholamines and are situated on the noradrenergic nerve endings. In view of these findings, an endeavour is made to interpret in a new way the role of the adrenergic mechanisms in the control of ovum transport through the oviduct.

During the last decade the role of the autonomic nervous system has acquired increased attention in reproductive biology. Thus, the importance of a balanced autonomic nervous function has been elucidated in several steps of the generative processes. This holds for a series of reproductive events from central functions like gonadotrophin-releasing mechanisms (Labhsetwar 1973b), through functions in the ovary (Ferrando & Nalbandov 1969; Virutamasen et al. 1971) to those

This work was supported by grants from the Swedish Medical Research Council (project B 73–04 x–3027–05) and from the Swedish Society of Medical Sciences.

16*

of the oviduct (Brundin 1965, 1969). Probably, both divisions of the autonomic nervous system – sympathetic and parasympathetic – are involved in governing oviductal functions. The role of the sympathetic division has been extensively studied in this respect (Marshall 1973), while the parasympathetic nervous system hithero has been of less interest (Marshall 1970, Polidoro 1974). Yet, the neuronal pre-requisites for parasympathetic interaction in oviductal physiology have been claimed to exist (Jacobowitz and Koelle 1965; Kubo, Kawano and Ishii 1970), although this was not confirmed (Owman and Sjöberg 1966). The present kowledge of how adrenergic mechanisms are involved in oviductal functions is based on observations done in a vast number of mammalian and avian species, but these mechanisms have been mostly studied in the rabbit and the human.

HISTOCHEMICAL OBSERVATIONS

It is nowadays generally accepted that the adrenergic innervation to the oviduct varies characteristically in intensity along the organ in all mammals studied so far, including the human (Brundin 1965; Woodruff and Pauerstein 1969; Marshall 1970, 1973). The heavy noradrenergic innervation to the isthmic muscular wall, especially at the ampullary-isthmic junction, the striking difference between this rich innervation of the intramural part of the isthmus and the scarce innervation of the surrounding myometrium (except in rats) and the poor innervation to the oviductal ampulla are some of these characteristics. In addition, the oviductal innervation constitutes to a considerable extent of "short adrenergic neurons" which possess specific physiological and pharmacological characteristics (Brundin 1965; Sjöberg 1967; Owman et al. 1974). It is natural that this specific neuronal architecture, observed constantly in so many species in such a reproductively important organ has gained considerable scientific interest. Consequently, increasing evidence and support for the possible importance of this innervation for intact reproductive function has been forthcoming, since it was first suggested by Brundin (1965).

VARIATIONS IN NOREPINEPHRINE (NE)

It is generally accepted that the activity of noradrenergic neurons is directly proportional to their content of NE (Euler 1956). This implies that any change of the norepinephrine content in the oviduct might influence oviductal functions and ovum transport. Attention has therefore been paid to fluctuations of the NE content in the oviduct during the influence of exogenous and/or endogenous ovarian steroids. The neuronal content of NE, examined histochemically, in the human oviduct could not be seen to vary under influence of estrogen and progesterone as in the rabbit uterus (Sjöberg 1967). Biochemical analysis of the NE content has shown that the amount of NE in the part of the rabbit isthmus adjacent to the ampulla increased under the influence of estrogen alone or in combination with progesterone (Bodkhe and Harper 1972a). Moreover, estrogen treatment caused at the same time retention of ova in the rabbit isthmus, but similar findings were observed after reserpine-induced depletion of the NE stores (Bodkhe and Harper 1972b). Pretreatment with reserpine also causes delay or arrest of mouse ova in the oviduct (Bennett and Kendle 1967) due to hypothermia, probably elicited in the central nervous system (Kendle and Bennett 1969a,b). In spite of this depletion of NE in the oviductal nerve endings ovum transport is reported not to be affected in the normothermic mouse (Kendle and Bennett 1969b). Reserpine is reported, however, to interrupt implantation in the rat (Chatterjee and Harper 1970). It is also interesting that pretreatment with a monoamine-oxidase-inhibitor, leading to high NE concentrations in the rabbit isthmus has been reported to accelerate ovum transport – identically to the effect of NE depletion – as reported by Bodkhe and Harper (1972b). It must be emphasized that the content of NE in the isthmus, namely the most important part of the oviduct (Polidoro et al. 1973), is significantly lowered during normal ovum transport in the rabbit (Bodkhe and Harper 1972a), while the amount of circulating estrogen is low (Eaton and Hilliard 1971).

It is known that 6-hydroxy-dopamine depletes NE stores in the noradrenergic nerves (Porter, Totaro and Stone 1963; Bennett, Malmfors and Cobb 1973) and has a destructive effect on noradrenergic nerves (Thoenen and Tranzer 1973). This has given us a tool for general and selective sympathectomy, which can also be performed unilaterally in the oviduct by transluminal perfusion of the organ (Eddy and Black 1973). When administered intraperitoneally to mice, however, this drug did not prevent a normal pregnancy rate (Johns, Chlumecky and Paton 1974). This was considered to indicate a minor noradrenergic role in oviductal function in the mouse, even though this drug causes a decreased litter size (Castrén, Airaksinen and Saarikoski 1973). In the rat 6-hydroxy-dopamine is an abortifacient (MacDonald and Airaksinen 1974), but in the rabbit pretreatment with 6-hydroxy-dopamine prevents pregnancy completely (Castrén, Airaksinen and Saarikoski 1973). It is not stated whether this effect is due to disruption of ovulation reflexes, disturbance of ovum transport or prevention of implantation, and this ought to be elucidated. The effect of selective, unilateral oviductal sympathectomy on ovum transport has been studied in the rabbit (Eddy 1973). Ovum transport was studied after unilateral, transluminal perfusion with 6-hydroxy-dopamine in a dose sufficient to deplete completely the neuronal NE in the oviductal wall. Remarkably, ovum transport was significantly retarded at 60 h post coitum, but not at 49 and 72 h post coitum. This effect was concluded to depend upon destruction of the noradrenergic control of ovum transport. It is not known whether these rabbits ever became pregnant.

NORADRENERGIC RECEPTORS IN THE OVIDUCT

Stimulation of the hypogastric nerves innervating the mammalian oviduct causes the circular muscles of the non-mated rabbit oviduct, and especially those of the isthmus, to contract (Brundin 1965). This is due to the presence of α-receptors in the muscle cell membrane. During the time of ovum transport this response is reduced (Brundin 1965). Electrical stimulation of supplying nerves has also revealed a separate α- and β-receptor activity in the rabbit oviduct in longitudinal and circular musles (Ueda et al. 1973). Stimulation of the hypogastric perivascular nerves to the human oviduct has also produced a similar type of response, which was reduced during pregnancy and in the post-menopausal woman, although no difference was recorded between isthmic and ampullary response (Nakanishi and Wood 1968). As in the rabbit most of these human nerves were postganglionic in nature.

The α-receptor stimulatory response in the rabbit can be mimicked by intra-venous injection of NE *in vivo* (Brundin 1965) or *in vitro* (Sandberg et al. 1960). Later the change in response, exhibited as a less pronounced reactivity to nerve stimulation after mating (Brundin 1965) and similarly in the human during pregnancy (Nakanishi and Wood 1968), has been explained. It is known that β-receptors are present in oviducts from rabbits (Longley et al. 1968; Martin et al. 1970) and humans (Rosenblum and Stein 1966; Seitchik et al. 1968; Cibils et al. 1971; Heilman et al. 1972). These receptors have been found to react in an anticipated manner to the appropriate stimulating and blocking compounds studied (Nakanishi and Wood 1968; Rosenblum and Stein 1966; Senior and Spencer-Gregson 1969; Levy and Lindner 1972; Hodgson et al. 1973; Howe and Black 1973). The β-receptors of rabbit oviducts are, however, not considered to be identical to either the B 1 or the B 2 type according to the Lands classification (Lands et al. 1967; Heilman et al. 1972; Coutinho et al. 1974). It is evident that the predominant α-receptor activity changes during various endocrine states and during ovum transport in favor of an increased β-receptor activity (Nakanishi and Wood 1968; Coutinho et al. 1970; Coutinho 1971; Coutinho et al. 1971; Levy and Lindner 1972; Howe and Black 1973; Higgs and Moawad 1974). It can then be empasized that estrogen was reported to cause an increased α-receptor activity through enhanced sensitivity, while progesterone should have the opposite effect by enhancing the β-sensitivity in the rabbit (Coutinho et al. 1971; Howe and Black 1973; Pauerstein et al. 1973). In previous studies on ovum transport (Chang 1966a,b; Harper 1961,

1964, 1965) estrogen has been committed to an essential role in ovum transport. However, the dual effect of estrogen capable of accelerating and/or delaying ovum transport (Greenwald 1961) has been difficult to explain (Greenwald 1968). Most of the conflicting data on the effect of estrogen and progesterone in ovum transport could probably be clarified, if the actual shifts in α- and β-receptors activities during the crucial time of ovum transport were taken into consideration when the hormonal effects are described. More spatially localized, and preferably cellular, effects have to be studied until the picture of the noradrenergic role in ovum transport is explicable.

CELLULAR EFFECTS

From studies in the sow we have learned that the size of the muscle fiber in the oviduct is increased under the influence of estrogen (Anopolsky 1928). Very little is, however, known on the cell metabolism under the influence of steroid hormones in the oviduct. It is generally claimed that β-adrenergic stimulation causes an accumulation of cyclic AMP and may act as an intracellular mediator of secretory processes in epithelial tissues (Sutherland and Robinson 1966). In the ampullary epithelium of the rabbit the transmembrane potential increases as well as the short circuit current upon β-receptor stimulation. This effect is identical to that of cyclic AMP or theophylline (Brunton 1972). From intracellular recordings it has been claimed that the muscular activity of the rabbit isthmus exhibits bursts of single action potentials while that of the ampulla shows a plateau type action potential, increased by prostaglandin (PG) $F_{2\alpha}$ and inhibited by PGE_1 (Nakajima and Nishimura 1972). From extracellular recordings of these potentials it has been reported that the propagation of the action potential is different in the isthmus when compared to that of the ampulla (Talo and Brundin 1971, 1973; Brundin and Talo 1972). Progesterone was recorded to disrupt the synchronized pattern of propagation along the isthmus that was recorded after estrogen pretreatment (Talo and Brundin 1971).

PROSTAGLANDINS (PGs)

A stimulatory effect on the human oviduct (Zetler et al. 1969; Coutinho and Maia 1971) and on the rabbit oviduct by $PGF_{2\alpha}$ and a recordable inhibition of muscular activity induced by PGE_1 has been known for some time (Horton et al. 1963; Brundin 1965, 1968; Spilman and Harper 1972, 1973). It has also been demonstrated that PGE_1 minimized or abolished the effect of hypogastric nerve stimulation in rabbit oviducts, suggesting a moderating role of

PGE$_1$ in the adrenergic response (Brundin 1968). Since then, it has been fully established that the prostaglandins are involved in the NE-releasing mechanisms in the mammalian adrenergic nerve endings (Hedqvist and Brundin 1969; Hedqvist 1970; Swedin 1971) and are released (E-series) from the autonomic effector cell upon nerve stimulation (Swedin 1971; Hedqvist and Euler 1972). The importance of prostaglandins in oviductal physiology has received additional support from the finding that oviductal secretion contains considerable amounts of PGF$_{2\alpha}$ (ewes) and that this amount varies with the influence of estrogen (Warnes et al. 1974); a similar high concentration was reported from studies in the human (Ogra et al. 1974). Stimulation by PGE$_1$ upon rabbit

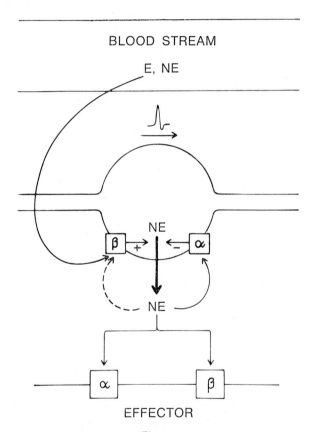

Fig. 1.
Schematic drawing of probable arrangement of receptors in the peripheral adrenergic nerve ending and events at the passage of action potential. Dashed line = low concentration. E = epinephrine. NE = norepinephrine. Solid line = higher concentration. + and −: positive and negative feedback on NE release, through activation via appropriate receptors. (Adapted from Stjärne 1975 with permission from Karolinska Institutet).

sperm transport has been reported (Mandl 1972), while $PGF_{2\alpha}$ has been reported to lack any effect upon the fertilizing capacity in the rabbit (Sorgen and Glass 1972) although a quite opposite effect has also been reported in rabbits (Spilman et al. 1973). Special receptors for prostaglandins with potent binding capacity allegedly exist in the oviduct (Wakeling and Spilman 1973; Fronduti and Archer 1974). Progesterone and – to some extent – estrogen are held to decrease the effects of exogenous PGE_1 and $PGF_{2\alpha}$ upon oviductal motility (Spilman 1974). Prostaglandin E_2 has been, in addition, reported to increase cyclic AMP synthesis in oviducts, particularly in the isthmus and intramural parts (Lerner et al. 1973) while PGE_1 and PGE_2 have been reported to induce delayed implantation in rats by oviductal retention of eggs, but $PGF_{2\alpha}$ lacks this effect (Labhsetwar 1973a). This is in line with observations in the rabbit where $PGF_{2\alpha}$ accelerates, while PGE_1 and PGE_2 delay, ovum transport (Chang et al. 1973; Ellinger and Kirton 1972; Aref et al. 1973).

THE PRESYNAPTIC RECEPTORS

Recently the question of α- and β-receptor control of smooth muscle activity has become more complex than previously. It has been reported from studies on various species and tissues that the adrenergic nerve-ending is equipped with its own receptors (Adler-Graschinsky and Langer 1975). These receptors are identical in nature to those of the effector cell as far as specific responses to stimulating and blocking compounds are concerned (Fig. 1). Different from the generally known situation on the effector in e. g., the oviductal muscles, these β-receptors act like "facilitators" of the release of NE from the varicosities of the nerve-endings during the passage of the action potential. On the other hand, the α-receptors act like "inhibitors" of NE-release from the nerves. This can be shown by estimating the amount of ^3H-(-)-NE released to the effluent per nerve-stimulation shock given *in vitro* to vasoconstrictor nerves preincubated with ^3H-(-)-NE. In studies of this release, similar inhibitory α-receptors have been demonstrated in human vasoconstrictor nerves (Stjärne and Brundin 1975a,b). In addition, these β-receptors are activated at extremely low concentrations (0.0016 μM) of catecholamines in the surrounding medium (Fig. 2).

This implies that the neuronal presynaptic β-receptors are sensitive to fluctuations of catecholamines around the concentrations found in the human peripheral circulation. It is noteworthy that this β-receptor activity can be elicited by addition of small amounts of the β-stimulant isoproterenol. The stimulation seen at "physiologic" concentrations of catecholamines is shifted into an inhibition when the concentration is increased to more than 0.008 μM. This switch of effect is probably elicited by activation of the less sensitive neuronal α-receptors when the surrounding NE-concentration is increased above

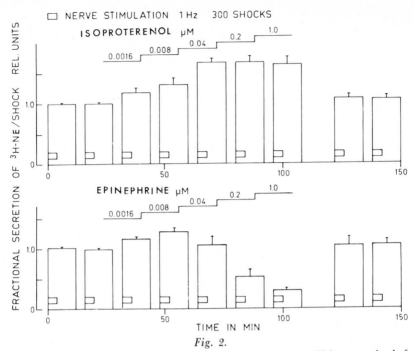

Fig. 2.

Fractional secretion of ^{3}H-norepinephrine (NE) per electric (1 Hz) nerve shock from strips of human omental arteries and veins (pooled data in relative units). Effects of isoproterenol and epinephrine. Means ± SE. (From Stjärne and Brundin 1975a with permission from Karolinska Institutet).

the threshold level. It is probable that the "short" adrenergic neurons behave identically to ordinary long ones in this respect since we have found, in collaboration with Dr. Stjärne, identical results from studies on the isthmus of human oviduct. In addition, prostaglandins of the E-series markedly reduce the iso-proterenol-induced stimulation. Moreover, blocking of the endogenous production of prostaglandins by eicosa-tetraenoic acid not only markedly increased the release of NE from the isthmus of the human oviduct but also increased simultaneously recorded mechanical response upon selective electrical nerve stimulation. As yet it is not known whether these neuronal receptors behave identically to those of the effector under different hormonal conditions. It will perhaps be possible to show that for instance, the effect of estrogen and progesterone is of importance in subordinating the neuronal receptor activity. If so, the role of the noradrenergic mechanisms in oviductal physiology will become still more complex.

Obviously, the most essential tools by which noradrenergic mechanisms handle the delicate governing of various processes are their receptors. Basic studies of these receptor activities – how they are brought in action, how they are blocked, what they look like, the chemistry involved, their dependence upon central nervous functions – are some of the most important questions to be solved. Until then our opportunities will be essentially limited to using the adrenergic mechanisms as a tool in the search for an effective contraceptive.

Finally, it may thus be emphasized that every endeavour to interpret the data, obtained from previous and present experiments without bringing receptor functions into consideration, is bound to make the results less valuable or even to confuse the true picture of how ovum transport is governed by the multipotent sympathetic nervous system.

REFERENCES

Adler-Graschinsky E. and Langer S. Z. (1975) Possible role of a beta-adrenoceptor in the regulation of noradrenaline release by nerve stimulation through a positive feed-back mechanism. *Brit. J. Pharmacol. 53*, 43–50.

Anopolsky D. (1928) Cyclic changes in the size of muscle fibers of the Fallopian tube of the sow. *Amer. J. Anat. 40*, 459–469.

Aref I., Hafez E. S. E. and Kamar G. A. R. (1973) Postcoital prostaglandins, *in vivo* oviductal motility and egg transport in rabbits. *Fertil. Steril. 24*, 671–676.

Bennett J. P. and Kendle K. E. (1967) The effect of reserpine upon the rate of egg transport in the Fallopian tube of the mouse. *J. Reprod. Fertil. 13*, 345–348.

Bennett T., Malmfors T. and Cobb J. L. S. (1973) A fluorescence histochemical study of the degeneration and regeneration of noradrenergic nerves in the chick following treatment with 6-hydroxydopamine. *Z. Zellforsch. 142*, 103–130.

Bodkhe R. R. and Harper M. J. K. (1972a) Mechanism of egg transport: changes in amount of adrenergic transmitter in the genital tract of normal and hormone treated rabbits. In: Segal S. J. et al., eds. *The Regulation of Mammalian Reproduction,* Chapter 26, pp. 364–374. C. C. Thomas, Springfield, Ill.

Bodkhe R. R. and Harper M. J. K. (1972b) Changes in the amount of adrenergic neurotransmitter in the genital tract of untreated rabbits, and rabbits given reserpine or iproniazid during the time of egg transport. *Biol. Reprod. 6*, 288–299.

Brundin J. (1965) Distribution and function of adrenergic nerves in the rabbit Fallopian tube. *Acta physiol. scand. 66*, Suppl. 259, 1–57.

Brundin J. (1968) The effect of prostaglandin E_1 on the response of the rabbit oviduct to hypogastric nerve stimulation. *Acta physiol. scand. 73*, 54–57.

Brundin J. (1969) Pharmacology of the Oviduct. In: Hafez E. S. E. and Blandau R. J., eds. *The Mammalian Oviduct,* pp. 251–269. The University of Chicago Press, Chicago.

Brundin J. and Talo A. (1972) The effects of estrogen and progesterone on the electric activity and intraluminal pressure of the castrated rabbit oviduct. *Biol. Reprod. 7*, 417–424.

Brunton W. J. (1972) Beta-adrenergic stimulation of transmembrane potential and short circuit current of isolated rabbit oviduct. *Nature New Biol. 236*, 12–14.

Castrén O., Airaksinen M. and Saarikoski S. (1973) Decrease of litter size and fetal monoamines by 6-hydroxydopamine in mice. *Experientia 29*, 576–578.

Chang M. C. (1966a) Effects of oral administration of medroxyprogesterone acetate and ethinyl estradiol on the transportation and development of rabbit eggs. *Endocrinology 79*, 939–948.

Chang M. C. (1966b) Transport of eggs from the Fallopian tube to the uterus as a function of estrogen. *Nature (Lond.) 212*, 1048–1049.

Chang M. C., Hunt D. M. and Polge C. (1973) Effects of prostaglandins (PGs) on sperm and egg transport in the rabbit. In: *Proc. Int. Conf. on Prostaglandins, Vienna* (1972). *Adv. Biosciences 9*, 805–810.

Chatterjee A. and Harper M. J. K. (1970) Interruption of implantation and gestation in rats by reserpine, chlorpromazine and ACTH: possible mode of action. *Endocrinology 87*, 966–969.

Cibils L. A., Sica-Blanco Y., Remedio M. R., Rozada H. and Gil B. E. (1971) Effect of sympathomimetic drugs upon the human oviduct *in vivo. Amer. J. Obstet. Gynec. 110*, 481–488.

Coutinho E. M. (1971) Physiologic and pharmacologic studies of the human oviduct. *Fertil. Steril. 22*, 807–815.

Coutinho E. M. and Maia H. (1971) The contractile response of the human uterus, Fallopian tubes and ovary to prostaglandins *in vitro. Fertil. Steril. 22*, 539–543.

Coutinho E. M., Maia H. and Adeodato Filho J. (1970) Response of the human Fallopian tube to adrenergic stimulation. *Fertil. Steril. 21*, 590–594.

Coutinho E. M., Maia H. and Adeodato Filho J. (1974) The inhibitory effect of ritodrine on human tubal activity *in vivo. Fertil. Steril. 25*, 596–601.

Coutinho E. M., de Mattos C. E. R. and da Silva A. R. (1971) The effect of ovarian hormones on the adrenergic stimulation of the rabbit Fallopian tube. *Fertil. Steril. 22*, 311–317.

Eaton L. W., Jr. and Hilliard J. (1971) Estradiol-17β and progestin released by the rabbit ovary from mating through implantation. *Biol. Reprod. 5*, 89 (abstr.).

Eddy C. A. (1973) Chemical sympathectomy of the rabbit oviduct and its effects on ovum transport. Ph. D. dissertation, Univ. of Massachusetts, pp. 1–93.

Eddy C. A. and Black D. L. (1973) Chemical sympathectomy of the rabbit oviduct using 6-hydroxydopamine. *J. Reprod. Fertil. 33*, 1–9.

Ellinger J. V. and Kirton K. T. (1972) Ovum transport in rabbits injected with prostaglandin E_1 or $F_{2\alpha}$. *Biol. Reprod. 7*, 106.

Euler U. S. v. (1956) *Noradrenaline*. C. C. Thomas, Springfield, Ill.

Ferrando G. and Nalbandov A. V. (1969) Direct effect on the ovary of the adrenergic blocking drug dibenzyline. *Endocrinology 85*, 38–42.

Fronduti R. L. and Archer D. F. (1974) Metabolism of estradiol-6,7-^{3}H by the human Fallopian tube. I. Effects of prostaglandin $F_{2\alpha}$ *in vitro. Fertil. Steril. 25*, 592–595.

Greenwald G. S. (1961) A study of the transport of ova through the rabbit oviduct. *Fertil. Steril. 12*, 80–95.

Greenwald G. S. (1968) Hormonal regulation of egg transport through the mammalian oviduct. In: Behrman S. J. and Kistner R. W., eds. *Progress in Infertility*, pp. 157–179. Churchill, London.

Harper M. J. K. (1961) Egg movement through the ampullar region of the Fallopian tube of the rabbit. *Proc. IVth Int. Congr. Anim. Reprod.* The Hague, pp. 375–380.

Harper M. J. K. (1964) The effects of constant doses of oestrogen and progesterone on the transport of artificial eggs through the reproductive tract of ovariectomized rabbits. *J. Endocr. 30*, 1–19.

Harper M. J. K. (1965) The effects of decreasing doses of oestrogen and increasing doses of progesterone on the transport of artificial eggs through the reproductive tract of ovariectomized rabbits. *J. Endocr. 31*, 217–226.

Hedqvist P. (1970) Studies on the effects of prostaglandins E_1 and E_2 on the sympathetic neuromuscular transmission in some animal tissues. *Acta physiol. scand. 79*, Suppl. 345, 1–40.

Hedqvist P. and Brundin J. (1969) Inhibition by prostaglandin E_1 of noradrenaline release and of effector response to nerve stimulation in the cat spleen. *Life Sci. 8*, 389–395.

Hedqvist P. and Euler U. S. v. (1972) Prostaglandin-induced neurotransmission failure in the field-stimulated, isolated vas deferens. *Neuropharmacol. 11*, 177–187.

Heilman R. D.. Bauer E. W., Hahn D. W. and DaVanzo J. P. (1972) A comparison of cardiovascular and oviduct beta adrenergic receptors. *Fertil. Steril. 23*, 221–229.

Higgs G. W. and Moawad A. H. (1974) The effect of ovarian hormones on the contractility of the rabbit oviductal isthmus. *Canad. J. Physiol. Pharmacol. 52*, 74–83.

Hodgson B. J., Sullivan K. B. and Pauerstein C. J. (1973) The role of sympathetic nerves in the response of uterus and oviduct to field stimulation. *Eur. J. Pharmacol. 23*, 107–110.

Horton E. W., Main I. H. M. and Thompson C. J. (1963) The action of intravaginal prostaglandin on the female reproductive tract. *J. Physiol. (Lond.) 168*, 54–55 P.

Howe G. R. and Black D. L. (1973) Autonomic nervous system and oviduct function in the rabbit. I. Hormones and contraction. *J. Reprod. Fertil. 33*, 425–430.

Jacobowitz D. and Koelle G. B. (1965) Histochemical correlations of acetylcholinesterase and catecholamines in postganglionic autonomic nerves of the cat, rabbit and guinea pig. *J. Pharmacol. exp. Ther. 148*, 225–237.

Johns A., Chlumecky J. and Paton D. M. (1974) Role of adrenergic nerves in ovulation and ovum transport. *Lancet 2*, 1079.

Kendle K. E. and Bennett J. P. (1969a) Studies upon the mechanism of reserpine-induced arrest of egg transport in the mouse oviduct. I. The effect of hormone replacement. *J. Reprod. Fertil. 20*, 429–434.

Kendle K. E. and Bennett J. P. (1969b) Studies upon the mechanism of reserpine-induced arrest of egg transport in the mouse oviduct. II. Comparative effects of some agents with actions on smooth muscle and tissue amines. *J. Reprod. Fertil. 20*, 435–441.

Kubo K., Kawano J. and Ishii S. (1970) Some observations on the autonomic innervation of the human oviduct. *Int. J. Fertil. 15*, 30–35.

Labhsetwar A. P. (1973a) Effects of prostaglandins E_1, E_2 and $F_{2\alpha}$ on zygote transportation in rats: induction of delayed implantation. *Prostaglandins 4*, 115–125.

Labhsetwar A. P. (1973b) Evidence for the involvement of a catecholaminergic pathway in gonadotrophin secretion for implantation in rats. *J. Reprod. Fertil. 33*, 545–548.

Lands A. M., Luduena F. P. and Buzzo H. J. (1967) Differentiation of receptors responsive to isoproterenol. *Life Sci. 6*, 2241–2249.

Lerner L. J., Carminati P. and Rubin B. L. (1973) Effects of prostaglandins PGE_2 and $PGF_{2\alpha}$ on the adenyl cyclase activity of various segments of the immature rabbit oviduct and uterus (37360). *Proc. Soc. exp. Biol. Med. 143*, 536–539.

Levy B. and Lindner H. R. (1972) The effects of adrenergic drugs on the rabbit oviduct. *Eur. J. Pharmacol. 18*, 15–21.

Longley W. J., Black D. L. and Currie G. N. (1968) Oviduct circular muscle response to drugs related to the autonomic nervous system. *J. Reprod. Fertil. 17*, 95–100.

MacDonald E. J. and Airaksinen M. (1974) The effect of 6-hydroxydopamine on the oestrous cycle and fertility of rats. *J. Pharm. Pharmacol. 26*, 518–521.

253

Mandl J. P. (1972) The effect of prostaglandin E_1 on rabbit sperm transport *in vivo*. *J. Reprod. Fertil. 31*, 263–269.

Marshall J. M. (1970) Adrenergic innervation of the female reproductive tract: anatomy, physiology and pharmacology. *Ergebnisse der Physiol. 62*, 6–67.

Marshall J. M. (1973) Effects of catecholamines on the smooth muscle of the female reproductive tract. *Ann. Rev. Pharmacol. 13*, 19–32.

Martin J. E., Ware R. W., Crosby R. J. and Pauerstein C. J. (1970) Demonstration of beta adrenergic receptors in the rabbit oviduct. *Gynec. Invest. 1*, 82–91.

Nakajima A. and Nishimura T. (1972) The effect of prostaglandin $F_{2\alpha}$ and E_1 on the electrical activity of the rabbit Fallopian tube. *Acta Obst. et Gynaec. Jap. 19*, 40–46.

Nakanishi H. and Wood C. (1968) Effects of adrenergic blocking agents on human Fallopian tube motility *in vitro*. *J. Reprod. Fertil. 16*, 21–28.

Ogra S. S., Kirton K. T., Tomasi T. B. and Lippes J. (1974) Prostaglandins in the human Fallopian tube. *Fertil. Steril. 25*, 250–255.

Owman C. and Sjöberg N.-O. (1966) Adrenergic nerves in the female genital tract of the rabbit. With remarks on cholinesterase-containing structures. *Z. Zellforsch. 74*, 182–197.

Owman C., Sjöberg N.-O. and Sjöstrand N. O. (1974) Short adrenergic neurons, a peripheral neuroendocrine mechanism. In: Fujiwara M. and Tanaka C., eds. *Amine Fluorescence Histochemistry*, pp. 47–67. Igaku Shoin Ltd., Tokyo.

Pauerstein C. J., Fremming B. D., Hodgson B. J. and Martin J. E. (1973) The promise of pharmacologic modification of ovum transport in contraceptive development. *Amer. J. Obstet. Gynec. 116*, 161–166.

Polidoro J. P. (1974) Recent advances in oviduct pharmacology. *J. Reprod. Med. 13*, 45–48.

Polidoro J. P., Howe G. R. and Black D. L. (1973) The effects of adrenergic drugs on ovum transport through the rabbit oviduct. *J. Reprod. Fertil. 35*, 331–337.

Porter C. C., Totaro J. A. and Stone C. A. (1963) Effect of 6-hydroxydopamine and some other compounds on the concentration of norepinephrine in the heart of mice. *J. Pharmacol. exp. Ther. 140*, 308–316.

Rosenblum I. and Stein A. A. (1966) Autonomic responses of the circular muscles of isolated human Fallopian tube. *Amer. J. Physiol. 210*, 1127–1129.

Sandberg F., Ingelman-Sundberg A., Lindgren L. and Rydén G. (1960) *In vitro* studies of the motility of the human Fallopian tube. Part I: The effects of acetycholine, adrenaline, noradrenaline and oxytocin on the spontaneous motility. *Acta obstet. gynec. scand. 39*, 506–516.

Seitchik J., Goldberg E., Goldsmith J. P. and Pauerstein C. (1968) Pharmacodynamic studies of the human Fallopian tube *in vitro*. *Amer. J. Obstet. Gynec. 102*, 727–735.

Senior J. B. and Spencer-Gregson R. N. (1969) The effects of sympathomimetic drugs and bradykinin on the human Fallopian tube *in vitro* using isometric recording methods. *J. Obstet. Gynaec. Brit. Cwlth 76*, 652–655.

Sjöberg N.-O. (1967) The adrenergic transmitter of the female reproductive tract: distribution and functional changes. *Acta physiol. scand. 67*, Suppl. 305, 1–32.

Sorgen C. D. and Glass R. H. (1972) Lack of effect of prostaglandin $F_{2\alpha}$ on the fertilizing ability of rabbit sperm. *Prostaglandins 1*, 229–233.

Spilman C. H. (1974) Oviduct response to prostaglandins: influence of estradiol and progesterone. *Prostaglandins 7*, 465–469.

Spilman C. H., Finn A. E. and Norland J. F. (1973) Effect of prostaglandins on sperm transport and fertilization in the rabbit. *Prostaglandins 4*, 57–64.

Spilman C. H. and Harper M. J. K. (1972) Effect of prostaglandins on oviduct motility in conscious rabbits. *Biol. Reprod. 7*, 106.

Spilman C. H. and Harper M. J. K. (1973) Effect of prostaglandins on oviduct motility in estrous rabbits. *Biol. Reprod. 9*, 36–45.

Stjärne L. (1975) Adrenoceptor mediated positive and negative feedback control of noradrenaline secretion from human vasoconstrictor nerves. *Acta physiol. scand.*, in press.

Stjärne L. and Brundin J. (1975a) Dual-adrenoceptor-mediated control of noradrenaline secretion from human vasoconstrictor nerves: facilitation by beta-receptors and inhibition by alpha-receptors. *Acta physiol. scand. 94*, 139–141.

Stjärne L. and Brundin J. (1957b) Affinity of noradrenaline and dopamine for neural alpha-receptors mediating negative feedback control of noradrenaline secretion in human vasoconstrictor nerves. *Acta physiol. scand. 95*, 89–94.

Stjärne L. and Gripe K. (1973) Prostaglandin-dependent and -independent feedback control of noradrenaline secretion in vasoconstrictor nerves of normotensive human subjects. *Naunyn-Schmiedeberg's Arch. Pharmak. 280*, 441–446.

Sutherland E. W. and Robison G. A. (1966) The role of cyclic $3',5'$ AMP in responses to catecholamines and other hormones. *Pharmacol. Rev. 18*, 145–161.

Swedin G. (1971) Studies on neurotransmission mechanisms in the rat and guinea-pig vas deferens. *Acta physiol. scand. 83*, Suppl. 369, 1–34.

Talo A. and Brundin J. (1971) Muscular activity in the rabbit oviduct: a combination of electric and mechanic recordings. *Biol. Reprod. 5*, 67–77.

Talo A. and Brundin J. (1973) The functional connections and contractile function of the upper reproductive tract in female rabbits. *Biol. Reprod. 9*, 142–148.

Thoenen H. and Tranzer J. P. (1973). The pharmacology of 6-hydroxydopamine. *Ann. Rev. Pharmacol. 13*, 169–180.

Ueda M., de Mattos C. E. R. and Coutinho E. M. (1973) The influence of adrenergic activation and blockade on the motility of the circular and longitudinal muscle layers of the rabbit oviduct *in vitro*. *Fertil. Steril. 24*, 440–447.

Virutamasen P., Hickok R. L. and Wallach E. E. (1971) Local ovarian effects of catecholamines on human chorionic gonadotropin-induced ovulation in the rabbit. *Fertil. Steril. 22*, 235–243.

Wakeling A. E. and Spilman C. H. (1973) Prostaglandin specific binding in the rabbit oviduct. *Prostaglandins 4*, 405–414.

Warnes G. M., Amato F. and Seamark R. F. (1974) Biochemical studies on Fallopian tube secretions. *J. Reprod. Fertil. 36*, 460–461.

Woodruff J. D. and Pauerstein C. J. (1969) *The Fallopian Tube*. The Williams & Wilkins Co., Baltimore.

Zetler G., Mönkemeier D. and Wiechell H. (1969) Stimulation of Fallopian tubes by prostaglandin $F_{2\alpha}$, biogenic amines and peptides. *J. Reprod. Fertil. 18*, 147–149.

Departments of Histology, Pharmacology, Obstetrics and Gynecology,
and Zoology, University of Lund, Lund;
and Primate Laboratory of the Department of Obstetrics and Gynecology,
University Hospital, Uppsala, Sweden

AUTONOMIC NERVES AND RELATED AMINE RECEPTORS MEDIATING MOTOR ACTIVITY IN THE OVIDUCT OF MONKEY AND MAN. A HISTOCHEMICAL, CHEMICAL AND PHARMACOLOGICAL STUDY

By

*Ch. Owman, B. Falck, E. D. B. Johansson,
E. Rosengren, N.-O. Sjöberg, B. Sporrong, K.-G. Svensson
and B. Walles*

ABSTRACT

The oviduct of rhesus monkey and man is extensively innervated by adrenergic nerves, particularly in the circular smooth muscle layer. The innervation is best developed in the ampullary end of the isthmic region, which possesses adrenergic sphincter functions. Part of the innervation belongs to the system of short adrenergic neurons, whose cell bodies form ganglia which are located in that part of the uterine cervix bordering the vagina. The neuronal level of norepinephrine transmitter during the secretory phase is almost twice that of the proliferative phase of the menstrual cycle, probably as a result of variations in the amount of circulating estrogen and progesterone. Preliminary pharmacological *in vitro* studies have shown that norepinephrine stimulates both the adrenergic α- and β-receptors to produce increased or decreased motor activity, depending on cyclic stage, and on the type of oviductal musculature (longitudinal *vs.* circular), as well as region (ampulla *vs.* isthmus) tested.

256

The cholinergic innervation appears to be less well-developed than the adrenergic.

The results indicate that the ovum transport function in the oviduct of monkeys and humans may be influenced by adrenergic mechanisms, involving *i. a.* changes in the activity of the adrenergic nerves and sensitivity of the smooth muscular adrenoceptors, caused by alterations in circulating steroid hormones.

In a series of studies on the sympathetic motor innervation of the genital tract in rabbits and cats, Langley and Anderson (1895a,b, 1896a,b) showed that the oviduct is supplied by sympathetic nerves running in the hypogastric nerves. The experiments further indicated that part of the fibers in these nerves was preganglionic, probably forming synapses in peripherally situated sympathetic ganglia, which were located near the effector organs. The results, which thus differed from the classical concept about the anatomy of the sympathetic innervation, were largely disregarded during the subsequent years, and the generally held opinion was that the hypogastric nerves carried only post-ganglionic sympathetic fibres to the genital tract. The development of the Falck-Hillarp histofluorescence technique (see Björklund et al. 1972), applied together with denervation experiments and chemical determinations of nor-epinephrine, provided new possibilities for a detailed mapping of the adrenergic innervation of the female genital organs. To-day, it has become established that the oviduct receives a well-developed innervation by way of a unique type of adrenergic nerves, whose arrangement in the smooth musculature suggests an important role in oviductal motor activity, including specialized sphincter functions, which is in agreement with the presence of adrenergic α- and β-receptors in its smooth musculature (for reviews, see Brundin 1965; Sjöberg 1967; Marshall 1970; Owman et al. 1974). It is thus possible that adrenergic mechanisms may influence the rate of ovum transport to the uterus (see Pauerstein 1974) and, accordingly, constitute one functional parameter of interest in the present extensive search for new types of chemical contraceptive compounds. For this reason, particular attention has been turned to the human oviduct in order to obtain information about a number of basic conditions: the exact distribution of autonomic nerves in the various parts of the smooth musculature, ultrastructural and functional aspects of the neuromuscular relations, identification and characterization of amine receptors mediating motor activity, and variations in amine-mediated motor functions during the normal menstrual cycle and the effects of hormones, sympathomimetics, and sympatholytics, etc. These are parameters which may provide points of attack when attempting to design pharmacologically active drugs which are able to alter ovum transport through the oviduct by an interference with the various autonomic neuro-receptor mechanisms in the oviductal smooth musculature.

257

Fluorescence histochemistry of catecholamines

Studies were performed with the Falck-Hillarp histofluorescence technique according to which primary catecholamines, such as dopamine and norepinephrine, in a reaction with gaseous formaldehyde are transformed into fluorescent isoquinolines which, under the histochemical and optical conditions used (see below), emit an intense green fluorescence. Immediately upon dissection the material is frozen in a propane-propylene mixture to the temperature of liquid nitrogen, freeze-dried, exposed to formaldehyde vapour at +80°C for 1 h, embedded in paraffin, sectioned at 6 μ, and mounted in Entellan® (Merck) for fluorescence microscopy. For further information on the methodology, see Björklund et al. (1972).

Human. – Seventeen oviducts were obtained from adult menstruating, non-pregnant patients (aged 31–53 years) subjected to abdominal hysterectomy because of pains, bleeding, uterine myoma, or preinvasive carcinoma of the cervix. Atropine (0.5 mg) and meperidine (50 mg) were administered as pre-anesthetic medication. Anesthesia was induced by Pentothal® administered intravenously, followed by inhalation of a mixture of dinitrous oxide and oxygen in a semiclosed system. All oviducts were studied *in toto,* and they included

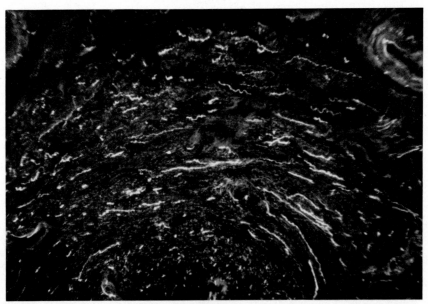

Fig. 1.

Fluorescence photomicrograph of cross section from human oviductal isthmus. The picture is dominated by the prominent circular smooth muscle layer, the mucosa is seen below in the middle. Numerous green-fluorescent adrenergic nerve fibres run in a direction parallel to the smooth muscle cells. × 200.

the intramural portion. The isthmic portion from 3 of the oviducts was divided into 3 pieces of equal length for special microscopic estimation of the thickness of the circular muscle layer.

The adrenergic innervation of the human oviduct (see Owman et al. 1967) – serially sectioned in 9 instances – was found to be organized principally in the same manner as in laboratory animals (Brundin 1965; Owman and Sjöberg 1966; Rosengren and Sjöberg 1967). Thus, some of the nerves ran along vessels in the entire organ, but the majority were distributed in the smooth muscles in numbers that varied characteristically in the 3 different portions of the oviduct: (a) In the ampulla, the thin muscle layer contained only relatively few nerves, the picture being dominated by vasomotor fibres. (b) The total number of nerves showed a distinct increase in the isthmus. It was obvious that the majority of fibres supplied the prominent circular muscle layer (Fig. 1). The number of nerves in this layer decreased slightly toward the intramural part of the oviduct. (c) In the smooth musculature of the intramural part, a further decrease in the number of fluorescent nerves was evident. However, the innervation was denser than that found in the surrounding smooth muscles of the uterine fundus.

On the basis of histochemical and functional studies in rabbits (Brundin 1965), the presence of an adrenergic sphincter mechanism in the isthmus of the oviduct has been proposed. Therefore, the thickness of the circular muscle layer – which receives most of the innervation – was measured microscopically on 3 transversly sectioned portions of the isthmus using an ocular micrometer. This offered a possibility to estimate the true degree of innervation (i. e., the

Table 1.
Fluorometric determinations of norepinephrine content in human oviductal isthmus divided into 3 portions of equal length.

Part of isthmus analyzed[a]	Norepinephrine[b]	
	Total amount (μg)	μg/g tissue weight
Nearest to ampulla	0.12 ± 0.02	0.63 ± 0.08
Intermediate	0.10 ± 0.01	0.77 ± 0.08
Nearest to intramural portion	0.11 ± 0.01	0.72 ± 0.08

[a] Three isthmic specimens from the same region were pooled for each assay (6 assays for each isthmic part). Differences between the 3 parts were not significant ($P > 0.05$).
[b] Mean ± SE.

259

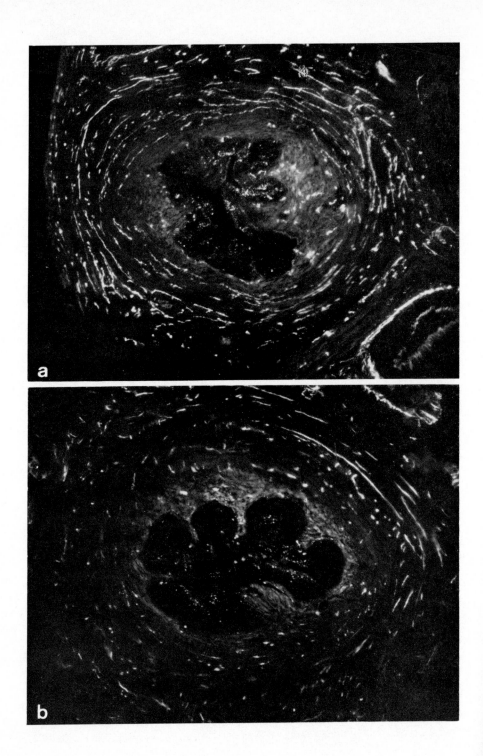

number of nerves related to the amount of smooth muscle innervated) in various parts of the isthmus. In a direction away from the ampulla, the circular layer showed a slight but distinct increase in thickness, followed by a decrease in that part nearest to the intramural portion. Although the slight variation in the number of nerves in the isthmic circular muscle layer could not be disclosed in the fluorometric assays (Table 1) the results taken together nevertheless provide strong evidence that the degree of innervation is highest in that part of the isthmus nearest the ampulla.

Monkey. – Material was obtained from one or both oviducts of 13 adult menstruating rhesus monkeys (*Macaca mulatta*) during Nembutal® anesthesia. Two of the oviducts were used for serial sectioning, and contained the uterotubal junction. Only small pieces from the isthmus, at 2 cm distal to the uterotubal junction, were taken from the remainder of the oviducts, which were then used in the chemical analyses (see below). The studies on the monkey material were concentrated on possibilities to reveal histochemically visible cyclic variations in the content of norepinephrine transmitter in the adrenergic nerve terminals. It is known that there is a linear relationship between fluorescence intensity and amine concentration within the range that can be expected for the adrenergic axons (Jonsson 1971). The cyclic stage was determined in either of the following ways: (a) relation to first day of last menstrual bleeding, (b) histological examination of the endometrium, and (c) radioimmunoassay of estradiol-17β (Edqvist and Johansson 1972) and progesterone (Thorneycroft and Stone 1972) in plasma.

Fluorescence microscopy of the serially sectioned monkey oviducts showed principally the same arrangement of adrenergic innervation as previously found in humans (Owman et al. 1967). On the basis of microscopic analysis of coded sections from the isthmus it was possible to demonstrate a clear variation in the fluorescence microscopic picture of the adrenergic innervation, most evident in the circular smooth muscle layer. Thus, during the proliferative stage the number of fluorescent nerve terminals was moderate and their fluorescence was less bright than during the secretory phase when the fibres were, in addition, more numerous (Fig. 2a and b). With regard to the fairly short time periods involved it is conceivable that this does not represent a true variation in the *number* of adrenergic nerves, but rather a change in norepinephrine *concentration* of the individual axons, which means that the transmitter level has been

---

Fig. 2.

Fluorescence photomicrographs of transversely sectioned monkey oviducts, isthmic region. The majority of fluorescent adrenergic nerve terminals run in the circular muscle layer, parallel to the smooth muscle cells. The number of fluorescent axons visible during (a) the secretory phase of the menstrual cycle is much larger than (b) during the proliferative phase, in agreement with the chemical determinations of norepinephrine (cf. Fig. 4 b).

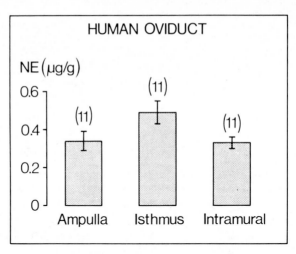

Fig. 3.
Fluorometric determination of norepinephrine concentration in the 3 anatomically distinct parts of the human oviduct. One organ was used for each determination. Values given are mean ± SE, number of determinations within parenthesis. Differences evaluated according to Student's *t*-test: ampulla *vs.* isthmus: $0.01 < P < 0.05$, isthmus *vs.* intramural part: $0.01 < P < 0.02$.

too low for histochemical detection in many of the nerves during the proliferative phase.

Chemical determinations of norepinephrine

The oviducts were homogenized in 0.4 N ice-cold perchloric acid and the catecholamines were determined fluorometrically according to Bertler et al. (1958) as modified by Häggendal (1963). Only norepinephrine was found in measurable amounts, which confirmed the identity of the primary catecholamine visualized histochemically in the oviductal nerves as described above.

Humans. – Eleven oviducts from patients (31–53 years old) were separated into the 3 anatomically distinct regions – ampulla, isthmus and intramural portion. In another series, the isthmic part from a further 18 oviducts was divided into 3 equally long portions, which were analyzed separately.

The mean values for the concentration of norepinephrine in the ampulla, isthmus, and intramural portion were in good agreement with the histochemical findings (Fig. 3). Comparison of the mean norepinephrine concentrations in the different regions showed a significantly higher concentration in the isthmus (Fig. 3). In order to minimize the influence due to variation in concentration between individual patients the amount of norepinephrine in each isthmus was expressed as the percentage of the concentration in each corresponding ampulla and intramural portion. The *t*-test showed the relative level of norepinephrine in the isthmus to be significantly higher than in both the ampulla ($0.001 < P < 0.01$ for 10 d. f.) and the intramural portion ($0.001 < P < 0.01$ for 10 d. f.). The norepinephrine concentration in the 3 isthmic portions did not, however, differ significantly from each other, as shown in Table 1.

The fluorometrically estimated levels of norepinephrine in the whole oviduct were also analyzed with special reference to any cyclic changes in the total amine content (*i. e.* in the level of transmitter of the oviductal nerve fibres). With regard to the stage of the menstrual cycle (based upon histologic examination of endometrial material) at which the oviducts were removed, the specimens could be grouped into proliferative and secretory phases, respectively. As shown in Fig. 4a the concentration during the secretory phase was almost twice that seen during the proliferative phase (Student's *t*-test: $P < 0.02$).

Monkeys. – The chemical determinations were performed on both oviducts and comprised the whole organ (except the small pieces taken for fluorescence microscopy) from eleven animals.

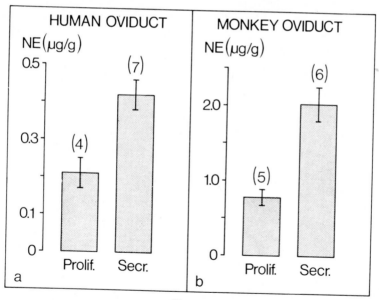

Fig. 4.

Fluorometric determinations of norepinephrine (NE) in the whole oviduct of (a) humans and (b) rhesus monkeys. One organ was used for each determination. The values given are mean ± SE, number of determinations within parentheses. There was in both humans and monkeys (cf. Fig. 2) a significantly higher (see text) transmitter concentration during the secretory compared with the proliferative phase.

Oviducts from the proliferative phase were obtained on days 4–12 of the cycle. The mean plasma estrogen values (78.3 pg/ml) were somewhat lower than during the secretory phase (99.8 pg/ml; oviducts obtained on days 19–26). The plasma concentration of progesterone was low in both groups (0.6 and 0.2 ng/ml), respectively). As shown in Fig. 4b there was, as in the human material, a significantly higher concentration of norepinephrine during the secretory phase as compared with that found during the proliferative phase (Student's t-test: $0.001 < P < 0.01$).

Comments. – A preliminary histochemical account on the adrenergic nerve supply of the human oviduct was presented by Brundin and Wirsén in 1964. Subsequently, a detailed fluorescence histochemical study, combined with chemical determinations of norepinephrine, was performed by Owman et al. (1967). Part of the study was repeated and confirmed by Kubo et al. (1970). The material now also includes an investigation on the oviduct of the rhesus monkey. The combined histochemical and chemical analysis has shown that the primate oviduct receives a well-developed supply of norepinephrine-containing adrenergic nerves. The most prominent innervation is found in the circular smooth muscle coat, particularly in the isthmic region. On the basis of histochemical and functional studies in rabbits, the presence of an adrenergic sphincter mechanism in the isthmus of the oviduct has been proposed (Brundin 1965). Judging from the conspicuously high concentration of neuronal norepinephrine found in this region it is likely that such a mechanism is to be found also in the human isthmus. It appears that the degree of adrenergic innervation is especially pronounced in that part of the isthmus nearest the ampulla, indicating that the isthmus may not be functionally uniform in its sphincter properties.

The results of electrical stimulation of perivascular nerves in the human oviduct (Nakanishi et al. 1967, 1970; Nakanishi and Wood 1968) and of transmural oviductal stimulation (Paton et al. 1975) have shown that the histochemically demonstrable adrenergic nerve supply represents a functional innervation capable of influencing the motor activity of its smooth musculature.

Only little is known about the cholinergic innervation of the human oviduct. On the basis of cholinesterase staining, Kubo et al. (1970) mention that the pattern of cholinesterase-positive nerves in the isthmus agrees with that of the adrenergic innervation, whereas stained fibres are only seldom present in the ampulla.

The amount and distribution of the adrenergic innervation of the primate oviduct agree with observations in the rabbit (Brundin 1965; Owman and Sjöberg 1966; Eddy and Black 1973), the cat (Rosengren and Sjöberg 1967), and the dog (Owman and Sjöberg 1972). As mentioned above, the sympathetic fibres innervating the oviduct of rabbit and cat and also of man run in the hypogastric nerve (Langley and Anderson 1895a,b, 1896a,b; Mitchell 1938).

264

Transection of this nerve causes, however, only a partial reduction in chemically measured norepinephrine in the oviduct (Brundin 1965; Owman et al. 1966; Rosengren and Sjöberg 1967), confirming the presence of a peripheral relay distal to the level of transection. The adrenergic ganglion formation could be traced by fluorescence microscopy and was found to be located in or near the utero-vaginal junction (Owman and Sjöberg 1966; Rosengren and Sjöberg 1967), where they have been demonstrated also in humans (Owman et al. 1967). Chemical determinations following hypogastric denervation have established that most, if not all, of the adrenergic innervation in the feline oviduct, and about one third to one half of the supply to the rabbit oviduct, consists of fibres belonging to the system of "short adrenergic neurons". In accordance with this, removal of the utero-vaginal ganglion formations produced an almost complete disappearance of fluorescent nerves in the oviduct of cats (Rosengren and Sjöberg 1967). These neurons differ from classical sympathetic nerves, originating in pre- and paravertebral ganglia, not only in their close topographic relation to the effector structure, but also in a number of functional aspects. The most interesting aspect in this context relates to the marked alterations in their transmitter level seen during pregnancy and under the influence of certain sex steroids (Owman and Sjöberg 1973; Owman et al. 1974). In the rabbit, for example, both estrogen treatment by 0.5 μg/kg of 17β-estradiol benzoate for 2 weeks (Owman and Sjöberg 1975) and pregnancy (Rosengren and Sjöberg 1968) doubles the level of norepinephrine in the oviductal adrenergic nerves. If progesterone (2 mg/kg) is added to the estrogen treatment (of non-pregnant rabbits) during the last week, the transmitter level becomes normalized (Owman and Sjöberg 1975). The changes in chemically determined norepinephrine correspond to an alteration in the number of adrenergic nerves visible by the formaldehyde histofluorescence technique (Owman and Sjöberg 1975) in a way similar to that described above for monkey and man.

Our studies on the primate oviducts have shown that marked alterations in the norepinephrine transmitter metabolism can be revealed also in connection with the endogenous hormonal fluctuations seen during the menstrual cycle. It is likely that the observed changes in oviductal norepinephrine constitute net results of hormone-induced alterations in the synthesis, breakdown, and/or release of the adrenergic transmitter. There is experimental evidence indicating that the turnover of transmitter in the short adrenergic neurons is slower than in classical sympathetic nerves (e. g. Euler and Lishajko 1966; Stjärne and Lishajko 1966; Owman and Sjöberg 1967; Sjöstrand and Swedin 1968). In view of this and of the mentioned effects of exogenous sex steroids on the rabbit's oviductal norepinephrine, it can be assumed that the plasma estrogen peak occurring before ovulation leads to the high norepinephrine concentration found in the human and monkey oviducts recorded during the secretory phase, whereas the transmitter level becomes reduced in the proliferative phase as a consequence of the preceding high concentration of progesterone (and estrogen) that is seen before menstruation (Midgley et al. 1973; Bosu et al. 1973a,b).

Pharmacology of amine receptors

Numerous studies have been carried out on the effect of various sympatho- and parasympathomimetic compounds on human oviductal motility, whereas no corresponding reports seem to be available for monkeys. Valuable – though for practical reasons limited – information has been obtained under *in vivo* conditions by methods such as that devised by Maia and Coutinho (1968). Such studies have indicated that the musculature of the human ampulla contains both α- and β-receptors, and that β-inhibitory responses are more pronounced during progesterone dominance (Coutinho et al. 1970; Coutinho 1971). On the other hand, Cibils et al. (1971) have claimed that the sensitivity of α- and β-agonists does not vary with hormonal state.

The pharmacological tests on human material can be made more extensive under *in vitro* conditions. Epinephrine and norepinephrine – like electric nerve stimulation – have in some investigations been found to increase the tone of the oviductal smooth musculature, and the effect is inhibited (or reversed) by α-antagonists, such as phenoxybenzamine and phentolamine (Sandberg et al. 1960; Hawkins 1964; Nakanishi et al. 1967; Nakanishi and Wood 1968). Also isoproterenol is reported to have a contractile effect (Rosenblum and Stein 1966). This seems strange in light of the finding that nerve stimulation in the presence of an α-antagonist produces relaxation, which can be inhibited by β-receptor blocking agents, *e. g.* propranolol, and isoproterenol dilates the ovi- duct in the presence of an α-blocker (Rosenblum and Stein 1966). It should be pointed out, though, that there is a considerable variability in the response (Sandberg et al. 1960; Seitchik et al. 1968), and some authors (*e. g.* Paton et al. 1975) have reported that the sympathetic system causes predominantly a de- crease in oviductal motor activity. The literature does not allow for any definite conclusion about the relation of the various amine-induced responses to cyclic stage.

Acetylcholine, like the catecholamines, stimulates contractile activity in the isolated human oviduct, and the effect is antagonized by atropine (Sandberg et al. 1960; Hawkins 1964).

Humans. – Available pharmacological data is far from sufficient to define and characterize the various autonomic receptor mechanisms mediating motor functions in the human oviduct. Therefore, a series of experiments was initiated with the intention to (a) define receptor types in different oviductal smooth muscle systems (longitudinal *vs.* circular) or anatomically separate portions (ampulla *vs.* isthmus), (b) compare quantitative differences in receptor sensitivity during various stages of the menstrual cycle, and (c) analyse, by electrical stimulation, quantitative variations in neuro-receptor activity in the two muscular layers of the ampulla and isthmus at various cyclic stages. The information thus far obtained from a limited amount of material (25 oviducts) is summarized below.

One or both oviducts have been removed from patients (27–54 years old) during abdominal hysterectomy (for menorrhagia, metrorrhagia, myomas, adenomyosis), salpingo-oophorectomy (for ovarian cysts, ovarian tumors, breast cancer), or salpingectomy (for sterilization). The cyclic stage was estimated on the basis of the patient's menstrual cycle as noted in the record, together with

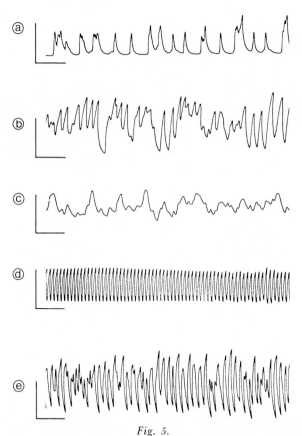

Fig. 5.

Various types of spontaneous motor activity in different human oviductal preparations *in vitro*. Calibration: vertical, 200 dyn; horizontal, 1 min. (a) isthmus, circular layer, pregnant; (b) isthmus, circular layer, menopause; (c) isthmus, longitudinal layer, menopause; (d) ampulla, circular layer, early secretory phase; (e) isthmus, circular layer, early secretory phase.

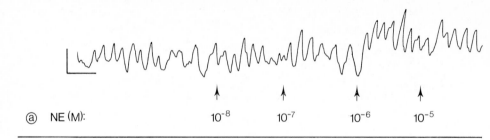

ⓐ NE (M): 10^{-8} 10^{-7} 10^{-6} 10^{-5}

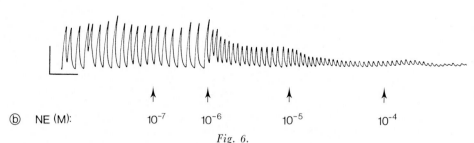

ⓑ NE (M): 10^{-7} 10^{-6} 10^{-5} 10^{-4}

Fig. 6.

Effects of various molar (M) concentrations of norepinephrine (NE) on isolated pieces of human oviducts. Calibration: vertical, 200 dyn; horizontal, 1 min. (a) increased motor activity is produced by NE in the longitudinal muscle layer of the ampulla (late proliferative stage). (b) Decreased motor activity is produced by NE shortly after ovulation (isthmus, circular layer).

histological examination of endometrial material obtained by curettage of the uterine cavity during the operation. After removal, the preparations were placed in ice-cold, previously aerated Krebs-Ringer buffer solution and transported to the laboratory. Rings (= circular muscle) and strips (= longitudinal muscle) were cut from defined parts of the ampulla and isthmus, and mounted between metal hooks in mantled organ baths maintained at $37\,^{\circ}C$ and containing a Krebs-Ringer buffer solution of the following composition (mM): NaCl 118, KCl 4.5, $CaCl_2. 2H_2O$ 2.5, $MgSO_4. 7H_2O$ 1.0, $NaHCO_3$ 25, KH_2PO_4 1.0, glucose 6.0. The bath and the stock solution were aerated by a mixture of 95 % O_2 and 5 % CO_2 to give a constant pH range of 7.40 ± 0.15, frequently checked in 50 μl samples by a pH Meter 27 with type E5021 electrode unit (Radiometer, Copenhagen). Isometric tension was recorded by Grass FT03C force-displacement transducers, and signals were amplified and written on a Grass Model 7 polygraph. The 4 preparations (as mentioned above) were run simultaneously in separate baths.. They were given a passive load of 500 dyn and allowed to accommodate for 60 min during which steady rhythmic activity was achieved. Although there was a tendency to decreasing amplitude of the spontaneous contractions after a few hours in the organ bath, changes in tone induced by various drugs could be studied during a whole day's experimentation. Fresh tissue could also be stored at +4°C in previously aerated Krebs-Ringer solution for 24 h without any alteration in response pattern.

As a routine procedure, the character of the spontaneous activity was always registered after the 1 h accommodation in the bath. Several types of activity, both in terms of frequency and amplitude, were seen (Fig. 5). A particularly low activity was revealed during pregnancy and in oviducts from patients taking oral contraceptives. The frequency was especially low in the circular muscle layers from both ampulla and isthmus in most of the oviducts (Fig. 5a). High activity, however, was observed in all parts of the organ immediately after ovulation (Fig. 5d,e).

In all 4 types of preparations tested, norepinephrine produced either contraction or relaxation: Contraction most often occurred in the longitudinal musculature (Fig. 6a), particularly intense before ovulation. The circular muscles appeared to contract only around ovulation; otherwise they dilated. A few days after ovulation, the circular isthmic musculature relaxed markedly (Fig. 6b) upon addition of norepinephrine, concomitant with a contraction in the longitudinal

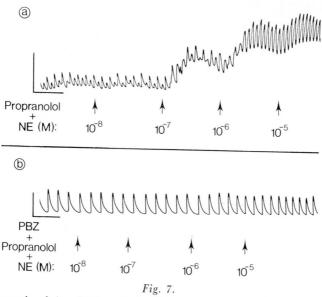

Fig. 7.
Effects of norepinephrine (NE) on isolated human oviduct. Calibration: vertical, 200 dyn; horizontal, 1 min. (a) Isthmus, longitudinal layer (early secretory phase); in the presence of 3×10^{-6} M of the β-receptor antagonist, propranolol, NE produces a contraction, irrespective of cyclic phase or region tested. (b) Ampulla, longitudinal layer (proliferative stage); after pretreatment with 10^{-6} M of the α-antagonist phenoxybenzamine (PBZ, exposure time 30 min, followed by washing) and in the presence of the β-antagonist propranolol (3×10^{-6} M), NE is without effect on the motor activity.

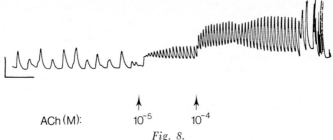

ACh (M): 10^{-5} 10^{-4}

Fig. 8.

Acetylcholine (ACh) increases the motor activity in this circular muscle preparation of human isthmus *in vitro* (early secretory stage). Calibration: vertical, 200 dyn; horizontal, 1 min.

musculature and dilation in the circular layer of the ampulla. In some of the circular muscle preparations, norepinephrine was without effect (equal sensitivity of contracting α- and relaxing β-receptors?). Blockade of the β-receptors with propranolol always resulted in a contractile response with norepinephrine (Fig. 7a); phenoxybenzamine inhibited that response (Fig. 7b). Isoproterenol caused dilation (or extinction of spontaneous contractions) in all 4 test preparations. A contraction, or no response at all, was obtained by acetylcholine in a few tests (Fig. 8). Prostaglandin $F_{2\alpha}$, studied in a couple of preparations, gave an intense contraction (Fig. 9).

Comments. The present preliminary results do, of course, not allow for any conclusion about the exact identity and characteristics of the various autonomic receptors in the human oviduct. However, they give strong reason to believe that the receptor mechanisms mediating motor activity in the oviductal smooth

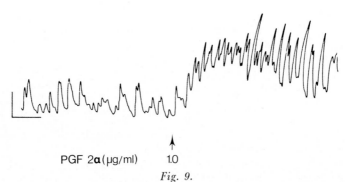

PGF 2α (μg/ml)   1.0

Fig. 9.

A pronounced increase in the motor activity is obtained by prostaglandin $F_{2\alpha}$ in the longitudinal muscle layer of a human ampulla from an early secretory phase. Calibration: vertical, 200 dyn; horizontal, 1 min.

musculature is far more complex than often realized: The amine-induced response in the circular and longitudinal muscle components from the same regions are not equal, and the ampullary and isthmic portions of the same oviduct behave differently. Moreover, distinct cyclic variation in the response pattern seems to exist. As could be expected, the norepinephrine transmitter stimulates both the α- and β-adrenergic receptors, and hence produces either a contraction or relaxation of the oviductal smooth musculature. It is therefore important that quantitative analysis of one of the receptor types must be carried out under conditions of efficient blockade of the other receptor in order to avoid interference. With regard to the effects of receptor activation during local norepinephrine release from the adrenergic nerves, it is likely that the change in sensitivity of either of the adrenoceptors under the influence of cyclic variations in the level of steroid hormones will be of considerable importance for the oviductal motor functions under physiological conditions.

General considerations

Only scarce information is available on the structure of the neuro-effector apparatus in the primate oviduct studied by electromicroscopy. The observations mentioned by Kubo et al. (1970) and Paton et al. (1975) indicate that it resembles the autonomic innervation of the uterus, in which there is a fairly large distance between the small axon bundles and the smooth muscle cells, and that further excitation spread occurs by apposition contacts between the individual muscle cells (see Bennett 1972). The close association between varicosities of adrenergic and non-adrenergic (probably cholinergic) axons in the rabbit myometrium suggests that, in addition to the neuro-muscular transmission mechanisms, also axo-axonal interaction may be involved in the autonomic control function (Hervonen and Kanerva 1973). Recently, a new type of connection between muscle cells and autonomic nerve terminals has been detected in the feline uterus, besides the above-mentioned long-distance relations (Sporrong 1975): The muscle cells seem to push out small stout processes, sometimes pedicular in shape, onto a small nerve fibre. The projections are supplied with a particularly dense concentration of myofilaments, and the membrane-to-membrane distance is only 20–25 nm. Such regions of close contacts are always found at the "end" of a muscle bundle, and projections from adjacent muscle bundles often form close contacts with the axonal varicosities. There is thus strong reason to suppose that the neuro-muscular apparatus in the oviduct also has a complex construction and, therefore, that detailed ultrastructural studies are required as a basis for proper understanding of autonomic neuro-muscular transmission functions in the primate oviduct.

A central question with regard to future possibilities of developing new types of antifertility compounds on the basis of the autonomic neuro-receptor mechanisms in the smooth musculature of the oviduct is, of course, whether such

271

mechanisms play a crucial role in the regulation of ovum transport. Experimental studies in this field have, for practical reasons, so far been limited to laboratory animals. Some of these experiments have recently been reviewed by Black (1974) and Pauerstein (1974): The studies show that sympathomimetic compounds, tested alone or in combination with specific antagonists, can *modify* the rate of ovum tranpsort in the oviduct. The effects appear to be highly dependent on dose and time of administration. There is evidence that the response is related to changes in receptor sensitivity resulting from varying levels of circulating ovarian steroids. The retardation of ovum passage caused by estrogen seems to involve two mechanisms, one that can be counteracted by progesterone and another that is antagonized by α-adrenergic blockade. On the basis of recent denervation experiments – performed either pharmacologically with 6-hydroxydopamine (Eddy and Black 1973) or surgically – it has been suggested that, although the action of ovarian steroids on the rate of ovum transport is partially mediated through adrenergic mechanisms, the adrenergic innervation is not of *crucial* importance in the regulation of the transport (Pauerstein et al. 1974; Johns et al. 1975). However, it is our opinion that the experimental approach hitherto used does not allow for a final answer to the question whether the above-mentioned modifying actions by the adrenergic mechanisms indeed have a more crucial importance in the control of ovum transport in humans: (a) it can be assumed that there are significant differences in the detailed construction of the oviductal adrenergic innervation between humans and laboratory animals, (b) the surgical denervation procedures used do not allow for selective removal of oviductal "short adrenergic neurons" which is the unique, and perhaps functionally most important, sympathetic system in the reproductive tract (see Owman et al. 1974), (c) it cannot be excluded that the pharmacological denervation procedures, in addition, have systemic effects – influencing amine functions in *e. g.* the ovary (see Svensson et al. 1975; Walles et al. 1975) or the median eminence (*e. g.* Hökfelt and Fuxe 1972; McCann et al. 1972), (d) the sympathectomy produces a considerable degree of denervation supersensitivity (see Johns and Paton 1974) that may mask expected deficiency symptoms, and (e) the denervation probably also affects the cholinergic system, either indirectly via the above-mentioned axo-axonal relations or directly in the surgical procedures. Thus, it is still an open question whether or not local adrenergic mechanisms are indispensable for normal ovum transport along the oviduct and, hence, for normal human fertility.

ACKNOWLEDGMENTS

Studies supported by the Ford Foundation, New York (grants No. 66–0405 and 680–0383A) and the World Health Organization.

REFERENCES

Bennett M. R. (1972) *Autonomic Neuromuscular Transmission.* Cambridge University Press, Cambridge.

Bertler Å., Carlsson A. and Rosengren E. (1958) A method for the fluorimetric determination of adrenaline and noradrenaline in tissues. *Acta physiol. scand.* 44, 273–292.

Björklund A., Falck B. and Owman Ch. (1972) Fluorescence microscopic and microspectrofluorometric techniques for the cellular localization and characterization of biogenic amines. In: Berson A. A., ed. *Methods of Investigative and Diagnostic Endocrinology,* Vol. 1, pp. 318–368. North-Holland Publ. Comp., Amsterdam.

Black D. L. (1974) Neuronal control of oviduct musculature. In: Johnson A. D. and Foley C. W., eds. *The Oviduct and its Function,* pp. 65–118. Academic Press Inc., New York and London.

Bosu W. T. K., Johansson E. D. B. and Gemzell C. (1973a) Ovarian steroid patterns in peripheral plasma during the menstrual cycle in the rhesus monkey. *Folia primat.* 19, 218–234.

Bosu W. T. K., Johansson E. D. B. and Gemzell C. (1973b) Peripheral plasma levels of oestrone, oestradiol-17β and progesterone during ovulatory menstrual cycles in the rhesus monkey with special reference to the onset of menstruation. *Acta endocr. (Kbh.)* 74, 732–742.

Brundin J. (1965) Distribution and function of adrenergic nerves in the rabbit Fallopian tube. *Acta physiol. scand.* 66, Suppl. 259, 1.

Brundin J. and Wirsen C. (1964) Adrenergic nerve terminals in the human Fallopian tube examined by fluorescence microscopy. *Acta physiol. scand.* 61, 505–506.

Cibils L. A., Sica-Blanco Y., Remedio M. R., Rozada H. and Gil B. E. (1971) Effect of sympathomimetic drugs upon the human oviduct *in vivo. Amer. J. Obstet. Gynec.* 110, 481–488.

Coutinho E. M. (1971) Tubal and uterine motility. In: Diczfalusy E. and Borell U., eds. *Nobel Symposium 15: Control of Human Fertility,* pp. 97–107. Almqvist and Wiksell, Stockholm.

Coutinho E. M., Maia M. and Filho J. A. (1970) Response of the human Fallopian tube to adrenergic stimulation. *Fertil Steril.* 21, 590–594.

Eddy C. A. and Black D. L. (1973) Chemical sympathectomy of the rabbit oviduct using 6-hydroxydopamine. *J. Reprod. Fertil.* 33, 1–9.

Edqvist L. E. and Johansson E. D. B. (1972) Radioimmunoassay of oestrone and oestradiol in human and bovine peripheral plasma. *Acta endocr. (Kbh.)* 71, 716–731.

Euler U. S. von and Lishajko F. (1966) A specific kind of noradrenergic granules in the vesicular gland and the vas deferens of the bull. *Life Sci.* 5, 687–691.

Häggendal J. (1963) An improved method for fluorimetric determination of small amounts of adrenaline and noradrenaline in plasma and tissues. *Acta physiol. scand.* 59, 242–254.

Hawkins D. F. (1964) Some pharmacological reactions of isolated rings of human Fallopian tube. *Arch. int. Pharmacodyn.* 152, 474–478.

Hervonen A. and Kanerva L. (1973) Fine structure of the autonomic nerves of the rabbit myometrium. *Z. Zellforsch.* 136, 19–30.

Hökfelt T. and Fuxe K. (1972) On the morphology and the neuroendocrine role of the hypothalamic catecholamine neurons. In: *Brain-Endocrine Interaction, Median Eminence: Structure and Function.* Int. Symp. Munich 1971, pp. 181–223. Karger, Basel.

273

Johns A., Chlumecky J., Cottle M. K. W. and Paton D. M. (1975) Effect of chemical sympathectomy and adrenergic agonists on the fertility of mice. *Contraception* 11, 563–570.

Johns A. and Paton D. M. (1974) Drug-induced changes in the sensitivity of the isthmus of rabbit oviduct to noradrenaline. *Brit. J. Pharmacol. 52*, 127 P.

Jonsson G. (1971) Quantitation of fluorescence of biogenic amines demonstrated with the formaldehyde fluorescence method. *Prog. Histochem. Cytochem. 2*, 299–334.

Kubo K., Kawano J. and Ishi S. (1970) Some observations on the autonomic innervation of the human oviduct. *Int. J. Fertil. 15*, 30–35.

Langley J. N. and Anderson H. K. (1895a) The innervation of the pelvic and adjoining viscera. Part 4. The internal generative organs. *J. Physiol. (Lond.) 19*, 122–130.

Langley J. N. and Anderson H. K. (1895b) The innervation of the pelvic and adjoining viscera. Part 5. Position of the nerve cells on the course of the efferent nerve fibres. *J. Physiol. (Lond.) 19*, 131–139.

Langley J. N. and Anderson H. K. (1896a) The innervation of the pelvic and adjoining viscera. Part 6. Histological and physiological observations upon the effects of section of the sacral nerve. *J. Physiol. (Lond.) 19*, 372–384.

Langley J. N. and Anderson H. K. (1896b) The innervation of the pelvic and adjoining viscera. Part 7. Anatomical observations. *J. Physiol. (Lond.) 20*, 372–406.

Maia H. and Coutinho E. M. (1968) A new technique for recording human tubal activity *in vivo*. *Amer. J. Obstet. Gynec. 102*, 1043–1047.

Marshall J. M. (1970) Adrenergic innervation of the female reproductive tract: anatomy, physiology and pharmacology. *Ergebn. Physiol. 62*, 2–67.

McCann S. M., Kalra P. S., Donoso A. O., Bishop W., Schneider H. P. G., Fawcett C. P. and Krulich L. (1972) The role of monoamines in the control of gonadotropin and prolactin secretion. In: *Brain-Endocrine Interaction, Median Eminence: Structure and Function*. Int. Symp. Munich 1971, pp. 224–235. Karger, Basel.

Midgley A. R., Jr., Gay V. L., Keyes P. L. and Hunter J. S. (1973) Human reproductive endocrinology. In: Hafez E. S. E. and Evans T. H., eds. *Human Reproduction: conception and contraception*. Harper and Row, Publishers, Inc., Haggerstown, Maryland.

Mitchell G. A. G. (1938) The innervation of the ovary, uterine tube, testis and epididymis. *J. Anat. (Lond.) 72*, 508–517.

Nakanishi H., Wansbrough H. and Wood C. (1967) Postganglionic sympathetic nerves innervating human Fallopian tube. *Amer. J. Physiol. 213*, 613–619.

Nakanishi H., Wansbrough H. and Wood C. (1970) Effect of temperature on sympathetic transmission in the human Fallopian tube. *Fertil. Steril. 21*, 329–334.

Nakanishi H. and Wood C. (1968) Effect of adrenergic blocking agents on human Fallopian tube motility *in vitro*. *J. Reprod. Fertil. 16*, 21–28.

Owman Ch., Rosengren E. and Sjöberg N.-O. (1967) Adrenergic innervation of the human female reproductive organs: a histochemical and chemical investigation. *Obstet. Gynec. 30*, 763–773.

Owman Ch. and Sjöberg N.-O. (1966) Adrenergic nerves in the female genital tract of the rabbit. With remarks on cholinesterase-containing structures. *Z. Zellforsch. 74*, 182–197.

Owman Ch. and Sjöberg N.-O. (1967) Difference in rate of depletion and recovery of noradrenaline in "short" and "long" sympathetic nerves after reserpine treatment. *Life Sci. 6*, 2549–2556.

Owman Ch. and Sjöberg N.-O. (1972) Adrenergic innervation of the female genital tract of the dog. *J. Reprod. Med. 8*, 63–66.

Owman Ch. and Sjöberg N.-O. (1973) Effect of pregnancy and sex hormones on the transmitter level in uterine short adrenergic neurons. In: Usdin E. and Snyder S., eds. *Frontiers in Catecholamine Research*, pp. 795–801. Pergamon Press, Oxford.

Owman Ch. and Sjöberg N.-O. (1975) Influence of sex hormones on the amount of adrenergic transmitter in the rabbit oviduct. Proc. Symp. Neuroendocrine Regulation of Fertility, Simla 1974. In press, Karger, Basel.

Owman Ch., Sjöberg N.-O. and Sjöstrand N. O. (1974) Short adrenergic neurons, a peripheral neuroendocrine mechanism. In: Fujiwara M. and Tanaka C., eds. *Amine Fluorescence Histochemistry*, pp. 47–67. Igaku Shoin Ltd., Tokyo.

Paton D. M., Johns A., Molnar S., Daniel E. E. and Beck R. P. (1975) Characteristics of responses of human and rabbit Fallopian tube to field stimulation and nor-adrenaline. *Proc. west. Pharmacol. Soc. 18*, 208–212.

Pauerstein C. J. (1974) *The Fallopian Tube: A Reappraisal.* Lea and Febiger, Philadelphia.

Pauerstein C. J., Hodgson B. J., Fremming B. D. and Martin J. E. (1974) Effects of sympathetic denervation of the rabbit oviduct on normal ovum transport and on transport modified by estrogen and progesterone. *Gynec. Invest. 5*, 121–132.

Rosenblum I. and Stein A. A. (1966) Autonomic responses of the circular muscles of the isolated human Fallopian tube. *Amer. J. Physiol. 210*, 1127–1129.

Rosengren E. and Sjöberg N.-O. (1967) The adrenergic nerve supply to the female reproductive tract of the cat. *Amer. J. Anat. 121*, 271–284.

Sandberg F., Ingelman-Sundberg A., Lindgren L. and Rydén G. (1960) *In vitro* studies of the motility of the human Fallopian tube. *Acta obstet. gynec. scand. 39*, 506–516.

Seitchik J., Goldberg E., Goldsmith J. P. and Pauerstein C. (1968) Pharmacodynamic studies of the human Fallopian tube *in vitro. Amer. J. Obstet. Gynec. 102*, 727–734.

Sjöberg N.-O. (1967) The adrenergic transmitter of the female reproductive tract: distribution and functional changes. *Acta physiol. scand.* Suppl. 305.

Sjöstrand N. O. and Swedin G. (1968) Effect of reserpine on the noradrenaline content of the vas deferens and the seminal vesicle compared with the submaxillary gland and the heart of the rat. *Acta physiol. scand. 72*, 370–377.

Sporrong B. (1975) Ultrastructural evidence for synaptic contacts between smooth muscle cells and adrenergic nerve terminals in the feline uterus. *Proc. 10th Int. Congr. of Anatomists*, Tokyo, in press.

Stjärne L. and Lishajko F. (1966) Comparison of spontaneous loss of catecholamines and ATP *in vitro* from isolated bovine adrenomedullary, vesicular gland, vas deferens and splenic nerve granules. *J. Neurochem. 13*, 1213–1216.

Svensson K.-G., Owman Ch., Sjöberg N.-O., Sporrong B. and Walles B. (1975) Ultra-structural evidence for adrenergic innervation of the interstitial gland in the guinea-pig ovary. *Neuroendocrinology 17*, 40–47.

Thorneycroft I. H. and Stone S. C. (1972) Radioimmunoassay of serum progesterone in women receiving oral contraceptive steroids. *Contraception 5*, 129–146.

Walles B., Edvinsson L., Falck B., Owman Ch., Sjöberg N.-O. and Svensson K.-G. (1975) Evidence for a neuromuscular mechanism involved in the contractility of the ovarian follicle wall: fluorescence and electron microscopy and effects of tyramine on follicle strips. *Biol. Reprod. 12*, 239–248.

The Department of Obstetrics and Gynecology,
University of Chicago
and The Department of Physiology,
Karolinska Institute, Stockholm

CORRELATION OF PLASMA ESTROGENS AND PROGESTERONE LEVELS WITH THE IN VITRO ADRENERGIC RESPONSES IN THE ISTHMUS OF THE HUMAN OVIDUCT

By

*Atef H. Moawad, Per Hedqvist and Moon H. Kim**

ABSTRACT

In 83 subjects correlation of the peripheral plasma levels of Estrone (E_1), Estradiol (E_2) and Progesterone (P) with the *in vitro* response of the isthmus of the human oviduct to transmural nerve stimulation (N. S.) was done using circular preparations. Tissues were classified according to the plasma hormone values into four groups: 1. Low estrogens and low progesterone. 2. High estrogens and low progesterone. 3. High progesterone. 4. Pregnant values. The responses were observed by measuring the change in frequency (F), tone (T) and area under the contractility curve (A). In groups 1 and 2 a positive correlation between the effective estrogen level ($E_1/10 + E_2$) and tissue contractile activity was demonstrated. The initial inhibition following N. S. in group 1 is gradually reversed to stimulation as the ($E_1/10 + E_2$) value rises to more than 48. In group 3, with progesterone values of 2 ng/ml or more, and in group 4, the response to N. S. is by inhibition of all parameters. The effect of epinephrine on the contractility of these tissues was investigated by constructing the

* Present address: Department of Obstetrics and Gynecology, Ohio State University, Columbus, Ohio.
Reprint requests: Atef H. Moawad, M. D., Department of Obstetrics and Gynecology, University of Chicago, 5841 South Maryland Avenue, Chicago, Illinois 60637. This research was supported by grants from The Rockefeller Foundation RF 70097, 72062, and The Biomedical Center for Population Research PHS-HD-07110-04.

cumulative dose response curve measuring the area with and without
α-adrenergic receptor activity blockade. In the follicular phase significant
reversal of the stimulation was achieved by α-receptor blockers. Similarly
in the luteal phase the tissue responded by inhibition.

I. M. injection of subjects with high doses of estradiol 12–24 hours prior
to surgery, did not change the expected responses.

In another set of experiments human and rabbit oviducts preincubated
with ^{3}H-NE were superfused with Tyrode's solution, the concentrations
were recorded and the superfusate was continuously collected. PGE_2
caused marked inhibition of the ^{3}H-NE release in response to N. S. This
depression occurred regardless of the species differences or the hormonal
status. In the rabbit, contractions caused by N. S. were depressed by
PGE_2 as well. On the other hand, PGE_2 affected N. S. contractions in the
human by either enhancement or inhibition, dependent on the hormonal
condition.

The musculature of the oviduct has been implicated in the mechanism of ovum
transport especially at the isthmic region (Greenwald 1961; Pauerstein et al.
1968; Boling 1969; Hodgson and Pauerstein 1974). At this site the fertilized
ovum is delayed in its journey towards its implantation site in the uterus. The
delay, which ranges between 48–72 hours in the human (Croxatto et al. 1972),
has been the subject of intensive investigations (Harper 1965a,b). In the human,
estrogens and progesterone have been implicated in influencing this mechanism
(Maia and Coutinho 1970). The correlation between physiological levels of
these ovarian steroids and the contractility of the *in vitro* human isthmic rings
is the subject of this report. We hope to offer a useful model to test the effects
of drugs on *in vitro* responses. We have limited this report to the investigation
of some of the adrenergic mechanisms, and a possible relationship with
prostaglandins.

MATERIAL AND METHODS

Tissues from the isthmic portion of the human oviducts were obtained from a
total of 83 subjects undergoing total abdominal hysterectomies or bilateral
partial salpingectomies for sterilization.

The hormonal status of these women was evaluated by measuring peripheral
plasma estrogens and progesterone at the time of surgery. Plasma levels of
total estradiol (E_2) and estrone (E_1) were measured by radioimmunoassay.
Water blank values for estradiol and estrone were less than 8 pg, and the
coefficients of variation between assays were 11 % and 17 % respectively. The
levels of progesterone in plasma were determined by a competitive protein
binding method which yields the coefficient of variation between assays of
14.5 % (Dupon et al. 1973).

277

The range of normal plasma hormone values for different phases of the menstrual cycle in our laboratory are as follows.

Table 1.

Phase	E_1 pg/ml	E_2 pg/ml	P ng/ml
Early follicular phase	15– 40	20– 50	1.5
Late follicular phase	40–150	80–500	1.5
Early or late luteal phase	30–105	32–110	1.5– 8
Mid luteal phase	40–150	60–300	7 –16

Circular segments from the isthmic portion of the oviduct of normal women in the reproductive years were taken 1–2 cm distal to the uterine insertion. The ring shaped sections were 3 mm in length and they were immediately incubated in modified Krebs Ringer. *In vitro* isometric contractions were measured as described previously (Higgs and Moawad 1974).

Transmural nerve stimulation was effected by 2 platinum wire electrodes applied on each side of, but not touching, the tissue. Leads from electrodes were passed to an Ael electronic stimulator delivering monophasic square wave pulses at various frequencies, durations and voltages.

Effect of transmural nerve stimulation. – The optimal dose which causes the maximal response has been arrived at empirically and is considered to be an electric current of 70 milliamperes, with a frequency of 7 pulses per sec and

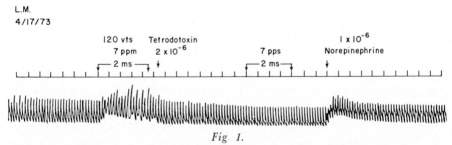

Fig. 1.

A record of the *in vitro* contractility of a tissue from the isthmic region. Transmural field stimulation resulted in an increased activity. This response was abolished when repeated following the application of tetrodotoxin (2×10^{-6} M concentration). On the other hand the tissue still responded by increased activity to the subsequent treatment with norepinephrine 10^{-6} M concentration.

a duration of 2 msec. This current on this preparation does not cause any direct effect on the muscle since this has been completely blocked by the application of tetrodotoxin (Fig. 1). It is obvious from this figure that application of transmural nerve stimulation caused an increase in tonus, amplitude, frequency and the area under the contractility curve. However, this effect was blocked with tetrodotoxin in the concentration of 2×10^{-6} molar (M).

An epinephrine cumulative dose response relationship was done on consecutive segments of each tissue with and without the addition of the α-adrenergic blocking agent phenoxybenzamine.

The contractility results were expressed in terms of percent change in 3 parameters: the area under the contractility curve, tone and frequency. This was measured for areas of 3 min duration immediately following the introduction of an agent comparing it to the preceding 3 min acting as a control.

This same protocol was followed throughout all the experiments. Contractility studies were done blind without prior knowledge of the phase of the menstrual cycle or the hormonal levels in the plasma. Consequently after the experiments were done the groups of patients were classified according to the plasma levels of hormones and the endometrial histology. It was felt that since estrone has approximately 1/10 the potency of estradiol on the receptor sites, a formula should be devised for the addition of both E_1 and E_2 values. This was arrived at by adding 1/10 the estrone value to the estradiol value ($E_1/10 + E_2$), and is referred to as the effective estrogen level.

Twenty-one subjects were injected intramuscularly with 5 mg of estradiol the afternoon before their planned surgical procedure (i. e. 14–24 h). They were randomly selected and the phase of their cycle was later determined by both the endometrial histology and the hormone levels in the plasma. The same protocol for the contractility studies was followed as described above.

Statistical analysis of the data was done using the Student t-test and the confidence limits set at the 0.05 level.

In another set of experiments where the release of norepinephrine (NE) was measured the following methodology was used. The isolated oviduct was incubated for $1\frac{1}{2}$ h in Tyrode's solution containing 10 μCi/ml of ^{3}H-1-NE (specific activity 5.4 Ci/mM) and was then thoroughly rinsed and continuously superfused in a 2 ml organ bath with NE-free Tyrode at a rate of 1 ml/min. The preparation was longitudinally mounted and electrically stimulated by means of platinum electrodes in the walls of the bath with a Grass stimulator delivering trains of pulses (5–10 Hz, 1 msec supramaximal voltage) for 30–60 sec. Contractions of the organ were recorded isotonically. The radioactivity in different superfusate samples was determined by counting 1 ml aliquots in a Packard liquid scintillation spectrometer. The details of the method, and the identification of norepinephrine and its metabolites have been described in a previous publication (Hedqvist 1974).

RESULTS

Tissues were classified mainly into two categories: the ones associated with low or no progesterone in plasma, i. e. less than 1.9 ng/ml, and those with progesterone values of 1.9 ng/ml or more. In the first category (insignificant progesterone), the relationship between the effective estrogen values ($E_1/10 + E_2$) and the change in contractility following N.S. were plotted as shown in Figs. 2, 3 and 4. These describe the effects on the frequency, tone and area under the contractility curve respectively.

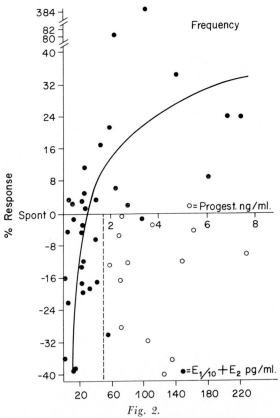

Fig. 2.

A graph showing the correlation between plasma hormone levels and the % change in frequency of contractions following transmural field stimulation. Solid points represent the tissues from the follicular phase (estrogen levels are represented as $E_1/10 + E_2$ in pg/ml in the lower scale). The broken line represents the estrogen level (48) beyond which stimulation is expected rather than inhibition. Tissues from the luteal phase with progesterone levels higher than 1.9 ng/ml are shown as open circles. (The progesterone level scale is the upper one). Notice the decrease in frequency following N. S. in all the tissues tested. Each point on this graph and the subsequent two others represent the average of three observations in one subject.

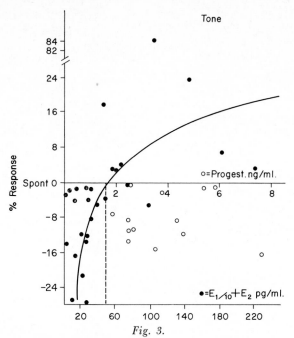

Fig. 3.

A graph showing the correlation between plasma hormone levels and % change in tone following N. S. Identification and labelling is similar to Fig. 2.

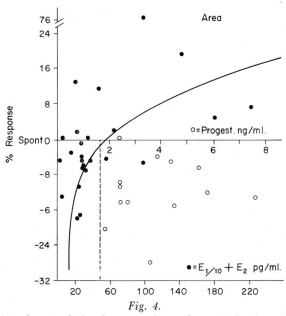

Fig. 4.

A graph showing the correlation between plasma hormone levels and % change in area under the contractility curve following N. S. Identification and labelling is similar to Fig. 2.

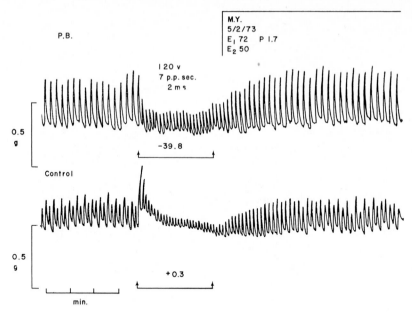

Fig. 5.

A record showing *in vitro* simultaneous contractility of two tissues from a subject in the follicular phase whose plasma hormone levels are charted. Transmural field stimulation resulted in an initial increase in activity (tone and amplitude). This response was blocked in the tissue exposed to phenoxybenzamine 10^{-7} M concentration (the upper record) and even reversed to inhibition.

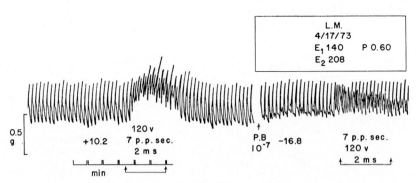

Fig. 6.

A record from a subject with very high estrogen and insignificant progesterone levels. N. S. stimulation was applied before and after blocking with phenoxybenzamine 10^{-7} M concentration.

A positive correlation was established between plasma estrogens and the stimulation of the contractility parameters. This was most clearly demonstrated by increased frequency (Fig. 2) and less so by increased tone (Fig. 3) and contractility area (Fig. 4).

It was also concluded after a further study of this relationship that a value for $E_1/10 + E_2$ in pg/ml of approximately 48 represents the turning point for reversal of the response. In other words a value higher than 48 is usually associated with stimulation of contractility rather than inhibition following N.S.

On the other hand the presence of significant amounts of progesterone pre-

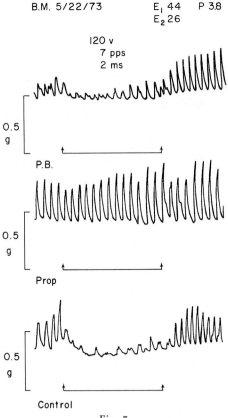

B.M. 5/22/73 E_1 44   P 3.8
                                E_2 26

120 v
7 pps
2 ms

0.5
g

P.B.

0.5
g

Prop

0.5
g

Control

Fig. 7.

A record of three consecutive tissues from a subject in the early luteal phase run simultaneously. The lower record shows the inhibition caused by N. S. The middle one shows the blocking of this response by pretreatment with propranolol. The upper one shows the tissue pretreated with phenoxybenzamine. Notice the marked similarity between this and the lower record (control).

vents this reversal of response regardless of the estrogen value. This is represented in Fig. 2, 3 and 4 by open circles. Studying these figures shows that these tissues usually respond by inhibition of all parameters.

Representative records showing these effects are shown in the following figures.

Fig. 5, shows the effects of N. S. on two consecutive tissues from a subject with estrogen values slightly higher $(E_1/10 + E_2 = 57.2)$ than 48, the turning point in the reversal of the response. There is an initial increase in amplitude and tone which was abolished by the pretreatment with the α-adrenergic blocking agent phenoxybenzamine.

Fig. 6 illustrates a record from a subject with very high (yet physiological) estrogen values and insignificant progesterone. All contractility parameters were clearly stimulated by N.S., a response blocked by pretreatment with phenoxybenzamine.

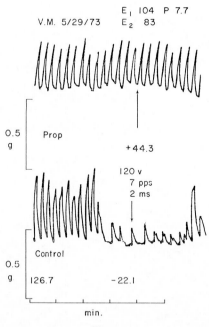

Fig. 8.

A record of *in vitro* contractility from two consecutive segments from the isthmus of a subject in the luteal phase of the cycle. Plasma hormone values are charted. The bottom tracing shows the response to field stimulation by relaxation. The top tracing illustrates the reversal of this response following the exposure to propranolol 10^{-7} M concentration.

284

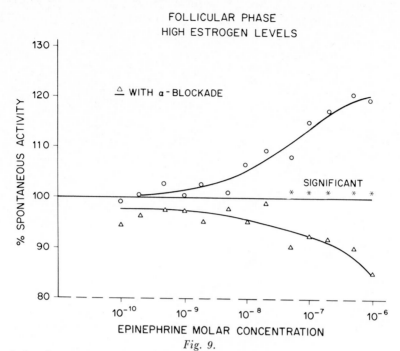

FOLLICULAR PHASE
HIGH ESTROGEN LEVELS

Fig. 9.

Cumulative dose relationship for epinephrine from follicular phase tissues with high estrogen levels, before and after α-adrenergic receptor blockade with phenoxybenzamine. * denotes the statistically significant difference.

Fig. 7 and 8 show the inhibitory response to N.S. in tissues with high progesterone values. This inhibition was blocked by the β-blocking agent propranolol.

Following this, we then classified our tissues into four groups. Group 1: low estrogens ($E_1/10 + E_2 =$ less than 48) and insignificant progesterone (P less than 1.9 ng/ml). There were 23 subjects. Group 2: high estrogens ($E_1/10 + E_2 = 48$ or more) and insignificant progesterone. There were 11 subjects. Group 3: significant progesterone (1.9 ng/ml or more). There were 14 subjects. Group 4: pregnancy. There were 13 subjects.

Statistical evaluation of the data between these groups showed that the differences in all parameters are significant at the 0.05 level, between the high estrogen (group 2) and the luteal (group 3), and also between the high estrogen and the pregnancy groups.

Epinephrine dose response relationship. – A cumulative dose response curve was constructed for the group with high estrogens (group 2) and the luteal group (group 3).

The high estrogen dose response curve is shown in Fig. 9. This was done simultaneously in 2 consecutive tissues from the same specimen with and without the presence of phenoxybenzamine. Stimulation was reversed by the α-adrenergic blocking agent phenoxybenzamine. The differences were significant in doses higher than 10^{-8} M epinephrine concentration.

In Fig. 10 dose response relationships of both group 2 and 3 tissues are represented. This shows the stimulation in the high estrogen group contrasted with the inhibition in the luteal group.

Statistical analysis of the contractility parameters in tissues obtained from subjects injected with estradiol prior to surgery, showed no significant difference between the luteal and follicular phases of the cycle.

Transmural stimulation of superfused human and rabbit oviducts for 30–60 sec periods (5–10 Hz, 1 msec, supramaximal voltage) consistently caused a marked and well reproducible increase in the release of ^{3}H, the bulk of which consisted of intact ^{3}H-NE (Moawad and Hedqvist 1975).

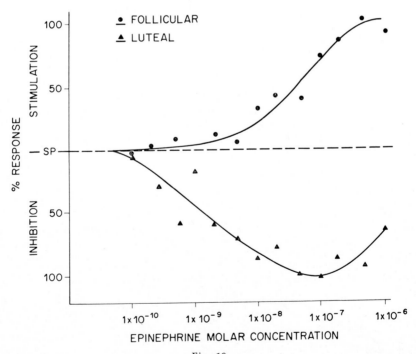

Fig. 10.

Comparison between the cumulative dose response curves of both follicular and luteal phase tissues.

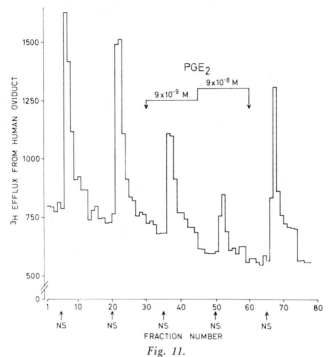

Fig. 11.

Human oviduct previously loaded with ³H-NE. Effect of PGE₂ on the outflow of
tracer in response to transmural stimulation (N. S.). 300 pulses at 5 Hz.
Time in min = fraction numbers.

In all hormonal conditions in the rabbit as well as the human, PGE₂ in
doses ranging from 9×10^{-9} M to 9×10^{-8} M inhibited the release of ³H-NE in
response to transmural nerve stimulation. The degree of inhibition was dose
dependent and the effect clearly reversible (Fig. 11).

In all hormonal conditions in the rabbit, PGE₂ inhibited spontaneous motility
as well as contractions resulting from transmural nerve stimulation. These
effects were dose dependent as well (Fig. 12).

On the other hand, contractions resulting from transmural nerve stimulation
in the human were modified by PGE₂ in a variety of ways. They were either
slightly depressed, not affected or even markedly enhanced. The latter response
is well demonstrated in Fig. 13. This tissue was obtained from a subject in the
immediate preovulatory period.

RABBIT OVIDUCT
FIELD STIM. 5 Hz 50 PULSES 1 ms

10 min

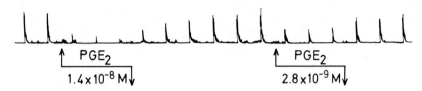

↑ PGE₂
1.4 × 10⁻⁸ M↓

↑ PGE₂
2.8 × 10⁻⁹ M↓

Fig. 12.
Effect of PGE₂ on the isotonic contractions of a rabbit oviduct *in vitro*. Transmural nerve stimulation delivered at equal intervals (every 5 min), 50 pulses at 5 Hz.

HUMAN OVIDUCT
FIELD STIM. 5 Hz 300 PULSES 1 ms

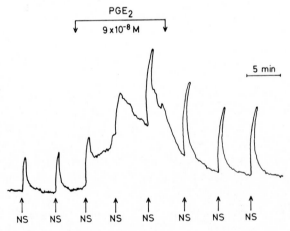

PGE₂
9 × 10⁻⁸ M

5 min

NS NS NS NS NS NS NS NS

Fig. 13.
Effect of PGE₂ on the *in vitro* isotonic contractions of a human oviduct in the late follicular phase. Transmural stimulation (N. S.), 300 pulses at 5 Hz, were delivered at 5 min intervals.

288

DISCUSSION

The effect of the ovarian hormones on oviductal muscular contractility has been the subject of intensive investigations in the laboratory animals and in the human, both *in vivo* and *in vitro*. In the rabbit definite patterns have been related to either estrogen or estrogen and progesterone dominance (Higgs and Moawad 1974).

Reports on this relationship in the human are conflicting. *In vivo*, the overall activity has been shown to diminish during the luteal phase (Maia and Coutinho 1970). On the other hand Sica-Blanco et al. (1971) found no correlation between human oviductal activity and the ovarian cycle. Also the response of human oviduct *in vivo* to adrenergic stimulation has been the subject of disagreement. Although Maia and Coutinho (1970) reported that during the luteal phase stimulatory effects of NE on oviductal activity is diminished. Cibils et al. (1971) failed to find any differences in the oviductal response to this agent.

In an effort to clarify this question by quantitating the response *in vitro* and properly classify the tissues, we presented earlier a report of our findings (Moawad 1973). Our classification was based on the endometrial histology. We found that transmural field stimulation inhibits spontaneous activity in the luteal phase and during pregnancy. On the other hand the follicular phase was characterized by a varied response, i. e. stimulation in some tissues and inhibition in others. This present report resolves the question of this varied response in the proliferative phase and adds further evidence to the notion that adrenergic receptors in the oviduct are cyclically affected by both hormones, estrogen and progesterone.

In cases from the menstrual or follicular phases of the cycle where estrogen levels are low, the response to the endogenous neurotransmitters is mainly an inhibition. This response can gradually be reversed to that of a stimulation as the estrogen levels rise, as is the situation in the latter part of the follicular phase. This response subsequently will be replaced by inhibition as the progesterone levels rise following ovulation. This, however, does not occur until progesterone levels exceed 1.9 ng/ml. This lag period may be a necessary one until the effect of progesterone on the adrenergic receptors is fully realized.

An estrogen level of $(E_1/10 + E_2)$ around 48 is necessary before the stimulatory responses becomes apparent. However, this level is only an approximation.

There seems to be a stronger correlation between the frequency of contractions and the hormonal levels than with the other parameters. This is understandable since it is difficult to quantitate objectively these parameters because of the active spontaneous motility of the oviduct. Also during field stimulation an initial response may be later attenuated as the N. S. continues, since the NE stores and resynthesis become exhausted.

The dose response curve for epinephrine in both phases and also after

289

α-adrenergic blockade is the expected one. This lends more support to the notion that estrogen enhances α-adrenergic receptor activity.

Although the effect of the exogenous injection of estradiol did not noticeably modify the response to N.S., we think this may be due to two reasons. First, the study lacked proper evaluation of the hormonal status of the patients, since plasma E_1, E_2 and P were not determined prior to the injections. Second, the estrogens most probably require a longer period of time (more than 14 h) to exert their effects on the adrenergic receptors.

To summarize our conclusions concerning the α- and β-adrenergic receptors in this organ, one has to relate the hormonal levels to the hypothetical model of these receptors as represented in Fig. 14. The α-receptors are of low activity near the beginning and the end of the ovulatory cycle. These become enhanced during the period where the estrogen levels rise and before the progesterone levels become significantly high, i. e. late follicular and very early luteal phases. The β-receptors' activity on the other hand becomes enhanced in the presence of significant progesterone levels in the luteal phase. Perhaps this latter phenomenon plays an important role in the relaxation of the circular muscle, and consequently, opening of the isthmic lumen for the passage of the fertilized ovum.

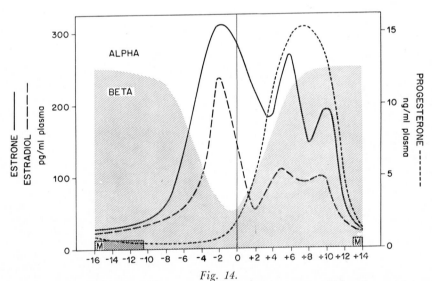

Fig. 14.

A graphic representation of the levels of estradiol (E_2), estrone (E_1) and progesterone in the ovulatory cycle. 0 day is day of ovulation. M = menstruation. The shaded area represents a hypothetical β-receptor predominance and the blank area represents the contribution of α-receptors.

In the experiments where we have measured ^{3}H-NE in the superfusate, we have shown that transmural nerve stimulation results in NE release in both the human and the rabbit. The inhibition of the NE release by the addition of PGE$_2$ is similar to the results obtained from other adrenergically innervated tissues, e. g. the vas deferens (Hedqvist 1974).

The response of the human oviduct to PGE$_2$ by enhancement of the N.S. induced contractions is unexpected. However this demonstrates the importance of species differences in the study of this organ. Also the resultant response might well be related to the hormonal background of the subject. Further detailed studies correlating the various responses to hormonal levels are therefore essential.

ACKNOWLEDGMENTS

This research was supported by grants from: The Rockefeller Foundation RF 70097, 72062; The Biomedical Center for Population Research PHS-HD-07110-04.

Correlation of the plasma levels of estrogens and progesterone with the *in vitro* responses to adrenergic stimulation was done in the Department of Obstetrics and Gynecology, University of Chicago. The radioimmunoassays of E$_1$, E$_2$ and P were done by Dr. Moon H. Kim. The recent experiments measuring the release of ^{3}H-NE and the effects of PGE$_2$ was done in the Physiology Department of the Karolinska Institute, Stockholm, in a collaborative effort between Dr. Atef H. Moawad and Dr. Per Hedqvist. The authors wish to thank Dr. Marc Bygdeman of the Karolinska Hospital for his help in making this study on human oviducts possible.

REFERENCES

Blandau R. J. (1969) Gamete transport – Comparative aspects. In: Hafez E. S. E. and Blandau R. J., eds. *The Mammalian Oviduct*, pp. 129–162. University of Chicago Press, Chicago.

Boling J. L. (1969) Endocrinology of Oviductal Musculature. In: Hafez E. S. E. and Blandau R. J., eds. *The Mammalian Oviduct*, pp. 163–181. University of Chicago Press, Chicago.

Cibils L. A., Sica-Blanco Y., Remedio M. R., Rozada H. and Gil B. E. (1971) Effect of sympathomimetic drugs upon the human oviduct *in vivo*. Amer. J. Obstet. Gynec. *110*, 481–488.

Croxatto H. B., Diaz S., Fuentealba B., Croxatto H. D., Carrillo D. and Fabres C. (1972). Studies on the duration of egg transport in the human oviduct. 1. The time interval between ovulation and egg recovery from the uterus in normal women. *Fertil. Steril. 23*, 447–458.

Dupon C., Hosseinian A. H. and Kim M. H. (1973) Simultaneous determination of plasma estrogens, androgens and progesterone during the human menstrual cycle. *Steroids 22*, 47–61.

Greenwald G. S. (1961) A study of the transport of ova through the rabbit oviduct. *Fertil. Steril. 12*, 80–95.

Harper M. J. K. (1965a) Transport of eggs in cumulus through the ampulla of the rabbit oviduct in relation to day of pseudopregnancy. *Endocrinology 77*, 114–123.

Harper M. J. K. (1965b) The effect of decreasing doses of estrogen and increasing doses of progesterone on the transport of artificial eggs through the reproductive tract of ovariectomized rabbits. *J. Endocrin. 31*, 217–226.

Hedqvist P. (1974) Prostaglandin action on noradrenaline release and mechanical responses in the stimulated guinea pig vas deferens. *Acta physiol. scand. 90*, 86–93.

Higgs G. and Moawad A. H. (1974) The effect of ovarian hormones on the contractility of the rabbit oviductal isthmus. *Canad. J. Physiol. Pharmacol. 52*, 74–83.

Hodgson B. J. and Pauerstein C. J. (1974) The effects of ovulation on the response of the rabbit oviduct to adrenergic agonists *in vitro*. *Biol. Reprod. 10*, 345–353.

Maia H. and Coutinho E. M. (1970) Peristalsis and antiperistalsis of the human Fallopian tube during the menstrual cycle. *Biol. Reprod. 2*, 305–314.

Moawad A. H. (1973) The effect of adrenergic drugs on the circular musculature of the isthmus of the human oviduct. Presented to the Society for Gynecologic Investigation, Twentieth Annual Meeting, Abstract # 59.

Moawad A. H. and Hedqvist P. (1975) Prostaglandin E$_2$ effect on noradrenaline release and mechanical responses to nerve stimulation in the rabbit and human oviduct. *Acta physiol. scand.*, in press.

Pauerstein C. J., Woodruff J. D. and Zachary A. S. (1968) Factors influencing physiologic activities in the Fallopian tube, the anatomy, physiology and pharmacology of tubal transport. *Obstet. gynec. Surv. 23*, 215–243.

Sica-Blanco Y., Cibils L. A., Remedio M. R., Rozada H. and Gil B. E. (1971) Isthmic and ampullary contractility of the human oviduct *in vitro*. *Amer. J. Obstet. Gynec. 111*, 91–97.

Department of Pharmacology, University of Alberta,
Edmonton, Alberta, Canada T6G 2H7

ADRENERGIC MECHANISMS IN RABBIT AND HUMAN OVIDUCTS

By

David M. Paton

ABSTRACT

Circular and longitudinal muscle of the ampulla and isthmus of rabbit oviduct always responded to transmural stimulation and to (–)-norepinephrine with a sustained contraction. Responses of the isthmus to (–)-norepinephrine were markedly potentiated by cocaine, desipramine and pretreatment with 6-hydroxydopamine suggesting that neuronal uptake of amine was the main route of inactivation. Longitudinal muscle of the isthmus was more sensitive to (–)-norepinephrine than circular muscle, and this differential sensitivity was abolished by cocaine and 6-hydroxydopamine. At 26°C, contractile responses of the circular muscle of the isthmus to transmural stimulation and to (–)-norepinephrine were very reproducible and were only slightly reduced by indomethacin. Responses to transmural stimulation were significantly reduced by prostaglandin E_2. At 37°C, spontaneous desensitization to both transmural stimulation and to (–)-norepinephrine occurred, and this desensitization was prevented by indomethacin. These findings suggest that the action of norepinephrine on the oviduct was not mediated through prostaglandin liberation, but that, at 37°C, spontaneous liberation of prostaglandins occurred and was responsible for the desensitization observed.

The response of all portions of the human oviduct to transmural stimulation and to (–)-norepinephrine was predominantly inhibitory (i. e., reduction in spontaneous contractility) during the mid and late phases of the menstrual cycles, whereas responses were more variable during the early phase of the cycle. These findings indicate that should the ampullary-isthmic junction indeed serve as a sphincter to regulate ovum transport, it would have to function quite differently in the human and rabbit oviducts.

Ova pass rapidly from the infundibulum to the ampullary-isthmic junction of the oviduct in all species studied, but their subsequent progression through the isthmic portion is very much slower (Pauerstein et al. 1974a). This delay in ovum transport appears to be required for subsequent implantation of the embryo. Elucidation of the mechanisms responsible for the regulation of ovum transport through the oviduct is, therefore, a very important priority for reproductive biologists.

The fluorescent histochemical technique for biogenic amines has demonstrated a dense adrenergic innervation to the circular muscle of the ampullary-isthmic junction of a number of species, including man and rabbit (Brundin 1965; Owman and Sjöberg 1966; Owman et al. 1967). The smooth muscle and blood vessels present in the rest of the isthmus receive adrenergic innervation, but to a lesser extent than at the junction. In the ampulla most adrenergic nerves are found in relation to the vasculature. The highest levels of norepinephrine are present in the distal isthmus of the rabbit oviduct and the lowest levels in the ampulla (Bodkhe and Harper 1972). These studies have thus provided evidence for a more dense adrenergic innervation to the isthmus and, in particular, to the circular muscle layer.

The presence of α excitatory and β inhibitory adrenergic receptors has been demonstrated in the oviducts of a number of species (for references see Brundin 1969; Pauerstein et al. 1974a). The studies of Pauerstein and his colleagues have shown that the activity of oviductal α- and β-receptors is subject to hormonal regulation (Pauerstein et al. 1973; Hodgson and Pauerstein 1974). As a result of these findings, it has been proposed that the adrenergic innervation of the isthmus functions as a sphincter under hormonal dominance and that this mechanism has an important role in the regulation of ovum transport (Brundin 1965; Pauerstein et al. 1974a).

In this paper, I have summarized the results of our studies of adrenergic mechanisms in rabbit and human oviducts. Further details are given in the following publications (Johns and Paton 1975[4], 1975a,b; Paton and Johns 1975a,b; Paton et al. 1975). Specifically we have examined the characteristics of the contractile responses of rabbit and human oviducts to field stimulation and to (–)-norepinephrine, the factors determining the magnitude of such responses in rabbit oviduct, and the influence of exogenous and endogenous prostaglandins on the responses of rabbit oviduct. In these studies, the isometric contractile responses of the circular and longitudinal muscle layers of ampulla and isthmus have been separately recorded under *in vitro* conditions.

MATERIALS AND METHODS

Preparation of rabbit oviduct and recording of contractile activity

New Zealand white rabbits (2.5–4 kg body weight) were injected daily with 100 μg 17β-estradiol subcutaneously for at least 5 days. Examination of vaginal smears showed that they were under estrogen dominance. After sacrifice, oviducts were placed in modified Krebs solution, the isthmic and ampullary portions of the oviduct identified and the surrounding connective and fatty tissue removed by fine dissection.

To record contractions of circular muscle, segments of the oviduct (approximately 2 mm) were cut and joined by thread, so as to form a chain. To record contractions of longitudinal muscle, the remainder of the oviduct was left intact. Tissues were mounted in 5 ml organ baths, maintained at 26°C unless otherwise stated, and bathed in a solution equilibrated with 95% O_2/5% CO_2. Contractions of both the longitudinally and circularly oriented smooth muscle preparations were recorded using force displacement transducers (Grass, model FT03C) connected to a Beckman RB dynograph or a Grass polygraph (Model 5D). A resting tension of 0.5 g was applied to all tissues.

The modified Krebs solution used had the following composition (mM): NaCl, 116; KCl, 5.4; $CaCl_2$, 0.5; $MgCl_2$, 2.4; NaH_2PO_4, 1.2; $NaHCO_3$, 22.0; D-glucose, 49.2. This medium and a temperature of 26°C was used because these conditions abolished spontaneous activity of the tissues.

Preparation of human oviduct and recording of contractile activity

Only macroscopically normal oviducts from women who had a history of regular menstrual cycles, were used. Segments of human oviduct were obtained from surgical specimens following oviductal ligations and abdominal hysterectomies at the time of surgery, and the tissues were placed in and transported in cooled Krebs solution. The tissues were carefully dissected free of any surrounding blood vessels and connective tissue, and the isthmic and ampullary portions of the oviduct identified. The isthmic and ampullary portion of the oviduct were then cut into three segments, measuring 2 mm ($\times$ 2) and 4 mm in length. To allow recording of circular muscle activity, the two smaller segments were joined with thread so as to form a chain. The third piece was left intact and was suspended longitudinally. Preparations of both isthmic and ampullary tissue were set up under 1.0 g tension in 5 ml organ baths perfused with Krebs solution. The solution was equilibrated with 95 % O_2/5 % CO_2 and maintained at 26°C, and had the following composition (mM): NaCl, 116; KCl, 5.4; $CaCl_2$, 2.5; $MgCl_2$, 1.2; NaH_2PO_4, 1.2; $NaHCO_3$, 22.0; D-glucose, 49.2. The isometric tension developed by each smooth muscle preparation was measured with force displacement transducers (Grass FT03C) and displayed on a polygraph (Grass 5D).

Determination of responses to agonists

Tissues were allowed to equilibrate for 30 min after being suspended before responses to agonists were studied. Second response curves to agonists were begun at least 20 min after completion of the first. Cocaine, desipramine and other agents were present throughout this period. Tissues were exposed to agonists until a maximal response to that concentration was obtained.

Non-cumulative concentration response curves to (−)-norepinephrine were determined using at least 5 rabbits for each study. The responses to different concentrations of (−)-norepinephrine were expressed as a percentage of the maximal response to the tissue. Log-concentration/response curves were plotted from the means of the results, and ED_{50} values calculated by interpolation on the mean log-concentration/response curves.

Determination of responses to transmural stimulation

Transmural stimulation was achieved using a Grass stimulator (model S6C) which supplied biphasic pulses of 1.0 msec duration and at supramaximal voltage and current of 150 mA for 60 sec (rabbit tissue) or 180 sec (human tissue). The tissues were placed between platinum electrodes at the top and bottom of the organ baths. The results are expressed as a percentage of the tissues' maximal response to either transmural stimulation or to a maximal concentration of (−)-norepinephrine, determined during the first determination of the response curve for the tissue.

Determination of accumulation of [³H](±)-metaraminol by rabbit and human oviducts

Portions of ampulla and isthmus from rabbit and human oviducts were prepared as described previously and exposed to 5×10^{-8} M [³H](±)-metaraminol for 30 min. At the end of this period, the total [³H] content of tissues was determinated by liquid scintillation spectrometry as described previously (Paton 1973).

RESULTS

A. *Characteristics of responses of rabbit oviduct to field stimulation*

Circular and longitudinal muscle of both the ampulla and isthmus of rabbit oviduct always responded to field stimulation with a sustained contraction. Responses to field stimulation resulted from release of norepinephrine and not from direct excitation of muscle since responses were abolished by 5×10^{-5} M guanethidine, 8.9×10^{-6} M phentolamine and 5×10^{-7} M tetrodotoxin, and by chronic pretreatment with 6-hydroxydopamine. Responses to field stimulation

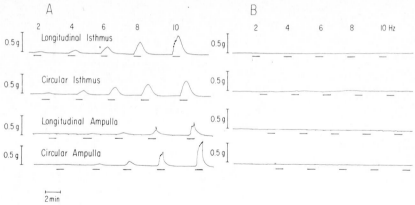

Fig. 1.

The effect of guanethidine (5×10^{-5} M) on the responses of rabbit oviduct to transmural stimulation. (A) shows the normal responses to differing frequencies of stimulation. (B) shows the responses in the presence of guanethidine.

From Johns and Paton (1975a), with the permission of the Publisher.

were maximal at 16–20 Hz. 3.9×10^{-6} M Propranolol did not modify responses to field stimulation showing that responses resulted almost entirely from an action on α-adrenergic receptors. Fig. 1 illustrates the nature of the response of estrogen-dominant tissue to field stimulation. The responses of progesterone-dominant tissue were not studied in detail, but again all portions of the oviduct responded to field stimulation with a sustained contraction.

B. *Characteristics of responses of human oviduct to field stimulation and sympathomimetic amines*

Field stimulation (5, 10 or 20 Hz) caused predominantly a decrease in the amplitude of spontaneous contractility of tissues obtained during the midcycle (Days 11–15) and late cycle (Day 15 on), and this was sometimes associated with a decrease in tension. Field stimulation of tissues obtained during the early phase of the cycle (Days 1–10) caused a more varied response. There was usually no response at 5 Hz, while at 10 or 20 Hz the most common response was a reduction in spontaneous contractility, but sometimes the response was excitatory. Inhibitory responses to field stimulation were blocked by 1.9×10^{-5} M propranolol and 5×10^{-5} M guanethidine. In general, longitudinal muscle was more responsive to field stimulation while the ampulla was more sensitive than the isthmus.

The response of all portions of the oviduct to $6 \times 10^{-7} - 3 \times 10^{-5}$ M (–)-nor-epinephrine was inhibitory in nature (i. e., a reduction in the amplitude of spontaneous contractility and/or tension), but tissues from the early phase of the cycle were less responsive. Such inhibitory responses were inhibited or reversed by 1.9×10^{-5} M propranolol. $6 \times 10^{-7} - 3 \times 10^{-5}$ M (–)-Phenylephrine generally had no effect or produced a very small contractile response at the highest concentrations used. Tachyphylaxis to such responses was noted. 4.7×10^{-6} M (±)-Isoproterenol always caused partial or total inhibition of spontaneous mechanical activity. 7.3×10^{-5} M p-Tyramine usually produced a biphasic response, consisting of initial excitation followed by a sustained contraction of both ampullary and isthmic tissue. Responses to p-tyramine were abolished or reduced by 5×10^{-5} M guanethidine. Certain of these features are illustrated in Figs. 2 and 3.

The finding that responses to field stimulation were inhibited by guanethidine and propranolol indicates that they resulted from the release of norepinephrine. Responses of all portions of the human oviduct, at all phases of the cycle, were predominantly inhibitory and these effects were reduced by propranolol showing that the responses were predominantly mediated through an action on β inhibitory adrenergic receptors.

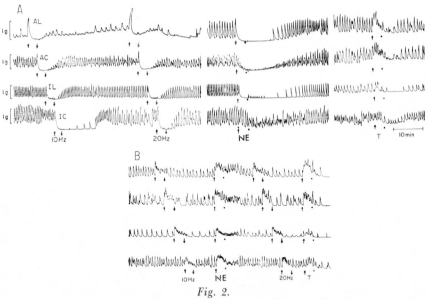

Fig. 2.

Effect of propranolol on responses to transmural stimulation and amines. Late phase of menstrual cycle. Responses were obtained to: transmural stimulation (10 Hz); 1.2×10^{-5} M (–)-norepinephrine (NE); 7.3×10^{-5} M p-tyramine (T). A: control responses; B: responses in the presence of 5×10^{-5} M guanethidine. ↑: start of transmural stimulation, or addition of drug; ↓: end of transmural stimulation; •: drug washed out. AL: longitudinal muscle of ampulla; AC: circular muscle of ampulla; IL: longitudinal muscle of isthmus; TC: circular muscle of isthmus.

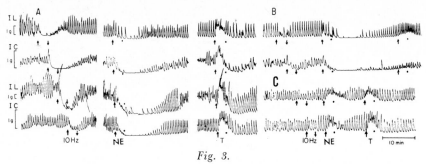

Fig. 3.

Effects of guanethidine and propranolol on response to transmural stimulation and drugs. Mid-phase of menstrual cycle. A: control responses; B: responses in presence of 5×10^{-5} M guanethidine; C: responses in presence of 1.9×10^{-5} M propranolol. Other details as in Fig. 2.

C. *Factors modifying the magnitude of the responses of the isthmus of the rabbit oviduct to (–)-norepinephrine and field stimulation*

Circular and longitudinal muscle of the isthmic portion of oviducts from estrogen-dominant rabbits responded to (–)-norepinephrine with a sustained contractile response. At 26°C, such responses were reproducible. Responses to (–)-norepinephrine were not altered by 3.9×10^{-6} M propranolol showing that the effect was almost entirely α in nature. Responses were markedly potentiated by 3×10^{-5} M cocaine and by chronic pre-treatment with 6-hydroxydopamine, and to a lesser extent by 10^{-7} M desipramine, but were not altered by 3×10^{-5} M hydrocortisone, 10^{-5} M U-0521 or 10^{-4} M oxytetracycline. These findings indicate that the magnitude of responses to (–)-norepinephrine was influenced by the neuronal uptake of amine since cocaine, desipramine and pre-treatment with 6-hydroxydopamine all inhibit the uptake of norepinephrine by adrenergic neurones and this is generally considered to account for the supersensitivity produced by these agents (Trendelenburg 1972). Extraneuronal uptake or binding of norepinephrine is not apparently an important determinant of the magnitude of responses to the amine since responses were not altered by hydrocortisone, U-0521 and oxytetracycline, agents that inhibit these processes (Kaumann 1970; Powis 1973). The results of these studies are summarized in Table 1.

Longitudinal muscle of the isthmus was more sensitive to (–)-norepinephrine than circular muscle. This difference was abolished by cocaine and 6-hydroxy-dopamine, providing evidence that the magnitude of responses of circular muscle was more influenced by neuronal uptake of amine. This is in keeping with the greater degree of adrenergic innervation to the circular muscle layer described by other workers.

Contractile responses of the circular muscle of the estrogen-dominant isthmus to field stimulation were not altered by 3.9×10^{-6} M propranolol. In marked

Table 1.

Effect of drugs on the sensitivity of the isthmus of rabbit oviduct to (–)-norepinephrine.

Drug treatment	ED_{50} values (M)			
	Circular muscle		Longitudinal muscle	
	Control	Treated	Control	Treated
—	4.7×10^{-6}	–	1.8×10^{-6}**	–
3.9×10^{-6} M propranolol	5.9×10^{-6}	4.7×10^{-6}	4.0×10^{-6}	2.6×10^{-6}
3×10^{-5} M cocaine	7.4×10^{-6}	5.6×10^{-7}*	1.4×10^{-6}	2.9×10^{-7}*
10^{-6} M desipramine	3.4×10^{-6}	1.2×10^{-6}*	1.6×10^{-6}	9.0×10^{-7}
3×10^{-5} M hydrocortisone $+ 3 \times 10^{-5}$ M U-0521	5.6×10^{-6}	6.0×10^{-6}	7.0×10^{-6}	7.0×10^{-6}
10^{-4} M oxytetracycline	5.6×10^{-6}	6.0×10^{-6}	7.0×10^{-6}	4.0×10^{-6}
6-hydroxydopamine	4.0×10^{-7}***	–	4.5×10^{-7}***	–
6-hydroxydopamine $+ 3 \times 10^{-5}$ M cocaine	4.0×10^{-7}	4.5×10^{-7}	4.7×10^{-7}	3.7×10^{-7}

Isometric contractions of circular and longitudinal muscle were recorded separately using estrogen-dominant tissue. Non-cumulative dose/response curves to (–)-norepinephrine were determined, using at least 5 animals in each study. ED_{50} values were calculated by interpolation on the mean log-concentration response curves. $P < 0.05$, compared to control* or to circular muscle**, or to untreated muscle***.

contrast to responses to (–)-norepinephrine, responses to field stimulation were not potentiated by $2 \times 10^{-6} - 3 \times 10^{-5}$ M cocaine and, in fact, at 3×10^{-5} M were partially inhibited. The inability of cocaine to potentiate such responses may have resulted from the local anaesthetic action of the drug and potentiated a inhibitory feedback on release, both causing a reduction in the amount of amine released. Following its release from adrenergic nerves, norepinephrine partially inhibits further release by an action on presynaptic a-receptors and it is likely that cocaine would greatly potentiate this effect by preventing the neuronal uptake of the transmitter (Langer 1974). The time required for relaxation after field stimulation was, however, significantly prolonged by 10^{-6} M cocaine.

D. *Characteristics of accumulation of [³H](±)-metaraminol by rabbit and human oviducts*

[³H](±)-Metaraminol was accumulated against the concentration gradient, in both the ampulla and isthmus of human and rabbit oviducts. In human tissue, accumulation was inhibited by 10^{-5} M (–)-norepinephrine, 3×10^{-5} M cocaine and

10^{-4} M ouabain but not by 10^{-5} M ($\pm$)-normetanephrine or 10^{-4} M oxytetracycline. The characteristics of accumulation of $[^3H](\pm)$-metaraminol by human ampulla and isthmus are thus similar to the accumulation of norepinephrine and metaraminol by adrenergic nerves in other tissues (Paton 1976). In rabbit tissue, accumulation was inhibited by 3×10^{-5} M cocaine and to a lesser extent by 10^{-7} M desipramine, but not by U-0521, hydrocortisone or oxytetracycline, providing additional evidence that cocaine and desipramine potentiated responses to (–)-norepinephrine by inhibiting neuronal uptake of the amine. $[^3H](\pm)$-Metaraminol was used in these studies because it has a high affinity for the membrane uptake site in adrenergic neurones utilized by noradrenaline, and does not undergo metabolic degradation as it is not a substrate for monoamine oxidase or catechol-O-methyl transferase (Paton 1976).

E. *Evidence for spontaneous liberation of prostaglandins by rabbit oviduct*

At 26°C, the contractile responses of the circular muscle of the isthmus of estrogen-dominant rabbit oviduct to field stimulation and to (–)-norepinephrine were very reproducible and consistent with little evidence of desensitization. Such responses were only slightly reduced by 5.6×10^{-5} M indomethacin. At 26°C, 10 ng/ml prostaglandin E_2 significantly reduced responses to field stimulation but had little effect on responses to (–)-norepinephrine.

At 37°C, spontaneous desensitization to both field stimulation and to (–)-norepinephrine occurred, but field stimulation was more inhibited. Addition of 2.8×10^{-6} M indomethacin prevented this desensitization (see Figs. 4 and 5).

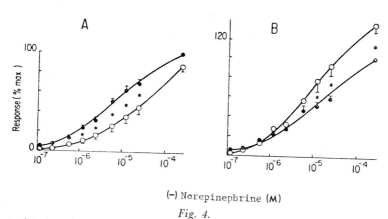

(–) Norepinephrine (M)

Fig. 4.

Effect of indomethacin on responses to (–)-norepinephrine at 37°C. First response curves (●——●) determined 45 min before the second curve (o——o). A, control. B, second response curve in the presence of 2.8×10^{-6} M indomethacin, n = 5. From Paton and Johns (1975b), with the permission of the Publisher.

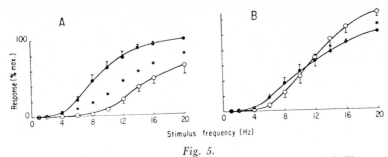

Fig. 5.

Effect of indomethacin on responses to transmural stimulation at 37°C. First response curves (●——●), determined 45 min before the second curves (o——o). A, control. B, second response curve in the presence of 2.8×10^{-6} M indomethacin, n = 5. From Paton and Johns (1975b), with the permission of the Publisher.

It has been suggested that, following its release from adrenergic nerves, norepinephrine activates α-receptors in the oviduct causing the release of prostaglandins of the F series which in turn stimulate the circular muscle of the oviduct (Spilman and Harper 1974). However, indomethacin, an inhibitor of prostaglandin synthesis (Ferreira and Vane 1974), did not abolish responses to (–)-norepinephrine or field stimulation suggesting that the action of norepinephrine on oviductal α-receptors is not mediated through prostaglandin liberation.

Adrenergic transmission to the oviduct was inhibited by exogenous prostaglandin E_2 and thus is similar to the situation in other adrenergically innervated preparations (Hedqvist 1974). The most striking observation was the marked desensitization that developed at 37°C to both field stimulation and to (–)-norepinephrine. The finding that this desensitization was completely abolished by indomethacin suggests that it resulted from the spontaneous generation of prostaglandins, presumably of the E series.

DISCUSSION

These studies have shown that the responses to exogenous (–)-norepinephrine and to field stimulation in rabbit oviduct are predominantly excitatory due to activation of α-receptors, whereas in the human oviduct, responses are predominantly inhibitory due to activation of β-receptors. In addition, the responses of ampulla and isthmus, and of circular and longitudinal muscle were always qualitatively similar and were not hormonally dependent. These findings are difficult to reconcile with any differential sphincteric mechanism at the ampullary-isthmic junction or in the isthmus, and certainly such a sphincter would have to function quite differently in the rabbit and human oviducts.

The responses of the rabbit oviduct we observed are qualitatively similar to those reported by other workers (Levy and Lindner 1972; Hodgson and Pauerstein 1974). However, the human oviduct has variously been reported to respond to norepinephrine with an excitatory response (Nakanishi et al. 1967), with excitation followed by inhibition (Senior and Spencer-Gregson 1969), or to be unresponsive (Zetler et al. 1969). Perivascular nerve stimulation produced a contraction of the mid-portion of the human oviduct (Nakanishi et al. 1967). This qualitative difference may possibly be accounted for by differences in experimental technique since these workers used a temperature of $36°C$, contractions were recorded isotonically and the stimulation period was usually 10 sec in duration.

A number of other studies have also cast doubt on the role of adrenergic transmission in ovum transport. Treatment with 6-hydroxydopamine to cause degeneration of peripheral adrenergic nerves, did not significantly modify fertility in mice and rats (MacDonald and Airaksinen 1974; Johns et al. 1975), and surgical denervation, produced by autotransplantation of the oviduct and ovary, did not prevent pregnancy in rabbits (Winston and McClure Browne 1974). Ovum transport in rabbits was not altered by pretreatment with 6-hydroxydopamine (Eddy and Black 1974; Pauerstein et al. 1974b) or by surgical denervation or systemic administration of reserpine (Bodkhe and Harper 1972; Pauerstein et al. 1974b). All of these different approaches have indicated that ovum transport and subsequent implantation can proceed apparently normally despite a very marked reduction in the adrenergic innervation to the oviduct. If should be noted, however, that after surgical and chemical denervation smooth muscle is supersensitive to norepinephrine (Trendelenburg 1972; Johns and Paton 1974). This postsynaptic effect may partially compensate for the loss of peripheral innervation since there will still be circulating norepinephrine and epinephrine, released from the adrenal medulla.

Our findings indicate that neuronal uptake is the most important route of inactivation for norepinephrine in the isthmus of the rabbit oviduct and this is also true of the ampulla (Johns and Paton, unpublished observations). The oviduct is thus similar to many other adrenergically innervated tissues in which neuronal uptake normally predominates: Extraneuronal uptake and metabolism usually only becomes the major route of inactivation for norepinephrine when neuronal uptake is impaired by drugs or is abolished by denervation (Trendelenburg 1972).

Prostaglandins have been demonstrated in the human oviduct (Ogra et al. 1974). Prostaglandins are spontaneously released from a number of smooth muscle preparations, and appear to be involved in the inherent smooth muscular activity of such tissues, e. g., rat uterus (Williams et al. 1974). It is particularly noteworthy therefore that the contractility of the isthmus of the rabbit oviduct, under estrogen dominance, appears to be inhibited by spontaneous generation

303

of prostaglandins. This is a particularly important observation in view of the suggestion that prostaglandins may be involved in the regulation of ovum transport (Spilman and Harper 1974). Further research is required to demonstrate conclusively that prostaglandins are indeed spontaneously liberated from the oviduct; to determine their effects on, and role in, the generations of spontaneous electrical and mechanical activity observed in human oviductal smooth muscle (Daniel et al. 1975), and to establish whether their synthesis and liberation is hormonally dependent.

ACKNOWLEDGMENTS

It is a pleasure to acknowledge the contributions of Dr. A. Johns and Drs. S. Molnar who were responsible for much of the work reviewed here. I also wish to thank Dr. E. E. Daniel for his collaboration in the studies of the contractile responses of human oviduct. These studies were supported by grants from the World Health Organization and the Medical Research Council of Canada (Grant MT 2472).

REFERENCES

Bodkhe R. R. and Harper M. J. K. (1972) Changes in the amount of adrenergic neurotransmitter in the genital tract of untreated rabbits and rabbits given reserpine or iproniazid during the time of egg transport. *Biol. Reprod. 6*, 288–299.

Brundin J. (1965) Distribution and function of adrenergic nerves in the rabbit Fallopian tube. *Acta physiol. scand. 66*, Suppl. 259, 1–57.

Brundin J. (1965) Pharmacology of the oviduct. In: Hafez E. S. E. and Blandau R. J., eds. *The Mammalian Oviduct*, pp. 251–270. University of Chicago Press, Chicago.

Daniel E. E., Lucien P., Posey V. A. and Paton D. M. (1975) A functional analysis of the myogenic control systems of the human Fallopian tube. *Amer. J. Obstet. Gynec. 121*, 1046–1053.

Eddy C. A. and Black D. L. (1972) Chemical sympathectomy of the rabbit oviduct using 6-hydroxydopamine. *J. Reprod. Fertil. 33*, 1–9.

Ferreira S. H. and Vane J. R. (1974) New aspects of the mode of action of non-steroid anti-inflammatory drugs. *Ann. Rev. Pharmacol. 14*, 57–74.

Hedqvist P. (1974) Restriction of transmitter release from adrenergic nerves mediated by prostaglandins and α-adrenoreceptors *Pol. J. Pharmacol. Pharmac. 26*, 119–125.

Hodgson B. J. and Pauerstein C. J. (1974) The effect of ovulation on the responses of the rabbit oviduct to adrenergic agonists *in vitro*. *Biol. Reprod. 10*, 346–353.

Johns A., Chlumecky J., Cottle M. K. W. and Paton D. M. (1975) Effect of chemical sympathectomy and adrenergic agonists on the fertility of mice. *Contraception 11*, 563–570.

Johns A. and Paton D. M. (1974) Drug-induced changes in the sensitivity of the isthmus of rabbit oviduct to noradrenaline. *Brit. J. Pharmacol. 52*, 127P.

Johns A. and Paton D. M. (1975a) Pharmacological characteristics of the responses of rabbit oviduct to transmural stimulation. *Arch. int. Pharmacodyn. Therap.*, in press.

Johns A. and Paton D. M. (1975b) Effect of cocaine and other drugs on sensitivity of the oestrogen-dominated isthmus of rabbit oviduct to noradrenaline. *Canad. J. Physiol. Pharmacol.*, in press.

Kalsner S. (1975) Role of extraneuronal mechanisms on the termination of contractile responses to amines in vascular tissue. *Brit. J. Pharmacol. 53*, 267–277.

Kaumann A. J. (1970) Adrenergic receptors in heart muscle: relations among factors influencing the sensitivity of the cat papillary muscle to catecholamines. *J. Pharmacol. exp. Ther. 173*, 383–398.

Langer S. Z. (1974) Presynaptic regulation of catecholamine release. *Biochem. Pharmacol. 23*, 1793–1800.

Levy B. and Lindner H. R. (1972) The effect of adrenergic drugs on the rabbit oviduct. *Eur. J. Pharmacol. 18*, 15–21.

MacDonald E. J. and Airaksinen M. M. (1974) The effect of 6-hydroxydopamine on the oestrus and fertility of rats. *J. Pharm. Pharmacol. 26*, 518–521.

Nakanishi H., Wansbrough H. and Wood C. (1967) Postganglionic sympathetic nerve innervating human Fallopian tube. *Amer. J. Physiol. 213*, 613–619.

Ogra S. S., Kirton K. T., Tomasi T. B. and Lippes J. (1974) Prostaglandins in the human Fallopian tube. *Fertil. Steril. 25*, 250–255.

Owman C., Rosengren E. and Sjöberg N.-O. (1967) Adrenergic innervation of the human reproductive organs; a histochemical and chemical investigation. *Obstet. Gynec. 30*, 763–773.

Owman C. and Sjöberg N.-O. (1966) Adrenergic nerves in the female genital tract of the rabbit. With remarks on cholinesterase-containing structure. *Z. Zellforsch. 74*, 182–197.

Paton D. M. (1973) Mechanism of efflux of noradrenaline from adrenergic nerves in rabbit atria. *Brit. J. Pharmacol. 49*, 614–627.

Paton D. M. (Editor) (1976) *The Mechanism of the Neuronal and Extraneuronal Trans of Catecholamines.* Raven Press (New York).

Paton D. M. and Johns A. (1975a) Characteristics of uptake of [³H] (±)-metaraminol by human Fallopian tube. *Res. Comm. Chem. Path. Pharmac. 10*, 267–272.

Paton D. M. and Johns A. (1975b) Effects of prostaglandin E_2 and indomethacin on responses of the isthmus of rabbit oviduct to norepinephrine and transmural stimulation. *Res. Comm. Chem. Path. Pharmacol. 11*, 15–24.

Paton D. M., Johns A., Molnar S., Daniel E. E. and Beck R. P. (1975) Characteristics of responses of human and rabbit Fallopian tube to field stimulation and noradrenaline. *Proc. West. Pharmac. Soc. 18*, 208–211.

Pauerstein C. J., Fremming B. D., Hodgson B. J. and Martin J. E. (1973) The promise of pharmacological modification of ovum transport in contraceptive development. *Amer. J. Obstet. Gynec. 116*, 161–166.

Pauerstein C. J., Hodgson B. J. and Kramen M. (1974a) The anatomy and physiology of the Fallopian tube. *Obstetrics & Gynecology Annual 1974*, 138–201.

Pauerstein C. J., Hodgson B. J., Fremming B. D. and Martin J. E. (1974b) Effects of sympathetic denervation on normal ovum transport and on transport modified by estrogen and progesterone. *Gynec. Invest. 5*, 121–132.

Powis G. (1973) Binding of catecholamines to connective tissue and the effect upon responses of blood vessels to noradrenaline and to nerve stimulation. *J. Physiol. (Lond.) 234*, 145–162.

305

Senior J. B. and Spencer-Gregson R. N. (1969) The effects of sympathomimetic drugs and bradykinin on the human Fallopian tube *in vitro* using isometric recording methods. *J. Obstet. Gynaec. Brit. Cwlth 76,* 652–655.

Spilman C. H. and Harper M. J. K. (1974) Comparison of the effects of adrenergic drugs and prostaglandins on rabbit oviduct motility. *Biol. Reprod. 10,* 549–554.

Trendelenburg U. (1972) Factors influencing the concentration of catecholamines at the receptors. In: Blaschko H. and Muscholl E., eds. *Catecholamines, Handb. exp. Pharmac.* N. S. Vol. 33, pp. 726–761. Springer-Verlag, Berlin and Heidelberg.

Williams K. I., Sneddon J. M. and Harvey P. J. (1974) Prostaglandin production by the pregnant rat uterus *in vitro* and its relevance to parturition. *Pol. J. Pharmacol. Pharm. 26,* 207–215.

Winston R. M. L. and McClure Browne J. C. (1974) Pregnancy following autograft transplantation of Fallopian tube and ovary in the rabbit. *Lancet 2,* 494–495.

Zetler G., Monkemeier D. and Wiechell H. (1969) Stimulation of Fallopian tubes by prostaglandin $F_{2\alpha}$, biogenic amines and peptides. *J. Reprod. Fertil. 18,* 147–149.

Shionogi Research Laboratory, Shionogi & Co., Ltd.,
Fukushima-ku, Osaka, Japan

ADRENERGIC MECHANISMS
AND HORMONAL STATUS OF THE OVIDUCT

By

Hiroshi Takeda and Masami Doteuchi

ABSTRACT

It has been confirmed that hormonal status and autonomic innervation
are major factors controlling oviductal motility. The oviduct from estrogen-dominated rabbits had greater mechanical activity compared with
that of progesterone-dominated or untreated castrated rabbits. The oviduct was densely innervated by the sympathetic nervous system. Results
from a series of pharmacological experiments indicated that a) the α-
adrenoceptors mediated oviductal contraction, b) the β-adrenoceptors
mediated oviductal relaxation, and c) there was no pharmacological evidence for cholinergic innervation. However, acetylcholine produced a
contractile response of the oviduct. With a view to investigating the
correlation of these two factors, the influence of hormonal status upon
adrenergic mechanism was studied relating to turnover, uptake, distribution etc. of catecholamine.

A number of studies have been made on the mechanisms controlling the motility
of the oviduct which, at least partially, regulates the rate of ova transport. The
histochemical technique (Falck and Owman 1965), which demonstrated the
presence of adrenergic neurons densely innervating the oviductal smooth muscle
(Brundin 1965; Owman et al. 1966; Takeda et al. 1968), allowed us to investigate
the adrenergic control of oviductal motility. In the present paper, we have
attempted to summarize our current studies of the adrenergic mechanisms and
hormonal influences on the mechanical activity of the rabbit oviduct.

1) *Autonomic control of oviductal motility*

The rabbit oviduct consists of two major smooth muscle layers, i. e. inner circular and outer longitudinal muscle. In addition to these, another longitudinal muscle layer (intraligamentary muscle) exists in the broad ligament layer connecting the uterine end of the oviduct and the ovary (Novak 1957; Takeda et al. 1968; Halbert and Conrad 1975). The nature of this muscle will be described later. Adrenergic innervations of the oviduct and their origins have been studied extensively (Owman et al. 1966; Takeda 1969), and the presence of adrenergic receptors was also evident from the responses of the oviduct to catecholamines (Nakanishi and Wood 1968; Howe and Black 1973). In *in vitro* experiments, oviducts show spontaneous rhythmical contractions, and are sensitive to adrenergic stimulation (Ueda et al. 1973).

Responses of the oviduct to nerve stimulation and autonomic drugs are summarized in Table 1. The concluding remarks from these results in regard to adrenergic mechanisms are as follows. In the oviduct there exist both α-(excitatory) and β-(inhibitory) adrenoreceptors, and under normal conditions the former usually mask the latter. The nature of perivascular and hypogastric nerves was found to be post- and pre-ganglionic respectively. Contrary to the excellent agreement between the rich adrenergic innervation based on histochemical data and the marked sensitivity of the oviduct to catecholamines, the cholinergic system appears to be complicated. The enhancement of mechanical activity of the oviduct due to adrenergic stimulation is characterized by increase of contraction-frequency, augmentation of contraction-amplitude, and elevation

Table 1.

Responses of the oviduct to nerve stimulation and autonomic drugs.

	Stimulation	Response	Pre-treatment	Influence
Sympathetic	Norepinephrine			
			Ganglion-blocker	(–)
			Ganglion-stimulant	(–)
	Perivascular nerve		Norepinephrine	Enhanced
		Contraction	α-blocker	Reverse to relax.
			α-blocker & β-blocker	No response
	Hypogastric nerve		Ganglion-blocker	Suppressed
Cholinergic	Perivascular nerve		Atropine	(–)
	Ach.			Suppressed
	Perivascular nerve		Physostigmine	(–)
	Ach.			Enhanced

of muscle tone. The details of these enhancement-patterns which varied according to the kind of muscular layer and hormonal content will be described in the next section.

2) *Hormonal influences on oviductal motility*

Hormonal status is also an essential factor which significantly affects oviductal motility. The mechanical activity of oviducts taken from rabbits treated with estrogen after ovariectomy was higher than the activity of those taken

OVARIECTOMIZED

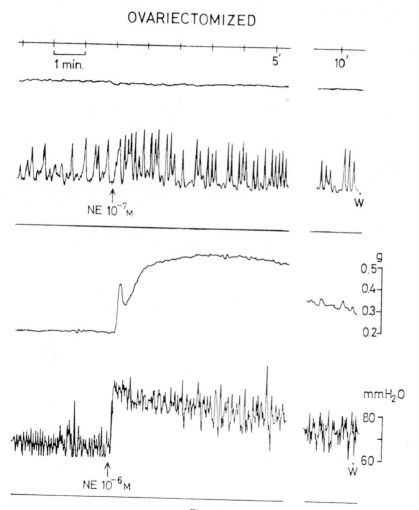

Fig. 1.

Effects of norepinephrine on the oviduct of ovariectomized rabbit.
upper trace: longitudinal muscle
lower trace: circular muscle

from progesterone-treated or castrated animals (Takeda 1969). However, Ichijo
(1960) observed spontaneous motility of the circular muscle in oviducts with
higher amplitude from progesterone-treated animals than estrogen-treated animals. Generally speaking, results varied from report to report. These differences
might be due to the kind of experiments, hormonal treatment, animal species
etc. We fixed the schedule of hormonal treatment as follows:

Estrogen-treated group: one week after ovariectomy, animals were given
intramuscularly 5 μg 17β-estradiol daily for five days.

Progesterone-treated group: one week after ovariectomy, animals were given
5 μg 17β-estradiol daily for three days, then 1.5 μg 17β-estradiol and 1 mg
progesterone daily for another five days.

Twenty-four h after the last injection of these hormones, the animals were
killed and tissues were isolated.

ESTROGEN

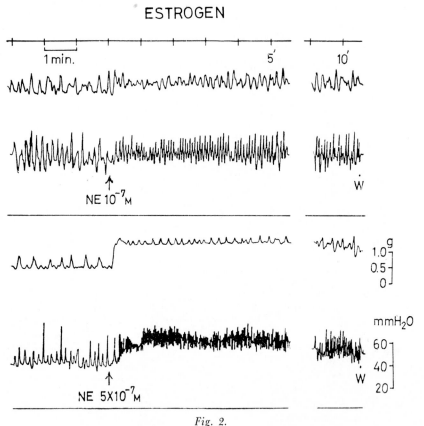

Fig. 2.
Effects of norepinephrine on the estrogen-dominated oviduct.
upper trace: longitudinal muscle
lower trace: circular muscle

PROGESTERONE

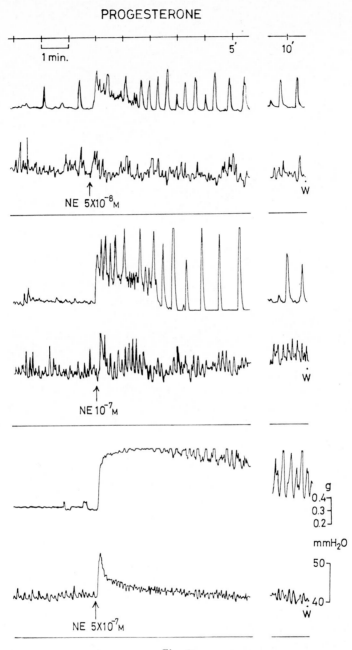

Fig. 3.
Effects of norepinephrine on the progesterone-dominated oviduct.
upper trace: longitudinal muscle
lower trace: circular muscle

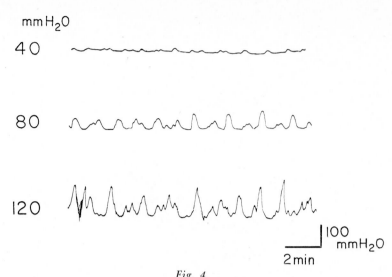

mmH$_2$O

40

80

120

|100 mmH$_2$O

2 min

Fig. 4.

Spontaneous motility of the oviductal circular muscle at various resting pressures.

Figs. 1, 2 and 3 show the simultaneous records of isometric contraction of oviductal longitudinal muscle and changes in intraluminal pressure caused by contraction of the circular muscle under various hormonal states *in vitro*. An initial intraluminal load of suitable pressure, i. e. resting tension, was necessary to obtain stable spontaneous contraction of both muscles. The correlation between resting tension and the pattern of contractions is illustrated in Fig. 4.

a) *Spontaneous activity.* – Spontaneous contractions of the longitudinal muscle were scarcely detectable from the oviducts of ovariectomized animals, whereas estrogen-dominated preparations showed rhythmical contractions with high frequency. The longitudinal oviductal muscle of progesterone-dominated animals showed intermittent contractions with fairly high amplitude.

Regarding the spontaneous contractions of the oviductal circular muscle, there were almost no differences between the three groups, except that some regularity was observed in the estrogen-dominated group as compared with the other two groups.

b) *Contractile responses to norepinephrine.* – Studies concerning the responses of the oviduct to norepinephrine have been well established, since norepinephrine is a neurotransmitter in mammalian oviducts (Brundin 1965; Nakanishi et al. 1967).

When 10^{-7} M norepinephrine was added *in vitro* to the oviducts of estrogen-dominated animals, the frequency of contraction of the circular muscle was markedly increased (Fig. 2), but response of the longitudinal muscle to concentrations of norepinephrine up to 5×10^{-7} M seemed rather weak and was no more than an elevation of muscular tone. The progesterone-dominated oviducts also responded to low concentrations of norepinephrine, but there were marked differences in the pattern of response between progesterone- and estrogen-dominated preparations. In progesterone-dominated cases, following a low concentration (5×10^{-8} M) of norepinephrine, a marked increase in frequency of contractions of the longitudinal muscle occurred simultaneously with an increase in amplitude. This is contrary to estrogen-dominated preparations. However, in the circular muscle, 5×10^{-7} M norepinephrine caused only an elevation of intraluminal pressure, and the response was found to be short-lasting.

Recently using the slope of the dose-response curve as an index of the reactivity it has been reported that the reactivity of adrenoreceptors of oviductal circular muscle is higher under estrogen-domination than under progesterone-domination (Hunter and Kendle 1974). If, however, the minimum dose of

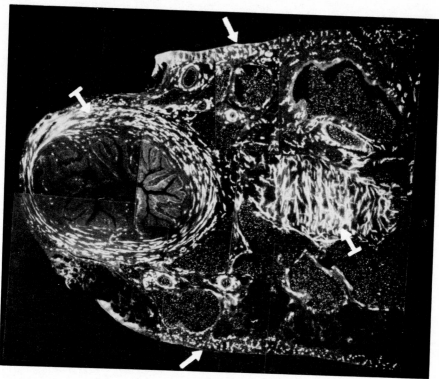

Fig. 5.
Photomontage of fluorescent fibers in peri-oviductal and oviductal smooth muscles.
↕: circular muscle layer
↑: intra-ligamentary muscle layer

313

norepinephrine required to produce a detectable response can be used as an index of sensitivity of receptor to neurotransmitter, the present data can be considered to indicate that there is no significant difference between estrogen- and progesterone-dominated groups. We still do not know the cause of the difference in norepinephrine-induced response due to hormonal states, but we can presume it to originate from the activity of smooth muscle, and not nervous activity or adrenoceptor.

3) *Histochemical and biochemical studies of norepinephrine in the oviduct*

Histochemical demonstration of the norepinephrine containing nerves in the oviduct revealed their distribution and origins (Brundin 1965; Owman and Sjöberg 1966; Sjöberg 1967). In this paper, we present evidence for the existence of adrenergic innervation of the intra-ligamentary muscle. As shown in Fig. 5, intensely fluorescent adrenergic fibers can be seen running along the smooth

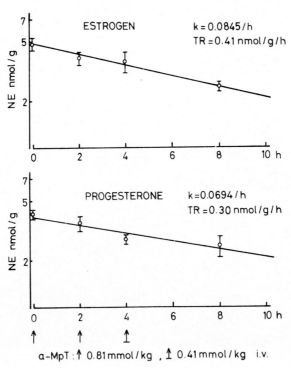

Fig. 6.

Decline of the oviductal norepinephrine at various times after intravenous injection of α-methyl-*p*-tyrosine methylester (α-M$_P$T) as indicated.

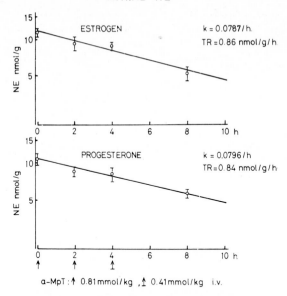

ATRIAL NE

Fig. 7.

Decline of atrial norepinephrine at various time after intravenous injection
of α-M$_P$T as indicated.

muscle cells, and the density of fluorescence is almost the same as that in the
circular muscle layer of the isthmus. We have not yet determined whether these
nerve fibers originate from the hypogastric or ovarian nerve.

Chemical estimation of norepinephrine in the oviduct has been widely studied
and hormonal influences on norepinephrine in the oviduct have been demonstrated to some extent (Brundin 1965; Rosengren and Sjöberg 1968). However, as
pointed out by several investigators, an estimation of the rate of catecholamine
turnover including norepinephrine provides more information about the neural
activity than a measurement of the amine concentration in the tissue (Oliverio
and Stjarne 1965; Gordon et al. 1966; Neff and Costa 1966; Sedvall and Kopin
1967).

In the present study, we attempted to estimate the norepinephrine turnover
rate in the oviducts of both estrogen- and progesterone-treated rabbits to see
if there was any difference in the rate of neural discharge under different
hormonal conditions.

Turnover rate of norepinephrine was determined by measuring its initial
rate of decline after blockade of its synthesis by α-methyl-p-tyrosine methylester
(Doteuchi and Costa 1973). In the oviduct of estrogen-dominated animals, the
rate of norepinephrine decline after synthesis blockade was slightly steeper

than that of progesterone-dominated animals (Fig. 6). Norepinephrine concentration at the steady state was also slightly higher in the oviducts of the estrogen group than those of the progesterone group. Therefore, it seemed that turnover rate of norepinephrine in the oviducts of the estrogen group was somewhat higher than that for the oviducts of the progesterone group. In order to compare the hormonal influence on oviducts with other tissues the norepinephrine turnover rate in atria and uterus was determined under different hormonal states.

In atria, as shown in Fig. 7, there was no difference of norepinephrine turnover rate between the two groups. However, in the uterus, turnover rate of estrogen treated animals was found to be more than six times as high as that of the progesterone group (Fig. 8). The differences found in various tissues can be explained by the types of adrenergic neurons innervating them (Owman et al. 1966; Sjöberg 1968). The atria is innervated by ordinary long adrenergic neurons and the uterus by short-adrenergic neurons, but the oviduct is inner-

UTERINE NE

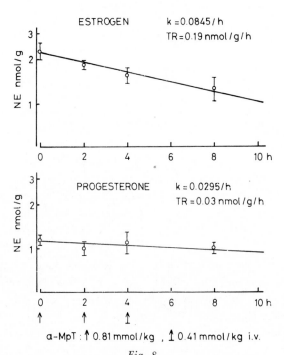

Fig. 8.
Decline of uterine norepinephrine at various time after intravenous injection of α-M$_P$T as indicated.

vated by both types of neurons, originating from the hypogastric and ovarian nerves. We believe the above experiments on determining the turnover rate in oviducts should be repeated, perhaps using still another method. Also the oviduct consists of several parts, i. e. isthmus, ampulla, infundibulum and peri-oviductal smooth muscle with varying density of innervation from different origins, and turnover rate should be estimated for each part separately prior to drawing a final conclusion.

4) *The correlation between oviductal motility and ova transport*

There are several kinds of oviductal movement, e. g. peristaltic, segmented, bending and torsional movement, and they are caused by the contraction of oviductal and peri-oviductal smooth muscles. Although ova transport is partially attributed to ciliary movement, it is a fact that oviductal movement is an indispensable factor for ova transport. However, several reports indicate that changes in oviductal motility are not always associated with the rate of ova transport, meaning that oviductal movement may occasionally contribute or obstruct ova transport depending upon its pattern.

The several kinds of oviductal movement are:

a) *Peristaltic movement.* – Peristaltic movement from the direction of the ampulla to the uterus generally seems to make the greatest contribution to ova transport, while that from the uterus to ampulla direction may obstruct transport.

b) *Segmented movement.* – Ova will shuttle with this movement.

c) *Spastic contraction of the circular muscle.* – This may obstruct ova transport completely like a sphincter.

d) *Bending movement.* – The motility of intra-ligamentary muscle, which is found in small amounts between the broad ligament layer, seems rather important for ova transport. In *in vitro* experiments, it contracted spontaneously and was responsive to norepinephrine in a way similar to proper oviductal smooth muscle (Fig. 9). Hormonal influences on the motility of this muscle are not distinct but contraction of the intra-ligamentary muscle causes the oviduct to bend. We feel this bending may occasionally obstruct or contribute to ova transport.

We also believe the reasons for discrepancy between ova transport and oviductal motility are: a) The motility of the oviduct is usually recorded under stimulated condition by intra-tubal balloon etc., so one should be aware of the influences and extent of such artificial factors: b) In *in vitro* experiments, peri-oviductal muscles, e. g. intra-ligamentary muscles were almost always removed. This must be one of the reasons which explains the difference between *in vitro* and *in vivo* patterns of oviductal activity.

317

INTRA-LIGAMENTARY MUSCLE

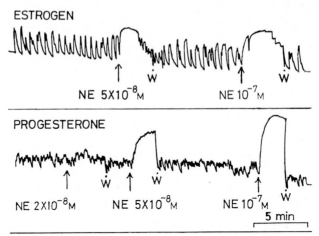

ESTROGEN

NE 5X10^{-8}M   NE 10^{-7}M

PROGESTERONE

NE 2X10^{-8}M   NE 5X10^{-8}M   NE 10^{-7}M

5 min

Fig. 9.

Spontaneous motility and contractile responses to norepinephrine of the intra-ligamentary muscle of estrogen- and progesterone-dominated rabbits recorded isotonically *in vitro*.

5) *Conclusion*

There are many problems awaiting solution concerning the controlling mechanisms of oviductal motility and ova transport, and the present paper is only an enumeration of our current studies. However, on the basis of what we have studied, we believe the rate of ova transport may be controlled artificially by means of combinations of ovarian hormones and autonomic drugs in the near future.

ACKNOWLEDGMENTS

Gratitude is expressed to H. Nakanishi, M. Ueda, K. Otani, H. Tanaka, F. Hirose and M. Sai for collaboration: to Prof. E. C. Wood, Department of Obstetrics and Gynecology, Monash University, Melbourne, Australia, and Prof. E. M. Coutinho, Maternidade Climerio de Oliveira, Univ. Fed. da Bahia, Salvador, Brazil for international cooperation.

REFERENCES

Brundin J. (1965) Distribution and function of adrenergic nerves in the rabbit Fallopian tube. *Acta physiol. scand. 66,* Suppl. 259, 1–57.

Doteuchi M. and Costa E. (1973) Pentylenetetrazol convulsions and brain catecholamine turnover rate in rat and mice receiving diphenylhydantoin or benzodiazepines. *Neuropharmacol. 12,* 1059–1072.

Falck B. and Owman C. (1965) A detailed methodological description of the fluorescence method for the cellular demonstration of biogenic monoamines. *Acta Univ. Lund*, Sec. II, 7, 5–23.

Gordon R., Reid J. V. O., Sjöerdsma A. and Udenfriend S. (1966) Increased synthesis of norepinephrine in the rat heart on electrical stimulation of the stellate ganglion. *Mol. Pharmacol.* 2, 606–613.

Halbert S. A. and Conrad J. T. (1975) *In vitro* contractile activity of the mesotubarium superium from the rabbit in various endocrine states. *Fertil. Steril.* 26, 248–256.

Howe G. R. and Black D. L. (1973) Autonomic nervous system and oviduct function in the rabbit. *J. Reprod. Fertil.* 33, 425–430.

Hunter D. S. and Kendle K. E. (1974) The influence of hormonal state on the response of the isolated rabbit oviduct to catecholamines. *J. Reprod. Fertil.* 41, 245–247.

Ichijo M. (1960) Studies on the motile function of the Fallopian tube. Report 1. Analytic studies on the motile function of the Fallopian tube. *Tohoku J. Exper. Med.* 72, 211–218.

Nakanishi H., Wansbrough H. and Wood C. (1967) Postganglionic sympathetic nerve innervating human Fallopian tube. *Amer. J. Physiol.* 213, 613–619.

Nakanishi H. and Wood C. (1968) Effects of adrenergic blocking agents on human Fallopian tube motility *in vitro. J. Reprod. Fertil.* 16, 21–28.

Neff N. H. and Costa E. (1966) Effect of tricyclic antidepressants and chlorpromazine on brain catecholamine synthesis. Proceedings of the First International Symposium on Antidepressant Drugs. *Excerpta Med. Int. Congr. Ser. 122*, 23–34.

Novak E. (1957) *Gynecologic and Obstetric Pathology*, W. B. Saunders Co., Philadelphia.

Oliverio A. and Stjärne L. (1965) Acceleration of norepinephrine turnover in mouse heart by cold exposure. *Life Sci. 4*, 2339–2343.

Owman C. and Sjöberg N.-O. (1966) Adrenergic nerves in the female genital tract of the rabbit. With remarks on cholinesterase-containing structures. *Z. Zellforsch. 74*, 182–197.

Owman C., Rosengren E. and Sjöberg N.-O. (1966) Origin of adrenergic innervation to the female genital tract of the rabbit. *Life Sci. 5*, 1389–1396.

Rosengren E. and Sjöberg N.-O. (1968) Changes in the amount of adrenergic transmitter in the female genital tract of the rabbit during pregnancy. *Acta physiol. scand. 72*, 412–414.

Sedvall G. C. and Kopin I. J. (1967) Acceleration of norepinephrine synthesis in the rat submaxillary gland *in vivo* during sympathetic nerve stimulation. *Life Sci. 6*, 45–51.

Sjöberg N.-O. (1967) The adrenergic transmitter of the female reproductive tract: Distribution and functional changes. *Acta physiol. scand. 72*, Suppl. 305.

Sjöberg N.-O. (1968) Consideration on the cause of disappearance of the adrenergic transmitter in the uterine nerves during pregnancy. *Acta physiol. scand. 72*, 510–517.

Takeda H. (1969) Physiology and clinic of Fallopian tube: Tubal movement. *Clin. Gynec. Obstet. 23*, 369–374.

Takeda H., Ueda M. and Doteuchi M. (1968) Motility of rabbit Fallopian tube and the autonomic nerve. *Jap. J. Smooth Muscle Res. 4*, 218–219.

Ueda M., de Mattos C. E. R. and Coutinho E. M. (1973) The influence of adrenergic activation and blockade on the motility of the circular and longitudinal muscle layers of the rabbit oviduct *in vitro. Fertil. Steril. 24*, 440–447.

Departments of Obstetrics and Gynaecology,
Al Azhar University School of Medicine, Cairo, Egypt*
and Wayne State University School of Medicine,
Detroit, Michigan 48201**

EFFECTS OF PROSTAGLANDINS
ON OVIDUCTAL CONTRACTILITY AND
EGG TRANSPORT IN RABBITS

By

I. Aref* and E. S. Hafez**

ABSTRACT

Variable doses of PGE_2 and $PGF_{2\alpha}$ were injected subcutaneously at 12, 24 and 36 h post-coitum (h p. c.) in rabbits. Variations in oviductal intraluminal pressure were monitored unilaterally *in vivo*. Egg transport was studied in the contralateral oviducts at 48 h p. c. Implantation was reported at 14 days post-coitum (d. p. c.). $PGF_{2\alpha}$ stimulated oviductal contractility, accelerated egg transport and reduced implantation significantly. The effect was maximal when the drug was injected at 36 h p. c. PGE_2 inhibited oviductal contractility and did not modify egg transport or interfere with implantation.

In the past few years great advances in the field of contraception have been achieved. Despite the availability of several methods of birth control, a radically new idea is needed, preferably one which involves less endocrinological insult than the present generation of hormonal contraceptives. The idea of post-coital contraception has much to commend it.

In most mammals, eggs reside in the oviduct for about three days (Blandau 1971). Throughout this interval, fertilization and concurrent cleavage of eggs takes place. Simultaneous with these developmental changes in embryos, the uterus undergoes several changes to facilitate their survival and subsequent implantation. Pharmacological disruption of this temporal and delicate relationship leads to the emergence of effective post-coital contraceptives. Several drugs have been tested in this way (reviewed by Duncan and Wheeler 1975). Large doses of estrogen and estrogen analogues were effective as post-coital contraceptives if administered within 72 h of unprotected mid-cycle intercourse (Haspels 1970, 1972; Kuchera 1971; Morris et al. 1967; Morris and Van Wagenen 1966, 1973). Blye (1973) has related the antifertility effects of post-coital estrogens to acceleration or retention ("tube-locking") of eggs in the oviduct. Morris and Wagenen (1973) have suggested the name *interception* for this approach. In view of the potential hazards of vaginal adenocarcinoma in offspring of women treated with these compounds (Greenwald et al. 1971; Robertson-Rintoul 1974). The Food and Drug Administration (FDA) has restricted their use to cases of rape and failure or neglect of prophylaxis.

The effectiveness of prostaglandins (PGs) in modifying the contractility of the genital organs *in vivo* (Coutinho and Maia 1971; Aref et al. 1973) and in altering steroidogenesis (Pharris and Wyngarden 1969) has encouraged us to test these compounds as adequate substitutes for available interceptives.

The aim of our experiment was to study the effect of variable doses of PGE_2 and $PGF_{2\alpha}$ at different hours post-coitum (h p. c.) on oviductal motility *in vivo*, egg transport and implantation in rabbits.

MATERIALS AND METHODS

Adult female New Zealand rabbits weighing $3\frac{1}{2}$–4 kg were divided into two groups. In the first group of 89 rabbits, the genital organs were exposed through a midline incision. Microballoons were pushed gently through the fimbriated end of the oviduct to the ampullary-isthmic junction of one oviduct. The free ends of the catheters were passed between the body wall and the skin to be exteriorized and fixed to the skin of the nape of the neck. The genital organs of the contralateral side were left untouched for the study of egg transport. Mating was allowed on the third post-operative day. PGE_2 or $PGF_{2\alpha}$ (6 or 9 mg) was injected subcutaneously (s. c.) 12, 24 or 36 h p. c. Oviductal motility was monitored before and following the injection of PGs. Contractility was recorded for 30 min and tracings were repeated every 2 h for 8 h. To monitor oviductal motility, the catheter was filled completely with saline and connected to a pressure transducer (Sanborn 267, B. C.) a carrier preamplifier (Sanborn 350, 1100 C) and Hewlett Packard 7700 recorder. Rabbits were autopsied at 48 h p. c. The number of corpora lutea in the corresponding ovary was counted and egg transport was studied in unmonitored oviducts by segmental flushing or by the freezing clearing technique.

321

In the second group of 49 rabbits, PGE₂ or PGF₂ₐ (6 or 9 mg) was injected subcutaneously at 12, 24 or 36 h p. c. Rabbits were sacrificed 14 days postcoitum, and the number of corpora lutea, implantation sites, living and degenerated embryos counted.

RESULTS

Oviductal motility

Cyclic variations in oviductal motility were observed in untreated rabbits. At 12 h p. c., outbursts of increased activity with remarkable variability of the resting pressure were recorded frequently. At 36 h p. c., the outbursts were infrequent and the changes in the resting pressure were minimal (Fig. 1). In prostaglandin-treated rabbits, PGE₂ inhibited and PGF₂ₐ stimulated oviductal motility (Fig. 2). The duration of response was directly related to the dose of prostaglandin injected. Similar responses, however, were observed when the drugs were injected at 12, 24 or 36 h p. c.

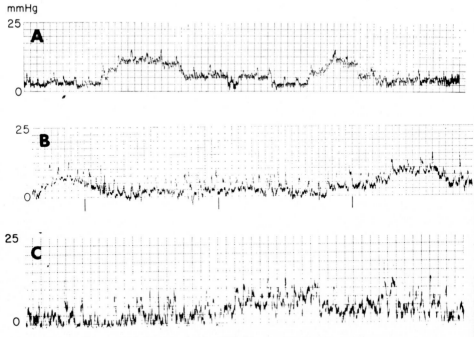

Fig. 1.

Cyclic changes in oviductal motility *in vivo* in untreated rabbits at 12 (A), 24 (B) and 36 (C) h p. c.

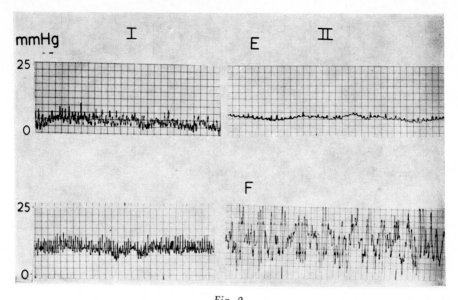

Fig. 2.

Effect of subcutaneous injection of PGE$_2$ and PGF$_{2\alpha}$ on oviductal motility *in vivo* in rabbits. PGE$_2$ inhibited and PGF$_{2\alpha}$ stimulated oviductal motility.
I Premedication tracing.   II Tracings following prostaglandin injection.

When 6 mg was injected, a latent period of 14–22 min was followed by a gradual decrease in the amplitude of concentrations. The suppressed pattern was observed for $2-2\frac{1}{2}$ h after the injection of PGE$_2$. Oviductal contractility returned to its initial level 4 h after the injection of PGE$_2$. When 9 mg PGE$_{2\alpha}$ was injected a latent period of 8–17 min was followed by a gradual decrease in contractility. Motility was inhibited at 2 and 4 h after the injection of PGE$_2$. It returned to initial values at 6 h after injection.

When 6 mg PGF$_{2\alpha}$ was injected, a latent period of 20–24 min was followed by a gradual increase in the amplitude and duration of contractions. The stimulated pattern was observed at 2 and 4 h after injection of PGF$_{2\alpha}$. After the injection of 9 mg PGF$_{2\alpha}$, a latent period of 15–18 min was followed by a remarkable increase in amplitude and duration of contractions. The stimulated pattern was observed at 2, 4, 6 and 8 h after the injection of PGF$_{2\alpha}$.

Egg transport

In 8 untreated rabbits, 95 % of eggs were recovered from oviducts and no eggs were recovered from uteri at autopsy 48 h p. c. When 6 mg PGE$_2$ was injected (s. c.) at 36 h p. c. in 8 rabbits, 89 % of eggs were recovered from oviducts and 8 % were recovered from uteri at autopsy 48 h p. c. When 6 mg

21*

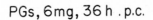

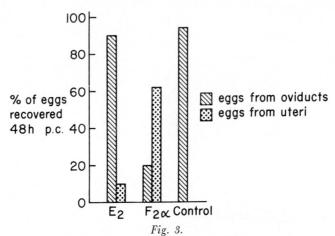

Fig. 3.

Effect of subcutaneous injection of 6 mg of PGE_2 or $PGF_{2\alpha}$ at 36 h p. c. on egg recovery at 48 h p. c.

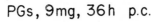

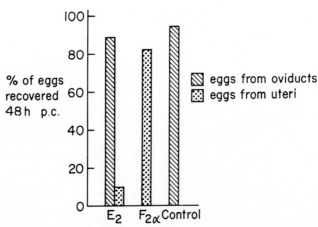

Fig. 4.

Effect of subcutaneous injection of 9 mg of PGE_2 or $PGF_{2\alpha}$ at 36 h p. c. on egg recovery at 48 h p. c.

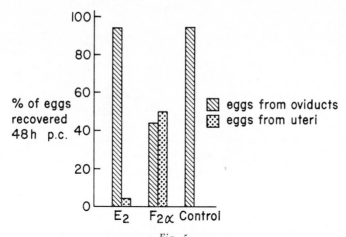

PGs, 6mg, 24h p.c.

% of eggs recovered 48h p.c.

▨ eggs from oviducts
▦ eggs from uteri

E₂ F₂α Control

Fig. 5.
Effect of subcutaneous injection of 6 mg of PGE₂ or PGF₂ₐ at
24 h p. c. on egg recovery at 48 h p. c.

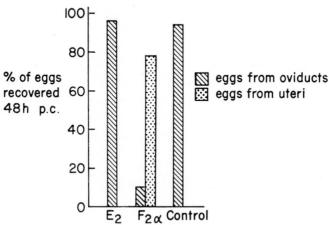

PGs, 9mg, 24h p.c.

% of eggs recovered 48h p.c.

▨ eggs from oviducts
▦ eggs from uteri

E₂ F₂α Control

Fig. 6.
Effect of subcutaneous injection of 9 mg of PGE₂ or PGF₂ₐ at
24 h p. c. on egg recovery at 48 h p. c.

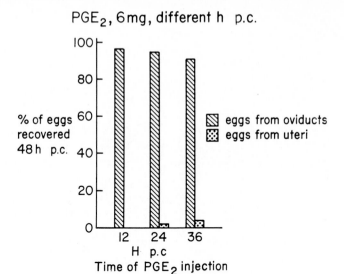

PGE$_2$, 6mg, different h p.c.

% of eggs recovered 48 h p.c.

⊠ eggs from oviducts
⊡ eggs from uteri

H p.c
Time of PGE$_2$ injection

Fig. 7.
Effect of subcutaneous injection of 9 mg of PGE$_2$ at different h p. c.
on egg recovery at 48 h p. c.

PGF$_{2\alpha}$ was injected (s. c.) at 36 h p. c. in 8 rabbits, 21 % of eggs were recovered from oviducts and 64 % were recovered from uteri at autopsy 48 h p. c. (Fig. 3). When 9 mg of either PGE$_2$ or PGF$_{2\alpha}$ was injected (s. c.) at 36 h p. c. and egg transport was studied at autopsy 48 h p. c., 86 % of eggs were recovered from the oviducts and 9 % were recovered from the uteri of 8 PGE$_2$-treated rabbits, but no eggs were recovered from the oviducts and 84 % of eggs were recovered from the uteri of 8 PGF$_{2\alpha}$-treated rabbits (Fig. 4).

When 6 mg PGE$_{2\alpha}$ was injected s. c. at 24 h p. c. in 9 rabbits, 95 % of eggs were recovered from the oviducts and 5 % were recovered from the uteri at autopsy 48 h p. c. When 6 mg PGF$_{2\alpha}$ was injected s. c. at 24 h p. c. in 8 rabbits, 46 % of eggs were recovered from the oviducts and 51 % were recovered from the uteri at autopsy 48 h p. c. (Fig. 5). When 9 mg of either PGE$_2$ or PGF$_{2\alpha}$ was injected at 24 h p. c. and egg transport was studied at autopsy 48 h p. c., 97 % of eggs were recovered from the oviducts and no eggs were recovered from the uteri of 8 PGE$_2$-treated rabbits while in eight PGF$_{2\alpha}$-treated rabbits, 10 % of eggs were recovered from the oviducts and 77 % from the uteri (Fig. 6). When 6 mg PGE$_2$ was injected (s. c.) at 12 h p. c. in 7 rabbits, 97 % of eggs were recovered from the oviducts and no eggs were recovered from the uteri at autopsy 48 h p. c. (Fig. 7). When 6 mg PGF$_{2\alpha}$ was injected (s. c.) at 12 h p. c. in 8 rabbits, 59 % of eggs were recovered from the oviducts and 35 % were recovered from the uteri at autopsy 48 h p. c. (Fig. 8).

326

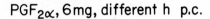

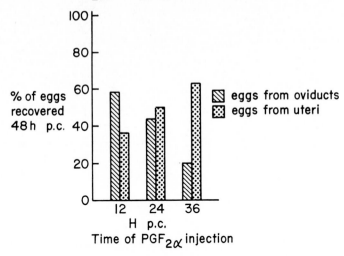

Fig. 8.
Effect of subcutaneous injection of 9 mg of $PGF_{2\alpha}$ at different h p. c.
on egg recovery at 48 h p. c.

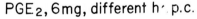

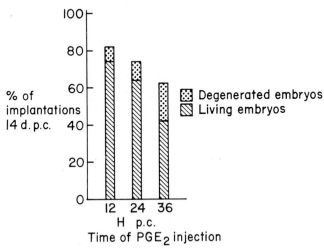

Fig. 9.
Effect of subcutaneous injection of 6 mg of PGE_2 at different h p. c.
on implantation 14 days p. c.

Implantation

When 6 mg PGE_2 was injected (s. c.) at 12 h p. c. in 8 rabbits, 83 % of eggs implanted and 75 % of embryos were living at autopsy 14 days p. c. When 6 mg PGE_2 was injected (s. c.) at 24 h p. c. in 9 rabbits, 75 % of eggs implanted and 65 % of embryos were living at autopsy 14 days p. c. When 6 mg PGE_2 was injected (s. c.) at 36 h p. c. in 8 rabbits, 62 % of eggs implanted and 43 % of embryos were living at autopsy 14 days p. c. (Fig. 9).

When 6 mg $PGF_{2\alpha}$ was injected (s. c.) at 12 h p. c. in 8 rabbits, 49 % of eggs implanted and 41 % of embryos were living. When 6 mg $PGF_{2\alpha}$ was injected (s. c.) at 24 h p. c. in 8 rabbits, 39 % of eggs implanted and 22 % of embryos were living. Implantations were reduced to 20 % when 6 mg $PGF_{2\alpha}$ was injected (s. c.) at 36 h p. c. in 8 rabbits. Six percent of implanted embryos were living at autopsy 14 days p. c. (Fig. 10).

DISCUSSION

In vivo monitoring of oviductal motility in restrained rabbits showed that PGE_2 and $PGF_{2\alpha}$ had antithetical effects on the smooth musculature of the oviduct. PGE_2 inhibited and $PGF_{2\alpha}$ stimulated oviductal motility dramatically. Several studies have reported similar effects in women and rabbits (Coutinho and Maia 1971; Spilman and Harper 1973; Aref and Hafez 1973). In women, a stimulatory response was observed following the intravenous injection of 100 mg $PGF_{2\alpha}$

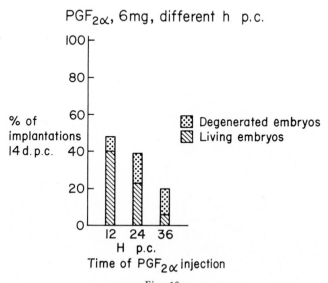

Fig. 10.
Effect of subcutaneous injection of 6 mg of $PGF_{2\alpha}$ at different h p. c. on implantation 14 days p. c.

(i. v.). Injection of 100 mg PGE_2 (i. v.), however, was followed by inhibition (Coutinho and Maia 1971).

In rabbits, Spilman and Harper (1973) reported suppression of oviductal contractility for 20–40 min following the injection of 0.5–1.5 mg PGE_2 (s. c.). Injection of 7.5 mg $PGF_{2\alpha}$ (s. c.) increased frequency and amplitude of contractions for 1–1.5 h. The intensity of the contractile response was related to the dose of prostaglandin administered. The effectiveness of prostaglandins to modify oviductal contractility, however, was independent of the time of administration. Similar responses were observed when the drugs were injected at 12, 24 or 36 h p. c.

$PGF_{2\alpha}$ accelerated egg transport. PGE_2, however, failed to modify the transport of eggs in oviducts. The effectiveness of $PGF_{2\alpha}$ to hasten the passage of eggs depended on the time of injection of the drug. Efficacy increased when $PGF_{2\alpha}$ was injected at 36 h p. c. compared to when it was injected at 12 or 24 h p. c. In rabbits, injection of 5 mg PGE_2, or $PGF_{2\alpha}$ hastened the transport of eggs to the uterus by approximately 40 h. PGE_2, however, failed to alter egg transport (Ellinger and Kirton 1972). Chang and his associates (1972, 1973) reported accelerated transport of eggs and disturbed implantation when 5 mg/kg $PGF_{2\alpha}$ was injected s. c. in rabbits. Despite the antagonistic effects of PGE_2 and $PGF_{2\alpha}$ on oviductal motility, the effects of the two prostaglandins on egg transport were not antithetical. In $PGF_{2\alpha}$-treated rabbits, stimulated oviductal motility in one oviduct was accompanied by accelerated transport of eggs in contralateral oviducts. Strong oviductal contractions may overcome distal antagonism and expel eggs prematurely to the uterus. In PGE_2-treated rabbits, however, the inhibition of oviductal motility was not accompanied by delayed transport of eggs. The relationship between oviductal contractility and egg transport is probably complex and other factors may be involved. Of particular significance is the sphincter-like mechanism at ampullary-isthmic and uterotubal junctions (Greenwald 1968; Brundin 1969). Since physiological levels of estrogen and progesterone are requisites for timed transport of eggs in rabbits (Harper 1965; Blandau 1971), prostaglandin-induced luteolysis and disturbed steroidogenesis may interfere with egg transport and implantation (Kirton 1972; Aref et al. 1974). Accelerated transport of embryos to the uterus was probably involved in the discrepancy between the number of corpora lutea and implantation sites in $PGF_{2\alpha}$-treated rabbits. On the contrary, PGE_2 failed to alter egg transport and to disturb implantation.

REFERENCES

Aref I. and Hafez E. S. E. (1973) Utero-oviductal motility with emphasis on ova transport. *Obstet. gynec. Surv. 28*, 679–703.
Aref I., Hafez E. S. E. and Kamar G. A. R. (1973) Postcoital prostaglandins *in vivo*. Oviductal motility and egg transport in rabbits. *Fertil. Steril. 24*, 671–676.

Aref I., Gottschewski G. H. M. and Hafez E. S. E. (1974) Antifertility effects of PGE$_2$ and PGF$_{2\alpha}$. *Contraception 10*, 291–298.

Blandau R. J. (1971) Normal egg transport through the oviduct of mammals. In: Sherman A. I., ed. *Pathways to Conception*, pp. 72–98. C. C. Thomas, Springfield, Ill.

Blye R. P. (1973) The use of estrogens as postcoital contraceptive agents. Clinical effectiveness and potential mode of action. *Amer. J. Obstet. Gynec. 116*, 1044–1050.

Brundin J. (1969) Pharmacology of the oviduct. In: Hafez E. S. E. and Blandau R. J., eds. *The Mammalian Oviduct*, pp. 251–269. The University of Chicago Press, Chicago.

Chang M. C. and Hunt D. M. (1972) Effect of prostaglandin F$_{2\alpha}$ on the early pregnancy of rabbits. *Nature (Lond.) 236*, 120–121.

Chang M. C., Hunt D. M. and Polge C. (1973) Effects of prostaglandins on sperm and egg transport in the rabbit. In: Raspe G. and Bernhard S., eds. *Adv. Biosciences 9*, 805–810.

Coutinho E. M. and Maia H. S. (1971) The contractile response of the human uterus, Fallopian tubes and ovary to prostaglandins *in vivo*. *Fertil. Steril. 22*, 539–544.

Duncan G. W. and Wheeler R. G. (1975) Pharmacological and mechanical control of implantation. *Biol. Reprod. 12*, 143–175.

Ellinger J. V. and Kirton K. T. (1972) Ovum transport in rabbits injected with prostaglandin E$_1$ or F$_{2\alpha}$. *Biol. Reprod. 7*, 106.

Greenwald G. S. (1968) Hormonal regulation of egg transport through the mammalian oviduct. In: Behrman S. J. and Kistner R. W., eds. *Progress in Infertility*, pp. 157–179. Little Brown, Boston, Mass.

Greenwald P., Barlow J. J., Nesca P. C. and Burnett W. S. (1971) Vaginal cancer after maternal treatment with synthetic estrogens. *New Engl. J. Med. 285*, 390–392.

Harper M. J. K. (1965) Transport of eggs in cumulus through the ampulla of the rabbit oviduct in relation to day of pseudo-pregnancy. *Endocrinology 77*, 114–123.

Haspels A. A. (1970) The morning after pill. Abstract No. 9, Sixth World Congress of Gynaecology and Obstetrics, N. Y.

Haspels A. A. (1972) Post-coital estrogen in large doses. *IPPF Medical Bulletin 6*, 2.

Kirton K. T. (1973) Prostaglandins and steroidogenesis. In: Raspé G. and Bernhard S., eds. *Adv. Biosciences 9*, 645–650.

Kuchera L. K. (1971) Post coital contraception with diethylstilboestrol. *J. Amer. med. Ass. 218*, 562–563.

Morris J. McL. and Van Wagenen G. (1966) Compounds interfering with ovum implantation and development III. The role of estrogens. *Amer. J. Obstet. Gynec. 96*, 804–815.

Morris J. McL. and Van Wagenen G. (1973) Interception: the use of post-ovulatory estrogens to prevent implantation. *Amer. J. Obstet. Gynec. 115*, 101–107.

Pharriss B. B. and Wyngarden L. J. (1969) The effect of prostaglandin F$_{2\alpha}$ on the progestogen content of ovaries from pseudopregnant rats. *Proc. Soc. exp. Biol. Med. 130*, 92–94.

Robertson-Rintoul J. (1974) Oral Contraception: Potential hazards of hormone therapy during pregnancy. *Lancet 31*, 515–516.

Spilman C. H. and Harper M. J. K. (1973) Effects of prostaglandins on oviduct motility in estrous rabbits. *Biol. Reprod. 9*, 36–45.

Ortho Research Laboratories, Ortho Pharmaceutical Corporation,
Raritan, New Jersey 08869, USA

EFFECTS OF ADRENERGIC DRUGS
OR DENERVATION
ON OVUM TRANSPORT IN RABBITS

By

J. P. Polidoro, R. D. Heilman, R. M. Culver
and R. R. Reo

ABSTRACT

The role of the adrenergic nervous system and its possible interaction
with the reproductive endocrine hormones in the regulation of ovum
transport was investigated. Using the "freezing-clearing" method (Orsini
1962), the effects of selective α- and β-adrenergic agonists on ovum
transport were evaluated at 60 and 72 h *post coitum* (p. c.) in rabbits.
Phenylephrine, a selective α-agonist, and norepinephrine, an agent possessing predominantly α-receptor stimulant activity, increased the mean
rate of ovum transport; isoproterenol, a selective β-receptor agonist, had
no effect.

The role of the adrenergic nervous system in estrogen-induced "tube-
locking" was investigated in rabbits in which the oviduct had been selectively pretreated with 6-hydroxydopamine (6-OHDA). Perfusion of the
oviduct with 6-OHDA did not alter the ability of estrogen to "tube-lock"
ova. However, tyramine, an agent known to release endogenous norepinephrine, produced contractions in 2 of 5 perfused rabbit oviducts after
pretreatment with 6-OHDA, thus suggesting that adrenergic influence
may be present in spite of chemical, adrenergic denervation. It is concluded that α-adrenergic receptor stimulation can increase the mean rate
of ovum transport (60 and 72 h p. c.) and that the neuroendocrine inter-
relationships which contribute to the regulation of ovum transport may
still exist following 6-OHDA treatment.

The potential pharmacologic modification of ovum transport, as a means of fertility control, is an area of considerable interest and research (Pauerstein et al. 1973; Polidoro 1974). The presence of a rich adrenergic innervation to the mammalian oviduct implies a probable role of the autonomic nervous system in the normal physiology of ovum transport. Utilizing the rabbit model, exogenously administered sympathomimetic drugs (Bodkhe and Harper 1972; Longley et al. 1968; Pauerstein et al. 1970a, 1970b; Polidoro et al. 1973) or selective adrenergic denervation of the oviduct with 6-hydroxydopamine (6-OHDA) (Eddy and Black 1973, 1974) appear to modify somewhat the normal rate of ovum transport; these effects, however, appear to be time and estrogen or progesterone dependent.

Polidoro et al. (1973) have shown that epinephrine, administered during a 12 h period preceding sacrifice at 60 or 72 h p. c., hastens the mean rate of ovum transport in rabbits. Epinephrine is a sympathomimetic amine that possesses both α- and β-adrenergic receptor stimulating activity. To determine if the effect of epinephrine on ovum transport is the result of its α (contractile) or β (relaxant) activity, the effects on ovum transport of phenylephrine, a selective α-agonist and isoproterenol, a selective β-agonist, were determined. The effect of norepinephrine, a dual α- and β-receptor stimulating agent with a propensity for α-receptor stimulation, was also investigated; norepinephrine is believed to be the natural neurotransmitter substance of the adrenergic nerves of the oviduct.

Since ovarian steroid hormones have been suggested to play a possible role in the modulation of the autonomic effects on the isthmus (Brundin 1965), an interaction between estrogen and the adrenergic nervous system might explain how the isthmus acts as a physiological sphincter and can induce oviductal retention of ova, i. e. "tube-locking" (Greenwald 1967). To further investigate the role of a neuroendocrine interrelationship in the regulation of ovum transport, and more specifically, the phenomenon of estrogen-induced "tube-locking", the effect on ovum transport, in the presence of exogenous estrogen, of selective adrenergic denervation of the oviduct with 6-OHDA, was also studied.

METHODS AND MATERIALS

Effect of adrenergic drugs on ovum transport

Mature, female Dutch-belted rabbits, obtained from commercial suppliers, were utilized in this investigation. The rabbits were isolated one week or more before experimentation and allowed free access to food and water. The effects of norepinephrine, phenylephrine or isoproterenol on the mean rate of ovum transport were studied seperately at both 60 and 72 h p. c. The results were then compared with the data of control and epinephrine-treated rabbits previously reported (Polidoro et al. 1973).

All drugs were injected subcutaneously in sterile, physiological saline (0.9 %), except isoproterenol, which was administered in sesame oil as a suspension. The following doses were used:

> norepinephrine – 1.0 or 2.0 mg/kg – 6 h intervals
> phenylephrine – 1.0, 2.0 or 4.0 mg/kg – 6 h intervals
> isoproterenol – 500 μg/kg – 2 h intervals.

Rabbits in each group were mated to one or two fertile males. Following mating and an intravenous injection of 50 IU of HCG, groups of 5 to 10 rabbits were killed (sodium pentobarbital overdose) at either 60 or 72 h p. c. Drugs were administered for a 12 h period immediately preceding death. The reproductive tracts were frozen *in situ* (liquid nitrogen – cooled isopentane), and upon thawing were removed and "cleared" according to a method previously described (Orsini 1962; Polidoro et al. 1973). In addition, the percentage recovery of ova was determined for each group by comparing the number of corpora lutea (CL) with the number of ova observed in the cleared oviducts and uteri. Statistical comparisons of the mean rate of ovum transport for the control and treated groups were analyzed by the Student's t-test (Steel and Torrie 1960). Percent recoveries of ova in the uteri at 60 and 72 h p. c. (Tables 2 and 3) were statistically analyzed by a two-sided Dunnett and Scheffe test for proportion.

An *in vivo* oviduct perfusion method described elsewhere (Heilman et al. 1972) was utilized to determine drug dosage and duration of action; the methodology, however, was slightly modified. The oviducts of adult, estrous Dutch-belted rabbits (non-vagotomized) were perfused at a rate of 53 μl/min utilizing a polyethylene cannula (PE50) ligated in position 1.0 cm into the isthmus. Following subcutaneous injections of either phenylephrine, norepinephrine or isoproterenol, changes in blood pressure and the mean "tone" of the oviduct were simultaneously recorded on a Grass polygraph. The duration of action for each drug was characterized by a gradual return of oviduct "tone" to pre-drug conditions.

6-Hydroxydopamine perfusion and effect of estrogen on ovum transport

In an additional study involving chemical adrenergic denervation of the oviduct, the mean rate of ovum transport was determined in intact and 6-OHDA perfused rabbit oviducts. Following sodium pentobarbital anesthesia and a mid-ventral laparotomy, one oviduct of each rabbit was perfused intraluminally with 6-OHDA according to the method of Eddy and Black (1973, 1974). The effectiveness of a 7.0 mg total dose of 6-OHDA, recommended by Eddy and Black (1973), in the selective destruction of the adrenergic nerves of the oviduct, was verified utilizing the fluorescent histochemical method for norepinephrine (Falck and Owman 1965) described in detail elsewhere (Polidoro et al. 1974). Subsequent to the confirmation of the denervation procedure, the oviducts (unilateral) of additional rabbits were similarly perfused with 6-OHDA and utilized in the ovum transport study.

One to four weeks following the 6-OHDA treatment, the rabbits were mated, injected with 50 IU of HCG and treated (17 h p. c.) with an intramuscular injection of 250 μg of *Depo-Estradiol Cypionate**, a dose previously tested and shown to induce oviductal retention of ova ("tube-locking"). The rabbits were killed at 72 h p. c. and the ovum transport rates determined in "cleared" reproductive tracts (described above). Direct comparisons were made between the intact and 6-OHDA treated oviducts from the same rabbit with special reference being made to the location of the ampullary-isthmic junction (AIJ).

6-Hydroxydopamine perfusion and effect of tyramine on oviductal contractility

To evaluate the functional effectiveness of the 6-OHDA perfusion on abolishing the adrenergic nervous system in the oviductal smooth musculature, the oviducts of rabbits pretreated with 6-OHDA were challenged with tyramine one week after perfusion. This sympathomimetic amine produces its effects indirectly, i. e. through the release of endogenous catecholamines. The tyramine study utilized the same perfusion technique described above except that vagotomized, estrous New Zealand rabbits were used. In addition, tyramine (in saline) was administered intravenously at 0.25, 0.5 and 1.0 mg/kg to obtain a three point dose response curve. Contralateral oviducts (6-OHDA-treated or nontreated) within the same animal were simultaneously monitored for contractile activity.

RESULTS

Effect of adrenergic drugs on ovum transport

The overall ovum recovery rate for the total experiment was 94 %. The effects of the adrenergic drugs norepinephrine, phenylephrine and isoproterenol on the mean rate of ovum transport at 60 and 72 h p. c. are shown in Table 1. The control and epinephrine ovum transport rates, shown here to facilitate the direct comparison of data, were previously published (Polidoro et al. 1973). Norepinephrine and phenylephrine increased ($P < 0.01$) the mean rate of ovum transport compared to controls at 60 and 72 h p. c.; the results are similar to those previously reported with epinephrine. Isoproterenol, at the dose studied,

---

* Trademark of The Upjohn Company.

Table 1.

Effect of adrenergic drugs on ovum transport rates at 60 and 72 h *post coitum* in rabbits.

Drug (mg/kg)	Hours *post coitum*			
	(n)	60 h	(n)	72 h
Control[x]	10	71.3 (1.18)	10	79.3 (1.17)
Epinephrine[x] (0.5)	10	82.3** (3.10)	10	95.4** (1.90)
Norepinephrine (1.0)	10	72.2 (1.29)	10	85.7* (2.76)
(2.0)	5	79.2** (2.02)	5	95.9** (4.06)
Phenylephrine (1.0)	10	69.9 (2.39)	10	84.1 (3.53)
(2.0)	7	75.7 (2.71)	5	89.5** (4.39)
(4.0)	5	79.0** (1.51)	5	92.3** (3.61)
Isoproterenol (0.5)	10	73.8 (1.34)	10	80.8 (4.10)

* ($P < 0.05$) from control.

** ($P < 0.01$) from control.

[x] Data from Polidoro et al., *J. Reprod. Fertil. 35,* 331 (1973). with permission of the journal editor.

Values expressed as mean % distance transported with SE in parentheses.

did not alter ovum transport rates at either 60 or 72 h p. c. but induced substantial fatality rates of 47 and 52 %, respectively. A 29 % incidence of mortality also occurred with each of the following dosages of α-adrenergic receptor drugs: norepinephrine 1.0 and 2.0 mg, phenylephrine 4.0 mg. Additional replacement rabbits were required to complete each series (Table 1).

In Tables 2 and 3, the influence of each drug on the percentage of ova recovered from the uteri at 60 and 72 h p. c. is presented. Although norepinephrine (2 mg/kg) and phenylephrine (4 mg/kg) increased the mean rate of ovum transport at 60 h p. c. (Table 1), the results in Table 2 indicate that the percentage of ova which were in the uterus at that time was not different from control values; none of the drugs appeared to mimic the effect of epinephrine.

Table 2.

The effect of adrenergic drugs on the percentage of ova recovered from the rabbit uterus at 60 h *post coitum.*

Drug (mg/kg)	(n)	Total No. of ova recovered	Total No. of ova in uterus	% of ova in uterus
Control	10	75	0	0
Epinephrine (0.5)	10	82	20	24.3*
Norepinephrine (1.0)	10	90	0	0
(2.0)	5	38	0	0
Phenylephrine (1.0)	10	78	0	0
(2.0)	7	50	2	4.0
(4.0)	5	41	2	4.8
Isoproterenol (0.5)	10	75	2	2.7

* $(P < 0.01)$ from control.

Table 3.

The effect of adrenergic drugs on the percentage of ova recovered from the rabbit uterus at 72 h *post coitum.*

Drug (mg/kg)	(n)	Total No. of ova recovered	Total No. of ova in uterus	% of ova in uterus
Control	10	90	5	5.5
Epinephrine (0.5)	10	79	52	65.8[b]
Norepinephrine (1.0)	10	70	11	15.7
(2.0)	5	29	17	58.6[b,c]
Phenylephrine (1.0)	10	77	17	22.0[a]
(2.0)	5	32	13	40.0[b,c]
(4.0)	5	29	14	48.2[b,c]
Isoproterenol (0.5)	10	80	25	31.2[b]

[a] $(P < 0.05)$ from control.
[b] $(P < 0.01)$ from control.
[c] *Not* statistically different from epinephrine.

The effect of the adrenergic drugs on increasing the percentage of ova in the uterus at 72 h p. c. (Table 3), however, was more apparent. The α-adrenergic stimulants, norepinephrine and phenylephrine, like epinephrine, increased ($P < 0.01$) the number of ova recovered from the uterus. Isoproterenol, which did not alter the mean transport rate at 72 h p. c. produced an increase in the percentage of ova in the uterus; this value, however, was statistically significantly less than that of epinephrine. The percentage recovery of ova for the higher doses of norepinephrine and phenylephrine were not statistically different from epinephrine.

6-Hydroxydopamine perfusion and effect of estrogen on ovum transport

Prior to studying the effects of estrogen on ovum transport in the 6-OHDA-perfused oviduct, the effectiveness of administering *Depo-Estradiol Cypionate* (250 μg) in inducing "tube-locking" at the ampullary-isthmic junction was confirmed in four rabbits. The mean percent distance ovum transport at 72 h p. c. was 51.3 % in these rabbits; the ampullary-isthmic junction was located at 53.5 % of the oviductal length.

The results of administering a single dose of estrogen to rabbits, in which one oviduct was previously perfused with 6-OHDA, are shown in Table 4. The mean percent distance ovum transport on the non-perfused and 6-OHDA-perfused sides was not significantly different; the mean percent distance of the ampullary-isthmic junction of the rabbits indicates that "tube-locking" occurred on both sides. The percent recovery of ova for the control and 6-OHDA sides was 106 % and 90 %, respectively.

6-Hydroxydopamine perfusion and effect of tyramine on oviductal contractility

The effect of tyramine on the contractility of the perfused rabbit oviduct, one week following 6-OHDA treatment, is shown in Fig. 1A, B, C. Pretreatment with 6-OHDA substantially reduced but did not always eliminate the response

Table 4.

The effect *Depo-Estradiol Cypionate* (250 μg) at 17 h *post coitum* on ovum position (72 h p. c.) in non-perfused and 6-hydroxydopamine-perfused oviducts (n = 4).

Oviduct	Location of AIJ (% distance)	Mean % distance ovum transport
Control side	46.6	45.5
6-OHDA side	50.1	50.9

337

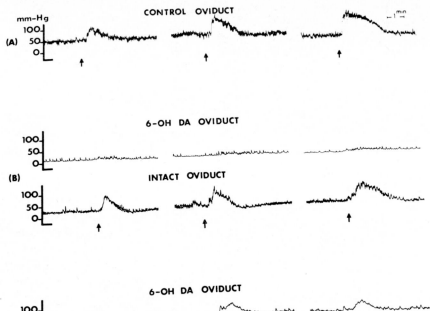

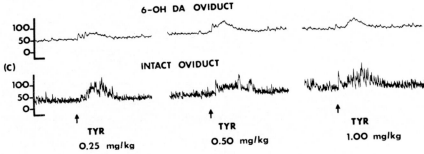

Fig. 1.

Contractile response of the perfused rabbit oviduct to tyramine (TYR) *in vivo.*
(A) Effect of tyramine in the estrous rabbit; (B) Effect of tyramine on oviductal
contraction one week following unilateral 6-ODHA perfusion (response was typical
of 3 of 5 rabbits recorded); (C) Effect of tyramine on oviductal contraction one
week following unilateral 6-ODHA perfusion (response was typical of 2 of 5 rabbits recorded). INTACT OVIDUCT refers to contralateral control (no 6-ODHA)
oviduct from the same rabbit. Arrows (↑) denote administration of tyramine.

of the oviduct to tyramine administration. Fig. 1A shows the response of the
oviduct following tyramine treatment to a normal estrous rabbit. Fig. 1B demonstrates the oviductal response to tyramine in a 6-OHDA-perfused and contralateral, non-treated oviduct. This typified the recorded pattern of 3 of 5
rabbits similarly monitored. The two additional rabbits responded differently
and showed a significant response to tyramine on the 6-OHDA-treated side.
These oviductal recordings are typified in Fig. 1C.

DISCUSSION

The ability of epinephrine to hasten ova into the uterus at 60 and 72 h p. c. (Polidoro et al. 1973) appears from the present study to be attributable to an α-stimulatory effect on the smooth musculature. The effects of the α-adrenergic agonists, norepinephrine and phenylephrine on ovum transport at 60 and 72 h p. c. resemble those noted with epinephrine. Similarly, Bodkhe and Harper (1972) have previously reported increased ovum transport rates when endogenous levels of norepinephrine are high in the oviduct. Isoproterenol, a β-receptor agonist, did not alter the mean rate of ovum transport at the dose studied. Higher doses of isoproterenol were not attempted since mortality rates were excessive at the one pharmacological dose studied.

The significant increase in ovum transport rates at 60 h p. c. with the α-adrenergic stimulants did not increase the percentage of ova recovered from the uterus (Table 2). While norepinephrine (2 mg/kg) significantly increased the transport rate at 60 h p. c., no ova were found in the uterus at that time. Treatment with both phenylephrine and isoproterenol resulted in a small number of ova being recovered for the uterus at 60 h p. c.; however, neither drug mimicked the pronounced increase in ovum recovery noted with epinephrine. The recovery of ova from the uterus of the 72 h treated groups (Table 3), was substantially increased, especially when one compares the percentage of ova recovered with that of the control group. An intriguing observation at 72 h p. c. was the percentage of ova in the uterus following isoproterenol treatment. Although isoproterenol did not alter the mean rate of ovum transport at 72 h p. c., a substantial number of ova (31.2 %) was recovered from the uterus at this time period. This percentage, however, was not as pronounced as that observed with the α-adrenergic stimulants (Table 3). No explanation for this effect of isoproterenol is presently available.

The results of the experiments involving the effects of the interaction of the adrenergic nervous system with estrogen on ovum transport rates in non-perfused and 6-OHDA-perfused oviducts raises questions concerning the role of adrenergic nerves in the physiology of the ampullary-isthmic junction (AIJ). Locking of ova at the AIJ on both the control and 6-OHDA-treated sides, suggests a minimal role, if any, of the adrenergic nervous system in eliciting estrogen-induced oviductal retention of ova. However, the demonstration of possible residual functional capacity of the adrenergic nervous system following 6-OHDA perfusion, as shown in Fig. 1C, suggests that the oviduct may retain the capacity to respond to autonomic stimulation in spite of the absence of intact, intrinsic, adrenergic innervation.

Supersensitization following denervation, as shown by Fleming and Westfall (1975), might explain the responsiveness of the oviduct following 6-OHDA treatment. Degeneration of the adrenergic nerve endings by 6-OHDA would eliminate neuronal reuptake of endogenous norepinephrine as a major deactivation process. This would tend to allow any norepinephrine at the receptor site to remain there longer. Postjunctional receptor supersensitivity may also result after adrenergic nerve destruction.

Tyramine may have induced a release of perivascular norepinephrine since blood vessels in the oviductal smooth musculature retain fluorescence following 6-OHDA perfusion (Eddy and Black 1973). The effects of tyramine-induced norepinephrine release from other tissues might also be responsible for eliciting the responses shown in Fig. 1C.

Blockade of the α-adrenergic receptor site with phenoxybenzamine was shown to antagonize estrogen-induced arrest of ovum transport (Pauerstein et al. 1970a, 1970b). This observation supports the concept of the control of oviductal ovum transport via an interaction of the adrenergic nervous system and estrogen. However, the results of Pauerstein et al. (1974), showing a similar effect following 6-OHDA treatment, are not consistent with our results. The reason for this discrepancy is not known; however, it may involve a difference in the 6-OHDA procedures used in the two studies.

In conclusion, the role of the sympathetic nervous system in the regulation of ovum transport, and the physiology of the isthmus remains unclear. It is difficult to understand how an adrenergic drug like norepinephrine can induce a sphinctering effect (Brundin 1965) of the isthmus and yet be responsible for increasing the rate of ovum transport through the uterotubal junction as noted in the present study.

The issue is further complicated by the recent report of successful pregnancies having been obtained in 2 rabbits following the complete autograft transplantation of the oviduct (Winston and Browne 1974). This preparation would most likely be free of adrenergic innervation; however, intrinsic "short adrenergic neurons" might remain functional.

ACKNOWLEDGMENTS

The authors wish to thank Miss Lucinda Jones for her excellent technical assistance. A special word of thanks is extended to Drs. D. W. Hahn and F. C. Greenslade for their comments and suggestions, to Mrs. Vicky Longo for typing the manuscript and to Mr. Ray Chen for assistance in the statistical analyses.

The drugs utilized in this study were: L-isoproterenol-3-bitartrate dihydrate (Winthrop Laboratories, New York, N.Y.); phenylephrine HCl (Sterling Winthrop, Rensselaer, N.Y.); levarterenol bitartrate, U.S.P. (Winthrop Laboratories, New York, N.Y.); tyramine HCl (Nutritional Biochemical Co., Cleveland, Ohio) and 6-hydroxydopamine HBr (Regis Chemical Co., Chicago, Illinois).

REFERENCES

Bodkhe R. and Harper M. J. K. (1972) Changes in the amount of adrenergic neurotransmitter in the genital tract of untreated rabbits, and rabbits given reserpine or iproniazid during the time of egg transport. *Biol. Reprod.* 6, 288–299.

Brundin J. (1965) Distribution and function of adrenergic nerves in the rabbit Fallopian tube. *Acta physiol. scand.* 66, Suppl. 259, 1–57.

Eddy C. A. and Black D. L. (1973) Chemical sympathectomy of the rabbit oviduct using 6-hydroxydopamine. *J. Reprod. Fertil.* 33, 1–9.

Eddy C. A. and Black D. L. (1974) Ovum transport through rabbit oviducts perfused with 6-hydroxydopamine. *J. Reprod. Fertil.* 38, 189–191.

Falck B. and Owman C. (1965) A detailed methodological description of the fluorescence method for the cellular demonstration of biogenic monoamines. *Acta Univ. Lund II* 7, 5–23.

Fleming W. W. and Westfall D. P. (1975) Altered resting potential in the supersensitive vas deferens of the guinea pig. *J. Pharmacol. exp. Ther.* 192, 381–389.

Greenwald G. S. (1967) Species differences in egg transport in response to exogenous estrogen. *Anatomical Record* 157, 163–172.

Heilman R. D., Bauer E., Hahn D. W. and DaVanzo J. P. (1972) A comparison of cardiovascular and oviduct β-adrenergic receptors. *Fertil. Steril.* 23, 221–229.

Longley W. J., Black D. L. and Currie G. N. (1968) Ovarian hormone control of ovum transport in the rabbit as influenced by autonomic drugs. *J. Reprod. Fertil.* 17, 579–581.

Orsini M. W. (1962) Technique of preparation, study and photography of benzyl-benzoate cleared material for embryological studies. *J. Reprod. Fertil.* 3, 283–287.

Pauerstein C. J., Fremming B. and Martin J. (1970a) Estrogen-induced tubal arrest of ovum: antagonism by alpha-adrenergic blockade. *Obstet. and Gynec.* 35, 671–675.

Pauerstein C. J., Fremming B. and Martin J. (1970b) Influence of progesterone and alpha-adrenergic blockade upon tubal transport of ova. *Gynec. Invest.* 1, 257–267.

Pauerstein C. J., Fremming B., Hodgson B. and Martin J. (1973) The promise of pharmacological modification of ovum transport in contraceptive development. *Amer. J. Obstet. Gynec.* 116, 161–166.

Pauerstein C. J., Hodgson B., Fremming B. and Martin J. (1974) Effects of sympathetic denervation of the rabbit oviduct on normal ovum transport and on transport modified by estrogen and progesterone. *Gynec. Invest.* 5, 121–132.

Polidoro J. P., Howe G. R. and Black D. L. (1973) The effects of adrenergic drugs on ovum transport through the rabbit oviduct. *J. Reprod. Fertil.* 35, 331–337.

Polidoro J. P. (1974) Recent advances in oviduct pharmacology. *J. Reprod. Medicine* 13, 45–48.

Polidoro J. P., Culver R., Thomas S. and Greenslade F. C. (1974) Selective sympathetic denervation of the rabbit ductus deferens using 6-hydroxydopamine. *J. Reprod. Fertil.* 39, 167–170.

Steel R. and Torrie J. (1960) *Principles and Procedures of Statistics*, pp. 43–44. McGraw Hill, New York.

Winston R. M. L. and Browne J. C. McClure (1974) Pregnancy following autograft transplantation of Fallopian tube and ovary in the rabbit. *Lancet* 2, 494–495.

341

Laboratory of Reproductive Physiology,
University of Massachusetts – Amherst, Mass. 01002

CHOLINERGIC MECHANISMS, OVIDUCTAL MOTILITY AND OVUM TRANSPORT*

By

G. R. Howe

ABSTRACT

Activity of the oviductal smooth muscle in the rabbit was evaluated by constant perfusion of the isthmus. Above threshold, intravenous injections of bethanechol chloride or pilocarpine at levels of 200–300 μg/kg resulted in elevated isthmic muscle tone. The stimulatory effect was approximately 17–24 % of that induced through adrenergic alpha stimulation with epinephrine. Comparable stimulation was induced by the administration of cholinergic agonists into the isthmic lumen *in vivo* or into an *in vitro* organ bath. Adrenergic alpha blockade with phenoxybenzamine inhibited cholinergic stimulation, whereas beta blockade with propranolol sometimes enhanced the action of cholinergic agonists. The introduction of atropine *in vivo* and *in vitro* also reduced the stimulatory effects of both cholinergic drugs. The results suggested that cholinergic agonists may act on the isthmic musculature via adrenergic alpha and/or cholinergic receptor stimulation.
Preliminary studies have shown that the systemic administration of cholinergic agonists or blockers to rabbits has little effect upon egg or sperm transport through the oviduct.

REVIEW OF LITERATURE

A number of investigators have reviewed the adrenergic nervous system as an oviductal regulatory mechanism (Pauerstein et al. 1968; Marshall 1970). There is sufficient evidence that the smooth muscle of the oviduct possesses

---

* This work was supported by NIH Grant HDO 4180-05.

342

alpha and beta receptors which are excitatory and inhibitory, respectively (Longley et al. 1968; Martin et al. 1970). Howe and Black (1973) have shown that estrogen and progesterone increase the sensitivity of alpha and beta receptors respectively in the rabbit oviduct. Eddy and Black (1973) were able to reduce the norepinephrine content of the oviductal musculature with 6-hydroxydopamine (6-OHDA). The same study as well as that by Goldman and Jacobowitz (1971) showed that 6-OHDA does not denervate vascular tissue.

The abundant adrenergic innervation of the oviductal musculature in conjunction with its response to adrenergic drugs has suggested that the sympathetic nervous system is involved in the regulation of ovum transport (Brundin 1965; Pauerstein et al. 1973). Adrenergic agonists, antagonists or denervation, however, appear to have little or no effect upon ovum transport (Bodkhe and Harper 1972; Eddy and Black 1973; Polidoro et al. 1973). Similarly, Johns et al. (1974) have shown that 6-OHDA does not alter fertility in mice.

Knowledge concerning the cholinergic innervation of the female genital tract is very limited due to the lack of a specific histochemical test for acetylcholine. No acetylcholinesterase activity is found in the ampulla of the rabbit or guinea pig (Jordon 1970). Owman et al. (1966) found small amounts of acetylcholinesterase in the isthmus, whereas Jacobowitz and Koelle (1965) observed numerous nerves containing cholinesterase in the cat oviduct. The latter authors noted that cholinesterase-active nerves corresponded with those exhibiting adrenergic fluorescence. More recently, Hervonen and Kanerva (1972), using the electron microscope, observed adrenergic and non-adrenergic (possibly cholinergic) terminals lying in close proximity to one another. Black (1974) found measurable amounts of acetylcholinesterase in all parts of the rabbit oviduct; however, there was little association between amounts and specific segments analyzed.

The present studies were designed to determine the influence of cholinergic mechanisms upon oviductal motility and hence ovum transport.

MATERIALS AND METHODS

Sexually mature rabbit does of the New Zealand variety were isolated 3 weeks prior to experimentation. Animals were anesthetized with Nembutal (37 mg/kg iv) and subjected to a midventral laparatomy.

Polyethylene tubing (PE90) was secured into the oviductal isthmus 1 cm above the uterotubal junction (UIJ) and directed towards the uterus. The cannula was attached to a Harvard constant perfusion pump and a Statham pressure transducer. Activity of the isthmic circular muscle was evaluated by measuring perfusion resistance on a Beckman recorder and quantified with a Resetting Integrator Coupler in terms of area (cm²) under the pressure curve. Saline

(0.9 %) was used as the perfusion medium at a rate of 103 μl/min. The effects of drug administration upon activity of the oviductal musculature were evaluated by comparing areas under the pressure curve 3 min prior to and 3 min post treatment.

All drugs were mixed in ascorbic saline (1 mg ascorbic acid/ml saline) and injected via the marginal ear vein.

RESULTS

In vivo cholinergic stimulation

Initial studies were directed towards the search for the proper cholinergic agonist, namely, an agent that is not metabolized rapidly, has minimal cardiovascular effects, and has specific action on smooth muscle. The cholinergic stimulators utilized in the studies were bethanechol chloride (Urecholine®; Merck Sharp and Dohme) and pilocarpine. The two parasympathetic agonists were administered in varying doses of 50–500 μg/kg and compared to ascorbic saline as the placebo control agent. Single or repetitive doses less than 100 μg/kg did not affect the muscular activity of the oviduct, whereas higher levels increased muscular perfusion resistance. The dose response data curve (post treatment) for bethanechol chloride and pilocarpine-treated animals are shown in Table 1. Both drugs increased perfusion resistance; however, a dose of 200–300 μg/kg was needed to induce a noticeable change. On the other hand, levels above 400 μg/kg did not appear to initiate additional muscular contraction. The stimulation from these two parasympathomimetic agents was far less than that induced by 5.0 μg/kg (iv) of epinephrine (+8.25 to +22.00, ave. +13.67 cm²).

Table 1.
The effect of cholinergic agonists on oviductal perfusion resistance.

Concentration of drug (μg/kg)	Change in area (cm²) under pressure curve 3 min prior to and post injection	
	Bethanechol cl. (7 does)	Pilocarpine (7 does)
50	−0.25 to +0.68 (+0.13)	+0.17 to +0.24 (+0.22)
100	+0.75 to +2.58 (+0.75)	+0.31 to +1.52 (+0.85)
300	+1.50 to +4.63 (+2.40)	+2.50 to +6.45 (+2.51)
400	+3.00 to +6.50 (+4.70)	+2.53 to +8.00 (+3.10)
600	+2.30 to +8.63 (+4.67)	+2.84 to +3.75 (+3.33)

Table 2.

Comparative effects of bethanechol chloride under varying pharmacologic states.

Concentration of beth. cl. (μg/kg)	Mean change in area (cm^2) under pressure curve 3 min prior to and post injection				
	Control	Phenoxy-benzamine[a]	Propranolol[b]	Atropine[c]	Reserpine[d]
100	+0.75	+0.06	+0.93	–	−0.06
300	+2.40	+0.13	+2.83	−0.60	−0.09
400	+4.70	+0.01	+3.85	−0.05	−0.25

[a] Phenoxybenzamine 10 mg/kg (complete alpha blocker); $1\frac{1}{2}$ h prior to beth. cl.
[b] Propranolol 7 mg/kg (incomplete beta block); $1\frac{1}{2}$ h prior to beth. cl.
[c] Atropine 2 mg/kg (complete cholinergic block); 2 h prior to beth. cl.
[d] Reserpine 2.5 mg/kg (complete NE depletion); 30–36 h prior to beth. cl.

Ovariectomy with or without hormonal replacement (regime reported earlier by Howe and Black 1973) had little effect upon the effects of the cholinergic agonists.

Subsequent studies were conducted in an attempt to determine if the moderate stimulation induced by the two cholinergic agonists was dependent upon adrenergic innervation to the oviduct. Phenoxybenzamine (iv) was utilized for adrenergic alpha blockade, and the degree of blockade was determined by drug challenge with epinephrine (5.0 μg/kg). Complete alpha inhibition of the oviduct was achieved with a dose level of 10.0 mg/kg, whereas smaller dosages (3–5 mg/kg) induced alpha blockade of the cardiovascular system. Phenoxybenzamine essentially inhibited the stimulatory response of the oviductal musculature to bethanechol chloride or pilocarpine. In contrast, adrenergic beta inhibition with propranolol at 7 mg/kg iv (blockade tested by challenge with 4.0 μg/kg iso-proterenol) enhanced the oviduct's response to cholinergic stimulation. These results suggested that the action of the parasympathetic agonists might be, in part, mediated indirectly via postganglionic adrenergic innervation.

In an attempt to determine if cholinergic agonists have any effect upon the oviductal muscle by direct stimulation of cholinergic receptors, 5 does were subjected to parasympathetic blockade with 2 mg/kg iv atropine. Surprisingly, atropine was as effective as phenoxybenzamine in inhibiting bethanechol-induced muscle stimulation. The comparative effects of bethanechol chloride (beth. cl.) under different pharmacological states are shown in Table 2. In an attempt to show the specific pathway of cholinergic-induced stimulation of the oviductal musculature, 5 does were given reserpine (2.5 mg/kg) 30–36 h prior to bethanechol challenge. Cholinergic stimulation was completely inhibited in these animals.

In vitro cholinergic stimulation

In an attempt to substantiate the specific effects of cholinergic agonists upon the circular muscle of the rabbit oviduct without circulatory and neural variables, experiments were conducted in an *in vitro* organ bath. The entire oviduct including the proximal uterine horn was suspended in Locke's solution aerated with 95 % O_2 and 5 % CO_2 and maintained at 37°C. The perfusion set-up was identical to that described for the *in vivo* studies, and a perfusion period of 30 min prior to drug treatment was allowed as a physiologic equilibration period. Drugs were added directly to the bathing medium (70 ml), washed out with two changes of Locke's solution, and the tissue allowed to recover from the drug treatment (approximately 15–20 min) prior to any subsequent treatment. Due to dilution factors increased drug levels were essential.

Both bethanechol chloride (30–75 μg/ml) and pilocarpine (150–4000 μg/ml) increased perfusion resistance with varying ranges in change under the pressure curve (cm²). The response was not dependent upon the concentration of the drug in the bathing medium. Both phenoxybenzamine (50–150 μg/ml)

Table 3.
In vitro effects of cholinergic agonists under different Pharmacological states.

Cholinergic agonist	Range and mean change in area (cm²) under pressure curve 3 min prior to and post-treatment			
	Control	Phenoxybenz-amine[a]	Propranolol[b]	Atropine[c]
Bethanechol chloride	10* −0.15 to +15.83 (+5.28)	6* −1.42 to +0.84 (−0.14)	–	6* −1.46 to +1.55 (+0.23)
Pilocarpine	16* −1.72 to +2.78 (+0.16)	14* −8.48 to +5.57 (−0.18)	10* −0.57 to +4.70 (+1.29)	8* −1.73 to +1.85 (−0.07)

* Number of oviducts under treatment.
a Phenoxybenzamine 100–150 μg/ml.
b Propranolol 200–300 μg/ml.
c Atropine 100–200 μg/ml.

and atropine (50–200 μg/ml) reduced or completely inhibited the stimulatory response of the oviductal musculature to both cholinergic agonists, whereas propranolol had little or no effect. Under *in vitro* conditions bethanechol chloride was more stimulatory than pilocarpine; phenoxybenzamine was more effective than atropine for inhibiting the stimulatory response. These data are summarized in Table 3.

DISCUSSION

Activity of rabbit oviductal circular muscle was increased by both bethanechol chloride and pilocarpine. This is in agreement with Sandberg et al. (1960) who observed acetylcholine to be stimulatory in the human, whereas Hawkins (1964) found pilocarpine to be ineffective at much smaller doses than the present study (20 μg/ml vs 150–4000 μg/ml). The stimulation in the present study was, however, much less than alpha activation induced by epinephrine (70 % or less than epinephrine response) in a previous study by Howe and Black (1973). In addition, drug levels about 20 times that of epinephrine was necessary to enhance perfusion resistance of the isthmus, which might explain the negative results of Longley (1967).

The present data suggest that the cholinergic drug stimulation of the isthmic musculature may be working indirectly via the adrenergic postganglionic release of norepinephrine acting on alpha receptors. To substantiate such a hypothesis, does were pretreated with phenoxybenzamine (alpha blocker) and challenged with epinephrine to evaluate the degree of blockade. Approximately 10 mg/kg (iv) was needed for complete oviductal blockade which is in contrast to 4 mg/kg reported by Longley et al. (1968). The latter authors used rabbits of the Dutch-belted variety whereas the present study utilized New Zealand whites. Adrenergic alpha blockade inhibited any cholinergic stimulation and this response was dependent upon the degree of blockade. Propranolol (beta blocker) in a dose of 7 mg/kg (iv) enhanced the activity of the cholinergic agonists; however, blockade was not complete as evaluated by drug challenge with isoproterenol. Such data strengthens the hypothesis of indirect cholinergic-adrenergic stimulation as Cibils et al. (1971) reported norepinephrine enhancement in the human oviduct after propranolol treatment.

Atropine at 2 mg/kg (iv) like phenoxybenzamine, resulted in the inhibition of any cholinergic stimulation. In contrast, Brundin (1965) reported that 20 mg/kg of atropine did not alter adrenergic nerve activity of the rabbit oviduct. It is possible that the present level of atropine was sufficient to inhibit ganglionic nerve transmission in that such activity has been documented as a pharmacological property of atropine.

347

In summary, the present results suggest that cholinergic stimulation of the rabbit oviduct may take place by the indirect adrenergic release of norepinephrine. Anatomical studies by Hervonen and Kanerva (1972) give plausibility to the indirect cholinergic-adrenergic theory. To strengthen such a theory, the present study shows the absence of cholinergic stimulation in reserpinized (NE depletion) rabbits. In an attempt to substantiate the action of atropine, cholinergic drug challenge must be carried out in animals subjected to ganglionic blockade.

REFERENCES

Black D. L. (1974) Neural control of oviduct musculature. In: Johnson A. D. and Foley C. W., eds. *The Oviduct and Its Functions,* pp. 65–118. Academic Press, New York.

Bodkhe R. R. and Harper M. J. K. (1972) Changes in the amount of adrenergic neurotransmitter in the genital tract of untreated rabbits, and rabbits given reserpine or iproniazid during the time of egg transport. *Biol. Reprod. 6,* 288–299.

Brundin J. (1965) Distribution and function of adrenergic nerves in the rabbit Fallopian tube. *Acta physiol. scand. 66,* 1–57.

Cibils L. A., Sica-Blanco Y., Remedio M. R., Rozada H. and Gil B. E. (1971) Effect of sympathomimetic drugs upon the human oviduct *in vivo. Amer. J. Obstet. Gynec. 110,* 481–488.

Eddy C. A. and Black D. L. (1973) Chemical sympathectomy of the rabbit oviduct using 6-hydroxydopamine. *J. Reprod. Fertil. 33,* 1–9.

Goldman H. and Jacobowitz D. (1971) Correlation of norepinephrine content with observations of adrenergic nerves after a single dose of 6-hydroxydopamine in the rat. *J. Pharmacol. exp. Ther. 176,* 119.

Hawkins D. F. (1964) Some pharmacological reactions of isolated rings of human Fallopian tube. *Arch. int. Pharmacodyn. 152,* 474–478.

Hervonen A. and Kanerva L. (1972) Adrenergic and noradrenergic axons of the rabbit uterus and oviduct. *Acta physiol. scand. 85,* 139–141.

Howe G. R. and Black D. L. (1973) Autonomic nervous system and oviduct function in the rabbit. I. Hormones and contraction. *J. Reprod. Fertil. 33,* 425–430.

Jacobowitz D. and Koelle G. B. (1965) Histochemical correlations of acetylcholinesterase and catecholamines in post ganglionic autonomic nerves of the cat, rabbit and guinea pig. *J. Pharmacol. exp. Ther. 148,* 225–237.

Johns A., Chlumecky J. and Paton D. M. (1974) Role of adrenergic nerves in ovulation and ovum transport. *Lancet 2,* 1079.

Jordon S. M. (1970) Adrenergic and cholinergic innervation of the reproductive tract and ovary in the guinea-pig and rabbit. *J. Physiol. (Lond.) 210,* 115.

Longley W. J. (1967) The role of the ovarian hormones and the autonomic nervous system in the transport of ova through the oviduct of the rabbit. Ph. D. Dissertation, University of Massachusetts.

Longley W. J., Black D. L. and Currie G. N. (1968) Oviduct circular muscle response to drugs related to the autonomic nervous system. *J. Reprod. Fertil. 17,* 95–100.

Martin J. E., Ware R. W., Crosby R. J. and Pauerstein C. J. (1970) Demonstration of beta adrenergic receptors in the rabbit oviduct. *Gynec. Invest. 1,* 82–91.

Owman C. and Sjöberg N. O. (1966) On short adrenergic neurons in the accessory male genital organs of the bull. *Experientia* 22, 759.

Pauerstein C. J., Fremming B. D., Hodgson B. J. and Martin J. E. (1973) The promise of pharmacological modification of ovum transport in contraceptive development. *Amer. J. Obstet. Gynec.* 116, 161–166.

Polidoro J. P., Howe G. R. and Black D. L. (1973) The effects of adrenergic drugs on ovum transport through the rabbit oviduct. *J. Reprod. Fertil.* 35, 331–337.

Sandberg F., Ingelman-Sundberg A., Lindgren L. and Rydén G. (1960) *In vitro* studies of the motility of the human Fallopian tube. Part I. The effects of acetylcholine, adrenaline, noradrenaline and oxytocin on the spontaneous motility. *Acta obstet. gynec. scand.* 39, 506–516.

Laboratory for Reproductive Physiology,
Department of Veterinary and Animal Science,
University of Massachusetts, Amherst, Massachusetts 01002

Discussion Paper

AUTONOMIC MECHANISMS IN OVUM TRANSPORT
SUMMARY AND CONCLUSION

By

D. L. Black

In summarizing this session on autonomic mechanisms in ovum transport, I want to point out certain well-established facts about the autonomic nerve supply to the oviduct, some of the deficiencies in our present knowledge, and some areas where I think future research is needed.

Anatomically, the distribution of adrenergic nerves within the oviduct of many animals, including the human, is well-established. Generally, a similarity in the pattern of nerve distribution exists. In the ampulla the nerves are mostly vasomotor with a few innervating the relatively thin muscle wall. Unlike the ampulla, there is a distinct increase in the number of nerves supplying the isthmic musculature. At the ampullary-isthmic junction, and in some animals at the uterotubal junction, there is a pronounced increase in adrenergic neurons. The adrenergic innervation to the female reproductive tract is unique. In addition to receiving nerves from pre- and paravertebral ganglia (long adrenergic neurons) it receives a portion from ganglionic formations in the uterovaginal area (short adrenergic neurons). The two types of neurons appear to differ physiologically as well as anatomically.

Information on the cholinergic component of the autonomic nervous system is sparse and the data available on its influence on the oviductal musculature are confusing. Histochemically very few cholinergic nerves can be demonstrated.

Pharmacologically, there also appear to be considerable similarities in the response of oviducts from various animals to adrenergic drugs. Both alpha and beta receptors have been found in the oviducts of all animals studied. The

350

alpha adrenoceptors are generally stimulatory whereas the beta are inhibitory. Currently, our concept of the role of adrenoceptors in the oviduct is primitive and probably overly simplistic. Dr. Brundin has presented data that show the presence of alpha and beta receptors on the neuron itself. These receptors influence the amount of norepinephrine released from the neuron and the relative activity of the two receptors may be dependent on the amount of neurotransmitter present.

The degree of response or the type of response elicited by adrenergic drugs depends to a certain degree on the endocrine state of the animal. In the rabbit, alpha response is increased by estrogens and decreased by progesterone. Progesterone production following ovulation appears to increase the beta response. Endocrine modification of neuronal activity is most pronounced in the human. As reported by Drs. Owman and Paton, norepinephrine can produce contraction or relaxation of the human oviduct depending on the hormonal status at the time. There also may be differences in the response of the ampulla and isthmus. These observations emphasize the danger of transferring data from laboratory animals to the human. Because of changes in autonomic activity under various hormonal conditions, an endocrine profile of the animal under investigation should be included in future experimentation.

From the physiological standpoint, it is difficult to establish a clearcut association between the autonomic nervous system and the reproductive process. In the first place we have not always defined what is meant by "significant" alteration of ovum transport. In many cases there is a distinct difference between a statistically significant and a physiologically significant alteration. While administration of the various adrenergic drugs will stimulate or depress oviductal activity, the influence of altered oviductal activity on ovum transport appears minimal. To my knowledge there is no definitive information that conception or pregnancy is prevented by alteration of autonomic activity during the gamete transport period. Indeed, after destruction of adrenergic nerves with 6-hydroxydopamine, depletion of norepinephrine with reserpine, or transplant of the reproductive tract, pregnancy is possible. The efficacy of present procedures for "denervating" the oviduct is unknown. Until adequate information is present to show that these methods are totally effective in depleting the neurotransmitter, care must be exercised in the interpretation of data.

From the information presented at this meeting it is clear that a great many factors are concerned in oviductal contractility – the autonomic nervous system being only one. While it is often necessary to remove the autonomic nervous system from other influences to simplify experimentation, one must ever be aware that the autonomic nervous system never acts unilaterally but in concert with other regulatory mechanisms. Many of these mechanisms have been discussed but the numerous interactions that occur have not been fully elucidated and require much additional research.

Much of the difficulty in assessing the role of the autonomic nervous system in ovum transport lies in the fact that the techniques used by researchers often vary. Contractility, the parameter used to assess the stimulatory or inhibitory effects of drugs or nerve stimulation on the oviduct, is usually determined by measuring changes in oviductal luminal diameter. As we have previously heard, methods employed to date have distinct shortcomings. The various techniques are in themselves apt to stimulate oviductal activity. In addition, they do not have the capability for providing a precise picture of the type of activity taking place. The oviduct, as pointed out earlier by Dr. Daniel, is a dynamic structure composed of many sites or compartments in which activity occurs. Methods now in use measure activity in a very small and often in a non-delineated area of the whole. Because of these methodological difficulties, little information concerning the type or degree of muscle activity modulation by the autonomic system is available.

Histochemical and biochemical methods for detection of the adrenergic neurotransmitter, norepinephrine, have been improved significantly in the last few years. These improved methods have proved extremely useful in anatomical studies designed to delineate the distribution of adrenergic nerves in the oviduct. In spite of their value in anatomical works, as commonly used, they leave much to be desired as a tool for studying the neurophysiology of the oviduct. Neither method distinguishes between the bound and more labile unbound neurotransmitter that participates in immediate physiological function. Data obtained by these methods must be evaluated, therefore, with this fact in mind. Likewise, these methods provide little information on the metabolic activity of the neurons; only the difference between the amount synthesized and the amount destroyed is measured. The fact that neuronal activity is altered by the endocrine state, as reported by Dr. Doteuchi, may be very significant. It is evident that an estimate of catecholamine turnover provides more information on neural activity than the measurement of the amine present in the tissue.

Unlike adrenergic nerves, there is no histochemical technique for the demonstration of the cholinergic neurotransmitter. At this time we still depend on the presence of acetylcholine esterase to demonstrate cholinergic nerves and the reliability of this method has been questioned. Dr. Howe has shown that pharmacological stimulation of the parasympathetic nervous system can excite the oviduct. This effect, however, is mediated via the action of drugs on the ganglia and secondary release of norepinephrine.

In most studies on ovum transport emphasis has been on the more dynamic aspects of ovum transport i. e. oviductal motility, ciliary action, and fluid dynamics. Without doubt, oviductal contractility and concomitantly luminal diameter can be altered by adrenergic drugs or nerve stimulation. It has been proposed that oviductal lumen constriction following drug administration has the dual effects of altering the fluid dynamics and propelling the ovum through the oviduct. Both effects have been deduced and not measured experimentally. The influence of adrenergic drugs on ciliary activity in the oviduct is not known. More attention should be paid to the less dynamic aspects, in particular, the tone of the isthmic portion of the oviduct. There is ample evidence to suggest that the rate of ovum transport is dependent on a balance between two forces: (1) a propulsive force supplied individually or collectively by muscular activity, cilia, and fluid flow, and (2) inhibitory forces such as constriction of the isthmic lumen. It is through the action of these two opposing forces that transport is controlled. Possibly, propulsive forces such as muscular and ciliary activity are generally adequate but fine tuning of transport depends on the size of the isthmic lumen. The size of the isthmic lumen may depend on either endocrine or neural mechanisms; or more likely, on a combination of the two.

Prostaglandins have been shown to modify the activity of the autonomic nervous system. PGE_1 and PGE_2 released by nerve stimulation inhibit the response of the effector tissue. Also, PGE_1 blocks the oviductal response to hypogastric nerve stimulation. Dr. Paton has evidence to suggest that prostaglandins may be spontaneously liberated from the oviduct; the role they play in normal oviductal function, however, is not clear. Evidence that there are temporal changes in the amount of prostaglandins in the oviduct suggest that they could play a significant role either by acting alone or by modifying the action of adrenergic nerves. Since prostaglandins have an effect on the rabbit oviduct that has been alpha and beta blocked indicates that in this species the nervous system is not essential for PG activity. Dr. Aref has shown that pharmacological doses of prostaglandin $F_{2\alpha}$ given to rabbits at 36 h *post coitum* markedly accelerates ovum transport and interferes with implantation. The fact that pregnancy is not adversely effected in the rabbit when indomethacin is given during the period of ovum transport indicates that prostaglandins may not be a prerequisite for satisfactory ovum transport in this species.

In the future, methods for accurately measuring the activity of the oviduct must be developed. In studies of adrenergic activity, more attention must be directed toward the synthesis, release, and uptake of norepinephrine by neurons in the oviduct. An attempt should be made to relate changes in these parameters to increasing and decreasing levels of steroid hormones and prostaglandins. Experiments should be conducted to see if the autonomic nervous system influences the constriction and ultimate relaxation of the isthmic musculature.

There is no information available at the present to indicate that the autonomic nervous system is essential for adequate ovum transport. In experiments conducted to date little effect on ovum transport has accompanied alteration of adrenergic or cholinergic activity. Conversely, we have no definitive knowledge that it is truly unimportant. Until we have more information based on experiments conducted with reliable methods, an intelligent evaluation of the importance of the autonomic nervous system in ovum transport is impossible.

353

SUMMARY OF DISCUSSIONS ON
AUTONOMIC MECHANISMS IN OVUM TRANSPORT

Reporter: *David M. Paton*

SUMMARY OF CURRENT KNOWLEDGE

There was general agreement that considerable information exists on the adrenergic innervation of the oviducts of several species, including the human. The oviduct, along with other reproductive organs, is partially supplied by "short" adrenergic neurons whose properties differ in certain respects from those of the more common "long" adrenergic neurons. Considerably less information is available on the detailed relationship of adrenergic nerve terminals to smooth muscle cells, especially in human tissues at different stages of the menstrual cycle.

The presence of alpha and beta adrenergic receptors has been demonstrated in several species, including the human. Results presented at this Symposium have indicated that, in the human, the sensitivity of the adrenergic receptors is influenced by the stage of the menstrual cycle and particularly by the presence of progesterone.

There is evidence that the oviductal content of norepinephrine is influenced by sex hormones. However, it was considered that measurements of amine content alone are not very useful but should be combined with turnover studies and with studies of other aspects of adrenergic transmission, e. g., changes in the sensitivity of receptors.

Considerable attention has been devoted to the results of denervation procedures on ovum transport and fertility in rabbits, rats and mice. In these studies, adrenergic "denervation" has been produced either surgically or chemically by using reserpine or pretreatment with 6-hydroxydopamine. These studies demonstrated that ovum transport and fertility are not greatly influenced by such procedures. The conclusions that can be drawn from such studies, were obviously a matter of dispute in different discussion groups. At one extreme were those who felt that the studies had convincingly demonstrated that the adrenergic innervation played little role in ovum transport and that therefore further research into adrenergic mechanisms was unlikely to result in the development of a clinically useful contraceptive. At the other extreme were participants who argued that the studies had not excluded a significant role for the adrenergic innervation since the degree of denervation achieved was not complete and because such procedures also altered processes outside the oviduct.

IDENTIFICATION OF NEEDED INFORMATION AND RESEARCH REQUIRED

If it is accepted that acceleration of ovum transport can form the basis of a contraceptive technique, certain conclusions flow from the assumption. There is experimental evidence indicating that interference with ovum transport can be contraceptive in lower animals, e. g., ovum transfer studies, but little conclusive evidence exists in women. It is possible that this is the mechanism of action of post-coital estrogens in women. It would be of value to establish that this is indeed their mechanism of action, e. g., by studies of ovum transport in women.

It is agreed that it is undesirable to retard ovum transport because of the potential danger of inducing ectopic pregnancy. Elucidation of the mechanism of ovum transport, and the factors responsible for its regulation, are important questions. However, long term studies will be required to determine the mechanisms involved, and such studies may not result in leads for contraception. It is considered, therefore, that such studies should receive lower priority in the WHO program, than those proposed below:

(a) An approach that could be used immediately is to utilize existing information on the pharmacological actions of known drugs. One such avenue is to test the hypothesis that drugs that increase oviductal motility, will prevent pregnancy. Agents of this type include: sympathomimetics acting on α-receptors, β-adrenergic receptor blocking agents, oxytocin and analogues, estrogens, antiestrogens, progestins, prostaglandins, and gonadotrophins.

Such a study would necessitate (1) a program to screen the effect of a variety of known agents on the motility of isolated human oviducts; and (2) a program to screen the effects of such agents on the fertility of lower species, e. g., rabbits, and, in promising cases, sub-human primates.

Attention should also be given to the potential use of drug combinations so as to reduce side effects.

23*

(b) The wide scale use of such agents will depend on the accurate detection of ovulation. High priority should be given to discovering a method for this that is simple to use, cheap, and reliable.

(c) Another area that might receive attention is the development of an electrical pacemaker for the oviduct. Such a method would have the advantage of potential reversibility, but would only be applicable to a small group of women. Because of this consideration, the methodology should be as direct and inexpensive as possible.

(d) Little is known about the role of cilia. It may be helpful to discover whether any known drugs can be used to increase or decrease ciliary action and the effects of these on fertility. It will be important, however, to ensure that such agents do not also impair ciliary action in other organs, e. g., the lungs.

The following specific studies were proposed by individual groups:
(1) to determine the effect of sympathetic overactivity on ovum transport. This could include, for example, chronic stimulation of the hypogastric nerves in conscious, restrained animals;

(2) to determine the effect of receptor blocking agents on the transport of artificial ova in women;

(3) a multicentre trial of the effects of autonomic drugs on the fertility of sub-human primates.

Most groups favoured additional studies of the interactions between norepinephrine and the adrenergic innervation, prostaglandins, cyclic nucleotides and ovarian steroids. All stressed that such studies should include details of the hormonal status of the patient or animal at the time measurements of oviductal function are made.

There was general agreement that there is comparatively little information on the role of the parasympathetic nervous system in oviductal function but it was felt that the cholinergic system is not a very significant factor in the regulation of ovum transport.

After reviewing the reports of each group, this reporter concluded that most participants believed that the adrenergic innervation was unlikely to play an important role in the regulation of ovum transport. Despite this, most participants favoured further rather basic studies into adrenergic mechanisms of the mammalian oviduct. This may simply reflect a feeling that there are very few other postulated mechanisms for the regulation of ovum transport that can be studied at present. It was recognized that these judgements are dependent on current knowledge and new information could significantly alter the scale of priorities of one approach versus another.

ASSESSMENT OF FEASIBILITY AND COSTS
OF SUCH APPROACHES

Such research must be viewed in the context of world population growth, the size of the total WHO budget, existing contraceptive techniques, the relative merits of different approaches to new techniques, etc.

A reasonably large number of relatively effective contraceptive methods are already available. Application of these would, in our opinion, greatly reduce the explosive growth in world population. Priority should therefore first be given to education of populations, and the provision of personnel and materials needed for large scale contraceptive programs in the third world.

There is, however, a need for other contraceptive techniques that would be more acceptable to certain groups, and/or have fewer side effects than existing methods, and/or be more effective, and/or be more applicable to certain developing countries. Decisions should be based on the relative merits of possible different approaches, the size of the total budget and an estimate of the time and funding required for each approach to yield a new contraceptive technique. The need and priority for research on methods for the regulation of ovum transport should be re-assessed by WHO with these considerations in mind.

It is considered that the urgency of the problem posed by the population explosion and the size of the WHO budget demands that only the most promising leads should be funded. This consideration would exclude many basic studies since they are unlikely to yield useable results in the near future. However, such studies would be important to establish the mechanism of drugs shown to act as contraceptives.

The studies proposed in women are unlikely to be costly and should take little time to obtain evidence for useful activity. Experiments in sub-human primates, by contrast, will be expensive given the scarcity of animals and the costs involved in quarantine, obtaining records of cycle data and fertility and routine maintenance. It should be noted that each such study will cost between $ 60,000–80,000/year. In other countries, costs may well be less but at the moment primate colonies suitable for research in lesser developed countries are very scarce or non-existent.

PERSONAL COMMENTS

I should like to conclude with a number of personal comments based on the papers presented at the Symposium and the discussion that followed. The available evidence has demonstrated that, in certain species, normal ovum transport can occur despite a very severe reduction in adrenergic innervation to the oviduct. It is very doubtful whether a similar degree of adrenergic denervation

357

could be achieved in women using available methods. The potential long-term side effects of 6-hydroxydopamine would have to be examined but in any event the lesion produced by this agent is not permanent. Systemic administration of agents such as reserpine or adrenergic neurone blocking agents is accompanied by important side effects that limit doses that can be administered systemically. Use of such agents would therefore be dependent upon the development of a local delivery system. Surgical denervation is, in my opinion, precluded by the magnitude of the surgery required. On practical grounds therefore adrenergic denervation of the human oviduct does not, at present, appear to be a practical proposition. In addition, it is important to remember that in other tissues adrenergic transmission is surprisingly well maintained despite a very severe reduction in norepinephrine content, e. g., after reserpine (Andén and Henning 1966). In addition, after chronic interruption of the innervation, postjunctional supersensitivity develops (Fleming et al. 1973) and this would tend to offset the effects of such procedures.

The alternative approach of increasing sympathetic activity to the oviduct could theoretically be achieved either by chronic stimulation of the nerves (but this would not be a practical proposition in humans) or by the administration of sympathomimetic amines. However, the administration of sympathomimetic amines has not had spectacular effects on ovum transport in lower animals, and as Dr. Polidoro's study demonstrated, is attended by significantly morbidity. Again it would seem that to be applied in humans, a local delivery system would need to be developed.

REFERENCES

Andén N. E. and Henning M. (1966) Adrenergic nerve function, noradrenaline level and noradrenaline uptake in cat nicitating membrane after reserpine treatment. *Acta physiol. scand.* 67, 498–504.
Fleming W. W., McPhillips J. J. and Westfall D. P. (1973) Postjunctional supersensitivity and subsensitivity of excitable tissues to drugs. *Ergebn. Physiol. Biol. Chem. Exp. Pharmakol.* 68, 56–119.

SECTION IV

Control of Ovum Transport
in the Oviduct

MODERATORS

J. P. BENNETT

and

E. S. E. HAFEZ

Department of Gynecology-Obstetrics
and Reproductive Physiology Laboratories,
C. S. Mott Center for Human Growth and Development,
Wayne State University School of Medicine,
Detroit, Michigan, USA

ANATOMICAL AND PHYSIOLOGICAL MECHANISMS OF OVUM TRANSPORT

By

E. S. E. Hafez

ABSTRACT

Several anatomical and physiological mechanisms have been implicated in the control of ova transport in the oviduct, e. g. the beat of kinocilia, the flow of oviductal secretions, contractions of oviductal musculature and the functional integrity of the ampullary-isthmic junction and the uterotubal junction. The relative importance of these mechanisms in ovum transport is unknown. Pharmacological and neural mechanisms are also involved. Future research is needed on a) contraction patterns of oviductal musculature as affected by the hormonal and pharmacological environments, b) currents and counter-currents of oviductal secretions, and c) ciliary beat in the isthmus and uterotubal junction.

Extensive investigations utilizing a variety of techniques have been undertaken to study the rate of ovum transport in laboratory mammals, primarily the rabbit (cf. Blandau 1969). Very little precise information is available on human or nonhuman primates. In the rhesus monkey ovum transport through the oviduct requires some 3 to 4 days (Mastroianni et al. 1967; Marston et al. 1969). The

Supported by the The Ford Foundation grant No. 710-0287 A and USPHS. National Institute of Child Health and Human Development grant No. HD 06234.

progress of ova through different segments of the oviduct has, however, not been established for primates, partly due to difficulties in determining the precise time of ovulation. Visualization *in vivo* by serial laparoscopy permits the monitoring of sequential changes in ovarian morphology which are more accurate for ovulation detection in primates, than other indirect methods, e. g. rectal palpatation and ferning or chloride concentration of cervical mucus. Noyes et al. (1966) reported that human ova were recovered from the oviducts up to 4 days after ovulation whereas Croxatto et al. (1972) recovered ova from the uterus 2 to 3 days after ovulation. Such a difference may be partly due to errors in determining the time of ovulation, and the possibility of displacing the ova from the oviduct to the uterus when using nonsurgical techniques.

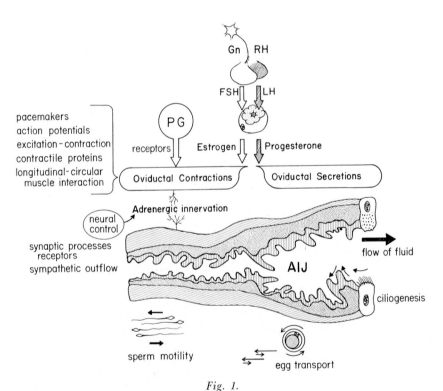

Fig. 1.

Diagrammatic illustration of the anatomical, physiological and pharmacological mechanisms affecting ovum transport, and possible approaches for fertility regulation.

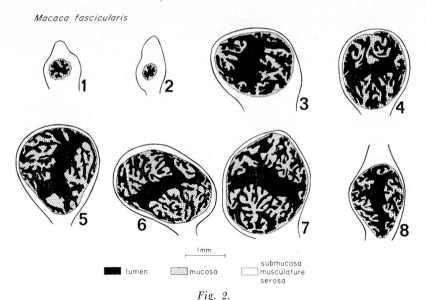

Macaca fascicularis

1 2 3 4

5 6 7 8

■ lumen	▨ mucosa	submucosa
		☐ musculature
		serosa

1 mm

Fig. 2.

Cross-section of different segments of the oviduct of crab-eating macaque (*Macaca fascicularis*), showing differences in the size of lumen and complexity of mucosal folds.

Several physiological and anatomical mechanisms have been implicated in the control of ova transport in the oviduct, e. g. the beat of kinocilia, the flow of oviductal secretions, contractions of oviductal musculature and the functional integrity of the ampullary-isthmic junction and the uterotubal junction (Fig. 1). The relative importance of these mechanisms in ovum transport is unknown. Pharmacological and neural mechanisms are also involved in ovum transport.

I. OVUM TRANSPORT IN THE MACAQUE

Ovum transport was studied in cycling crab-eating macaques (*Macaca fasicularis*) during regular menstrual cycles. The time of ovulation was determined by serial laparoscopy, and ovum transport was evaluated by segmental flushing of the oviducts and uterus. Oviductal structure, as observed by scanning electron microscopy, was correlated with the location of ova. Ovulated ova, Sephadex beads and rabbit ova were transported to the ampullary-isthmic region by 48 h, retained in the isthmus between 48 and 96 h, and entered the uterus between 96 and 120 h after ovulation (Jainudeen and Hafez 1973). Structural characte-

363

ristics of different regions of the oviduct may play specific roles in ovum transport (Fig. 2). For example, the ampullary-isthmic junction, as observed by scanning electron microscopy, has a characteristic muscosal fold. During the initial stages of our experiments, an attempt was made to study the transport of ovulated ova. This approach was abandoned because the number of ova recovered was significantly reduced. This reduction was probably related to a disturbance in the relationship of the fimbriae to the ovary during laparoscopy manipulation.

II. POSSIBLE ROLE OF AMPULLARY-ISTHMIC JUNCTION

Several mechanisms have been suggested to account for the closure of the isthmus or ampullary-isthmic junction which is responsible for the retention of ova within the oviduct before they are rapidly transported into the uterus (Blandau 1969). However, no structural basis for an isthmic block has been demonstrated by histological techniques. Electron microscopic studies in the mouse (Nilsson and Reinius 1969) have shown long mucosal folds protruding through the isthmic opening into the ampullary lumen. In the crab-eating macaque there is no evidence suggesting retention of ova in the ampullary-isthmic region, but the ova are retained in the extramural segment of the isthmus (Jainudeen and Hafez 1973). In the human oviduct, microspheres are retained in the ampullary-isthmic junction for 72 h (Avendano et al. 1971). This study was, however, conducted on excised oviducts deprived of their blood and nerve supply.

In rabbits, the ampullary-isthmic junction is biochemically characterized by high acid phosphatase activity as compared to the isthmus or ampulla, but during passage of the ova a "surge" of activity of this enzyme is noted uniformly throughout the oviduct (Gupta et al. 1970). Acid phosphatase may play a role in ova denudation, and removal of denuded cumulus and corona cell debris.

Ovarian hormones control the activity of an electric pacemaker which is localized in a discrete area around the ampullary-isthmic junction (Talo and Brundin 1971; Larks et al. 1971). In goats a pronounced activity and groups of positive pulses are recorded during estrus. In diestrus, the activity is abolished and groups of negative pulses are dominant. The electric pulses and the changes in their directions are probably involved in the underlying control of ovum transport in the isthmus.

The failure rate associated with reconstructive surgery is high, despite demonstration of postoperative oviductal patency in a large number of cases. This may be due to malfunction of the ampullary-isthmic junction or to unbalanced numbers of ciliated and secretory cells.

364

III. POSSIBLE ROLE OF UTEROTUBAL JUNCTION

The uterotubal junction may exert a regulatory influence on ova entry into the uterus. In rabbits, this junction opens only on days 3, 4 and 30 of pregnancy, when the ova are transported into the uterus, and at the time of parturition (Hafez 1963). In sheep estrogen-induced edema and flexure of the uterotubal junction causes a valve-like action which prevents movement of fluid and presumably ova, from the oviduct into the uterus (Edgar and Asdell 1960). The presence of a relatively thick tunica propria in the pig-tail macaque (Hafez and Black 1969), or the prominent layer of connective tissue surrounding the oviductal lumen of the rhesus macaque (David and Czernobilsky 1968) in the uterotubal junction may be of physiological significance in ovum transport. The human uterotubal junction is marked by a noticeable abundance of ciliated cells.

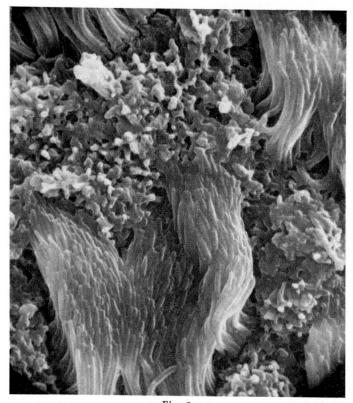

Fig. 3.
Scanning electron micrograph of oviductal epithelium showing ciliated cells with kinocilia and secretory cells covered with microvilli (Hafez 1973).

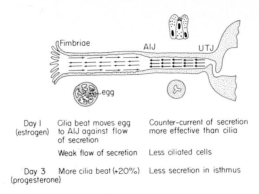

Day I (estrogen)	Cilia beat moves egg to AIJ against flow of secretion	Counter-current of secretion more effective than cilia
	Weak flow of secretion	Less ciliated cells
Day 3 (progesterone)	More cilia beat (+20%)	Less secretion in isthmus

Fig. 4.

Diagram showing forces in oviduct which may be involved in gamete transport. The arrows in the ampulla (wide lumen) represent ciliary beat toward the ampullary-isthmic junction (AIJ) and the flow of oviductal fluid toward the fimbriae. The arrows in the isthmus (narrow lumen) represent flow of oviductal fluid from the uterotubal junction (UTJ); note differential effect of estrogen and progesterone on forces in ampulla and isthmus (Hafez 1973).

Fluid movement of oviductal secretions

Very little attention has been given to fluid dynamics in the highly convoluted oviductal lumen. Several physiological factors may be involved in creating currents and counter-currents (Figs. 3, 4):

1. quantitative and qualitative changes in oviductal secretions throughout the menstrual cycle and in response to contraceptives,

2. beat of kinocilia in oviductal compartments of variable sizes and shapes,

3. constant change in the diameter of the oviductal lumen in different segments as a result of muscle contraction and re-orientation of mucosal folds (Hafez 1973).

The directional movement of oviductal secretions may contribute to ovum transport to the uterus. In sheep most of the oviductal secretions passes out of the oviductal ostium early in the estrous cycle (Belve and McDonald 1968). On day 4, however, the time when ova usually enter the uterus, fluid flow through the uterotubal junction remarkably increases. Similar observations have been recorded in the monkey (unpublished data). Ova are transported prematurely into the uterus from ligated oviducts in the rabbit, probably as a result of the passage of oviductal fluid into the uterus (Sharp and Black 1975).

IV. PHYSIO-PHARMACOLOGICAL MECHANISMS

Several mechanisms influence ovum transport in the oviduct, e. g., (a) muscular contractions of the tunica muscularis; (b) volume changes of the lamina propria; (c) secretory activity of the lamina epithelialis; and (d) the beating of kinocilia (Blandau 1969). Unlike intestinal peristalsis, oviductal peristalsis instead of transporting the ovum tends to delay slightly its progression. Oviductal contraction facilitates mixing of oviductal contents, promotes fertilization and helps to denude ova. Adrenergic nerve fibers are implicated in the control of muscular activity of the oviduct. There is more norepinephrine in the isthmus than in the ampulla of the rabbit (Bodkhe and Harper 1972) and the human oviduct (Owman et al. 1967).

During menstruation and the proliferative phase of the cycle, the human oviduct responds with outbursts of increased oviductal activity to intravenous infusions of epinephrine or norepinephrine (Coutinho et al. 1970). In the rabbit, such outbursts are observed at 36 h p. c., when the majority of ova are in the oviduct. A drop in oviductal motility occurs at 72 h p. c., when most ova are in the uterus (Aref and Hafez 1973). This decrease in oviductal motility is presumably due to a postovulatory drop in norepinephrine levels and relaxation of oviductal musculature (Bodkhe and Harper 1972). The patterns of ovum transport are correlated with cyclical changes in the contractions of the oviduct in rabbits (Mattos and Coutinho 1971; Salomy and Harper 1971; Aref and Hafez 1973) and women (Maia and Coutinho 1968).

Myosalpingeal contraction mediated by adrenergic innervation to the circular muscle of the oviductal isthmus is believed to be involved in delay of ovum transport at the isthmus (Chatkoff and Pauerstein 1975). The mechanisms underlying this phenomenon, including modulation of adrenergic factors by ovarian steroids are unknown.

V. PROSTAGLANDINS AND OVUM TRANSPORT

Subcutaneous injection of prostaglandin $F_{2\alpha}$ prevents pregnancy in hamsters and blocks implantation in rats and rabbits. Subcutaneous injection or intravenous infusion of PGE_2 and $PGF_{2\alpha}$ terminates pregnancy in the rhesus monkey (Kirton et al. 1970). Little is known about the mode of action. Prostaglandins have a remarkable effect on the smooth musculature of the oviducts and the uterus (see review by Horton 1972). The formation and release of prostaglandins is brought about by nerve activity. The human uterus and oviducts contain a network of adrenergic nerves, the highest concentrations of these nerves being present in the oviductal isthmus and uterine cervix.

A. Prostaglandins and postcoital contraceptives

The mechanism of action of PGE_2 and $PGF_{2\alpha}$ as antifertility agents varies with the time of their injection. Following ovulation, the effectiveness of $PGF_{2\alpha}$ is related to its capacity to stimulate oviductal contractility and to accelerate ovum transport. When injected *in utero* in rabbits 4 days post coitum, the effectiveness of PGE_2 and $PGF_{2\alpha}$ to interrupt pregnancy may be related to their capacity to stimulate uterine contractility and to expel the embryos from the uterus to the vagina (Aref et al. 1974). Disruptions of hormonal synthesis also may be involved and further studies are needed to estimate associated hormonal changes.

B. Prostaglandins and oviductal motility

In vitro studies in women showed that PGE_1 and PGE_2 exert a characteristic effect on the longitudinal musculature of the oviduct: an increase in tonus of the proximal part and relaxation of the rest of the organ. However, PGE_3 relaxes the whole oviduct (Sandberg et al. 1963, 1964). On the other hand, $PGF_{1\alpha}$, $PGF_{1\beta}$, and $PGF_{2\alpha}$ act as stimulators, the strongest effect being exerted by $PGF_{2\alpha}$ with no apparent change in sensitivity or action throughout the menstrual cycle. $PGF_{2\beta}$ has a relaxing effect on the whole oviduct. *In vitro* studies by Zetler et al. (1969) showed that strips of the infundibular segment of human and rabbit oviducts are highly responsive to stimulation by $PGF_{2\alpha}$. *In vitro* (Sandberg et al. 1965; Zetler et al. 1969) and *in vivo* studies (Coutinho and Maia 1971) in women have shown that $PGF_{2\alpha}$ stimulates and PGE_2 inhibits oviductal motility. *In vivo* human recordings of intraluminal pressure fluctuations in the oviduct are beset with obvious difficulties.

Following intravenous injection of PGE_1 or PGE_2 in rabbits, the spontaneous motility of the oviduct is suppressed with a large decrease in tone and frequency of contractions. On the other hand, $PGF_{1\alpha}$ and $PGF_{2\alpha}$ evoke a sustained increase in oviductal muscular tone (Spilman and Harper 1972). Thus it would appear that the prostaglandins are antithetically involved in the regulation of oviductal function. Ellinger and Kirton (1972) reported that both PGE_1 and $PGF_{2\alpha}$ hasten ovum transport through the rabbit oviduct.

The effect on oviductal and uterine contractility of intravenous administration of PGE_1 and $PGF_{2\alpha}$ was studied in non-pregnant women at various stages of the menstrual cycle (Roth-Brandel et al. 1971). The individual response to prostaglandins varies considerably from one case to another (Roth-Brandel et al. 1970).

PGE_2 appears more potent than $PGF_{2\alpha}$ on the human myometrium, whereas the two prostaglandins have opposing effects on the oviduct. $PGF_{2\alpha}$ stimulates whereas PGE_2 inhibits oviductal motility *in vivo* (Countinho and Maia 1971). It was proposed that relaxation of the isthmus induced by seminal PGE_2 is a prerequisite for sperm penetration into the oviduct. Little is known about the mode of action of prostaglandins at the cellular and subcellular levels.

VI. NEURAL MECHANISMS OVUM TRANSPORT

Little is known about the neural control of ovum transport in the oviduct. In the rabbit, adrenergic innervation of the oviduct is derived from postganglionic fibers which originate in the inferior mesenteric ganglia (long adrenergic neurons), and others that originate in ganglia located near the cervix, at the level of the cervicovaginal junction (short adrenergic neurons) (cf. Pauerstein et al. 1974).

Pauerstein et al. (1973, 1974) depleted oviducts of endogenous sympathetic neurotransmitter by either surgical denervation, or intraluminal infusion of 6-hydroxydopamine or systemic administration of reserpine. Their data suggest that the effects of steroid hormones on ovum transport are partially mediated by the sympathetic nerves of the myosalpinx (Brundin 1969; Pauerstein et al. 1973, 1974). The amount of norepinephrine in the isthmus is hormonally dependent (Bodkhe and Harper 1973) whereas the response of the myosalpingeal adrenoceptors to adrenergic agonists changes with hormonal status (Bennett and Kendle 1967).

The adrenergic nerves of the oviduct can be destroyed surgically or chemically. The administration of 6-hydroxydopamine (2,4,5-trihydroxyphenylethylamine) causes the degeneration of adrenergic nerve endings within 2–3 days after administration. This chemical denervation is associated with depletion of local norepinephrine, and reduction in tyrosine hydroxylase. 6-Hydroxydopamine does not alter the cell bodies of sympathetic ganglia, the Schwann cells, the cholinergic nerve endings, or the smooth musculature (Thoenen and Tranzer 1968; Thoenen et al. 1970). Depleting the adrenergic nerves of norepinephrine with reserpine causes functional adrenergic denervation. The extent of the depletion induced by reserpine is species-, organ- and time-dependent (Carlsson 1966). One intravenous injection of reserpine causes catecholamines to disappear more slowly and recover more quickly from organs innervated by short adrenergic neurons such as the oviduct, than from organs innervated exclusively by long adrenergic neurons as in the ovary (Owman and Sjöberg 1967).

VII. STEROID CONTRACEPTIVES AND OVUM TRANSPORT

Extensive studies have been undertaken to clarify the mode of action of steroid contraceptives. Combined therapy with progestins and estrogens alters the hypothalamo-pituitary-ovarian function and suppress ovulation with several

369

side effects (cf. Hafez and Evans 1973). It is imperative to develop other contraceptives with a high efficiency and without undesirable side effects. Since the introduction of continuous progestin therapy without estrogens as an effective contraceptive, it has become apparent that suppression of ovulation is not essential for contraception. Continuous microdose progestin therapy does not inhibit ovulation in about 60 % of cycles (1600 cycles in over 40 women) as judged by culdoscopy, ovarian biopsy, pregnanediol levels, endometrial biopsy and physico-chemical properties of cervical mucus. Recently attention has been focused on other possible contraceptive mechanisms, such as inhibition of sperm transport. Progestins exert their contraceptive effect by reducing the secretion of cervical mucus and sperm penetration through the cervix (Martinez-Manautou et al. 1966; Gutierrez-Najar et al. 1969; Lebech et al. 1970; Moghissi and Marks 1971).

There is no information on the effect of contraceptives on ovum transport in nonhuman primates. However, more is known about the effect of steroid contraceptives on ovulation (Kraemer et al. 1969; Harrison and Dukelow 1971), spermatogenesis (Setty and Kar 1969), ovum development implantation and (Morris et al. 1967), sexual receptivity (Michael 1969; Everitt and Herbert 1971), thyroid function (Roy et al. 1966), and endometrial enzymes of nonhuman primates (Wan et al. 1970; Manning et al. 1971).

VIII. FUTURE RESEARCH AND FERTILITY
REGULATION

Little is known about the relative importance of physiological, anatomical and pharmacological mechanisms in ovum transport through the isthmus: a) contraction patterns of oviductal musculature as affected by the hormonal and pharmacological environments, b) currents and counter-currents of oviductal secretions, and c) ciliary beat in the isthmus and uterotubal junction. Future research is also needed to evaluate the effect of contraceptives on fertilization, ovum transport, sperm transport or sperm survival in the oviduct. Although interference with oviductal transport or embryonic development in the oviduct provides an attractive method of fertility control, little is known about the physiological mechanisms of ovum transport in the oviduct. Theoretically, it should be possible to develop safer and more effective contraceptive agents which would act by hastening ovum transport through the isthmus, by causing degeneration of the fertilized ovum, or by preventing sperm transport to the ampullary-isthmic junction.

It is highly desirable to use nonhuman primates to study the mode of action of steroid contraceptives. Gamete transport in the female reproductive tract of these species can be effectively studied in relation to cyclical changes in ovarian morphology, serum levels of ovarian steroids and quantity and physico-chemical properties of cervical mucus. Microspheres and Sephadex beads provide excellent 'surrogate' ova and may therefore be employed to study ovum transport. This experimental model could be utilized in future studies on the effects of various contraceptives or hormonal therapy upon ovum transport. It should be possible to develop animal models mimicking the human situation as nearly as possible which could be used in future screening programs looking for new and different contraceptive effective agents.

REFERENCES

Aref I. and Hafez E. S. E. (1973) Oviductal contractility in relation to egg transport in the rabbit. *Obstet. Gynec. 42*, 165–171.

Aref I., Gottschewski G. H. M. and Hafez E. S. E. (1974) Prostaglandins and early pregnancy in rabbits. *Contraception 10*, 291–298.

Avendaño S., Pelaez J. and Croxatto H. B. (1971) Transport of microspheres by the human oviduct. *in vitro* and the effect of treatment with megestrol acetate. *J. Reprod. Fertil. 27*, 261–264.

Belve A. R. and McDonald M. F. (1968) Directional flow of Fallopian tube secretion in the Romney ewe. *J. Reprod. Fertil. 15*, 357–364.

Bennett J. P. and Kendle K. E. (1967) The effect of reserpine upon the rate of egg transport in the Fallopian tube of the mouse. *J. Reprod. Fertil. 13*, 345–348.

Blandau R. J. (1969) Gamete transport – comparative aspects. In: Hafez E. S. E. and Blandau R. J., eds. *The Mammalian Oviduct*, pp. 129–162. University of Chicago Press, Chicago.

Bodkhe R. R. and Harper M. J. K. (1972) Changes in the amount of adrenergic neuro-transmitter in the genital tract of untreated rabbits, and rabbits given reserpine or iproniazid during the time of egg transport. *Biol. Reprod. 6*, 288–299.

Bodkhe R. R. and Harper M. J. K. (1973) Mechanisms of egg transport: Changes in amount of adrenergic transmitter in the genital tract of normal and hormone treated rabbits. In: Segal S. J. et al., eds. NIH Symp. *The Regulation of Mammalian Reproduction*, Chapter 26, pp. 364–374. C. C. Thomas, Springfield, Ill.

Brundin J. (1969) Pharmacology of the oviduct. In: Hafez E. S. E. and Blandau R. J., eds. *The Mammalian Oviduct*, pp. 251–307. University of Chicago Press, Chicago.

Carlsson A. (1966) Drugs which block the storage of 5-hydroxytryptamine and related amines. *Handbuch exp. Pharmakol. 19*, 529–592.

Chatkoff M. L. and Pauerstein C. J. (1975) Biochemistry of adrenergic receptors in ovum transport. *Gynec. Invest. 6*, 43–44.

Coutinho E. M. and Maia H. S. (1971) The contractile response of the human uterus, Fallopian tubes and ovary to prostaglandins *in vivo*. *Fertil. Steril. 22*, 539–543.

Coutinho E. M., Maia H. and Filho J. A. (1970) Response of the human Fallopian tube to adrenergic stimulation. *Fertil. Steril. 21*, 590–594.

Croxatto H. B., Diaz S., Fuentealba B., Croxatto H. D., Carrillo D. and Fabres C. (1972) Studies on the duration of egg transport in the human oviduct. I. The time interval between ovulation and egg recovery from the uterus in normal women. *Fertil. Steril. 23*, 447–458.

371

David A. and Czernobilsky B. (1968) A comparative histological study of the uterotubal junction in the rabbit, rhesus monkey and human female. *Amer. J. Obstet. Gynec.* **101**, 417–421.

Edgar D. G. and Adsell S. A. (1960) Spermatozoa in the female genital tract. *J. Endocr.* **21**, 321–326.

Ellinger J. V. and Kirton K. T. (1972) Ovum transport in rabbits injected with prostaglandin E_1 or $F_{2\alpha}$. *Biol. Reprod.* **7**, 106 (Abstr.).

Everitt B. and Herbert J. (1971) The effects of dexamethasone and androgens on sexual receptivity of female rhesus monkeys. *J. Endocr.* **51**, 575–588.

Gupta D. N., Karkun J. N. and Kar A. B. (1970) Biochemical changes in different parts of the rabbit Fallopian tube during passage of ova. *Amer. J. Obstet. Gynec.* **106**, 833–837.

Gutierrez-Najar A., Giner-Velazquez J. and Martinez-Manautou J. (1969) Role of cervical mucus in contraception with the continuous chlormadinone acetate method. In: Sobrero A. and Lewit S., eds. *Advances in Planned Parenthood* **4**, 97–112. Excerpta Medica Found., New York.

Hafez E. S. E. (1963) The uterotubal junction and the luminal fluid of the uterine tube in the rabbit. *Anat. Rec.* **145**, 7–12.

Hafez E. S. E. (1973) Gamete transport. In: Hafez E. S. E. and Evans T. N., eds. *Human Reproduction Conception and Contraception*, pp. 85–118. Harper & Row, New York, N. Y.

Hafez E. S. E. and Black D. L. (1969) The mammalian uterotubal junction. In: Hafez E. S. E. and Blandau R. J., eds. *The Mammalian Oviduct*, pp. 85–126. University of Chicago Press, Chicago.

Harrison R. M. and Dukelow W. R. (1971) Megestrol acetate: Its effect on inhibition of ovulation in squirrel monkeys, *Saimiri sciureus*. *J. Reprod. Fertil.* **25**, 99–101.

Horton E. W. (1972) Female reproductive tract smooth muscle. In: Horton E. W., ed. *Prostaglandins*, Monographs on Endocrinology **7**, 87–104. Springer Verlag, New York.

Jainudeen M. R. and Hafez E. S. E. (1973) Egg transport in the crab-eating macaque (*M. fascicularis*). *Biol. Reprod.* **9**, 305–308.

Kirton K. T., Pharriss B. B. and Forbes A. D. (1970) Some effects of prostaglandin E_2 and $F_{2\alpha}$ on the pregnant rhesus monkey. *Biol. Reprod.* **3**, 163–168.

Kraemer D. C., Hendricks A. G. and Kriewaldt F. H. (1969) Experiences with norethindrone-mestranol, human gonadotropins (HMG + HCG) and clomiphene citrate in baboons. In: Vagtborg H., ed. *Use of Nonhuman Primates in Drug Evaluation*, pp. 118–128. University of Texas Press, Austin, Texas.

Larks S. D., Larks G. G., Hoffer R. E. and Charlson E. J. (1971) Electrical pacemaker of oviductal activity. *Nature (Lond.)* **234**, 556–557.

Lebech P. E., Svendsen P. A. and Ostergaard E. (1970) The effect of small doses of megestrol acetate on the cervical mucus. *Int. J. Fertil.* **15**, 65–75.

Maia H. and Coutinho E. M. (1968) A new technique for recording human tube activity *in vivo*. *Amer. J. Obstet. Gynec.* **102**, 1043–1047.

Manning J. P., Tornaben J. A. and Schwartz E. (1971) Influence of quinestrol on the histology and phosphatase activity of the simian uterus. *Fertil. Steril.* **22**, 194–203.

Marston J. H., Kelly W. A. and Eckstein P. (1969) Effect of an intrauterine device on uterine motility in the rhesus monkey. *J. Reprod. Fertil.* **19**, 321–330.

Martinez-Manautou J., Cortez V., Giner J., Aznar R., Casasola J. and Rudel H. W. (1966) Low dose progestogen as an approach to fertility control. *Fertil. Steril.* **17**, 49–57.

Mastroianni L., Suzuki S., Manabe Y. and Watson F. (1967) Further observations on the influence of the intrauterine device on ovum and sperm distribution in the monkey. *Amer. J. Obstet. Gynec. 99*, 649–661.

Mattos C. E. R. and Coutinho E. M. (1971) Effects of the ovarian hormones on tubal motility of the rabbit. *Endocrinology 89*, 912–917.

Michael R. P. (1969) Behavioral effects of gonadal hormones and contraceptive steroids in primates. In: Salhanick H., Kipnis D. M. and VandeWiele R. L., eds. *Metabolic Effects of Gonadal Hormones and Contraceptive Steroids*, pp. 706–721. Plenum Press, New York.

Moghissi K. S. and Marks C. (1971) Effects of microdose norgestrel on endogenous gonadotropic and steroid hormones, cervical mucus properties, vaginal cytology and endometrium. *Fertil. Steril. 22*, 424–434.

Morris J. M., van Wagenen G., McCann T. and Jacob D. (1967) Compounds interfering with ovum implantation and development. II. Synthetic estrogens and antiestrogens. *Fertil. Steril. 18*, 18–34.

Nilsson O. and Reinius S. (1969) Light and electron microscopic structure of the oviduct. In: Hafez E. S. E. and Blandau R. J., eds. *The Mammalian Oviduct*, pp. 57–83. University of Chicago Press, Chicago.

Noyes R. W., Clewe T. H., Bonney W. A., Burrus S. B., DeFeo V. J. and Morgenstern L. L. (1966) Searches for ova in the human uterus and tubes. I. Review, clinical methodology and summary. *Amer. J. Obstet. Gynec. 96*, 157–167.

Owman C., Rosengren E. and Sjöberg N.-O. (1967) Adrenergic innervation of the human female reproductive organs: A histochemical and chemical investigation. *Obstet. Gynec. 30*, 763–773.

Owman C. and Sjöberg N.-O. (1967) Difference in rate of depletion and recovery of noradrenaline in 'short' and 'long' sympathetic nerves after reserpine treatment. *Life Sci. 6*, 2549–2556.

Pauerstein C. J., Fremming B. D., Hodgson B. J. and Martin J. E. (1973) The promise of pharmacological modification of ovum transport in contraceptive development. *Amer. J. Obstet. Gynec. 116*, 161–166.

Pauerstein C. J., Hodgson B. J., Fremming B. D. and Martin J. E. (1974) Effects of sympathetic denervation of the rabbit oviduct on normal ovum transport and on transport modified by estrogen and progesterone. *Gynec. Invest. 5*, 121–132.

Roth-Brandel U. (1971) Response of pregnant human uterus to low and high doses of prostaglandin E_1 and E_2. *Acta obstet. gynec. scand. 50*, 159–166.

Roth-Brandel U., Bygdeman M. and Wiqvist N. (1970) Effect of intravenous administration of prostaglandin E_1 and $F_{2\alpha}$ on the contractility of the non-pregnant human uterus *in vivo*. *Acta obstet. gynec. scand. 49*, 19–25.

Roth-Brandel U., Wiqvist N. and Bygdeman M. (1971) Effect of prostaglandins on the contractility of the non-pregnant human uterus *in vivo*. *Acta obstet. gynec. scand. 50*, 35–49.

Roy S. K., Kar A. B. and Setty B. S. (1966) Effect of progestational steroids on thyroid function in rhesus monkeys. *Indian J. exp. Biol. 4*, 173–174.

Salomy M. and Harper M. J. K. (1971) Cyclical changes of oviduct motility in rabbits. *Biol. Reprod. 4*, 185–194.

Sandberg F., Ingelman-Sundberg A. and Rydén G. (1963) The effect of prostaglandin E_1 on the human uterus and the Fallopian tubes *in vitro*. *Acta obstet. gynec. scand. 42*, 269–278.

Sandberg F., Ingelman-Sundberg A. and Rydén G. (1964) The effect of prostaglandin E_2 and E_3 on the human uterus and the Fallopian tubes *in vitro. Acta obstet. gynec. scand. 43*, 95–102.

Sandberg F., Ingelman-Sundberg A. and Rydén G. (1965) The effect of prostaglandin $F_{1\alpha}$, $F_{2\alpha}$ and $F_{2\beta}$ on the human uterus and the Fallopian tubes *in vitro. Acta obstet. gynec. scand. 44*, 585–594.

Setty B. S. and Kar A. B. (1969) Antispermatogenic effect of norgestrel in rhesus monkeys. *Indian J. exp. Biol. 7*, 49–51.

Sharp D. C. & Black D. L. (1975) The effects of tubal ligation on ovum transport in rabbits. *J. Reprod. Fertil. 42*, 23–28.

Spilman C. H. and Harper M. J. K. (1972) Effect of prostaglandins on oviduct motility in conscious rabbits. *Biol. Reprod. 7*, 106 (Abstr.).

Talo A. and Brundin J. (1971) Muscular activity in the rabbit oviduct; a combination of electric and mechanic recordings. *Biol. Reprod. 5*, 67–77.

Thoenen H. and Tranzer J. P. (1968) Chemical sympathectomy by selective destruction of adrenergic nerve endings with 6-hydroxydopamine. *Arch. Pharmakol. exp. Path. 261*, 271–288.

Thoenen H., Tranzer J. P. and Hausler G. (1970) Chemical sympathectomy with 6-hydroxydopamine. In: Schuemann H. J. and Kroneberg G., eds. *New Aspects of Storage and Release Mechanisms of Catecholamines*, pp. 130–142. Springer-Verlag, New York.

Wan L. S., Hilf R., Shah M., Lerner L. J. and Balin H. (1970) Enzymatic characteristics of the monkey endometrium during ovulatory and anovulatory cycles and under hormonal contraception treatment. *J. Reprod. Med. 4*, 127–136.

Zetler C. H., Mönkmeier D. and Wiechell H. (1969) Stimulation of Fallopian tubes by prostaglandin $F_{2\alpha}$, biogenic amines and peptides. *J. Reprod. Fertil. 18*, 147–149.

374

Department of Human and Animal Physiology,
University of Stellenbosch, Stellenbosch, South Africa

RETENTION OF UNFERTILIZED OVA
IN THE OVIDUCTS OF MARES

By

C. H. Van Niekerk

ABSTRACT

Immediately after ovulation the ovum was found to be without a corona radiata but enclosed in a large, irregular gelatinous mass of follicular origin.

As many as ten different ova in all stages of cytolysis were encountered in the oviducts of mares. As the follicles of the mare were consistently found to be monovular, it is concluded that unfertilized ova do not, as a rule, pass out of the oviducts, but, contrary to all accepted data on the migration of ova, may remain there up to seven and a half months or longer. During this time they undergo gradual disintegration characterized by the following order of changes: deutoplasmic condensation, deutoplasmic extrusion, cytoplasmolysis, deutoplasmic fragmentation and comminution of yolk granules. The final stage identified is a fluid-filled, collapsed vesicle (zona vesicle) surrounded by the zona pellucida only.

It had been generally accepted that in mammals the ova, whether fertilized or not, migrate through the oviducts into the uterus until Van Niekerk and Gerneke (1966) first proved that unfertilized ova are selectively retained in the oviducts of mares for several months while fertilized ova pass unimpeded into the uterus within six days after ovulation. This unusual phenomenon has subsequently been confirmed by several investigators (Betteridge and Mitchell 1972, 1974; Steffenhagen et al. 1972; Oguri and Tsutsumi 1972).

This report presents a review of my own published and unpublished work as well as an appraisal of other work in the same field.

MATERIALS AND METHODS

The ovaries of thirty five and the oviducts of twenty mares, slaughtered at different stages of the estrous cycle and early pregnancy, were obtained. Sexual activity was monitored by teaser stallions for several months prior to slaughter. The ovaries were examined daily per rectum but more frequently in late estrous to establish the time of ovulation. Ten of the twenty mares from which the oviducts were collected had been served by fertile stallions, but otherwise mares and stallions were kept strictly apart.

For the purpose of this study Graafian follicles from a few days before until just after ovulation were collected for histological studies on the ova, follicular walls and the mucoid layer. The walls of the follicles were fixed in Zenker-formol. Paraffin wax sections were prepared and stained with haematoxylin and eosin, and where indicated with Hale's colloidal iron for mucopolysacchari-des. The oviducts of the twenty mares were dissected out immediately after slaughter and flushed with normal saline. These flushings were examined for ova by means of a stereoscopic dissecting microscope. The ova were mounted on drop centre slides in dilute glycerine coloured slightly with safranin or cresyl violet.

Follicular fluid and saline flushings of six Graafian follicles of six mares were examined separately for ova.

RESULTS AND DISCUSSION

Mucoid substance

Approximately three days before ovulation the wall of the largest follicle was clearly divided into three layers. The enlarged polyhedral thecal cells appeared to be very active, probably secreting estrogens (Short 1961; Van Rensburg and Van Niekerk 1968; Bjersing and Younglai 1972).

Thereafter these cells underwent degeneration which by 24 h after ovulation was nearly complete. By the third day before ovulation the tightly packed granulosa cells had ceased to divide and appeared inactive with their small dark nuclei surrounded by a small amount of cytoplasm. No mucoid substance covered the membrana granulosa at this stage. In the mature follicle on the point of ovulation the granulosa cells had changed from a compact to an open lace-like layer. At this stage, the granulosa cells which had become stellated, secreted a basophilic filamentous mucoid substance which formed a compact lining around the antrum and stained strongly positive for mucopolysaccharides. This mucous lining was also noticeable after spontaneous ovulation and became more and more homogeneous, dense and sticky as the corpus luteum aged. At ovulation this mucoid substance is pushed into the oviducts and the recently ovulated ovum was always seen embedded in a filamentous mucoid mass which was completely transparent, sticky, elastic and contained blood specks and corona radiata cells. A similar mass was detached from a 4 cell stage ovum 30 h after ovulation whereas both a 16 cell and morular stage zygote were devoid of this mucoid mass. As the mucoid mass aged in the oviducts it became more homogenous, and globular gelatinous bodies were attached to a central more compact sticky mass by short strands. These masses were consistently observed in the washings of oviducts in which ova were discovered. None was found in the tubes of mares from whose corresponding ovary no ovulation had yet occurred. In the interval since Van Niekerk and Gerneke (1966) described the presence of these mucoid masses in the oviducts of mares their role in fertilization, ovum transport and ovum retention has not been explained.

Oviductal sojourn of ova

From one to ten ova in different stages of cytolysis were encountered in the oviducts of the mare (Table 1 and Fig. 1).

Daily rectal examination of the ovaries before ovulation correlated with post mortem examinations revealed that during each estrous period only a single

Table 1.
Number and approximate ages (in days) of ova found in oviducts.

Mare No.	Left oviduct	Age of ova	Right oviduct	Age of ova
1	1	± 60	not exam.	
2	6	2; 20; 37; 120–150	not exam.	
3	2	5; 29	not exam.	
4	not exam.		2	$1^1/_4$; 45 +
5	2	5; 30	not exam.	
6	1	50	1	68 +
7	4	99; 117; 137; 157	3	137; ± 150; ± 150
8	0		3	1; 20; 40
9	1	?	6	?
10	0		1	54
11	2	14; 120–150	4	35; ?
12	2	27; 70–80	2	8; 50
13	1	± 120	3	2–4 h; 19; 58
14	0		1	± 90
15	4	44; 63; 150 & 170	4	90; 105 ?
16	4	$1^1/_2$; 22; 107; 147	6	1; 46; 63; 129; 180; 225
17	0		2	± 105; ± 120
18	4	71; 95; 115; 135 +	2	115 +; 135 +
19	0		1	84 +
20	2	7 ?; ± 210	2	6; 28

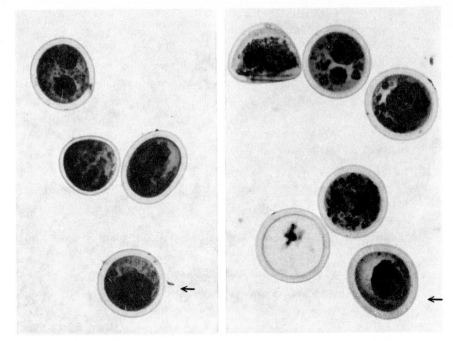

Fig. 1.
Ten ova recovered from the left (A) and right (B) oviducts of mare no. 16. The ova
from a double ovulation 1 and 1.5 days old, respectively (arrows) reveal a condensed
cytoplasm and a distinct vitelline membrane. Slight deutoplasmic extrusions can be
seen. The two-cell parthenogenetic stage at the top of A was 22 days old.
The different morphological changes involving deutoplasmic extrusions, deutoplasmic
fragmentation and comminution of yolk granules are visible in the rest of the ova,
which in the left oviduct were 107 and 147 days old, and those in the right oviduct
were 46, 63, 129 and 180 days old. The bottom left ovum in B, visible as a clear vesicle
surrounded by a zona pellucida, was at least 7.5 months old.
The cresyl violet stain gives a darker than normal appearance to the deutoplasm.

follicle ovulated except in mare no. 16 where a double ovulation 1.5 days apart
was diagnosed and confirmed on autopsy. Furthermore only a single ovum
was found in each of the six Graafian follicles examined before ovulation.
These observations established beyond doubt that only a single ovum is set free
at each ovulation and is in agreement with the findings of Betteridge and
Mitchell (1972); Steffenhagen et al. (1972) and Onuma and Ohnami (1975).
The statement of David (1975), that some of the atretic follicles situated near
the ovarian fossa may rupture at the same time as the mature follicle and shed
their ova in various stages of degeneration into the oviduct, has been disproved
by the excellent work of Betteridge and Mitchell (1974, 1975), which gives
direct evidence of retention of unfertilized ova in the oviducts of the mare.

378

When the number of ova recovered was related to the ovulation dates and corpora lutea and corpora albicans in the ovaries, as well as the state of degeneration of the ova themselves, it became possible to estimate their ages as given in Table 1.

Maturation and degeneration of ova

Flushings of Graafian follicles revealed that the first maturation division occurs before ovulation and that the ovum is shed with a very distinct vitelline membrane and one polar body in the perivitelline space. The zona pellucida was found to be tightly enclosed in a mucous mass described previously, with no corona radiata cells surrounding the zona pellucida. Previously it was always believed that, in the mare, the first maturation division took place only after ovulation (Hamilton and Day 1945) but it may well be that, unaware of the phenomenon of persistence of oviductal ova, these authors were dealing mainly with ova in the early stages of degeneration.

Examination of the oviductal ova of known or estimated age enabled us to arrange them in series representing typical stages of degeneration. These morphological changes involve the following:

(a) *Deutoplasmic condensation.* – The cytoplasm shortly after ovulation condenses into a more compact mass (Fig. 1).

As condensation of deutoplasm is also an early phenomenon of a normal process which is undergone by fertilized ova preparatory to the first cleavage it is difficult to determine the stage at which degeneration sets in.

(b) *Parthenogenetic division or deutoplasmic extrusions.* – Shortly after condensation of the deutoplasm in unfertilized ova either parthenogenetic cleavage may occur (Fig. 1), which may continue up to the eight cell stage (as found in a mare twenty days after ovulation which had not been served), or deutoplasmic protrusions from the central mass may extrude into the perivitelline space. These protrusions become more numerous up to day 50 and eventually break up into scattered granules.

(c) *Deutoplasmic fragmentation.* – The central part of the deutoplasm of the above ova as well as those that had first undergone parthenogenetic cleavage, eventually undergoes fragmentation and the deutoplasm eventually breaks up into small fragments from days 60 to 70 after ovulation.

(d) *Comminution of yolk granules.* – This process takes place very gradually and as soon as the granules are fine enough they can be seen passing through the pores in the zona pellucida. As the yolk granules gradually decrease in number this eventually results in a vesicle surrounded only by the zona pellucida (Fig. 1). The later stages of degenerated ova, after three months, lose their globular shape and may become disc-shaped or collapse to a tri-radiated form.

379

The question arises as to what causes fertilized ova to descend into the uterus before day 6, while unfertilized ova remain in the oviduct for varying periods up to at least 7.5 months. The role which the mucoid masses may play in this retention remains an open question and the mechanism which leads to a differential transport of fertilized ova remains obscure. Betteridge and Mitchell (1974) speculated on the role of enzymes associated with steroid synthesis produced by the zona pellucida, such as found in the blastomere of the rat four days after fertilization (Oguri and Tsutsumi 1972). Several workers cited by Perry et al. (1973) have found that the early uterine blastocyst of several mammals contains enzyme systems capable of synthesizing various steroids which may play a role in maternal recognition of pregnancy. It may be that in the mare as well as in other mammals, including the human, these steroids are already produced in the morula and early blastocyst stages while still in the oviducts and may play an important role in the transport of the fertilized ovum.

REFERENCES

Betteridge K. J. and Mitchell D. (1972) Retention of ova by the Fallopian tube in mares. *J. Reprod. Fertil. 31*, 515.
Betteridge K. J. and Mitchell D. (1974) Direct evidence of the retention of unfertilized ova in the oviduct of the mare. *J. Reprod. Fertil. 39*, 145–148.
Betteridge K. J. and Mitchell D. (1975) A surgical technique applied to the study of tubal eggs in the mare. *J. Reprod. Fertil., Suppl. 23* (in press).
Bjersing L. and Younglai E. V. (1972) Steroid hormones and ultrastructure of the equine Graafian follicle. *Z. Zellforsch. mikrosk. Anat. 132*, 357–364.
David J. S. E. (1975) A survey of eggs in the oviducts of mares. *J. Reprod. Fertil., Suppl. 23* (in press).
Hamilton W. J. and Day F. T. (1945) Cleavage stages of the ova of the horse, with notes on ovulation. *J. Anat. (Lond.) 79*, 127–130.
Oguri N. and Tsutsumi Y. (1972) Non-surgical recovery of equine eggs, and an attempt at non-surgical egg transfer in horses. *J. Reprod. Fertil. 31*, 187–195.
Onuma H. and Ohnami Y. (1975) Retention of tubal eggs in mares. *J. Reprod. Fertil., Suppl. 23* (in press).
Perry J. S., Heap R. B. and Amoroso E. C. (1973) Steroid hormone production by pig blastocysts. *Nature (Lond.) 245*, 45–47.
Short R. V. (1961) Steroid concentrations in the follicular fluid of mares at various stages of the reproductive cycle. *J. Endocr. 22*, 153–163.
Steffenhagen W. P., Pineda M. H. and Ginther O. J. (1972) Retention of unfertilized ova in uterine tubes of mares. *Amer. J. Vet. Res. 33*, 2391–2398.
Van Niekerk C. H. and Gerneke W. H. (1966) Persistence and parthenogenetic cleavage of tubal ova in the mare. *Onderstepoort J. Vet. Res. 33*, 195–232.
Van Rensburg S. J. and Van Niekerk C. H. (1968) Ovarian function, follicular oestradiol-17β and luteal progesterone and 20α-hydroxypregn-4-en-3-one in cycling and pregnant equines. *Onderstepoort J. vet. Res. 35*, 301–318.

Animal Pathology Division, Health of Animals Branch,
Agriculture Canada, Animal Diseases Research Institute (E),
P. O. Box 11300, Station H, Ottawa, Ontario, K2H 8P9.

POSSIBLE ROLE OF THE EMBRYO
IN THE CONTROL
OF OVIDUCTAL TRANSPORT IN MARES

By

K. J. Betteridge, P. F. Flood* and D. Mitchell

ABSTRACT

Evidence for differential oviductal transport of fertilized and unfertilized
ova in mares is reviewed. The possibility that morphological surface differences are involved in this phenomenon has been investigated by light
– and transmission electron-microscopy of ova recovered from the oviduct.
Six freshly ovulated ova (including two that were fertilized) and six old,
retained ova have been compared. No marked differences between the
surfaces of fertilized and unfertilized ova within six days of ovulation
were apparent but both categories of fresh ova differed from those that
had been retained in the oviduct for 29 days or longer. Whether non-
morphological surface characteristics or metabolic differences between
fertilized and fresh unfertilized ova could account for differential transport is discussed with reference to other species. It is postulated that the
equine embryo may influence its own passage through the oviduct by the
production of a humoral agent.

Finding the oviducts of the mare to contain as many as ten ova in varying
stages of degeneration, Van Niekerk and Gerneke (1966) suggested that unfertilized ova accumulated there and that only fertilized ova entered the uterus.

---

* Permanent address: Department of Anatomy, University of Bristol, Bristol, BS1 5LS,
England.

These observations have been confirmed (Webel et al. 1970; Steffenhagen et al. 1972; Oguri and Tsutsumi 1972a) and the recovery of sperm-marked, degenerating ova 30 and 58 days after isolated matings has provided direct evidence of oviductal retention of unfertilized ova (Betteridge and Mitchell 1974). Differential transport of fertilized and unfertilized ova is not peculiar to Equidae. Rasweiler (1972) has shown that empty zonae pellucidae and unfertilized ova of the bat *Glossophaga soricina* are retained in the ampulla of the oviduct while fertilized ova enter the uterotubal junction where they implant. In this species however, the zona pellucida is shed before the blastocyst leaves the ampulla, while in the horse the zona is still present when the blastocyst enters the uterus about six days after ovulation (Oguri and Tsutsumi 1972b).

In this paper, an ultrastructural comparison of fertilized and unfertilized oviductal ova is discussed in relation to possible mechanisms underlying their differential transport.

MATERIALS AND METHODS

Six freshly ovulated ova and six unfertilized old ova were recovered as previously described (Betteridge and Mitchell 1975). They were aged with respect to the time of ovulation as determined by rectal palpation of the ovaries. Time zero was taken to be midway between the examinations before and after ovulation. Of the fresh ova, two were fertilized (aged $3\frac{1}{2} \pm \frac{1}{2}$ and $5 \pm \frac{1}{2}$ days), two were from unmated mares ($4\frac{1}{2} \pm \frac{1}{2}$ and 5 ± 1) one was an unfertilized ovum from a mated mare ($3\frac{1}{2} \pm \frac{1}{2}$) and one a possibly fertilized ovum that failed to develop (4 ± 1). Three of the old ova were of unknown age and the others were 29, 58 and 33 days of age.

The eggs were photographed, then fixed in 2.5 % glutaraldehyde in 0.1 M cacodylate buffer. After postfixation in 1 % osmium tetroxide they were dehydrated through ethanol and embedded in either Epon or Spurr's medium. Sections were stained in uranyl acetate and lead citrate (Stempak and Ward 1964; Venable and Coggeshall 1965) and examined with a Hitachi HU12A electron microscope.

RESULTS

The zona pellucida

In both fertilized and unfertilized ova collected within 6 days of ovulation the zona appeared as a band of fine filamentous material approximately 5 μ thick pierced by numerous channels, presumably once occupied by the processes of the granulosa cells and the oocyte. In the outer third of the zona these channels tended to be more oblique and numerous than in the inner two thirds which may account for the bilaminar appearance often seen in the zona of fresh ova by light microscopy (Figs. 1 and 2). It may have been these channels that caused the outer surface of the zona to appear slightly roughened. These deductions are supported by preliminary observations on follicular oocytes in which cellular processes seem to be most abundant in the outer third of the zona.

In degenerating ova that had been retained in the oviduct for long periods, the zona often appeared extremely smooth by light microscopy and consisted of only a single layer. The smooth outer surface was confirmed in electron micrographs which also showed the zona material to be condensed, largely obliterating the channels (Figs. 3 and 4).

The perivitelline space

In the morulae, large numbers of lipid bodies, degenerating mitochondria and fragments of membrane were lying free in the perivitelline space (Fig. 5), probably accounting for the granular appearance often noted in the unfixed ovum. Similar material was frequently seen to have been engulfed by the blastomeres in which it formed large spherical vacuoles.

The cell surface

The cell surfaces of both fertilized and unfertilized fresh ova bore many finger-like microvilli which were more irregular and numerous in the unfertilized ones. In old ova the cell membrane had broken down completely thus allowing cellular debris to disperse throughout the zonal cavity. In recently ovulated unfertilized ova a few cortical granules were present beneath the cell surface but none could be recognized in either the fertilized or old ova (Fig. 6).

The cytoplasm

In the morulae, cells contained the usual organelles including elongated mitochondria with dense matrices, well developed Golgi complexes, granular endoplasmic reticulum and free ribosomes. Numerous lipid bodies and a few yolk bodies were also recognizable. The lipid bodies were usually closely associated with mitochondria and many showed signs of coalescence; some were almost as large as the nucleus and tended to distort other structures.

In the freshly ovulated unfertilized ova the bulk of the cytoplasm consisted of a flocculent material of moderate electron density. Within this matrix, lipid and yolk bodies and mitochondria were prominent (Fig. 7). The mitochondria, though sometimes degenerate, were often well preserved but were not associated with the lipid bodies which, in turn, showed less tendency to coalesce. Neither

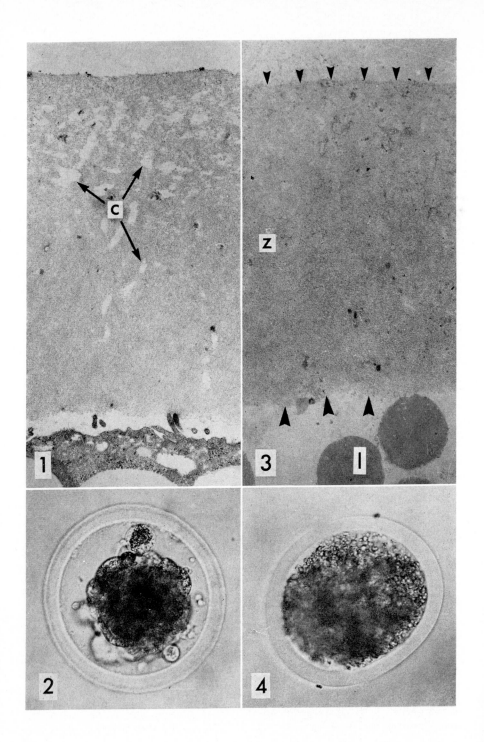

Golgi complex nor endoplasmic reticulum was positively identified though collections of membrane vesicles were occasionally seen. The degree of fragmentation of the vitellus was variable, ranging from a single large cytoplasmic mass with a little debris in the perivitelline space to complete division of the cytoplasm into numerous fragments superficially resembling a morula. However, the fragments were not closely applied to one another as the cell surfaces were in morulae. Nuclear material was visible in only one fragmented ovum which had possibly begun to degenerate following fertilization.

In the old ova the zonal cavity was loosely packed with lipid bodies interspersed with membrane-bound dense granules and membrane fragments (Fig. 8).

DISCUSSION

The fact that mares' oviducts can retain several unfertilized ova while allowing passage of fertilized ones suggests that early embryos in some way influence their own transport. How this is accomplished remains unresolved. From the present studies, there is as yet no indication of any marked morphological difference between the surfaces of the fertilized ovum which is destined to enter the uterus and the unfertilized ovum that will remain in the oviduct. However, as there was some latitude in the timing of ovulation and since the method of ovum recovery did not provide information on the position of the ovum in the oviduct, it remains possible that the fertilized ova examined had not reached the critical stage when a morphological difference might be manifest. In this connection, nothing corresponding to "... a thin coat of material resembling the albumin of the rabbit egg" (Hamilton and Day 1945) could be recognized and it seemed that the bilaminar appearance often seen in the zona was determined prior to ovulation. It remains possible that other surface characteristics of the zona, and hence the potential for oviductal transport, are altered by

---

Figs. 1–4.

1. The zona pellucida and a small part of one blastomere of a $5 \pm \frac{1}{2}$ day old morula. Channels (c) are most numerous in the outer third of the zona. × 12,500.

2. A photomicrograph of a 4 ± 1 day old ovum showing the bilaminar appearance of the zona. The narrow inner bright band is an optical artifact but the differences in texture between the inner $^2/_3$ and the outer $^1/_3$ are real and characteristic of both fertilized and unfertilized ova of this age. On electron microscopy this ovum showed nuclear material but did not seem to be cleaving normally. Bright field, unstained. × 305.

3. Part of an unfertilized ovum of > 33 days of age. The inner and outer surfaces of the zona (z) are indicated by the large and small arrows respectively. Lipid bodies (l) are recognizable but the channels in the zona are almost completely obliterated. This ovum was passed in the oviduct by a fertilized ovum. × 12,500.

4. A photomicrograph of the ovum seen Fig. 3. The zona appears very smooth and lacks the bilaminar structure seen Fig. 2. Bright field, unstained. × 305.

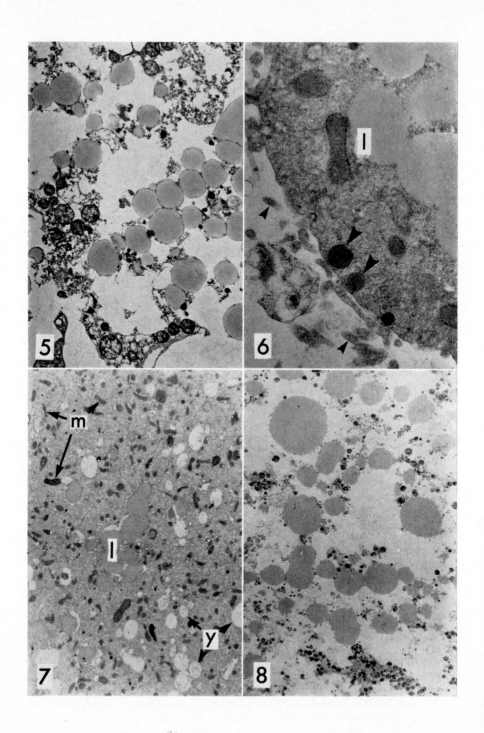

fertilization and the release of the cortical granules as, for example, zona solubility is affected by fertilization in mice (Inoue and Wolf 1974). Though cortical granule release without passage into the uterus eventually occurs in unfertilized ova as they degenerate, this does not necessarily exclude a role for the cortical granules in oviductal transport because other characteristics of the ovum and oviduct prevailing at fertilization and at degeneration may not be comparable. The shapes and surfaces of old retained ova examined in the present study, for example, were clearly different from those of newly ovulated ones whether or not the latter were fertilized.

If differential oviductal transport cannot be accounted for by morphological surface differences, the fertilized ovum may exert its influence through its metabolism, either systemically or locally. Early differences in steroid and gonadotrophin production by pregnant and non-pregnant animals suggest that the developing embryo may provoke a systemic response on the part of the mother at as early as six days of gestation in the cow (Henricks et al. 1972), six days in the sow (Tillson et al. 1970), five days in the rabbit (Fuchs and Beling 1974) and eight days in the mare (Holtan et al. 1975), though the differences in mares were not statistically significant. Such hormonal effects could stimulate oviductal transport and it is again possible that only the freshly ovulated ovum would respond owing to the marked structural differences between fresh and old ova.

Alternatively, the effect of the early embryo's metabolism may be entirely local. The degenerate state of the cytoplasmic organelles in unfertilized ova emphasizes the differences in general metabolic activity that must exist between fertilized and unfertilized ova and poses the question of whether oviductal transport could be influenced by local changes in simple parameters such as pH, pO_2 and/or pCO_2. Perhaps more pertinent in this regard is the increasing body of evidence suggesting that very young embryos are capable of hormone production. Gonadotrophins have been demonstrated in blastocysts and maternal plasma 5–6 days after mating in rabbits (Haour and Saxena 1974) and human chorionic gonadotrophin has been demonstrated in maternal plasma 6–8 days after fertilization in man (Saxena et al. 1974) though the reliability of the assays used has been questioned (Catt et al. 1975). Oviductal embryos of the rat,

---

Figs. 5–8.
5. Lipid bodies and membrane fragments in the perivitelline space of a $3\frac{1}{2} \pm \frac{1}{2}$ day old fertilized ovum. × 5,800.
6. The cell surface of an unfertilized ovum $3\frac{1}{2} \pm \frac{1}{2}$ days after ovulation showing cortical granules (▼), microvilli (▲) and lipid (l). × 17,500.
7. Area of cytoplasm from an unfertilized ovum $4\frac{1}{2} \pm \frac{1}{2}$ days after ovulation. Mitochondria (m), lipid bodies (l) and yolk bodies (y) are visible. × 4,000.
8. Lipid bodies and membrane fragments in the zonal cavity of an old ovum. × 3,000.

rabbit, mouse and hamster contain enzymes normally associated with steroidogenesis (see Dickmann et al. 1975) and 6-day rabbit blastocysts are capable of metabolizing steroids (Huff and Eik-Nes 1966). Localized responses to stimuli arising within the lumen are common in the uterus and include the induction of pontamine blue permeability in the endometrial capillaries of the rat by the preimplantation blastocyst (Psychoyos 1960), the asymmetrical suppression of myometrial activity by unilaterally administered progesterone in the rabbit (Porter 1968), and the appearance of steroid metabolizing enzymes in the uterine epithelium adjacent to the filamentous blastocyst in the sow (Flood 1974). Likewise, Blandau (1969) reports that the contractility of the rabbit oviduct is greatest in the region containing the ovum. These findings in other species suggest the possibility that the equine embryo may influence its own passage through the oviduct by the production of a humoral agent.

ACKNOWLEDGMENTS

We thank Miss S. Becker for skilled electron-micrographical assistance, Mrs. J. Hierlihy, Messrs. R. Bériault, J. Shackleton, G. Raby and Y. Barbeau for technical help, Miss E. Cathcart, Mr. G. Hogan and Mr. S. Shearer for their help with animals. This work was in part supported by a post-doctoral fellowship awarded to P.F.F. by the National Research Council of Canada.

REFERENCES

Betteridge K. J. and Mitchell D. (1974) Direct evidence of the retention of unfertilized ova in the oviduct of the mare. *J. Reprod. Fertil. 39*, 145–148.

Betteridge K. J. and Mitchell D. (1975) A surgical technique applied to the study of tubal eggs in the mare. *J. Reprod. Fertil., Suppl. 23* (in press).

Blandau R. J. (1969) Gamete transport – comparative aspects. In: Hafez E. S. E. and Blandau R. J., eds. *The Mammalian Oviduct*, pp. 129–162. University of Chicago Press, Chicago.

Catt K. J., Dufau M. L. and Vaitukaitis J. L. (1975) Apperance of hCG in pregnancy plasma following initiation of implantation of the blastocyst. *J. clin. Endocr. Metab. 40*, 537–540.

Dickman Z., Dey S. K. and Gupta S. J. (1975) Steroidogenesis in rabbit preimplantation embryos. *Proc. nat. Acad. Sci., Wash. 72*, 298–300.

Flood P. F. (1974) Steroid-metabolizing enzymes in the early pig conceptus and in the related endometrium. *J. Endocr. 63*, 413–414.

Fuchs A.-R. and Beling C. (1974) Evidence of early ovarian recognition of blastocysts in rabbits. *Endocrinology 95*, 1054–1058.

Hamilton W. J. and Day F. T. (1945) Cleavage stages in the ova of the horse, with notes on ovulation. *J. Anat. (Lond.) 79*, 127–129.

Haour F. and Saxena B. B. (1975) Detection of gonadotrophin in rabbit blastocyst before implantation. *Science 185*, 444–445.

Henricks D. M., Dickey J. F., Hill J. R. and Johnston W. E. (1972) Plasma estrogen and progesterone levels after mating, and during late pregnancy and postpartum in cows. *Endocrinology 90*, 1336–1342.

Holtan D. W., Nett T. M. and Estergreen V. L. (1975) Plasma progestins in pregnant, postpartum and cycling mares. *J. Animal Sci. 40*, 251–260.

Huff R. L. and Eik-Nes K. B. (1966) Metabolism *in vitro* of acetate and certain steroids by six-day-old rabbit blastocysts. *J. Reprod. Fertil. 11*, 57–63.

Inoue M. and Wolf D. P. (1974) Comparative solubility properties of the zonae pellucidae of unfertilized and fertilized mouse ova. *Biol. Reprod. 11*, 558–565.

Oguri N. and Tsutsumi Y. (1972a) Studies on lodging of the equine unfertilized ova in Fallopian tubes. *Res. Bull. Livestock Farm, Hokkaido Univ. 6*, 32–43.

Oguri N. and Tsutsumi Y. (1972b) Non-surgical recovery of equine eggs, and an attempt at non-surgical egg transfer in horses. *J. Reprod. Fertil. 31*, 187–195.

Porter D. G. (1968) The local effect of intra-uterine progesterone treatment on myometrial activity in rabbits. *J. Reprod. Fertil. 15*, 437–445.

Psychoyos A. (1961) Perméabilité capillaire et décidualization utérine. *C. R. hebd. Séanc. Acad. Sci. (Paris) 252*, 1515–1517.

Rasweiler J. J. (1972) Reproduction in the long tailed bat, *Glossophaga soricina*. 1. Preimplantation development and histology of the oviduct. *J. Reprod. Fertil. 31*, 249–262.

Saxena B. B., Hasan S. H., Haour F. and Schmidt-Gollwitzer (1974) Radioreceptorassay of HCG: Detection of early pregnancy. *Science 184*, 793–795.

Steffenhagen S. P., Pineda M. H. and Ginther O. J. (1972) Retention of unfertilized ova in uterine tubes of mares. *Amer. J. vet. Res. 33*, 2391–2398.

Stempak J. G. and Ward R. T. (1964) An improved staining method for electron microscopy. *J. Cell Biol. 22*, 697–701.

Tillson S. A., Erb R. E. and Niswender G. D. (1970) Comparison of LH and progesterone in blood and metabolites of progesterone in urine of domestic sows during estrus and early pregnancy. *J. Animal Sci. 30*, 795–805.

Van Niekerk C. H. and Gerneke W. H. (1966) Persistence and parthenogenetic cleavage of tubal ova in the mare. *Onderstepoort J. vet. Res. 33*, 195–232.

Venable J. H. and Coggeshall R. (1965) A simplified lead citrate stain for use in electron microscopy. *J. Cell Biol. 25*, 407–408.

Webel S. K., Ellicott A. R. and Dziuk P. J. (1970) Control of ovulation (HCG) and maturation of pony eggs. *J. Animal Sci. 31*, 1036 (Abstr.).

389

*From the Center for Research and Training
in Reproductive Biology and Voluntary Regulation of Fertility
(supported by the Rockefeller Foundation)
Department of Obstetrics and Gynecology and Physiology,
The University of Texas Health Science Center at San Antonio,
7703 Floyd Curl Drive, San Antonio, Texas 78228

OVUM TRANSPORT IN NON-HUMAN PRIMATES*

By

Carlton A. Eddy, Raul G. Garcia[1]
Duane C. Kraemer[2] and Carl J. Pauerstein[3]

ABSTRACT

The normal time course of ovum transport was studied in two species of non-human primate, *Macaca mulatta* and *Papio anubis*. Plasma estrogen values were determined daily by radioimmunoassay commencing on day 8 of the rhesus menstrual cycle and approximately at the midpoint of the sexual turgescence period of the baboon in order to provide predictive indication of impending ovulation. After detection of a well-defined pre-ovulatory increase in estrogen production (levels in excess of 200–300 pg/ml of plasma) serial laparoscopies were performed every 12 to 24 h in order to monitor ovarian follicular development and to visually confirm and time ovulation. Alternatively in half of the baboons studied, timing of ovulation was accomplished on the basis of corpus luteum histology, cycle data, and periovulatory estrogen values in lieu of serial laparoscopy.

Laparotomies were performed approximately 24, 48 or 72 h after ovulation and the reproductive tracts were flushed *in situ* to recover ova. The

[1] Rockefeller Foundation Post-Doctoral Fellow in Reproductive Biology.
[2] Present address: College of Veterinary Medicine, Department of Veterinary Physiology and Pharmacology, Texas A & M University, College Station, Texas 77843.
[3] Recipient of NICHHD Research Career Development Award K04 HD47279.

ampulla, isthmus and uterus were flushed separately allowing the position of ova within the tract to be determined. Ova were consistently recovered from the ampulla at 24 h after ovulation in both species. At 48 h after ovulation ova were still in the rhesus ampulla but the majority had been transported into the baboon isthmus. By 72 h after ovulation all baboon ova were found in the uterus as were the majority of rhesus ova.

On the basis of these data it would appear that the non-human primate constitutes a potentially valuable animal model for the evaluation and pre-clinical investigation of contraceptive techniques affecting oviductal function.

The continued rapid increase in world population despite the availability of effective methods for fertility regulation affirms the need to evolve additional contraceptive techniques. With the exception of surgical intervention, no current contraceptive technique is specifically designed to alter oviductal function.

Knowledge of the normal time course of ovum transport is basic to an understanding of oviductal function and is a prerequisite to development of contraceptive techniques operative on the oviduct. Although the detailed time course of ovum transport has been determined for various laboratory species, similar information for primates is either lacking or incomplete. This lack of knowledge reflects the inherent complexities associated with utilization of primates, including humans, in ovum transport studies, chief among which are difficulty in accurately determining the time of ovulation and in recovery of the single ovulated ovum. Attempts to characterize the process of ovum transport in man have achieved variable but incomplete success in overcoming these difficulties. With few exceptions most studies have relied upon indirect and often subjective criteria retrospectively to time ovulation. Recovery rates, whether from *in vivo* procedures or from excised material, have been universally low. The availability of an animal model in which the pattern and duration of ovum transport approximates that of man and in which more precise means of timing ovulation and recovering ova may be employed is therefore highly desirable. Because of its anatomic, endocrinologic and physiologic similarity to man, the non-human primate is a potentially valuable model with which to investigate oviductal transport phenomena. The few reports of ovum transport in the spontaneously ovulating primate have generally dealt with overall time of transport from ovary to uterus, and have not been based on accurate knowledge of the time of ovulation. Hartman (1944) used rectal palpation to time ovulation and determined ovum transport through the rhesus' oviduct to require "somewhat over three days" based on recovery of ova from the uterus. Mastroianni et al. (1967) used ferning of cervical mucus to time ovulation and recovered ova from the oviducts of spontaneously ovulating rhesus monkeys 24 h after presumed ovulation. Marston et al. (1969) used morphologic dating of the corpus luteum and found that ova were retained in the rhesus oviduct for as long as 4 days after ovulation while ova were recovered from the uterus 4 to 7 days after ovulation.

Periovulatory changes in gross ovarian follicular morphology have been observed in various species of non-human primates using serial laparotomy (*Macaca mulatta:* Johansson et al. 1968; Betteridge et al. 1970) and laparoscopy (*Macaca fascicularis:* Dukelow et al. 1972; Jewett and Dukelow 1973; Rawson and Dukelow 1973; Jainudeen and Hafez 1973; and *Saimiri sciureus:* Harrison and Dukelow 1971). Such serial observations provide the opportunity to time accurately the occurrence of ovulation in the primate. However, serial laparoscopic timing of ovulation in conjunction with studies of the detailed time course of ovum transport has been employed only in *Macaca fascicularis* (Jainudeen and Hafez 1973). Difficulty in recovery of natural ova dictated the substitution of surrogate ova (Sephadex beads and rabbit ova) early in the study. Thus the time course of ovum transport of natural primate ova remains largely undefined.

It has been suggested that frequent and repeated laparoscopic manipulation of the reproductive tract interferes with ovum pick up (Jainudeen and Hafez 1973). Because the primate ovulates spontaneously, an excessive number of serial laparoscopic observations may be required if laparoscopy is initiated prematurely. In the rhesus monkey the preovulatory surge of LH is preceded by a gradual increase in circulating estrogen of approximately three days duration (Hotchkiss et al. 1971). Estrogen levels then rise sharply, peak 9–15 h prior to the LH surge, then decline prior to ovulation. Ovulation follows the estrogen peak by approximately 37 h (Weick et al. 1973). A similar peak is also observed in the baboon (Stevens et al. 1970). Utilizing the predictive value of the preovulatory peak in circulating estrogen the number of laparoscopies required to verify ovulation may be minimized. Similarly, the combination of such estrogen data with histologic dating of the corpus luteum can be used in lieu of serial laparoscopy to time ovulation with reasonable accuracy.

We have examined the detailed time course of ovum transport in two species of primate, *Macaca mulatta* (Eddy et al. 1975a), and *Papio anubis* (Eddy et al. 1975b). By comparing the detailed time course and pattern of ovum transport in these non-human primates with that of the human, the validity of such primates as animal models of human ovum transport may be evaluated.

MATERIALS AND METHODS

Sexually mature female rhesus monkeys (*Macaca mulatta*) weighing 3.3–5.3 kg were individually caged under controlled conditions of 24°C and 50 per cent relative humidity and exposed to a 14 h fluorescent light photo-period. Commercially prepared pelleted monkey chow was supplemented twice weekly with fresh fruit and vegetables. Tap water was available *ad lib*. Vaginal swabs were taken each morning and examined for menses. The first day of menstrual bleeding was designated day 1 of the cycle.

Sexually mature female baboons (*Papio anubis*) weighing 11.96–14.72 kg were individually caged under ambient conditions and exposed to natural lighting. An unsupplemented diet of commercially formulated baboon chow was provided. Tap water was available *ad lib*. The degree of perineal turgescence of each animal was evaluated daily and rated on a scale of 0–4 (lack of turgescence = 0, maximum turgescence = 4) in order to monitor menstrual cycle activity (Hagino and Goldzieher 1970).

Each animal was allowed to establish regular, spontaneous, cyclic menstrual activity prior to use. Daily blood samples (2–3 ml) were drawn each morning beginning on day 8 of the cycle (rhesus) or at the midpoint of the period of maximum turgescence (baboon) by femoral puncture following phencyclidine tranquilization. The heparinized blood was centrifuged and the plasma assayed for estrogen. Blood was drawn through day 16 (rhesus), until the onset of deturgescence (baboon), or until a preovulatory estrogen peak was detected.

Estrogen assay

Total plasma estrogen levels were determined by radioimmunoassay as described by Wu et al. (1973) with minor modification. Absolute ethanol was used in place of methanol for precipitation of plasma proteins. The estrogen antibody was prepared and made available by Dr. Burton V. Caldwell.

Laparoscopy

Following the detection of a preovulatory peak in estrogen (levels in excess of 200–300 pg/ml), serial laparoscopies were initiated in order to monitor sequential changes in follicular morphology. Under general anesthesia (phencyclidine, 3–5 mg/kg body weight, rhesus; halothane-oxygen, baboon) the entire surface of both ovaries was visualized using a pediatric (rhesus) or standard size (baboon) laparoscope. The time of ovulation was arbitrarily designated as the midpoint between two successive laparoscopic observations, the former preovulatory and the latter postovulatory. Using this rationale, the time of ovulation was accurately defined within a range of ± 6–15 h for the rhesus and ± 12 h for the baboon.

Corpus luteum dating

In the baboons not previously monitored by serial laparoscopy, the corpus luteum was excised following *in situ* flushing of the reproductive tract, fixed in buffered formalin and histologically dated (Corner 1945).

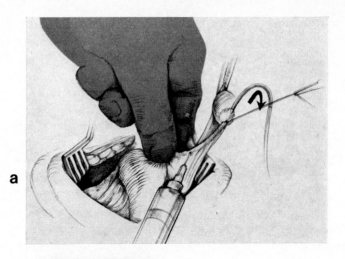

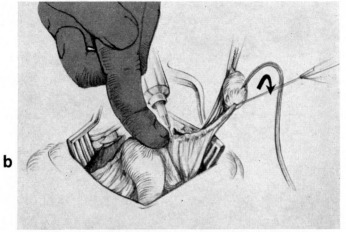

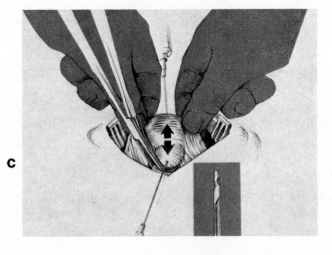

Ovum recovery

Midventral laparotomies were performed under general anesthesia 24, 48 or 72 h after ovulation and the reproductive tracts flushed *in situ* to recover ova (Fig. 1). In the majority of cases a polyethylene cannula (P. E. 60, i. d. 0.030 in., o. d. 0.048 in.) was inserted into the ampulla to a point just beyond the infundibulum and ligated in place. In the remaining cases, the oviduct was flushed directly into a receptacle (Mastroianni and Rosseau 1965). The ampullary-isthmic junction (AIJ) was located and a short, 30 gauge needle mounted on a syringe filled with normal saline was inserted into the lumen of the ampulla at the level of the AIJ or several millimeters to the ovarian side of it. The uterotubal junction (UTJ) was digitally occluded and 3–10 ml of saline was flushed through the ampulla. The needle was then introduced into the isthmus as close to the UTJ as possible. The isthmus, excluding the intramural portion and a 3–5 mm proximal segment, was flushed with 3–5 ml of saline, and the effluent collected through the ampulla.

To flush the uterus, an 18 gauge polyethylene catheter fenestrated at the tip was introduced through the uterine fundus into the uterine cavity. A second catheter was inserted through the ventral aspect of the uterus into the uterine cavity at a point several mm above the internal cervical os. Syringes were attached to each catheter and successive 6 ml quantities of saline were flushed through the uterine cavity from alternating syringes. At each flushing the effluent was collected in the corresponding empty syringe. The use of a cervical clamp prevented transcervical leakage of fluid during uterine flushing. Alternatively the baboon uterus was flushed transfundally through the cervical os using a single 30 ml syringe fitted with an 18 gauge needle and the effluent collected from the vagina via a polished glass tube fitted snugly against the cervix. In the 72 h group, the uterus was flushed first, with the UTJ occluded, to avoid artifactual dislocation of ova located in the proximal isthmus into the uterus during oviductal flushing. Oviductal and uterine effluents were examined for the presence of ova with a binocular dissecting microscope.

Fig. 1.

In situ flushing technique for the recovery of ova from various portions of the non-human primate reproductive tract.

a) Ampullary flush.

b) Isthmic flush.

c) Uterine flush (insert: details of fenestrations applied).
(Reprinted from Biology of Reproduction).

Timing of ovulation

Detection of a preovulatory peak in peripheral plasma estrogen constituted a consistent and accurate means of predicting impending ovulation in the primate (Fig. 2 and 3). In all cycles in which ova were recovered, a well defined preovulatory peak of estrogen in excess of 200 pg/ml (range 200–325 pg/ml in rhesus, 200–300 pg/ml in baboons) preceded ovulation by 24–48 h. As a result, the number of laparoscopies required to time ovulation was minimized; 60 per cent of timed ovulations required two laparoscopies, 27 per cent required three and 13 per cent required four.

During the initial observation the ovary containing the Graafian follicle was easily distinguished from the contralateral non-ovulatory ovary in both species. The former was much larger, the entire ovary assuming a fluid-filled, bluish-pink opaque appearance which could occasionally be localized to a specific area which subsequently proved to be the site of ovulation. In agreement with Betteridge et al. (1970) we uniformly failed to observe persistent, well defined, protuberant Graafian follicles with preovulatory stigmata (Johansson et al. 1968). Instead, final follicular maturation and ovulation, visually observed as the transition from poorly defined Graafian follicle to protuberant, hemor-

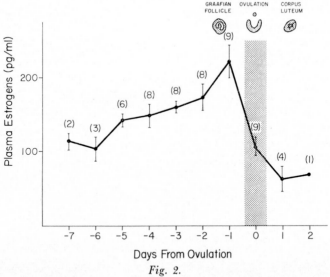

Fig. 2.

Mean plasma estrogen pattern of nine ovulatory menstrual cycles in which ova were recovered in *Macaca mulatta*. Values are normalized to the day of ovulation. Vertical lines about each point represent the standard error of the mean. Numbers in parentheses represent the number of observations. Hatched area defines the average interval of time during which ovulation occurred (range ± 6–15 h).

(Reprinted from Biology of Reproduction).

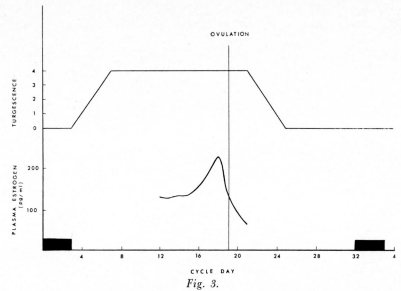

Fig. 3.

Menstrual cycle of *Papio anubis*. Upper tracing: mean pattern of turgescence of fifteen randomly selected ovulatory menstrual cycles in eight animals. Lower tracings: periovulatory plasma estrogen pattern associated with the above tracing.

rhagic, raw, postovulatory corpus luteum (CL), generally encompassed a period of only 12–24 h. Although variety in periovulatory follicular morphology was encountered, the diagnosis of ovulation was always unequivocal, due primarily to the opportunity to view progressive changes, before and after ovulation.

Ovum transport

A total of twenty-four *in situ* flushings was performed in the rhesus following laparoscopic timing of ovulation and resulted in the recovery of 9 ova (Table 1)

Table 1.

Ovum recovery rates following *in situ* flushing of the reproductive tract of *Macaca mulatta*.

Time after ovulation (h)	Number of flushings	Number of ova recovered	Per cent recovery
24	4	3	75
48	8	3	37.5
72	12	3	25
Total	24	9	37.5

397

Table 2.

Results of *in situ* flushing of the reproductive tract following timed ovulation
in *Macaca mulatta*.

Animal Number	Time after ovulation (h)	Oviductal flush	Uterine flush	Location of ovum
323	23 ± 11.5	+	−	Ampulla
843	24 ± 6	+	−	Ampulla
843	24 ± 6	+	−	Ampulla
563	48 ± 15	+	−	Ampulla
839	48 ± 6	+	−	Ampulla
843	48 ± 12	+	−	Ampulla
A11	72 ± 15	−	+	Uterus
A13	72 ± 12	+	−	Oviduct
A17	72 ± 12	−	+	Uterus

yielding an overall recovery rate of 37.5 per cent. In contrast, recovery rates
for individual time groups ranged from 75 per cent to 25 per cent.

The location of ova recovered through *in situ* flushing of the reproductive
tract at various times after ovulation is summarized in Table 2. Ova were consistently recovered from the ampulla at both 24 and 48 h after ovulation. By
72 h after ovulation, ova were entering the uterus. Two ova were recovered
from this site whereas a third was flushed from the oviduct. In the latter
recovery, the precise location of the ovum within the oviduct was not determined
with certainty.

In the baboon, thirty nine *in situ* flushings were performed and resulted in
the recovery of ten ova (Table 3) yielding an overall recovery rate of 26 per

Table 3.

Ovum recovery rates following *in situ* flushing of the reproductive tract
of *Papio anubis*.

Time after ovulation (h)	Number of flushings	Number of ova recovered	Per cent recovery
24	8	2	25
48	10	4	40
72	21	4	19
Total	39	10	26

Table 4.

Results of *in situ* flushing of the reproductive tract following timed ovulation in *Papio anubis*.

Animal Number	Time after ovulation (h)	Oviductal flush	Uterine flush	Location of ovum
X167	24 ± 12	+	−	Ampulla
B621	24 ± 12	+	−	Ampulla
X184	48 ± 12	+	−	Isthmus
X180	48 ± 12	+	−	Oviduct
0221	48	+	−	Ampulla
X179	48	+	−	Isthmus
X179	72 ± 12	−	+	Uterus
0221	72 ± 12	−	+	Uterus
X182	72	−	+	Uterus
X180	72	−	+	Uterus

cent. As in the rhesus, recovery rates for individual time groups were variable, ranging from 40 per cent to 19 per cent.

Ova recovered 24 h after ovulation were located in the ampulla as was a single ovum recovered 48 h after ovulation. However, unlike the rhesus, ova had passed beyond the ampulla by 48 h in the baboon, two being located in the isthmus while the precise location of a fourth egg within the oviduct was not determined. All ova recovered at 72 h after ovulation were located in the uterus (Table 4).

DISCUSSION

With few exceptions the overall time course of ovum transport appears to be remarkably similar in all mammalian species examined, 3 to 4 days being required for ova to travel from the ovary to the uterus. Major differences concern the details of entrance into and transit through various portions of the oviduct. These differences are at least partially a reflection of anatomic and endocrinologic differences between species.

Much of the available data on normal and pharmacologically modified ovum transport have been obtained in the rabbit. While the rabbit has been of great value in this regard, extrapolation of results to man may not be fully warranted. Although the overall time course of ovum transport is similar in the rabbit and human, the details of transport are quite dissimilar.

The periovulatory hormonal patterns are similar in man and the non-human primates, but differ from those in the rabbit. In the rabbit estrogen and progestin levels are elevated immediately prior to ovulation but are undetectably low during the period of ovum transport (Hilliard et al. 1971). Ovum transport in the rabbit thus occurs under conditions of ovarian hormonal withdrawal. In man and non-human primates, estrogen and progestin levels also exhibit a preovulatory elevation and decline, but estrogen levels are not as depressed while progestin levels rise throughout the period of transport. In the primate, then, ovum transport occurs under conditions of increasing ovarian hormonal support.

Because of the lack of accuracy in timing the occurrence of ovulation in the human and the use of recovery techniques which do not discriminate between various portions of the oviduct, the bulk of data concerning ovum transport in humans describes the overall transport rate rather than the detailed time course (Rock and Hertig 1944; Noyes et al. 1966; Clewe et al. 1971; Croxatto et al. 1972; Noriega and Oberti 1973). From these data, it is generally believed that 3 to 4 days are required for transport in the human.

The utilization of additional criteria including LH and estrogen determinations to time more accurately ovulation, combined with differential flushing of various portions of the reproductive tract, has heralded the emergence of a more detailed description of the time course of ovum transport in the human. Human ova have been found to be slowly transported through the ampulla. Approximately 30 h are required to reach the ampullary-isthmic junction. Following an additional 30 h at the junction, human ova enter the isthmus and are rapidly transported to the uterus since recovery of ova is lowest from the proximal isthmic segments of excised human oviducts (Croxatto and Ortiz 1975).

Preliminary results of human oviductal ovum transport studies in our laboratories support the observation of slow ampullary transport and retention of ova at the ampullary-isthmic junction. Women of high fertility seeking surgical sterilization who were not taking oral contraceptives and were not fitted with an IUD were monitored to determine the occurrence of ovulation. Peripheral plasma estrogen levels were measured daily during the follicular phase of the menstrual cycle by radioimmunoassay. Following detection of a preovulatory peak in estrogen, surgery was performed at selected postovulatory intervals. At laparotomy both oviducts were divided into three equal segments by placing ligatures at the fimbria, uterotubal junction and at two equidistant points between. The tract was then flushed *in situ* or excised, segmented and flushed. Two ova have been recovered in four attempts. On the basis of estrogen profile and dating of the endometrium and corpus luteum, ovulation occurred approximately 48 h prior to recovery in both cases. As confirmed from histology of the segments from which they were recovered, both ova were located in the ampulla, one at or near the ampullary-isthmic junction.

The potential value of the non-human primate as an animal model in the study of reproductive physiology has long been recognized. However, confirmation of the non-human primate as a valid model for ovum transport studies awaits further study. Our results suggest that the time course of ovum transport in *Macaca mulatta* and *Papio anubis* are similar in duration but different in detail. Baboon ova do not appear to reside in the ampulla for as long a period as do rhesus or human ova. Baboon ova reach the isthmus at a time when rhesus and human ova are still in the ampulla (48 ± 15 h after ovulation) although eggs in all three species require approximately equal times to be transported to the uterus. Thus it appears that the baboon presents a transport pattern characterized by an overall 3 day period of transport during which approximately equal periods of time are spent in the ampulla and isthmus. In contrast, transport in the rhesus appears to require approximately 3 days during most of which time ova reside in the ampulla, and then rapidly pass through the isthmus into the uterus.

The results of Jainudeen and Hafez (1973) are largely predicated upon the movement of artificial ova which were not proved to mimic accurately the transport of natural ova. They did, however, observe the location of 3 natural ova at 24, 48 and 72 h after ovulation. The ovum recovered at 24 h after ovulation was located in the ampulla, that at 48 h in the middle third or ampullary-isthmic region of the oviduct and that at 72 h was found in the isthmus. The detailed pattern of ovum transport in *Macaca fascicularis* therefore appears to combine the slow ampullary transport characteristic of the rhesus with slow isthmic transport perhaps more characteristic of the baboon. Thus, it appears that *Macaca mulatta* and *Papio anubis* constitute more faithful models of human ovum transport than does *Macaca fascicularis* with *Macaca mulatta* the more valid of the two.

ACKNOWLEDGMENTS

The authors gratefully acknowledge the excellent technical assistance of Thomas G. Turner and Elizabeth Menchaca, Department of Obstetrics and Gynecology.

This work was supported by the Agency for International Development, Subcontract PARFR-56 from the University of Minnesota.

REFERENCES

Betteridge K. J., Kelly W. A. and Marston J. H. (1970) Morphology of the rhesus monkey ovary near the time of ovulation. *J. Reprod. Fertil.* 22, 453–459.
Clewe T. H., Morgenstern L. L., Noyes R. W., Bonney W. A. Jr., Burrus S. B. and DeFeo V. J. (1971) Searches for ova in the human uterus and tubes. II. Clinical and laboratory data on nine successful searches for human ova. *Amer. J. Obstet. Gynec.* 109, 313–334.

401

Corner G. W. (1945) Development, organization and breakdown of corpus luteum in the rhesus monkey. *Contr. Embryol. 31*, 117–165.

Croxatto H. B., Diaz S., Fuentealba B., Croxatto H. D., Carrillo D. and Fabres C. (1972) Studies on the duration of egg transport in the human oviduct. I. The time interval between ovulation and egg recovery from the uterus in normal women. *Fertil. Steril. 23*, 447–458.

Croxatto H. B. and Ortiz M. S. (1975) Egg transport in the Fallopian tube. *Gynec. Invest. 6*, 215–225.

Dukelow W. R., Harrison R. M., Rawson J. M. R. and Johnson M. P. (1972) Natural and artificial control of ovulation in nonhuman primates. *Medical Primatology Proc. 3rd Conf. exp. Med. Surg. Primates,* Lyon 1972, Part I, pp. 232–236.

Eddy C. A., Garcia R. G., Kraemer D. C. and Pauerstein C. J. (1975a) Detailed time course of ovum transport in the rhesus monkey *(Macaca mulatta). Biol. Reprod. 13*, 363–369.

Eddy C. A., Turner T. T., Kraemer D. C. and Pauerstein C. J. (1975b) Pattern and duration of ovum transport in the baboon *(Papio anubis). Obstet. Gynec.,* in press.

Hagino N. and Goldzieher J. W. (1970) Regulation of gonadotrophin release by the corpus luteum in the baboon. *Endocrinology 87*, 413–418.

Harrison R. M. and Dukelow W. R. (1971) Megestrol acetate: Its effect on the inhibition of ovulation in squirrel monkeys, *Saimiri sciureus. J. Reprod. Fertil. 25*, 99–101.

Hartman C. G. (1944) Recovery of primate eggs and embryos. Methods and data on the time of ovulation. *West. J. Surg. Obstet. Gynec. 52*, 41–61.

Hilliard J. and Eaton L. W. Jr. (1971) Estradiol-17β, progesterone and 20α-hydroxy-pregn-4-en-3-one in rabbit ovarian venous plasma. II. From mating through implantation. *Endocrinology 89*, 522–527.

Hotchkiss J., Atkinson L. W. and Knobil E. (1971) Time course of serum estrogen and luteinizing hormone concentrations during the menstrual cycle of the rhesus monkey. *Endocrinology 89*, 177–183.

Jainudeen M. R. and Hafez E. S. E. (1973) Egg transport in the macaque *(Macaca fascicularis). Biol. Reprod. 9*, 305–308.

Jewett D. A. and Dukelow W. R. (1973) Follicular observation and laparoscopic aspiration techniques in *Macaca fascicularis. J. med. Primatology 2*, 108–113.

Johansson E. D. B., Neill J. D. and Knobil E. (1968) Peri-ovulatory progesterone concentration in the peripheral plasma of the rhesus monkey with a methodologic note on the detection of ovulation. *Endocrinology 82*, 143–148.

Marston J. H., Kelly W. A. and Eckstein P. (1969) Effect of an intra-uterine device on gamete transport and fertilization in the rhesus monkey. *J. Reprod. Fertil. 19*, 149–156.

Mastroianni L. and Rosseau C. H. (1965) Influence of the intrauterine coil on ovum transport and sperm distribution in the monkey. *Amer. J. Obstet. Gynec. 93*, 416–420.

Mastroianni L., Suzuki S., Manabe Y. and Watson F. (1967) Further observations on the influence of the intrauterine device on ovum and sperm distribution in the monkey. *Amer. J. Obstet. Gynec. 99*, 649–661.

Noriega C. and Oberti C. (1973) Studies of the human unfertilized tubal ovum. *Fertil. Steril. 24*, 595–601.

Noyes R. W., Clewe T. H., Bonney W. A. Jr., Burrus S. B., Defeo V. J. and Morgenstern L. L. (1966) Searches for ova in the human uterus and tubes. I. Review, clinical methodology, and summary of findings. *Amer. J. Obstet. Gynec. 96*, 157–167

Rawson J. M. R. and Dukelow W. R. (1973) Observation of ovulation in *Macaca fascicularis*. *J. Reprod. Fertil. 34*, 187–190.

Rock J. and Hertig A. T. (1944) Information regarding the time of human ovulation derived from a study of 3 unfertilized and 11 fertilized ova. *Amer. J. Obstet. Gynec. 47*, 343–356.

Stevens V. C., Sparks S. J. and Powell J. E. (1970) Levels of estrogens, progestogens and luteinizing hormone during the menstrual cycle of the baboon. *Endocrinology 87*, 658–666.

Weick R. F., Dierschke D. J., Karsch F. J., Hotchkiss J. and Knobil E. (1973) Periovulatory time course of the circulating gonadotropin and ovarian hormones in the rhesus monkey. *The Endocrine Society Meetings* (Abstr.), July 1973, Chicago.

Wu C.-H., Lundy L. E. and Lee S. G. (1973) A rapid radioimmunoassay for plasma estrogen. *Amer. J. Obstet. Gynec. 115*, 169–180.

26*

Laboratorio de Endocrinología y Departamento de Radiología
de la Universidad Católica de Chile and
Departamentos de Obstetricia y Ginecología del Hospital Sótero
del Rio y del Hospital San Juan de Dios,
Santiago, Chile

TRANSPORT OF OVUM SURROGATES
BY THE HUMAN OVIDUCT

By

J. Díaz, J. Vásquez, S. Díaz, F. Díaz
and H. B. Croxatto

ABSTRACT

The uptake and transport of foreign particulate matter by the human oviduct *in situ* was studied in 36 women scheduled for surgical sterilization. Dextran spheres with a diameter of 150 μ were injected into the peritoneal cavity in 3 women during the mid-follicular phase, in 3 women around the time of ovulation, and in 3 women during the puerperium. Oviducts were removed 24 h after the injection and were segmentally flushed to determine the uptake and distribution of spheres. The greatest uptake was observed in women injected in the ovulatory period and no uptake was observed in puerperal women.

Five to 15 copper spheres with a diameter of 300, 600 or 1200 μ were introduced into the ampulla of one oviduct in 20 women during laparotomy. The distal end was ligated and radiopaque markers were placed alongside the oviduct. Retention and transport of spheres to the uterus were assessed at various intervals thereafter by X-ray examinations. 300 and 600 μ spheres were transported batchwise in few weeks, whereas 1200 μ spheres were retained. The relationship between physiologic conditions and transportation to the uterus was studied in seven patients in whom copper or silver spheres were introduced into the oviduct. Passage in close proximity to ovulation was observed in five out of seven cycles studied. Transport temporarily unrelated to ovulation was observed in two cycles and in one non-cycling woman.

It was concluded that such ovum surrogates might be useful for studying the physiology and pharmacology of the human oviduct.

404

Studies on the physiology and pharmacology of ovum transport in women have been very limited in number and unrewarding, because of the difficulties in timing ovulation and locating the single ovulated ovum in the genital tract. In order to circumvent the latter problem, it would appear desirable to develop ovum surrogates, that is foreign particles, which could be transported like ova by the oviduct and which could be followed or located easily in the genital tract.

The ability of the oviduct to transport particles different from natural ova has been demonstrated in several species (rabbit: Harper et al. 1960; Croxatto et al. 1973; sheep: Wintenberger-Torres 1961; monkey: Jainudeen and Hafez 1973; and human: Decker 1954; Avendaño et al. 1971; Ascenzo et al. 1974). Earlier work has been reviewed by Pauerstein (1968).

Most of the investigators who experimented in women utilized dyes (Orsini 1974), oil droplets (Sheffery 1954; Fernström 1971) or solid particles much smaller than a human ovum. The main objective of these studies was to develop clinical tests to detect functional failures of transport in infertile women with patent oviducts. The information available from such clinical reports is limited and, in many cases, of doubtful meaning, in the light of the knowledge that very small particles do not follow the same pattern of transport as ova (Croxatto et al. 1972; Hodgson et al., unpublished).

For these reasons, it was considered of interest to explore further the behaviour of solid particles of various sizes and materials in the human oviduct *in situ*.

This report presents preliminary results obtained with both light and heavy particles. Dextran spheres, which are readily available in large numbers, were used to study uptake from the peritoneal cavity. Heavy metallic spheres were used with the aim of following their movements through the oviducts by serial X-ray examinations.

MATERIALS AND METHODS

Dextran microspheres

Dextran spheres were used to test the ability of the oviduct to take up and transport light spheres of a size similar to that of a denuded ovum under various physiologic conditions. Spheres were obtained after sifting Sephadex G 100 (Pharmacia, Sweden) through a set of sieves (A. H. Thomas & Co. cat. # 8323–P61–97, Philadelphia, Pa.). One g of the material retained between sieves with openings of 0.063 and 0.075 mm was suspended in sterile saline after several washings. The volume of the suspension was adjusted until a concentration of 2×10^5 spheres per ml was obtained. Aliquots of 5 ml were placed in ampoules and autoclaved. The average diameter of these spheres in saline was 150 μ, with a range between 120 and 180 μ.

Varying numbers of spheres from 5×10^4 to 1×10^6 were injected through the cul de sac into the Douglas pouch in 9 women, who were scheduled for surgical sterilization. The volume of the injection was adjusted to 5 ml by diluting with saline. Six of these patients had been cycling regularly and the others had delivered or aborted during the previous 20 days. The injection was done in the mid-follicular phase in 3 of the cyclic cases and 48 or 72 h after the estrogen peak in the others. The phase of the cycle was assessed from the menstrual history and confirmed by ovarian inspection during laparotomy. In addition, 10 ml of blood were drawn daily at 09:00 am, beginning on day 10 of the cycle, to measure estrogen concentration by radioimmunoassay (RIA), as described below.

Surgery was performed under spinal anesthesia 24 h after the injection of spheres. After laparotomy, five ligatures were placed on each oviduct so as to divide it in four equal segments before subtotal salpingectomy. After this, the ovaries were inspected for signs of recent ovulation and a search was made in Douglas pouch for clumps of spheres, as evidence that the injection had been correctly placed.

The excised oviducts were transected at the site of the ligatures and each segment was flushed separately with saline. The flushings were examined under a microscope and the number of spheres counted.

Copper and silver spheres

Copper and silver spheres of different sizes were used to test the ability of the oviduct to transport heavy particles under various physiologic conditions. Copper spheres of various sizes were supplied by Instituto Technológico del Cobre (Santiago, Chile). Spheres of 300, 600, and 1200 μ used in this study were selected with the aid of a microscope equipped with an eyepiece scale. Pure silver spheres of 300 and 600 μ were supplied by a jeweler.

Spheres were introduced in the distal third of the ampullary portion of one oviduct during laparotomy in patients operated on for surgical sterilization. Capillary glass tubes, fitted with slightly longer stainless steel barrels, were preloaded with the spheres and autoclaved (Fig. 1). The tip of a capillary tube was introduced gently through the ostium and the spheres were discharged by pushing the barrel.

Prior to introduction of the spheres, radiologic markers were placed in the mesosalpinx for subsequent identification of the position and course of the oviduct in X-ray pictures. Three types of markers were used in this study: silver clips, surgical 5–0 multifilament steel, and a radiopaque thread. In some cases, two of these markers were combined, but most of the study was done using the radiopaque thread alone, which proved to be the best. An example of this marker in place is shown in Fig. 2. After placing the markers, and having introduced the spheres, the distal end of the oviduct was ligated and fimbriectomy was performed.

406

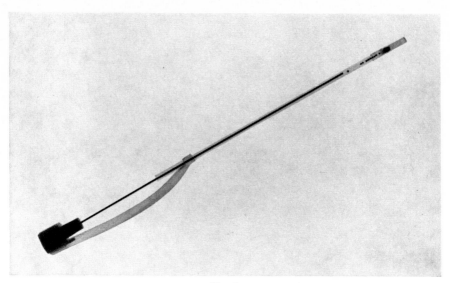

Fig. 1.

Inserter for metallic spheres. The barrel is obtained from disposable spinal needles and it is held by a silastic loop to the glass capillary tube.

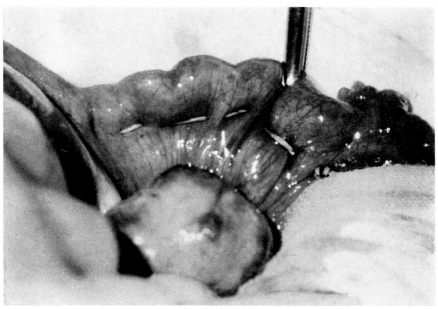

Fig. 2.

Radiophaque thread placed in the mesosalpinx alongside the oviduct. A knot served to identify the position of the fimbriated-end in X-ray pictures.

Serial X-ray examinations were done after surgery in order to determine the presence, number, and location of the spheres. The first X-ray examination was done within the first week after surgery. Subsequent examinations were done at intervals described below.

After gaining some experience in surgical and radiologic techniques, two studies were carried out. The first was designed to assess the relationship between size of spheres and their retention by the oviduct. For this purpose, copper spheres of 300, 600, or 1200 μ in diameter, were used.

The number of spheres inserted in each oviduct, the number of patients, and the frequency of radiologic examinations are indicated in Table 2. All patients in this study were cycling at the time of surgery. Results were expressed as percentage of spheres remaining in the oviduct at various time-intervals after surgery.

The second study was designed to explore the relationship between physiologic conditions and transport to the uterus. For this purpose, copper or silver spheres of 300 or 600 μ in diameter were inserted in one oviduct in six patients at different times of the menstrual cycle and in one patient during lactation amenorrhea. Radiologic markers, as described above, were used to trace the course of the oviduct in radiographs, which were taken at variable intervals after surgery.

The occurrence of ovulation was assessed either by a change of cervical mucus to a progestational type, or by a rise of progesterone levels in blood. Blood samples were drawn each time an X-ray was taken and progesterone was measured by RIA, as described below.

Hormone assays in plasma

Estrogen was measured by RIA as described by Edqvist and Johansson (1972), except that the chromatographic step to separate estrone from estradiol was omitted. The antiserum to estradiol 17-beta-succinyl BSA used was a gift from Dr. E. Johansson (Uppsala, Sweden).

Progesterone was measured by RIA as described by Thorneycroft and Stone (1972) using an antiserum to 4-pregnen-11-alpha-ol-3,2-dione hemisuccinyl BSA prepared in rabbits.

RESULTS

Uptake and transport of dextran spheres

The number of spheres taken up by the oviducts under various physiologic conditions is shown in Table 1. No spheres were taken up in puerperal patients and in two out of six cycling women. No spheres were found in the peritoneal cavity of these two cycling women.

In the four patients who had spheres in their oviduct, the number recovered

408

Table 1.

Table 1.
Uptake of dextran microspheres injected in the Douglas pouch.

Case	Physiologic condition	Number of spheres	
		Injected	Recovered from oviducts
IDS	Follicular phase	4×10^5	50
DRO		5×10^4	57
JS		5×10^4	0
EMF	Luteal phase	1×10^6	> 1000
MCL		2×10^5	> 4000
GMP		5×10^4	0
MMC	Puerperium	2×10^5	0
BLD		1×10^5	0
RVP		5×10^4	0

was less than 3 % of the number injected, and within the range studied, the proportion recovered was unrelated to the number injected.

Patients operated on in the luteal phase had taken up much larger numbers than patients operated on in the follicular phase. Marked differences in the uptake between the right and left oviducts were noted in each of the four cases. In both patients in the luteal phase, the side with the greater uptake corresponded with that of the ovary with the corpus luteum.

Spheres were found in all segments of the oviduct. Approximately 75 % of spheres recovered from patients in the luteal phase were in the distal middle quarter, whereas in the follicular phase, between 80 and 90 % were in the proximal middle quarter.

Table 2.
Percentage of copper spheres remaining in the oviducts.

Number of spheres inserted in each patient	Size of spheres (μm)	Number of patients	Weeks after insertion				
			I	II	III	VIII	XII
15	300	8	71	60	43	28	14
5	600	3	100	60	–	–	17
10	1200	9	99	–	98	97	77

Table 3.
Transport of copper and silver spheres to the uterus during ovulatory cycles.

| Case | Insertion | | Transport | | Ovulation |
	Spheres*	Day of cycle	Number	Days after insertion	Days after insertion
LCA	15 Cu 300	4	15	23–27	23–25
RTC	10 Ag 300	8	10	8–20	8–20
GGG	10 Ag 600	8	6 2	1– 7 10–21	10–24
MAG	10 Ag 600	9	3	34–41	34–45
VTR	10 Ag 600	14	6 4	11–15 28–35	1– 6 28–35
NDC	10 Ag 600	28	0	–	16–20

* Number, material and diameter in μ.

Relationship between size of copper spheres and their retention by the oviduct

The percentages of spheres remaining in the oviducts at various times after insertion are shown in Table 2.

Copper spheres of 300 μ decreased in number progressively from insertion until the last examination at the 12th week, in which 14 % still remained in the

Table 4.
Passage of spheres to the uterus and blood progesterone levels in patient VTR.

| Days after insertion | Number of spheres in | | Progesterone (ng/ml) |
	Oviduct	Uterus-Vagina	
3	10	0	
6	10	0	5.2
11	10	0	4.6
15	4	0	2.2
16 Menses			
20	4	0	1.7
28	4	0	2.3
35	0	3	13.0
40	0	0	4.2

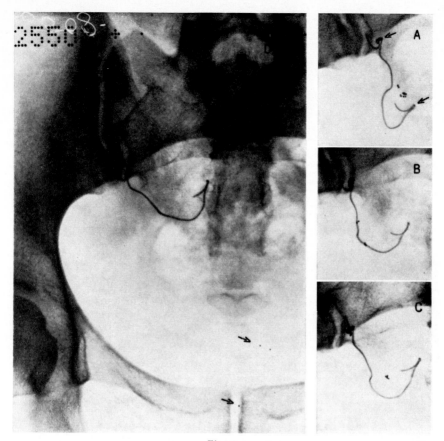

Fig. 3.
Transport of silver spheres in patient VTR.
A – X-ray picture taken 11 days after surgery. 10 spheres are present in the middle third of the oviduct. The upper arrow indicates the fimbriated-end and the lower arrow points to the uterotubal junction.
B – X-ray picture taken 15 days after surgery. Only 4 spheres remain in the oviduct. They are separated into two groups in the middle third.
C – X-ray picture taken 28 days after surgery. The 4 spheres are now gathered together in the middle third of the oviduct.
D – X-ray picture taken 35 days after surgery. No spheres are present in the oviduct and 3 spheres indicated by the arrows are present in the area corresponding to the uterus and vagina.

oviduct. About 50 % had been lost between the second and fourth weeks. Spheres of 600 μ followed a similar trend, whereas those of 1200 μ tended to be retained throughout the period of observation. A decrease in the number of spheres occurred in all patients in the first two groups, whereas in only one patient were 1200 μ spheres transported.

411

Relative changes of position of spheres within the oviduct were observed in successive X-ray pictures in most patients, including those in which transport did not take place.

Relationship between physiologic conditions and transport of metallic spheres

The occurrence of transport during ovulatory cycles is shown in Table 3. A total of seven cycles was studied in six patients. In four out of the seven cycles studied, transport occurred only in close temporal proximity to ovulation. In one cycle, transport took place on two different occasions, one preceding and the other coinciding with the ovulatory period. Transport near the end of the

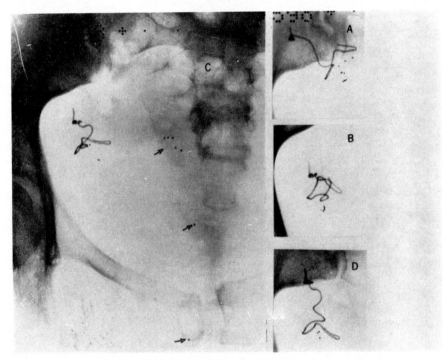

Fig. 4.

Transport of silver spheres in a non-cycling woman.

A – X-ray picture taken 4 days after surgery. 10 spheres are dispersed along the middle and proximal thirds of the oviduct.

B – X-ray picture taken 14 days after surgery. The spheres are grouped close together in the middle third of the oviduct.

C – X-ray picture taken 21 days after surgery. Arrows indicate spheres in uterus and vagina. 3 spheres remain in the oviduct.

D – X-ray picture taken 24 days after surgery. 3 spheres in the oviduct.

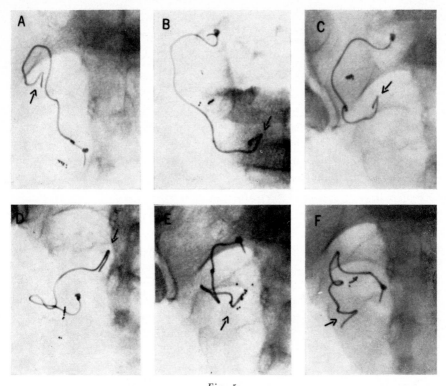

Fig. 5.

A to F – X-ray pictures taken of patient NDC 4, 7, 13, 19 and 33 days respectively after surgery. The arrow points to the uterotubal junction. Note changes in the position of spheres and in the position and course of the oviduct.

luteal phase occurred in one cycle and no transport was effected in another.

All 300 μ spheres were transported at one time in both cases in which they were tested. In no instance were all 600 μ spheres inserted transported at once. This situation allowed us to study the transport of spheres during a second cycle in patient VTR. Details of the study carried out in this patient are shown as an example, in Table 4 and in Fig. 3.

A sequence of 4 X-ray pictures showing transportation of spheres in the amenorrheic patient is presented in Fig. 4. In her case, 7 out of 10 spheres were transported between 14 and 21 days after surgery, and in addition, marked changes in the location of spheres within the oviduct were observed in successive X-ray pictures, preceding passage to the uterus. Similar changes in the position of spheres were seen also in the cycling women, including patient NDC, in whom transport did not occur. These changes, as well as changes in the position of the oviduct, are illustrated in Fig. 5.

DISCUSSION

The present results confirm that the human oviduct is able to take up and transport to the uterus foreign particulate matter of a size and density quite different from that of natural ova.

The uptake and transport of these foreign materials seem to be more dependent upon the physiologic conditions of the patient than upon the physical properties of the particles. The influence of size did not become evident until very large particles were used. The almost complete retention of 1200 μ spheres observed in this study is in close agreement with observations made in rabbits by Hodgson et al. (unpublished) using plastic microspheres.

Uptake and transport of these foreign materials were observed at various stages of the menstrual cycle, but both processes seemed to be enhanced around the time of ovulation. This supposition is supported by the greater uptake of dextran spheres injected 48 to 72 h after the estrogen peak compared to the minor uptake of spheres injected in the mid-follicular phase. In addition, there is a positive correlation between passage of metallic spheres to the uterus and ovulation. In 5 out of 7 ovulatory cycles, transport to the uterus and ovulation took place in the period between the same two radiologic examinations. Whether or not passage to the uterus occurred before, during, or after ovulation, cannot be inferred from the present data, and additional work with shorter intervals between examinations will be necessary to obtain this information.

A noticeable feature in the transport of metallic spheres was their batchwise passage to the uterus in successive cycles. Exceptionally, the smaller size spheres were transported all at one time.

Usually, by the first examination after surgery, 300 and 600 μ spheres had a tendency to occupy the middle and proximal thirds of the oviduct. Of great interest was the fact that they kept moving back and forth, almost reaching the uterotubal junction at times and then returning again to the middle third. Dispersion throughout portions of the oviduct alternated with close grouping in one of the middle quarters. These features indicate that retention of particles in the oviduct is not necessarily associated with quiescence of the organ. Moreover, passage into the proximal isthmus is not necessarily followed by transportation to the uterus. From these observations, it would appear that the main gate preventing ovum transport in the human oviduct is at the level of the uterotubal junction. Whether or not the same concept applies to the transportation of natural ova cannot be decided at the present time.

It is very likely that transport of metallic particles results exclusively from mechanical energy supplied by the smooth muscles of the oviduct, since it is difficult to conceive that cilia could move these heavy spheres.

Possible artifacts in the results obtained could derive from several factors. Ligation of the distal end may cause fluid accumulation and distension of the oviduct. The use of several spheres with up to four times the diameter of a denuded egg could act as an abnormal stimulus to the walls of the oviduct. Last but not least, copper is known to release ions which interfere with some biological processes essential to reproduction. These limitations need to be properly evaluated in the future for the correct interpretation of the data. Notwithstanding, the techniques described here may become a useful tool in the investigation of the physiology and pharmacology of the oviduct.

ACKNOWLEDGMENTS

The authors wish to acknowledge the cooperation of the Department of Radiology of Hospital Sótero del Rio in the radiologic study of patients with 1200 μ spheres. We are grateful to Miss Carmen Llados for performing the progesterone assays, and Mr. Daniel Godoy for his assistance in the coordination of the study.

These investigations were supported by the Expanded Programme of Research, Development and Research Training in Human Reproduction of the World Health Organization.

REFERENCES

Ascenzo-Cabello J., Hoyle-Cox J. and Ascenzo A. E. (1974) Prueba de captación y transporte. *Proceedings VIII World Congress on Fertility and Sterility*, Buenos Aires. Abstract No. 376.

Avendaño S., Peláez J. and Croxatto H. B. (1971) Transport of microspheres by the human oviduct *in vitro* and the effect of treatment with megestrol acetate. *J. Reprod. Fertil. 27*, 261–264.

Croxatto H. B., Vogel C. and Vásquez J. (1973) Transport of microspheres in the genital tract of the female rabbit. *J. Reprod. Fertil. 33*, 337–341.

Decker A. and Decker W. H. (1954) A tubal function test. *Obstet. Gynec. 4*, 35–38.

Fernström I. (1971) A new method for studying the motility of the Fallopian tubes. *Acta obstet. gynec. scand. 50*, 129–133.

Harper M. J. K., Bennett J. P., Boursnell J. C. and Rowson L. E. (1960) An autoradiographic method for the study of egg transport in the rabbit Fallopian tube. *J. Reprod. Fertil. 1*, 249–267.

Jainudeen M. R. and Hafez E. S. E. (1973) Egg transport in the Macaque (*Macaca fascicularis*). *Biol. Reprod. 9*, 305–308.

Orsini W., Bianchi J. C., Tambussi F., D'Angelo A. R. and Paesa E. (1974) Investigación de la permeabilidad tubaria. Prueba de Rivanol. *Proceedings VIII World Congress of Fertility and Sterility*, Buenos Aires. Abstract No. 418.

Pauerstein C. J., Woodruff J. D. and Zachary A. S. (1968) Factors influencing physiologic activities in the Fallopian tube: the anatomy physiology and pharmacology of tubal transport. *Obstet. Gynec. Survey 23*, 215–243.

Sheffery J. B. (1954) A method of determining tubal patency and tubal ciliary activity. *N. Y. State J. Medicine 54*, 3092–3094.

Wintenberger-Torres S. (1961) Mouvements des trompes et progression des oeufs chez la brebis. *Ann. Biol. anim. Bioch. Biophys. 1*, 121–133.

Laboratorio de Endocrinología y Anatomía Patológica,
Universidad Católica, Chile,
Centro de Estudios en Biología de la Reproducción (CEBRE),
Universidad de Chile, and
Instituto Latinoamericano de Fisiología de la Reproducción (ILAFIR),
Buenos Aires, Argentina

OVUM TRANSPORT IN WOMEN

By

Sergio Cheviakoff, Soledad Díaz, Mirta Carril,
Nilsa Patritti, Héctor D. Croxatto,
Carmen Llados, María E. Ortíz and Horacio B. Croxatto

ABSTRACT

The time course of ovum transport in normal fertile women was studied
either by recovering ova from the oviducts in patients subjected to laparotomy or by transcervical flushing of the endometrial cavity in volunteers
in whom surgery was not indicated. Each procedure was performed at
various intervals after the estrogen preovulatory peak, which was determined by radioimmunoassay.

Twenty six patients were operated on between 2 and 184 h after the
estrogen peak. No patient had ovulated earlier than 40 h, and all patients
had ovulated within 63 h after the estrogen peak. Eight ova were recovered from the oviducts between 40 and 97 h. Four ova localized in the
distal middle quarter of the oviducts were obtained between 40 and 94 h
and 3 of them, localized in the proximal middle quarter, were recovered
between 63 and 97 h. One ovum was recovered at 48 h but its location
within the oviduct was not determined.

Six ova were recovered in 20 patients submitted to uterine flushings between 72 and 216 h after the estrogen peak. Two ova were obtained out
of 9 flushings performed at 120 h, and 4 ova were recovered out of 8
flushings performed at 144 h. No ova were recovered from 17 flushings
performed at shorter or longer intervals.

416

The interpretation of these results was that, in women, ovulation takes place between 40 and 63 h after the estrogen peak and that the minimum time spent by ova in the oviduct lies somewhere between two and three days.

The time course of ovum transport in the human has not been well established. Based on recovery of ova from the oviducts or uterus of patients operated on in the luteal phase of the menstrual cycle, several authors have suggested that the duration of ovum transport in the human oviduct is 3 to 4 days (Rock and Hertig 1944; Hertig et al. 1956; Noyes et al. 1966; Clewe et al. 1971). Using a non surgical technique, Croxatto et al. (1972a) recovered ova from the uterine cavity at various intervals after ovulation. Ovulation dating was based on basal body temperature, cervical mucus score, urinary pregnanediol determinations, endometrial dating and the concentration of luteinizing hormone (LH) in urine. They concluded that ovum transport in the human oviduct could take 2 to 3 days. These different estimations of the duration of ovum transport could be ascribed to the use of different criteria for dating ovulation.

In order to determine the time course of ovum transport precise timing of ovulation is required. Until this can be achieved in women it seems appropriate to relate ovum recovery to the hormonal parameters of the menstrual cycle. The hormonal events known to occur most constantly before ovulation are the plasma peaks of estradiol and LH. The time relationship between LH peak and follicular rupture is known to be constant in several species (Cumming et al. 1973; Gay et al. 1970; Harper 1961; Phemister et al. 1973). In the human, ovulation can occur as early as 15 h after the LH peak (Croxatto et al. 1974) but, the constancy of this interval has not been proved. The time interval between the estradiol and LH peaks is variable and can take from a few h to three days (Korenman and Sherman 1973).

As a result of these considerations the location of ova in the genital tract of women was investigated at various times after these hormonal events. This report presents preliminary data on the time course of ovum transport in women related to the preovulatory estrogen peak.

MATERIAL AND METHODS

The recovery of ova from the genital tract was attempted by means of either a surgical or a non surgical procedure which will be described separately.

Surgical procedure

Normally menstruating women in whom elective laparotomy was indicated were invited to participate in the study. The data presented below were obtained from 25 patients who requested sterilization and from one infertile patient.

417

Blood samples were drawn every 6 h beginning 3 days before the expected day of ovulation and ending on the day of surgery. Serum was separated by centrifugation, stored at –15°C and shipped at a later date to another laboratory for radioimmunoassay (RIA) of estradiol-17 beta.

In the first 13 patients, the day of surgery was decided on the basis of a change of cervical mucus to a progestational type. Later, a short RIA for estrogens, described below, was set up locally and, in the next 13 patients, surgery was decided on the basis of the preovulatory estrogen peak. Serum samples obtained between 08:30 and 09:30 a. m. were analyzed the same day and used for this purpose.

Surgery was done under spinal or general anesthesia. After laparotomy, five ligatures were placed on each oviduct in such a way that the oviduct was divided into four segments of approximately equal length. Bilateral salpingectomy was done by excising each oviduct approximately 5 mm distal from the external surface of the uterus. Both ovaries were inspected for signs of recent ovulation and a biopsy was taken from ruptured follicles or corpora lutea. Finally, a transfundal flushing of the uterine cavity was performed. In the infertile patient the oviducts were flushed *in situ*.

Excised oviducts were divided into four segments by transecting at the level of each ligature. Each segment was flushed separately and flushings were screened under a dissecting microscope for ova. The criteria used to establish ovulation were the finding of a fresh corpus luteum confirmed by histopathologic examination and/or the finding of an ovum within the oviducts. Oviductal segments containing ova were examined by routine histologic techniques.

Non surgical procedure

Twenty normal women consented to be subjected to a search for ova in the uterine cavity by the non-surgical procedure. All patients were instructed to refrain from unprotected intercourse during the study. Blood samples were drawn at daily intervals between 08:30 and 09:30 a. m. beginning 5 days before the expected day of ovulation and ending 4 days after the estrogen peak. Estrogen determinations were performed daily by a short RIA described below. The endometrial cavity was flushed with saline through the cervical canal, as previously described (Croxatto et al. 1972b), between 3 and 9 days after the estrogen peak. In each patient 1 to 3 flushings were performed at daily intervals. Flushings were examined to determine the presence of ova.

Estradiol-17 beta was measured by RIA as described by Edqvist and Johansson (1972). The same method was used in the short RIA for estrogens except that the chromatographic step to separate estrone from estradiol was omitted. The antiserum to estradiol-17 beta succinyl BSA used was a gift from Dr. E. Johansson (Uppsala).

Table 1.

Interval from estrogen peak to surgery (h)	Number of patients operated	Number of patients ovulating	Number of ova recovered
0– 24	3	0	0
24– 48	9	3	3
48– 72	7	4	2
72– 96	4	4	2
96–120	1	1	1
120–144	0	0	0
144–168	1	1	0
168 or more	1	1	0
Total	26	14	8

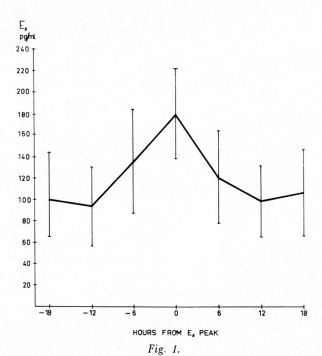

Fig. 1.

Estradiol-17 beta preovulatory values in 13 patients. Each point corresponds to mean ± SD of 9 to 13 samples.

419

27*

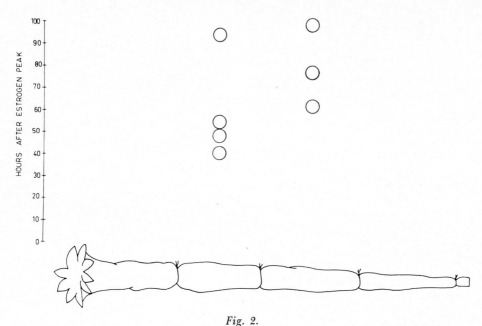

Fig. 2.

Segmental distribution of 7 ova recovered from excised human oviducts. Each oviduct was divided into 4 segments of approximately the same length. The time interval between the estrogen peak and surgery is indicated on the vertical axis.

RESULTS

Surgical procedure

Fourteen out of 26 cases showed signs of recent ovulation (Table 1). No ovulation was observed in the 3 patients operated on within 24 h after the estrogen peak. Three out of 9 patients operated on between 24 and 48 h, and 4 out of 7 patients operated on between 48 and 72 h had ovulated. All patients operated on after 72 h had ovulated. Preovulatory estradiol-17 beta values measured every 6 h in 13 patients are shown in Fig. 1.

One ovum was recovered from the oviduct in each of 8 patients out of 14 who had ovulated. No ova were recovered from the uterine cavity. The relationship between location of ova and time of surgery after the estrogen peak is shown in Fig. 2. Four ova were recovered from the distal middle quarter of the oviducts 40, 48, 52 and 94 h respectively after the estrogen peak. Three ova were recovered from the proximal middle quarter at 63, 78 and 97 h respectively. One ovum was recovered at 48 h from one oviduct flushed *in situ*. The segment in which this ovum was located could not be established. No ova were recovered from the proximal and distal quarters of the oviducts. In one case (time interval 78 h) a fertilized four cell ovum was recovered. All other ova were unfertilized.

Ova recovered between 24 and 72 h after the estrogen peak were surrounded by cumulus. The fertilized ovum recovered at 72 h and one ovum recovered at 94 h were partially denuded. The ovum recovered at 97 h was completely denuded.

Non surgical procedure

Fig. 3 shows the results of the uterine flushings performed in 20 patients and their temporal relation to estrogen values. Two ova were obtained out of 9 flushings performed 120 h after the estrogen peak and 4 ova were recovered out of 8 flushings performed at 144 h. No ova were recovered at shorter or longer intervals. All ova were unfertilized except one morula recovered at 144 h. Most unfertilized ova showed varying degrees of cytolysis or fragmentation.

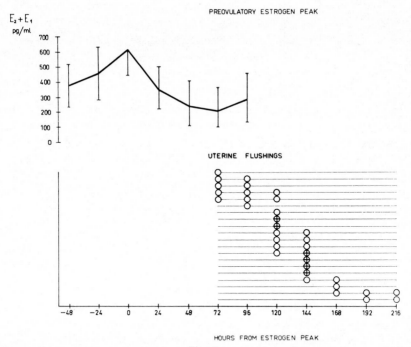

Fig. 3.

Results of uterine flushings performed in 20 patients and their temporal relation to preovulatory estrogen peak. Time 0 corresponds with the maximum estrogen value in each case. Each circle depicts an uterine flushing while each cross means the finding of an ovum. Circles placed in the same horizontal line represent uterine flushings performed in the same patient.

DISCUSSION

The present data are far from sufficient to arrive at a definite assessment of the time course of ovum transport in women. First, the most proximal portion of the oviduct was not studied. Second, the number of patients allocated to each interval in the surgical procedure is too small, especially after 96 h; and third, the total of 14 ova recovered from 34 women who had ovulated, represents a small absolute number and a rate of recovery of only 41 per cent. Therefore, whatever trends emerge from these results, should be regarded with caution.

Peak values of estradiol-17 beta observed in the first 13 patients were, on the average, lower than those reported in the literature by other investigators. This is probably due to inadequate handling of the samples during trans-shipment, which can cause degradation of estradiol-17 beta. Samples analyzed locally for total estrogens showed peak values around 600 pg/ml. This difference between the two sets of data does not rule out the validity of pooling them for the purpose of setting time zero, as used in these studies. On the other hand, in individual cases, estrone and estradiol-17 beta peaks, measured independently, may not coincide (Lundy et al. 1974) but when the plasma concentrations of both hormones are added, the resulting peak coincides with the estradiol-17 beta peak. If these criteria are accepted, the use of the short RIA of estrogens as a guide to decide the day of surgery or of uterine flushing appears to be adequate for this type of study.

The average and normal limits of variation of the time interval between the estrogen peak and follicular rupture in women have not been established. In the present series, the shortest interval did not exceed 40 h, and 100 % of the women operated on from 63 h onwards, but not before, had ovulated. Therefore, the length of the interval extended from at least 40 to 63 h. This is in agreement with other reports which indicate a variation of 1 or 2 days for the interval between the estrogen peak and the LH surge which precedes ovulation (Ferin et al. 1973).

Assuming that ovum transport begins readily after extrusion of the ovum, and taking 52 h as the average interval between the estrogen peak and ovulation, the data support the following concepts:

(1) Ova seem to spend most of the first 45 h after ovulation in the two middle quarters of the oviduct. According to histologic examination, the distal middle quarter corresponded with the proximal ampulla and the proximal middle quarter corresponded with the ampullary-isthmic junction. Overlapping of the intervals for ova recovered from these two segments is apparent in Fig. 2. This could result from individual variations or inaccuracy in the timing of ovulation and/or localization of ova. Back and forth movements of ova while they reside in the ampulla could also produce a similar picture.

(2) Transport through the ampulla seems to be slower than in other mammals, since the ova recovered from the distal middle quarter had presumably not reached the ampullary-isthmic junction several hours after ovulation.

(3) Ova were recovered from the uterine cavity at least 68 h after ovulation and from the oviducts up to 45 h after ovulation. Since no ova were recovered from uterine flushings done 24 h earlier, the conclusion is drawn that the most rapidly transported ova entered the uterus between 45 and 68 h after ovulation. These figures have a margin of error of approximately $\pm$ 12 h.

(4) The maximum time spent by ova in the oviducts cannot be assessed until more subjects are examined by the surgical procedure after 96 h from the estrogen peak. However, if one assumes that the first ova arriving at the uterus were those ovulated between 40 and 52 h after the estrogen peak, then the maximum time they spent in the oviduct lies between 68 and 80 h.

(5) Denudation of human ova seems to be completed when they are about to enter the uterus.

Gathering information on human ovum transport is an appealing challenge which can be met with some success using the presently available hormonal tests to detect impending ovulation. This presentation will accomplish its objective if it serves to encourage other investigators to search for human ova and explore their behaviour in the female genital tract. The research efforts of several groups will be necessary before we learn how to control the transport of ova.

ACKNOWLEDGMENTS

The dedication of Mrs. Elizabeth Nuñez for performing the short RIA for estrogens, is gratefully acknowledged.

These investigations were supported by the Expanded Programme of Research, Development and Research Training in Human Reproduction of the World Health Organization and by the Contraceptive Development Research Program sponsored and coordinated by the International Committee for Contraception Research of The Population Council, New York.

REFERENCES

Clewe T. H., Morgensten L. L., Noyes R. W., Bonney W. A., Burrus S. B. and De Feo V. J. (1971) Searches for ova in the human uterus and tubes. II. Clinical and laboratory data on nine successful searches for human ova. *Amer. J. Obstet. Gynec. 109*, 313–334.

Croxatto H. B., Diaz S., Fuentealba B., Croxatto H. D., Carrillo D. and Fabres C. (1972a) Studies on the duration of egg transport in the human oviduct. I. The time interval between ovulation and egg recovery from the uterus in normal women. *Fertil. Steril.* 23, 447–458.

Croxatto H. B., Fuentealba B., Diaz S., Pastene L. and Tatum H. J. (1972b) A simple nonsurgical technique to obtain unimplanted eggs from human uteri. *Amer. J. Obstet. Gynec. 112*, 662–668.

Croxatto H. B., Carril M., Cheviakoff S., Patritti N., Pedroza E., Croxatto H. D., Gomez-Rogers C. and Rosner J. M. (1974) Time interval between LH peak and ovulation in women. *Proceedings VIII World Congress of Fertility and Sterility*, Buenos Aires. Abstract No. 158.

Cumming I. A., Buckmaster J. M., Blockey M. A. de B., Goding J. R., Winfield C. G. and Baxter R. W. (1973) Constancy of interval between luteinizing hormone release and ovulation in the ewe. *Biol. Reprod. 9*, 24–29.

Edqvist L. E. and Johansson E. D. B. (1972) Radioimmunoassay of oestrone and oestradiol in human and bovine peripheral plasma. *Acta endocr. (Kbh.) 71*, 716–731.

Ferin J., Thomas K. and Johansson E. D. B. (1973) Ovulation detection. In: Hafez E. S. E. and Evans T. N., eds. *Human Reproduction*, pp. 260–283. Harper and Row, New York.

Gay V. L., Midgley A. R. and Niswender G. D. (1970) Patterns of gonadotrophin secretion associated with ovulation. *Fed. Proc. 29*, 1880–1887.

Harper M. J. K. (1961) The time of ovulation in the rabbit following the injection of luteinizing hormone. *J. Endocr. 22*, 147–152.

Hertig A. T., Rock J. and Adams E. C. (1956) A description of 34 human ova within the first 17 days of development. *Amer. J. Anat. 98*, 435–494.

Korenman S. G. and Sherman B. M. (1973) Further studies on gonadotropin and estradiol secretion during the preovulatory phase of the human menstrual cycle. *J. clin. Endocr. Metab. 36*, 1205–1209.

Lundy L. E., Lee S. G., Levy W., Woodruff J. D., Wu C-H. and Abdalla M. (1974) The ovulatory cycle. A histologic, thermal, steroid and gonadotropin correlation. *Obstet. Gynec. 44*, 14–25.

Noyes R. W., Clewe T. H., Bonney W. A. Jr., Burrus S. B., De Feo V. J. and Morgenstern L. L. (1966) Searches for ova in the human uterus and tubes. I. Review, clinical methodology and summary of findings. *Amer. J. Obstet. Gynec. 96*, 157–167.

Phemister R. D., Holst P. A., Spano J. S. and Hopwood M. L. (1973) Time of ovulation in the beagle bitch. *Biol. Reprod. 8*, 74–82.

Rock J. and Hertig A. T. (1944) Information regarding the time of human ovulation derived from a study of 3 unfertilized and 11 fertilized ova. *Amer. J. Obstet. Gynec. 47*, 343–356.

424

A. R. C. Unit of Reproductive Physiology and Biochemistry,
University of Cambridge

EGG SURVIVAL RELATIVE
TO MATERNAL ENDOCRINE STATUS

By

C. E. Adams

ABSTRACT

In experimental animals either the estrogen or progesterone dominated uterus constitutes an unfavourable, even hostile environment such that short exposure may prove fatal to the egg, either through expulsion or damage *in situ*. In contrast cleavage and initial blastulation of rabbit eggs restricted by ligation to the oviduct appear to be unaffected by the host's endocrine status, except for showing some retardation in estrous or estrogen and/or progesterone treated does.

In man the occurrence of ectopic (oviductal) pregnancy is common. Equally, claims of successful pregnancy following Este's operation suggest that the precocious arrival of the human egg in the uterus may still be compatible with its survival. Potentially these two conditions have far reaching consequencies for the development of contraceptive methods depending on interference with egg transport mechanisms.

The evolution of viviparity in mammals has necessitated the development of highly intergrated systems and this is especially evident in the case of pre-implantation events. The dominant role played by ovarian hormones during this period is now well established. Of greatest significance relative to the initiation of pregnancy is the transformation of the Graafian follicle into the corpus luteum and, concomitant with that change, the switch from estrogen to progesterone secretion. These hormones, acting in concert, control the fate of the egg, governing the rate of its transport to the uterus and the preparation of that organ for its reception and further wellbeing.

In the account that follows emphasis will be placed upon observations derived from experimental studies, most of which have employed laboratory animals and involved the use of the egg transfer technique. With this technique it is possible to vary at will the age and position of the embryo relative to ovulation.

Chang (1950) was the first to investigate systematically the development and fate of eggs or blastocysts in relation to the ovulation time of the recipient. Working with the rabbit, he firmly established the significance of synchronizing the stage of development with the luteal phase of the recipient. Subsequently, the need for synchronization has been demonstrated in every species so far investigated, including the mouse (McLaren and Michie 1956; Doyle et al. 1963), the rat (Noyes and Dickmann 1960), sheep, (Moore and Shelton 1964; Rowson and Moor 1966), cow (Rowson et al. 1969), ferret (Chang 1969) and pig (Webel et al. 1970). Taking the time of ovulation as the reference point, for successful pregnancy the limits of tolerance between the donor and recipient animals are usually ± 1 to 2 days, and are equally demanding in species with a long pre-implantation interval as in those where that period is very brief.

With few exceptions the investigation of synchronization requirements has been concentrated upon establising the optimal 'donor-recipient' combinations so that degrees of asynchrony which might be expected to be incompatible with success generally have been avoided. Consequently, comparatively little is known of the fate of eggs transferred asynchronously except for certain observations on the rabbit (Chang 1950; Adams 1965a, 1967, 1969, 1971), rat (Dickmann and Noyes 1960), mouse (Doyle et al. 1963) and ferret (Chang 1969). In farm animals, in particular, almost no attempts have been made to evaluate the fate of eggs shortly after transfer, either due to cost or other considerations, e. g. an over-riding interest in corpus luteum function.

EGG TRANSFER TO THE UTERUS

(1) *In the follicular phase*

In experimental animals it has been recognised for some time that the estrogen dominated uterus constitutes an unfavourable environment for early eggs, not only due to expulsion but also on account of adverse effects *in situ* (see reviews by Adams 1967, 1969; Chang 1969). For example, Chang (1955) reported that when recently ovulated unfertilized rabbit eggs were transferred to the uteri of does which had been mated 12 h earlier the recovery rate 24 h later was very low (11 out of 82) due, it was suggested, to the eggs having "probably disintegrated". Eggs recovered 6 h after transfer were "fertilized but in poor shape with the zona pellucida swollen and their cytoplasm not in healthy condition". Chang also observed that the swelling and disintegration of the zona pellucida

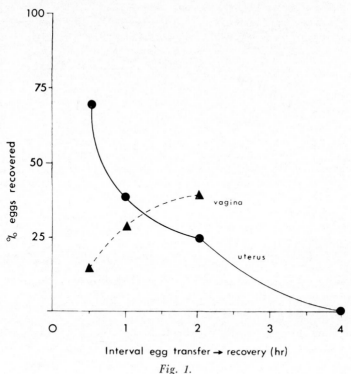

Fig. 1.

Fate of newly ovulated eggs transferred to the uterus of estrous does.

occurred when newly fertilized rabbit eggs were cultured in rabbit uterine fluid *in vitro*.

Adams (1969) transferred newly ovulated denuded eggs (cumulus removed with hyaluronidase) to the uterine horns of estrous does in which the vagina was ligated at the time of transfer. Autopsy took place 0.5, 1, 2 or 4 h after transfer, when the uterine horns and vaginae were searched for eggs. The findings are illustrated in Fig. 1. Some eggs (8/60) were recovered from the vagina only 0.5 h after transfer and the proportion increased threefold over the next 1.5 h (23/57). Of the eggs that were unaccounted for, i. e. neither recovered from the uterus nor vagina (17 %, 32 % and 36 % at 0.5, 1 and 2 h resp.), it seems likely that some must have been destroyed *in utero* since others were recovered which showed damage to the zona pellucida.

Under estrogen dominance, therefore, the uterus is doubly hostile both via the endometrium and the myometrium. Hitherto, I believe there has been a tendency to neglect the role of the myometrium in early pregnancy, except possibly in relation to sperm transport. Even endometrial function, particularly

Table 1.

Recovery of eggs 3 days after transfer to the uteri of does in which the number of corpora lutea was reduced to 0 by spaying, or 2, 4 or 8 by semi-spaying 15 h post coitum.

No. of corpora lutea	No. of eggs		Recovery (%)
	transferred	recovered	
0	89	4	4.5
2	123	49	39.8
4	125	62	49.6
8	121	100	82.6

the secretions, has been comparatively neglected until very recently. Uterine function is deserving of special attention both in relation to infertility problems and contraceptive development.

In the rabbit there is a marked difference in the amount of luteal tissue which suffices to stimulate endometrial proliferation (Corner 1928; Brouha 1934) and early egg development (Adams 1965b) on the one hand, or to render the myometrium quiescent so as to ensure retention of the eggs, on the other. This latter function seems to require the full complement of corpora lutea, as shown in Table 1. It can be visualized that reduced secretory activity of the corpus luteum may produce the same effect.

Corner (1942) wrote as follows: "I believe that one of the most important functions of the oviduct is to hold back the eggs until the uterus is ready for them . . . I have long thought that we ought not to emphasize the oviduct solely as an organ for transporting the ova, but rather as a means of delaying their transportation. The uterus must have time to get ready for its exigent tenant".

ESTES' OPERATION

In man there are reports that pregnancy may follow Estes' operation in which the ovaries are transplanted into the uterus. However, it is difficult to evaluate the level of success that has attended this operation. Whilst it is believed to be low, one is nevertheless cautioned to consider man as yet another exception regarding the possibility of egg survival in the estrogen-dominated uterus. Certainly, further investigation of this problem would appear to be well justified.

(2) *In the luteal phase*

Fig. 2 (Adams 1967) will serve to illustrate the adverse effects of transferring eggs asynchronously, when the combination is 'endometrium in advance of egg'. It is based upon 60 h eggs and recipient rabbits in which ovulation was either synchronous with, or 24 or 48 h in advance of the donors. Autopsy took place 3 days after transfer. It will be noted that with increasing asynchrony (1) the proportion of transferred eggs recovered fell steeply, (2) the proportion of normal blastocysts fell even more sharply and (3) there was a corresponding increase in the proportion of degenerate morulae and blastocysts. Blastocyst size (surface area) was also reduced by asynchrony, being 18.2 mm² (60 → 60), 9.3 mm² (60 → 84) and 4.3 mm² (60 → 108).

With advancing pseudopregnancy the rabbit uterus becomes increasingly hostile to the fertilized egg so that by days 9 to 11 practically no eggs survive 24 h exposure. It is noteworthy that eggs may show evidence of this effect

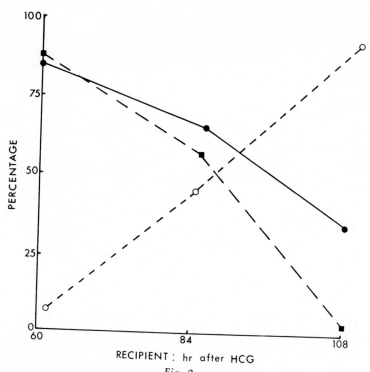

Fig. 2.

Fate of $2\frac{1}{2}$ day eggs transferred to the uteri of does given HCG 60, 84 or 108 h before transfer. ●——● egg recovery; ■——■ normal blastocysts; ○——○ degenerate morulae and blastocysts.

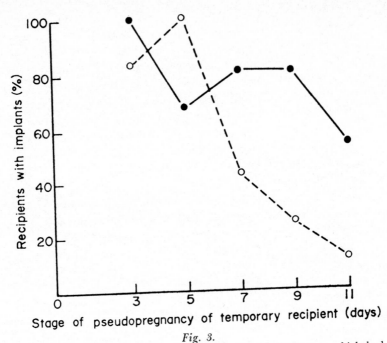

Fig. 3.

The proportion of recipients becoming pregnant after receiving eggs which had spent either 6 h (●) or 24 h (○) in the uteri of pseudopregnant rabbits.

within a few hours ($<$ 6) both in terms of morphology and viability, (Figs. 3 and 4). A deleterious uterine effect has also been reported to occur in the rat on day 5 (Dickmann and Noyes 1960), in the spayed, progesterone-treated rat (Dickmann 1970) and in the mouse about day 4 (Doyle et al. 1963).

THE OVIDUCT

Ectopic (Oviductal) Pregnancy

In man approximately 96 % to 98 % of extra uterine pregnancies are oviductal in type (Benirschke 1969; Reid et al. 1972). Though attachment may occur in any part of the oviduct, by far the most common positions are the ampullary (60 %) and isthmic portions (30 %) as shown in Fig. 5 (Pauerstein 1974). The usual incidence of oviductal pregnancy is listed from 0.25 to 1 % of all pregnancies but where pelvic inflammatory disease is prevalent the incidence rises to about 3 % (Reid et al. 1972). According to Pauerstein (1974) the incidence of ectopic pregnancy is rising in the United States.

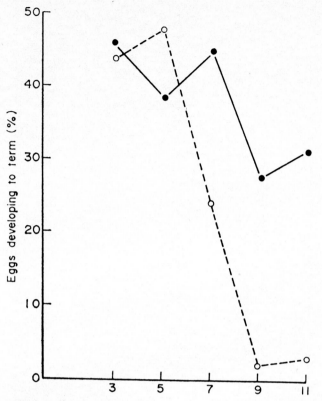

Stage of pseudopregnancy of temporary recipient (days)

Fig. 4.

The proportion of eggs developing to term in recipients to which they were transferred after spending 6 h (●) or 24 h (o) in the uteri of pseudopregnant rabbits.

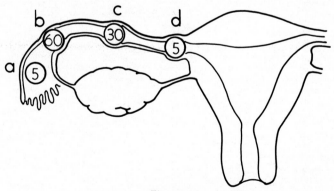

Fig. 5.

Proportion (%) of pregnancies found in various portions of the oviduct.
a = fimbriated end; b = ampulla; c = isthmus; d = interstitial portion
(after Pauerstein 1974).

431

Table 2.

The development of 30 h 2- and 4-cell rabbit eggs transferred to the ligated oviducts of estrous, 1-day, or 9- to 11-day pseudopregnant rabbits.

Temporary recipient		Time eggs spent in temporary recipient (h)	No. eggs		Stage of egg development			No. young born/no. eggs re-transferred (%)
Condition	No.		transferred	recovered	morulae	Early blastocysts		
						unexpanded	expanded	
Estrous	2	24	55	41	41	–	–	2/37 (5)
Early luteal	3		65	63	63	–	–	3/31 (10)
Mid-luteal	2		55	49	49	–	–	1/38 (3)
Estrous	5	48	142	116	92	24	–	31/77 (40)
Early luteal	4		85	75	39	45	–	16/69 (23)
Mid-luteal	4		118	101	30	62	–	19/96 (20)
Estrous	2	72	36	34	13	16	5	5/29 (17)
Early luteal	2		60	49	2	7	40	1/36 (3)
Mid-luteal	1		27	24	1	23	0	4/23 (17)

In man it appears that if the fertilized egg is prevented from leaving the oviduct a significant proportion can develop and lead to complications. Implicit in this fact is that any therapy that may cause the eggs to be retained, unless it also inhibits fertilization or cleavage, is virtually ruled out in practice because of the unacceptable risk of oviductal pregnancy.

From a comparative standpoint the common occurrence of oviductal pregnancy in man is quite exceptional; the condition is very rare in monkeys and apparently non-existent in domestic animals (Benirschke 1969). Pauerstein (1974), quoting Woodruff and Pauerstein (1969) and Thibault (1972), notes that only 3 ectopics have been recorded among nearly 3000 primate pregnancies.

Oviductal pregnancy has not been induced experimentally in any of the animal species so far tested. Both within and between species egg development fails at the early blastocyst stage (for references see Adams 1973a), indicating that at this point the oviductal environment fails to satisfy blastocyst requirements. Whether the human blastocyst is less fastidious or the human oviduct better equipped to satisfy its demands is not known.

Within species the loss of viability of eggs "tube-locked" by ligation has only been investigated in the sheep (Wintenberger-Torres, 1956), rabbit (Adams, 1958, 1973) and mouse (Weitlauf, 1971). In veterinary practice, "tube-locking" brought about by estrogen therapy has long been exploited as a means of terminating undesired pregnancies in the dog and cat. Interestingly, in these two species the fate of eggs "tube-locked" by ligation as opposed to estrogen treatment appears not to have been investigated.

Egg transfer to the oviduct under different endocrine conditions

In the rabbit, Adams (1973a) has investigated the fate of 2 and 4 cell eggs, recovered 30 h p. c. and transferred to the ligated oviducts of estrous, early luteal (synchronous) or mid-luteal (Day 9) recipients for periods of up to 72 h. The results are presented in Table 2. After 72 h (indeed the effect was already showing at 48 h) egg development was retarded in the estrous recipients where 13/34 (38.2 %) were still at the morular stage compared with only 2/49 (4.1 %) and 1/24 (4.2 %) in the luteal phase does, in which the majority of the eggs had reached the blastocyst stage. Nevertheless, the viability of the eggs recovered from the estrous does, as tested by re-transfer to synchronous recipients, equalled or even surpassed that of the other groups. In the case of 60 h morulae transferred to the oviducts of estrous or day 9 to day 11 recipients, neither the rate of egg development nor viability was significantly affected by the endocrine status of the temporary recipient. In a further investigation sponsored by WHO, Abbott (unpublished observations), also using the rabbit, has confirmed that the development of 26 h eggs, evaluated 3 days after transfer to the ligated oviduct, was retarded in estrous does as compared with that in day 1, day 8 or

Table 3.

Development of 26 h eggs transferred to the ligated oviducts of rabbits in various endocrine states. Eggs recovered for examination 3 days after transfer. (Percentages in parentheses).

Group	Condition of temporary recipient	No. of recipients	No. eggs transferred	No. eggs recovered	No. and condition of eggs recovered				
					8 cell	morulae	Blastocysts		
							unexpanded	expanded
1	Day 1 (control)	11	202	110 (54)	0	5 (4)	12 (11)	93 (85)
2	Day 8 (luteal)	2	34	30 (88)	0	0	1 (3)	29 (97)
3	Estrous	3	79	62 (78)	0	0	40 (65)	22 (35)
4	Spayed	12	243	123 (51)	11 (9)	0	29 (24)	83 (67)
5	Spayed + estradiol benzoate	8	231	182 (79)	9 (5)	23 (13)	30 (16)	120 (66)
6	Spayed + progesterone	16	314	205 (65)	8 (4)	13 (6)	21 (10)	163 (80)
7	Spayed + estradiol benzoate + progesterone	8	181	118 (65)	0	22 (19)	11 (9)	85 (72)

Table 4.

Development of 16 h eggs transferred to the ligated oviducts of spayed or Day 1 recipients. Eggs recovered for examination 3 days after transfer. (Percentages in parentheses).

Condition of temporary recipient	No. recipients	No. eggs transferred	No. and condition of eggs recovered			Blastocysts	
			total	8 cell	morulae	unexpanded	expanded
Spayed	5	64	27 (42)	0	0	9 (33)	18 (67)
Day 1	4	136	81 (60)	4 (5)	5 (6)	15 (19)	57 (70)

spayed recipients. Notably, throughout these four groups only 16/325 (4.9 %) of eggs failed to reach the blastocyst stage. In similar animals spayed for 3 to 6 weeks and then treated for one week before transfer with high doses of estradiol benzoate (10 μg/kg/day) or progesterone released from silastic capsules (3.3–5.8 mg/kg/day) either alone or in combination, 80 to 90 % of the transferred eggs developed into blastocysts, the majority of which underwent some slight expansion (Table 3).

Abbott also examined the development of pronuclear eggs recovered 16 h p. c. and transferred for 3 days to the oviducts of either spayed or day 1 recipients. The results are shown in Table 4. As with the later stages, 80 to 100 % of the pronuclear eggs developed into blastocysts.

Thus, it is clear that whilst the rabbit egg remains in the oviduct the cleavage and blastulation processes, except for some degree of retardation under the influence of estrogen are little affected even by marked changes in endocrine status. However, the question of developmental potential of the egg is another matter since morphological criteria alone are inadequate. For example, Table 5 which gives the results obtained from re-transferring the products of the pronuclear eggs, shows that only 4 to 6 % of the eggs implanted and none developed to term. To what extent this failure may be attributable to the vulnerability of the pronuclear stage, lack of an adequate mucin layer or to other factors is not known.

'DELAYED SECRETION'

In the rabbit estrogen treatment applied shortly after mating causes retardation in endometrial proliferation (Courrier and Kehl, 1932) and so called delayed secretion in which, *inter alia,* the appearance of the uterine protein, uteroglobin, is delayed (Beier et. al., 1971). Thus when two injections of 100 μg estradiol benzoate are given at 6 and 30 h p. c. the secretory pattern of the day 8 uterus

Table 5.
Development in Day 3 recipients of 16 h eggs which had spent 3 days in the ligated oviducts of spayed or Day 1 temporary recipients. (Percentages in parentheses).

Condition of temporary recipient	No. recipients	No. eggs re-transferred	No. implantations	No. young born
Spayed	3	26	1 (4)	0
Day 1	7	65	4 (6)	0

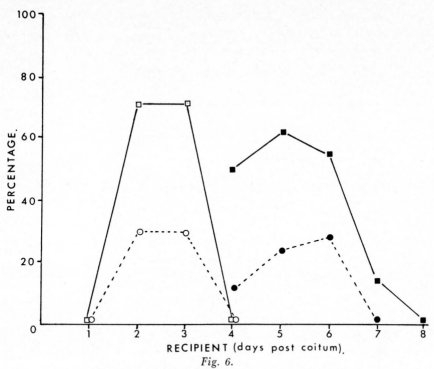

Fig. 6.

Transfer of 2 day eggs to the uterus of normally synchronized recipient rabbits (Chang 1950) and of 2½ day eggs to recipients treated with estradiol benzoate (Adams 1973b). ——— pregnancy rate; – – – eggs developing to term. ○ □ Chang; ● ■ Adams.

resembles that of the normal day 4 stage. In turn this affects synchronization requirements, (Beier et al., 1972; Adams, 1973b), as illustrated in Figs. 6 and 7. Increasing the number of estradiol injections to 4 (6, 30, 48 and 72 h p.c.) causes further delay so that 60 h morulae can survive in 'day 9 or 10' recipients. It is of considerable interest that the whole profile of uterine response is apparently equally affected, individual components not responding differentially. Apparently the estrogen acts directly at the uterine level and not indirectly via corpus luteum function because luteal development (corpus luteum weights at autopsy) and function (levels of progesterone in peripheral blood) are consistent with post-ovulatory age (Adams, 1973b). Therefore, by means of the appropriate estrogen treatment it is possible to effect a controlled dissociation of the synchrony that normally exists between the developing corpora lutea and endometrium. Combining this technique with egg transfer, which permits the selection of any developmental stage, we now have the ability to permutate at will the three major components of pregnancy, corpus luteum,

437

endometrium and embryo. This advance should benefit the investigation of early pregnancy.

ACKNOWLEDGMENTS

The author acknowledges permission to reprint figures from the following sources:

>*Journal of Reproduction and Fertility*
>Vol. 26, No. 1, 1971.
>*The Fallopian Tube – – a Reappraisal*
>Carl J. Pauerstein, Lea & Febiger:
>Philadelphia, 1974.
>*Advances in the Biosciences 4*
>Friedr. Vieweg & Sohn: Germany, 1969.
>*Advances in the Biosciences 13*
>Friedr. Vieweg & Sohn: Germany, 1974.

>Specific citations appear in the text.

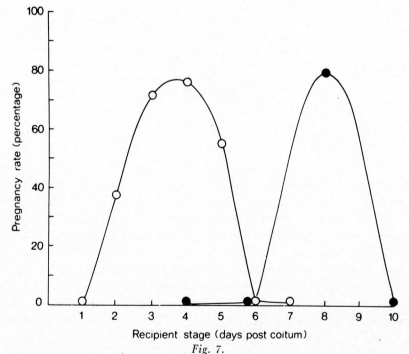

Fig. 7.

Pregnancy rate after transfer of 4 day blastocysts into normally synchronized recipient rabbits (Chang 1950) and transfer into estrogen treated rabbits (Beier 1972) (after Beier 1974). o——o Chang; ●——● Beier.

REFERENCES

Adams C. E. (1958) Egg development in the rabbit: The influence of post coital ligation of the uterine tube and of ovariectomy. *J. Endocr. 16,* 283–293.

Adams C. E. (1965a) The influence of maternal environment on preimplantation stages of pregnancy in the rabbit. In: Wolstenholme G. E. W. and O'Connor Maeve, eds. *Preimplantation Stages of Pregnancy,* pp. 345–373. Churchill, London.

Adams C. E. (1965b) Influence of the number of corpora lutea on endometrial proliferation and embryo development in the rabbit. *J. Endocr. 31,* 29–30.

Adams C. E. (1967) Ovarian control of early embryonic development within the uterus. In: Lamming G. E. and Amoroso E. C., eds. *Reproduction in the Female Mammal,* pp. 532–546. Butterworths, London.

Adams C. E. (1969) Egg-uterus interrelationships. In: Raspé G., ed. *Adv. Biosciences 4,* 149–162.

Adams C. E. (1971) The fate of fertilized eggs transferred to the uterus or oviduct during advancing pseudopregnancy in the rabbit. *J. Reprod. Fertil. 26,* 99–111.

Adams C. E. (1973a) The development of rabbit eggs in the ligated oviduct and their viability after re-transfer to recipient rabbits. *J. Embryol. exp. Morph. 29,* 133–144.

Adams C. E. (1973b) Asynchronous egg transfer in the rabbit. *J. Reprod. Fertil. 35,* 613–614.

Beier H. M. (1972) Die hormonelle Steuerung der Uterussekretion und frühen Embryonalentwicklung des Kaninchens. *Habil-Schrift. Med.,* Fakult. Univ., Kiel.

Beier H. M. (1974) Ovarian steroids in embryonic development before nidation. In: Raspé G., ed. *Hormones and Embryonic Development. Adv. Biosciences 13,* 199–219.

Beier H. M., Kühnel W. and Petry G. (1971) Uterine secretion proteins as extrinsic factors in preimplantation development. In: Raspé G., ed. *Adv. Biosciences 6,* 165–189.

Beier H. M., Mootz V. and Kühnel W. (1972) Asynchrone Eirtransplantationen während der verzögerten Uterussekretion beim Kaninchen. *Proc. VIIth Int. Congr. on Animal Reprod. & A. I., Munich, 3,* 1891–1896.

Benirschke K. (1969) Pathologic processes of the oviduct. In: Hafez E. S. E. and Blandau R. J., eds. *The Mammalian Oviduct,* Ch. 11, pp. 271–307. University of Chicago Press, Chicago.

Brouha A. (1934) Études des rapports entre les modifications pregravidiques de la muqueuse utérine et les hormones ovariennes. *Arch. Biol. (Paris) 45,* 571–609.

Chang M. C. (1950) Development and fate of transferred rabbit ova or blastocyst in relation to the ovulation time of recipients. *J. exp. Zool. 114,* 197–216.

Chang M. C. (1955) Développement de la capacité fertilisatrice des spermatozoides du lapin a l'interieur du tractus génital femelle et fécondabilité des oeufs de lapine. In: Funck-Brentano P., ed. *La fonction tubaire et ses troubles,* pp. 40–52. Masson, Paris.

Chang M. C. (1967) The reaction of uterine endometrium on spermatozoa and eggs. In: Lamming G. E. and Amoroso E. C., eds. *Reproduction in the Female Mammal,* pp. 459–476. Butterworths, London.

Chang M. C. (1969) Development of transferred ferret eggs in relation to the age of the corpora lutea. *J. exp. Zool. 171,* 459–464.

Corner G. W. (1928) Physiology of the corpus luteum. 1. The effect of very early ablation of the corpus luteum upon embryos and uterus. *Amer. J. Physiol. 86,* 74–81.

Corner G. W. (1942) *The Hormones in Human Reproduction.* Princeton University Press.

439

Courrier R. and Kehl R. (1933) Sur l'existence de sevils differentiels endocriniens dans les réactions utérines de la phases luteinique. *C. R. Soc. Biol. (Paris) 113*, 607–609.

Dickmann Z. (1970) Effects of progesterone on the development of the rat morula. *Fertil. Steril. 21*, 541–548.

Dickmann Z. and Noyes R. W. (1960) The fate of ova transferred into the uterus of the rat. *J. Reprod. Fertil. 1*, 197–212.

Doyle L. L., Gates A. H. and Noyes R. W. (1963) Asynchronous transfer of mouse ova. *Fertil. Steril. 14*, 215–225.

McLaren A. and Michie D. (1956) Studies on the transfer of fertilized mouse eggs to uterine foster mothers. 1. Factors affecting implantation and survival of native and transferred eggs. *J. exp. Biol. 33*, 394–416.

Moore N. W. and Shelton J. N. (1964) Egg transfer in sheep: Effect of degree of synchronization between donor and recipient, age of egg, and site of transfer on the survival of transferred eggs. *J. Reprod. Fertil. 7*, 145–152.

Noyes R. W. and Dickmann Z. (1960) Relationship of ovular age to endometrial development. *J. Reprod. Fertil. 1*, 186–196.

Pauerstein C. J. (1974) *The Fallopian Tube: A Reappraisal.* Lea & Febiger, Philadelphia.

Reid D. E., Ryan K. J. and Benirschke K. (1972) *Principles and Management of Human Reproduction.* W. B. Saunders, Philadelphia.

Rowson L. E. A. and Moor R. M. (1966) Embryo-transfer in sheep; the significance of synchronizing oestrus in the donor and recipient animal. *J. Reprod. Fertil. 11*, 207–212.

Rowson L. E. A., Moor R. M. and Lawson R. A. S. (1969) Fertility following egg transfer in the cow; effect of method, medium and synchronization of oestrus. *J. Reprod. Fertil. 18*, 517–523.

Thibault C. (1972) Some pathological aspects of ovum maturation and gamete transport in mammals and man. *Acta endocr. (Kbh.)* Suppl. *166*, 59–66.

Webel S. K., Peters J. B. and Anderson L. L. (1970) Synchronous and asynchronous transfer of embryos in the pig. *J. Animal Sci. 30*, 565–568.

Weitlauf H. M. (1971) Protein synthesis by blastocysts in the uteri and oviducts of intact and hypophysectomized mice. *J. exp. Zool. 176*, 35–40.

Wintenberger-Torres S. (1966) Les rapports entre l'oeuf en segmentation et le tractus maternel chez la brebis. *IIIrd Int. Congr. Anim. Reprod. & A. I.*, Cambridge, *1*, 62–64.

Woodruff J. D. and Pauerstein C. J. (1969) *The Fallopian Tube.* The Williams & Wilkins Co., Baltimore.

Syntex (USA) Inc., Hillview Avenue, Palo Alto, California

Discussion Paper

DRUG REGULATION OF EGG TRANSPORT

By

J. P. Bennett

ABSTRACT

Studies and hypotheses on the natural regulation of egg transport are followed by a review of attempts to develop novel contraceptives by alteration of the rate of egg transport by administration of hormones, synthetic chemicals and natural substances. These include the steroidal estrogens and anti-estrogens, gonadotropins, prostaglandins, autonomic drugs and a large number of synthetic non-steroids which act to accelerate or retard the rate of egg transport in the female reproductive tract. The potential of new contraceptives producing chemical occlusion of the oviduct is included.

The egg transport phase in the oviduct of most species occupies the first three or four days after ovulation. During the first day, while under estrogen domination, the eggs move quickly through the thin walled ciliated ampulla. Under a delicate balance of endogenous estrogen and progesterone, the eggs are held at the ampullary-isthmic junction until fertilized and then descend through the muscular ampulla to enter the uterus via the uterotubal junction. The eggs then move freely in the uterus until attachment, the time of which of course varies from one species to another. Many different hormones, synthetic chemicals and natural substances have been used with the aim of altering the delicate hormonal balance required for natural egg transport, to produce a novel contraceptive approach (see Bennett 1974b). Such contraceptives may function by ovicidal action, alteration of the rate of egg transport, inhibition of fertilization or a combination of these effects in the reproductive tract.

Fig. 1 lists groups of chemical compounds which have been studied with a view to developing new contraceptiives acting upon egg transport. Until recently, most of this work was done in rodents, rabbits and monkeys. There has been little research in women, mainly due to the difficulty of locating sufficient numbers who would elect to use mechanical contraceptives only, except during and shortly after the mid-cycle test period, when coitus was followed by a drug acting upon egg transport.

The mechanism of action of these compounds in animals remains speculative possibly involving changes in oviductal secretions, altered oviductal muscular activity and isthmic resistance to passage of the egg. A generally held theory is that changes in the rate of egg transport are produced by a drug-induced alteration of the endogenous estrogen level, producing a desynchronization of the biochemical and transport relationships between the egg and the reproductive tract, with consequent degeneration of the egg. A similar explanation for the activities of such compounds in women is probable.

Koester (1969, 1970) discounts oviductal muscular activity as a regulator of egg transport and postulates that the speed of oviductal ciliary action and flow of oviductal secretions interact to control the rate of egg transport. The theory includes increased ciliary beating on the 3rd day after ovulation.

Pauerstein (1974) suggests another explanation for the mechanism of egg transport, particularly of the isthmic delay of egg passage. He hypothesizes that estrogen enhances alpha adrenergic activity and thus isthmic constriction. The stimulus of ovulation results in production of progesterone. On the third day after ovulation progesterone has enhanced beta receptor activity sufficient to relax the isthmic constriction and allow the egg to move into the uterus.

Acceleration and arrest ("tube-locking") of the rate of egg transport has been observed with some compounds administered to laboratory animals (Fig. 1). However, only acceleration of the rate of egg transport would be acceptable as a contraceptive method in women, since arrest of an egg within the oviduct might lead to an ectopic pregnancy with dangerous consequences.

The use of many of the compounds studied produces increased estrogenic activity, resulting in possible unpleasant side effects in women and has led chemists to seek compounds which retain their effects upon the rate of egg transport, without an increased estrogenic activity.

STEROIDAL ESTROGENS

Chang and Yanagimachi in 1965 concluded that "any compound with estrogenic activity may have antifertility activity if taken at a particular time soon after mating". The work of Parkes and Bellerby (1926), Smith (1926), Courrier and Raynaud (1934), Pincus and Kirsch (1936), Heckel and Allen (1939), Segal and Nelson (1958), Greenwald (1959), Chang and Harper (1966) and others listed in Fig. 1 confirm this statement.

Fig. 1.
Some compounds affecting the rate of egg transport in the oviduct of common laboratory mammals.

Compound	Effect on egg transport	Species	References
Synthetic and steroidal estrogens	accelerate or arrest	rabbit	Greenwald (1961, 1963, 1965, 1967)
	accelerate or arrest	mouse	Burdick & Pincus (1935)
	accelerate or arrest	guinea pig	Deanesly (1961) Greenwald (1967)
	accelerate or arrest	hamster	Greenwald (1961, 1967)
	accelerate only	rat	Greenwald (1961) Gardner et al. (1964) Bennett et al. (1969)
Synthetic non-steroidal estrogens	accelerate	rat	Duncan et al. (1962) Greenwald (1965) Harper & Walpole (1967) Jensen (1968)
Synthetic progestins	accelerate	rabbit	Chang & Bedford (1961) Chang (1964a, 1964b) Bennett et al. (1969)
	accelerate	rat	Davis (1963) Wakeling (1965)
Gonadotropins	accelerate	rabbit	Wislocki & Snyder (1933)
	accelerate	mouse	Harrington (1965)
	accelerate	monkey	Bennett (1967)
Prostaglandin $PGF_{2\alpha}$ PGE_1	accelerate	rabbit	Ellinger & Kirton (1972, 1974)
PGE_1	arrest	mouse	Liu et al. (1974)
PGE_2	arrest	rat	Eliasson (1959) Horton et al. (1965) Nutting & Cammarata (1969)
Reserpine	arrest	mouse	Bennett & Kendle (1967)
Chlorpromazine	arrest	mouse	Bennett & Kendle (1967)
Tetrabenazine	arrest	mouse	Kendle & Bennett (1969a, 1969b)
Oviductal occludents	arrest	rabbit	Richart et al. (1972)
		monkey	Dafoe et al. (1972)

Table 1.

The effect of single injections of estradiol cyclopentylpropionate[a], given to animals shortly after mating, upon rate of egg transport in the oviduct.

Species	Dose accelerating rate of egg transport (μg)	Dose "tube-locking" eggs at ampullary-isthmic junction (μg)	Dose interrupting pregnancy in +80 % of animals (μg)
Mouse	> 1	1	1
Rabbit	25	100	50
Rat	> 10	–	10
Guinea pig	50–100	250	10
Hamster	100	250	25

[a] Estradiol cyclopentylpropionate is estra-1,3,5(10)-triene-3,17β-cyclopentyl-propionate.

Source: Compiled from Greenwald (1967).

The effect of exogenous estrogens upon egg transport varies with the species and the dose used (Fig. 1, Table 1). Greenwald (1967) showed that a suitable dose of a given estrogen produced an accelerated rate of egg transport in the oviduct of mouse, rabbit, rat, guinea pig and hamster. In contrast, relatively high unphysiological doses of estrogen in the rabbit, guinea pig or hamster produced an arrest of egg transport at the sphincter-like ampullary-isthmic junction (Greenwald 1968). The use of concurrent massive doses of 17a-hydroxyprogesterone caproate (100 mg for four days) did not prevent the arrest of egg transport, leading to the belief that regulation of egg transport in this region was estrogen- rather than progestin-dominated. Greenwald (1961, 1963, 1965) further concluded that premature or delayed relaxation of the egg transport control mechanism at the ampullary-isthmic junction, was responsible for the regulation of egg transport and not changes in oviductal motility.

Pauerstein et al. (1970) confirmed Greenwald's observation that 250 mg estradiol arrests egg transport in the rabbit, but observed that a phenoxybenz-amine-induced a-adrenergic blockade, counteracted the effect, but did not accelerate egg transport in non-steroid treated rabbits. They suggested that the effect of the estrogen dose on egg transport was mediated via the adrenergic nerves as described earlier.

The successful transfer of eggs from estrogen treated donor rabbits (Green-wald 1962; Ketchel and Pincus 1964) and rats (Pincus et al. 1964) to undosed recipients suggest that the hormone is not directly ovicidal. The drug acce-

Table 2.

Effect of topical application of steroidal agents on implantation in rats.

Agent[a]	Dose per rat	Treatment (days of pregnancy)	No. of rats		Total no. of corpora lutea		Total no. of implantations	
			Total	Pregnant	Mean	Range	Mean	Range
Ethanol (control rats)	0.1 ml	1–5	18	18	7.6	5–10	6.6	3–9
Estrone	20 μg	1	12	0	7.2	4–11	0.0	0–0
Estradiol-17β	20 μg	1	8	0	5.7	4–8	0.0	0–0
3-cyclopentyl ether of 17α-ethynyl estradiol	20 μg	1	8	0	6.1	3–7	0.0	0–0
17α-ethynyl estradiol	20 μg	1	9	0	6.6	2–9	0.0	0–0

[a] Compounds were dissolved in 0.1 ml absolute ethanol.

Source: Adapted from Kar, Setty and Kamboj (1968) (Table 1).

Table 3.

Prevention of pregnancy in the rabbit by subcutaneous implantation of silastic tube containing estrogen.

Compounds in a silastic tube kg per rabbit	No. of animals used	No. of females ovulating after mating	No. of females ovulating after human chorionic gonadotrophin (HCG)	Day of examination after mating or insemination and injection of HCG								
				Day 2			Day 6			Day 12		
				No. of rabbits	Total corpora lutea	Total eggs fertilized	No. of rabbits	Total corpora lutea	Total normal blasto-cysts	No. of rabbits	Total corpora lutea	Total embryos
Progesterone, 20 mg	12	6	6	5	57	$51-4^a$ (90%)	5	65	$56+3^b$ (86%)	2	24	$23+1^c$ (96%)
Chlormadinone acetate, 20 mg	8	1	7	2	31	31 (100%)	3	33	$27+2^b$ (82%)	3	43	$29+4^c$ (68%)
Ethinyl estradiol, 2 mg	13	7	$4+2^d$	3	11	$7+3^e$ (91%)	6	39	2^f (0%)	2	13	$0+12^f$ (0%)
Ethinyl estradiol, 0.5 mg	8	3	$4+1^d$	2	5	1 (20%)	3	20	4^f (0%)	2	14	0 (0%)
Control, empty tube implanted	10	4	6	3	20	20 (100%)	4	44	$38+1^f$ (87%)	3	39	34 (87%)

aUnfertilized eggs. bSmall blastocysts. cDegenerated embryos. dFailed to ovulate after HCG. eFrom the uterus. fDegenerated small blastocysts.
Source: Chang, Casas and Hunt (1970) (Table 1).

Table 4.
Some steroidal antiestrogens with effects upon egg transport and fertility.

Compound	Species	Effective dose/day	Dose route	Effect upon rate of egg transport	Author
1. 10275-S	Rat	0.25–0.5 mg (D1–6)	sc	arrest	Miyake & Takeda (1967)
2. Norethindrone	Rat	0.9 mg (D2)	sc	arrest	Davis (1963)
	Rabbit	10 mg/kg (D1–3)	oral	arrest	Bennett & Vickery (unpubl.)
		8 mg/kg (D1)	oral	arrest	
3. D-Norgestrel	Human	0.4 mg (D12, 10 & 12, 8, 10 & 12 cycle. D2, 4 & 2, 4 & 6 after LH peak)	oral	unknown	Spona et al. (1974)
4. Sch-10015*	Rat	5 mg/kg/day (D2 & D3)	oral	accelerate	Watnick et al. (1966)
5. Norethynodrel	Rat	0.2 mg/rat/day (D1 or D1–4)	sc	accelerate	Wakeling (1965)
	Rat	5 mg/kg (D1–3)	topical	accelerate	Kar et al. (1968)
	Rabbit	10 or 20 mg/rabbit (D1–3)	oral	undecided	Chang (1964b)
6. Ethynodiol diacetate	Rat	2.5 mg/kg (D1–3)	topical	accelerate	Kar et al. (1968)
7. Progesterone	Rabbit	1–4 mg/rabbit (D2, D1 and D0)	sc	accelerate	Chang (1967)
8. Chlormadinone acetate	Rabbit	0.09 mg/kg (D2 to D0)	oral	accelerate	Vickery & Bennett (1969)

* 10β-hydroperoxy-17α-ethynyl-4-estren-17β-ol-3-one = Sch. 10015.

Table 5.

Some orally active non-steroids which act upon the rate of egg transport.

Compound group	Examples	Effective antifertility dose per day mg/kg (day dosed)	Species	Author
Triarylalkenes	Clomiphene (MRL 41) Tamoxifen (ICI-46474)	0.3 (D1–4) 0.03 (D2–4)	Rat Rat	Segal & Nelson (1961) Harper & Walpole (1966)
Triarylalkanes	Ethamoxytriphetol (MER 25)	25.0 (01–4)	Rat	Lerner et al. (1958), Segal & Nelson (1958), Pincus (1965)
Stilbene derivatives	Diethylstilbestrol	1–25 mg* (D1–6) 25 mg* (4–5 days) postcoital	Monkey Human Human	Morris & Van Wagenen (1966, 1967a,b) Haspels (1969, 1970) Kuchera (1971)
Methoxy phenyl-β-nitro-styrylphenoxyethyl pyrrolidine	CN-55945-27	0.025 (D1–7) 0.5 (Single D1)	Rat	Callantine et al. (1966)
Diphenylindenes	U-11555A	0.5 (D1–6) 10.0 (Single dose)	Rat	Duncan et al. (1962)

448

Dihydronaphthalenes	U-11100A	0.025 (D1–6)	Rat	Duncan et al. (1963)
Benzofurans	2,3-diphenyl benzofuran	4–16 (D1–5)	Rat	Grover et al. (1965)
Coumarins	3,4-diphenyl coumarin	0.4 (D1–6)	Rat	Lednicer et al. (1965)
Chromenes	3,4-diphenyl chromenes	0.02 (D1–5)	Rat	Bencze et al. (1965)
Diazocine	U-10293	0.5 mg* (D1–7)	Rat	Duncan et al. (1965)
Oxazolidinethiones	U-11634	2.5 mg (D1–7)	Rat	Duncan et al. (1965)
Diphenylsulfoxide	p-p'-diamino diphenyl sulfoxide	100–200 (D1–5)	Rat	Kamboj & Kar (1966)
Naphthofurans	NF or 66/179	1–5 (D1–3)	Rat	Kamboj et al. (1970)
Cyclohexene carboxylic acids	ORF 3858 (Fenestrel)	0.05 (D1–3)	Rabbit	Morris & Van Wagenen (1967a)
		2.0 (D1–6)	Monkey	Morris et al. (1967b)
		0.01 (D0, 2; 1, 2; 2, 3)	Rat	Blye (1969)
Doisynolic acids	RS2874	0.027 oil (D1, 2 or 3)	Rat	Rooks et al. (1971)
		0.0125 (D1–6)	Rat	Rooks et al. (1971)
		2.0 (D1–6)	Rabbit	Morris & Dorfman (1971)

* mg per animal dosed per day.

449

lerated entry of the eggs in the uterus results in their degeneration, due to the premature stage of the eggs' development with respect to that of the uterus.

Among estrogenic steroids synthesized to produce separation of antifertility and estrogenic activity were a number of A-norandrostanes (Pincus et al. 1964), some 17α-butadiynyl-17β-hydroxyesterene derivatives (Gardner et al. 1964) and a series of halogenated 17-ethinyl compounds (Bennett et al. 1966) in which 17α-trifluorethynyl-3,17β-dihydroxyestra-1,3,5(10)-triene (BDH 6146) showed a ratio of antifertility to estrogenic activity in the rat of 30:1.

Estrogenic steroids have prevented pregnancy in rats during the egg transport phase when administered topically (Table 2, Kar et al. 1968) and when contained in a silastic tube implanted subcutaneously (Table 3) or within the uterus (Casas and Chang 1970; Chang et al. 1970).

Morris and Van Wagenen (1966, 1967a,b) prevented implantation of the egg in rhesus monkeys by administration of 10 mg ethinyl estradiol orally for six days after proven matings, and also claimed antifertility activity in women given 0.5–2.0 mg ethinyl estradiol orally per day for four or more days after mid-cycle intercourse. These results were confirmed by Haspels (1969, 1970) using 1 mg ethinyl estradiol, given twice daily for five days, 48 h postcoitally, to raped women or where condoms had failed.

ANTI-ESTROGENS

Emmens (1965) observed that many antiestrogens (e. g. dimethyl-stilbestrol) are estrogenic at high doses and that this explained their contraceptive effect. Some of the antiestrogens found to be effective in altering the rate of egg transport are shown in Table 4.

Most of 19 nor-progestins produce their antifertility effect by conversion to estrogens (Petrow 1966). However, recently D-norgestrel, which is more stable, was found to active during the egg transport phase in women given 400 mg orally on day 12, or days 10 and 12, or days 8, 10 and 12 of the cycle, or on the 2nd and 4th day and on the 2nd, 4th and 6th day after the LH peak (Spona et al. 1974).

The 17 acetoxy-progestins have been shown to cause an accelerated egg transport in rabbits (Table 4) when given before ovulation and/or continued during the egg transport phase. Chang (1967) suggested that the accelerated rate of egg transport was produced from a rebound estrogen level after cessation of progestin dosing at ovulation. However, Vickery and Bennett (1969) continued to observe accelerated egg transport in rabbit dosed days –2 to +8 of pregnancy with chlormadinone acetate. Thus further explanation is required.

A variety of non-steroidal compounds have been tested in laboratory animals for effects upon the egg transport phase with the aim of discovering a non-toxic antifertility agent (see Bennett 1974b, Ch. 6). Most of the examples shown in Table 5 produce their effects by acting as estrogens or antiestrogens, or they initiate an alteration in the rate of egg transport from direct or indirect changes in the hormonal balance, which results in degeneration of eggs in the uterus.

Superovulation by gonadotropin injections causes accelerated egg transport in mice (Harrington 1965), rabbits (Wislocki and Snyder 1933), sheep (Robinson 1951), cattle (Rowson 1951) and monkey (Bennett 1967). The endogenous estrogen level is elevated after dosing, with consequent acceleration of egg passage through the oviduct into the uterus.

Substances which act upon the smooth muscle of the oviduct have also been effective in altering the rate of egg transport, e. g. ergot alkaloids, autonomic drugs (e. g. reserpine) and the prostaglandins.

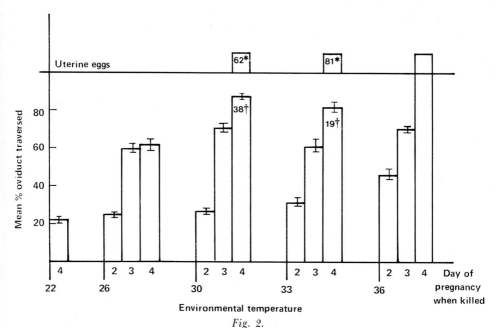

Fig. 2.

The rate of egg transport in groups of ten mated mice given 4 mg/kg reserpine on Day 1 of pregnancy and maintained at various environmental temperatures.

* Percentage of total eggs recovered from uterus.

† Percentage of total eggs observed in the oviduct.

From: Kendle & Bennett (1969a).

As early as 1957, Shelesnyak observed antifertility effects of the ergot alkaloids ergocornine and ergocristine, upon injecting rats once during days 1–7 of pregnancy. Agroclavine was active in rats when given orally during the first 5 days of pregnancy (Edwardson 1968), but was inactive when injected intraperitoneally for the same period. The Czech workers Rezabek et al. (1969) discovered that a single oral postcoital dose of 10 mg/kg D-6-methyl-8-cyanomethylergoline (6605-VUFB) was an effective, non-toxic oral contraceptive in rats. A dose of 1 mg/kg repeated 5 times was more effective than a single dose. The toxic dose was 110 times higher than the antifertility dose.

There is growing evidence in reviews by Boling (1969), Brundin (1969) and Pauerstein (1974) that egg transport is modulated by sympathetic innervation and the adrenoreceptors of the isthmus in the oviduct, under hormonal control. Reserpine, chlorpromazine and tetrabenazine have produced a reversible arrest of egg transport in mice (Bennett and Kendle 1967, Kendle and Bennett 1969a,b, Kendle 1969), when dosed intraperitoneally on D1 or D1–3 of pregnancy. Prevention of the drug induced body hypothermia, obtained by placing the treated animal in an environmental cage, reversed the effects upon egg transport. The minimal environmental temperature which completely pre-

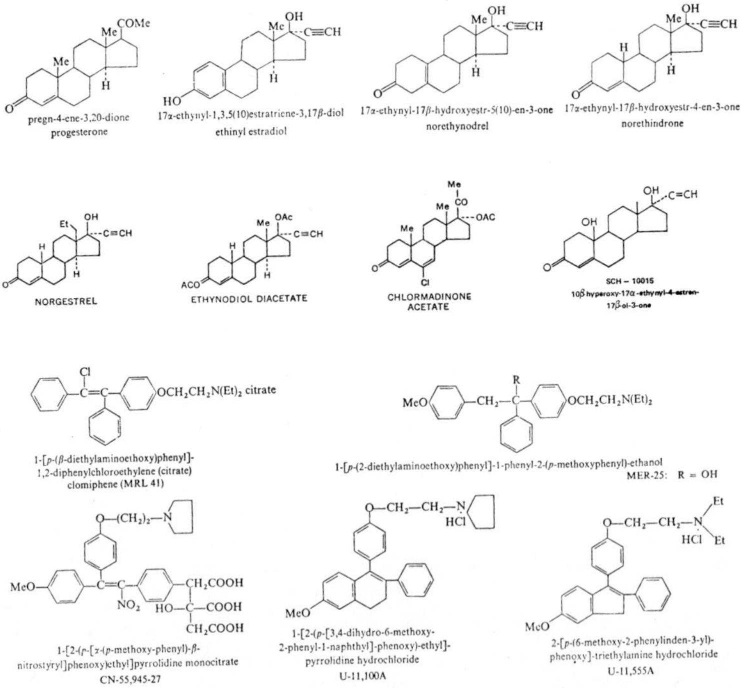

Fig. 3.
Formulae of drugs affecting egg transport.

vented retardation of egg transport was 36°C (Fig. 2) and was also the minimum which prevented the lowering of body temperature by reserpine on any day of autopsy. There was some indication of retarded egg transport associated with decreased norepinephrine levels in the isthmus of reserpine treated rabbits given 0.25 or 1 mg/kg/day sc from D1 to D2, D3 or D7 of pregnancy (Bodkhe and Harper 1972). In contrast, in the same study, iproniazid (25 mg/kg/day sc D1 to D2, D3 or D7) marginally accelerated the rate of egg transport while the norepinephrine levels were elevated. They did not observe any effects upon body temperature such as noted by Kendle and Bennett (1969b), but the dose administered was much lower because of toxicity in this species.

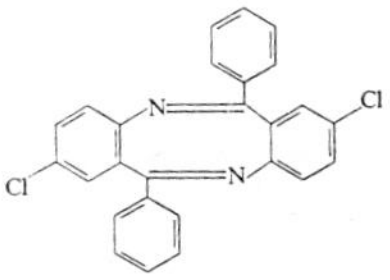

2,8-dichloro-6,12-diphenyl-dibenzo-[b,f][1,5]diazocine
U-10,293

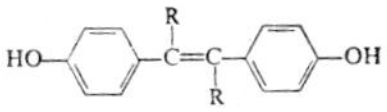

dimethyl stilbestrol: R = Methyl
diethyl stilbestrol: R = Ethyl

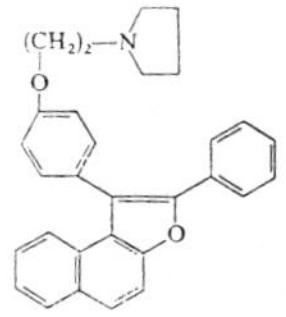

2-phenyl-3-p-(β-pyrrolidinoethoxy)-phenyl-(2:1,b)naphthofuran
NF or 66/179

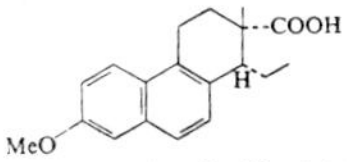

dl-cis-bisdehydrodoisynolic acid methyl ether
RS-2874

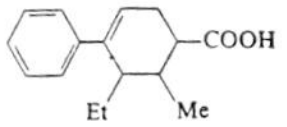

2-methyl-3-ethyl-4-phenyl-Δ4-cyclohexenecarboxylic acid
ORF-3858

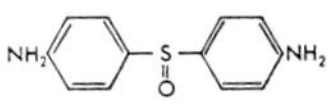

p, p'– diamino diphenyl sulfoxide

prostaglandin E2
(11α,15α-dihydroxy-9-ketoprosta-5,β-dienoic acid)

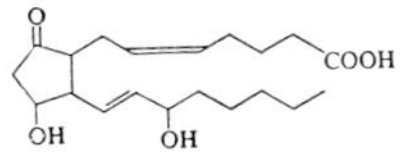

2,3-Diphenyl benzofuranes

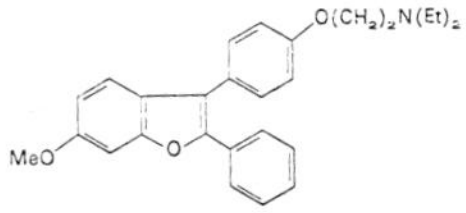

3,4-Diphenyl-coumarins

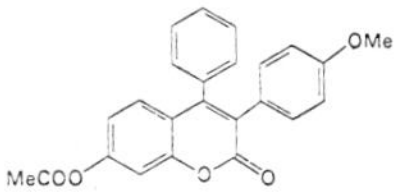

prostaglandin F2α
(9α-11α,15α-trihydroxyprosta-5,β-dienoic acid)

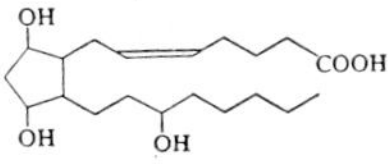

3,4-Diphenyl-chromenes

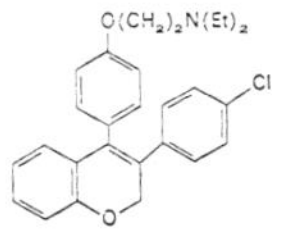

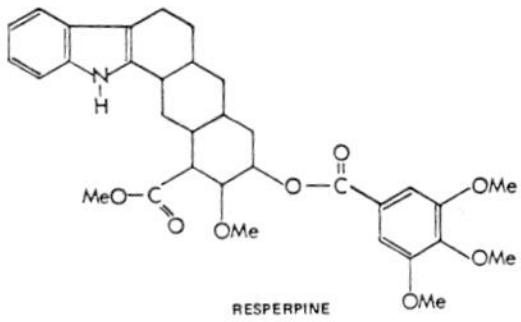

RESERPINE

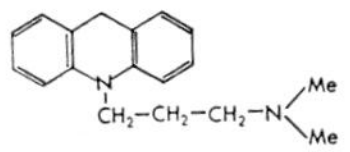

Chlorpromazine

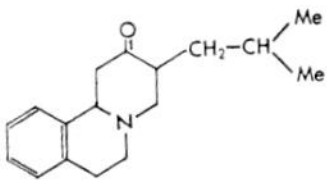

Tetrabenazine

453

Table 6.

Effect of prostaglandins (sc) on the rate of egg transport in the oviduct of various species.

Species	Prostaglandin	Dose	Effect on rate of egg transport	Author
Mouse	$PGF_{2\alpha}$	0.3 mg × 2, D1, D2 or D2 & D3	None	Liu et al. (1970)
	PGE_2	0.25, 0.5 mg × 2, D2, D3 & D4	Arrest	Liu et al. (1970)
Mouse	PGE_1	1 mg/kg D1 & D2, D3 & D4, D5	None	Horton & Marley (1969)
Rat	PGE_2	0.5 mg × 2 D1–6	Arrest	Nutting & Cammarata (1969)
	PGE_1	0.2 mg × 2 D1–3	Arrest	
	PGE_2	1.0 mg × 2 D1–3	Arrest	Labhsetwar (1973)
	$PGF_{2\alpha}$	0.2 mg D1–3	None	
Hamster	$PGF_{2\alpha}$	50 mg D4 or D4–6	None	Labhsetwar (1972)
Rabbit	PGE_2		None	Nutting (1969)
	$PGF_{2\alpha}$	5 mg/kg D4 or D4–6	Accelerate	Chang & Hunt (1972)
	$PGF_{2\alpha}$	5 mg/kg D1		Chang et al. (1973),
	PGE_1	1–5 mg/kg D1	Accelerate	Ellinger & Kirton (1974)

Pauerstein et al. (1970) and Hodgson et al. (1974) showed that estrogen-induced "tube-locking" of eggs and progesterone-accelerated rate of egg transport were antagonized by blockade or depletion of neurotransmitter from the intrinsic adrenergic nerves of the oviduct, suggesting that the effects of sex steroids on egg transport are partially mediated through adrenergic processes.

The prostaglandins (PG) are a group of hydroxy-acidic lipids with marked effects on smooth muscle contractility, which have been shown to disturb the rate of egg transport in several species (Table 6). The mechanisms of action which produce these effects are presently unknown, but a specific relationship has been established between prostaglandins and the altered smooth muscle contractility of the oviduct (Horton et al. 1965, Spilman and Harper 1972, Hafez and Aref 1974). In the mouse and rat PGE_2 produces an arrest of egg transport while $PGF_{2\alpha}$ and PGE_2 had no effect (Table 6). In contrast, Chang and Hunt (1972) and Chang et al. (1973) showed that 1–5 mg/kg of $PGF_{2\alpha}$ given subcutaneously on day 1 of pregnancy accelerated the rate of egg transport in rabbits.

CHEMICAL OCCLUSION OF THE OVIDUCT

There is increasing interest in the search for a suitable chemical substance which will reversibly occlude the lumen of the oviduct and thus prevent egg transport or fertilization. Some substances producing irreversible occlusion in women include ethanol-formalin (Zipper et al. 1969) and quinacrine sulphate (Zipper et al. 1970). In other tests in rabbits, zinc chloride, silver nitrate, phenol, salicylic acid and a variety of strong acids and bases all produced consistent and severe necrosis of the tubal epithelium and the muscular wall (Richart et al. 1972). Despite massive necrosis, in many instances the damaged but intact oviduct, was found to have a patent lumen 6 to 8 weeks following the original chemical-induced injury. Treated monkeys were also able to reconstitute the tubal lumen after similar chemical injury.

This area of study has promise but as yet experience is small. Certainly such a localized contraceptive technology would obviate many difficulties associated with prolonged drug absorption from chemical contraceptives interfering with the normal physiological and biochemical reproductive processes.

CONTRACEPTIVE USE OF COMPOUNDS
AFFECTING EGG TRANSPORT

Many of the compounds previously described have been categorised, perhaps mistakenly, as postcoital contraceptives, when they might better be defined as postovulatory contraceptives. This has occurred because nearly all the work has been done in laboratory animals where coitus and ovulation occur about the same time. In women coitus and ovulation are not necessarily synchronized. An improved contraceptive method affecting the regulation of egg transport in women requires a knowledge of the time of ovulation so that the treatment may be administered only during the egg transport phase. Without a method for detecting ovulation and with the known variance in ovulation time between women, and in the same women between cycles, the chemical contraceptive would be less effective unless taken daily. However, daily dosing with such compounds would probably produce all the disadvantages of the continuously administered combination, sequential or minipill hormonal contraceptive regimens. In addition, the drug regulatory agencies may be willing to ease the lengthy toxicological requirement for a contraceptive given only once or twice post ovulation rather than daily. Similar easing of the requirements may be forthcoming for a reversible oviductal occlusive chemical. Failing this, it is very doubtful whether such contraceptives will be available in the next decade.

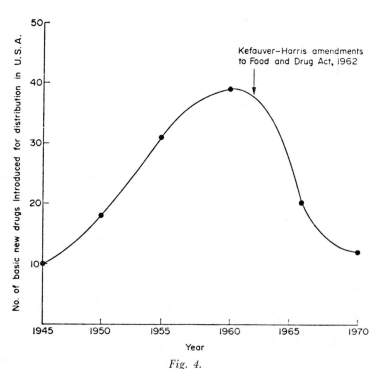

Fig. 4.
Numbers of basic new drugs introduced/year of distribution in the United States.
From: Bennett (1974a).

ADDITIONAL COMMENTS

I would like to amplify the reasons for the slow introduction of new contraceptives.

Since the introduction in 1962 of the Kefauver-Harris Amendment to the Food and Drug Act, under which the Food and Drug Administration (FDA) derive their authority, there has been a progressive decline in new drug introductions (Fig. 4). The regulations in many developed countries, but particularly in the United States, have become increasingly complex and demanding for the introduction of new chemical contraceptives given to healthy women on a continuous basis for prolonged periods.

Table 7 shows the regulatory requirements for an oral or parenteral drug treatment in human disease. Species to be used in toxicology are unnamed and clinical requirements of reasonable duration. When these requirements are compared to those needed for introduction of a new chemical contraceptive the time and cost constraints upon development become apparent. The extremely high cost in manpower, facilities, materials, patients and the duration required to develop this enormous mass of data (Table 8, Fig. 5) has severely slowed

Table 7.
Animal toxicology required by the FDA for oral or parenteral use of a new drug in the clinic. (From: Bennett 1974a).

Duration of human administration	Clinical phase tested[1]	Subacute or chronic toxicity[3] – two species by route used clinically
Several days	I up to NDA[2]	2 weeks
Up to 2 weeks	I	2 weeks
	II	Up to 4 weeks
	III, NDA	Up to 3 months
Up to 3 months	I, II	4 weeks
	III	3 months
	NDA	Up to 6 months
6 months and more	I, II	3 months
	III	6 months *or longer*
	NDA	12 months non-rodent
	IV	18 months rodent

[1] Definitions described in § 130 of New Drug Regulations, FDA.
[2] NDA = New Drug Application.
[3] Acute toxicity determined in three or four species.

Table 8.

Some regulatory agency requirements for animal toxicity studies for non-steroidal and steroidal contraceptives. (From Bennett 1974a).

Clinical use	FDA	U. K. committee on safety of medicine
Small nos. of patients Few days No reproductive risk	90-days rats, dogs, monkeys	90-day rat, non-rodent
With reproductive risk (equiv. phase I)	Plus teratology in rodent and fertility and reproductive performance female rodent	Plus teratology in rat and rabbit
Controlled no. up to three cycles (equiv. phase II)	1-year rat, dog, monkey	6-months rat, non-rodent
Unlimited no. patients (equiv. phase III)	2-year rat (carcinogenesis) 7-year dog (in progress 2 years) 10-year monkey (in progress 2 years) Peri- and post-natal fertility rodent Fertility and reproductive performance male rodent	2-year rat 18-months mouse (carcinogenesis)

new contraceptive development. If we had an active postcoital compound now it would probably take 8 to 10 years and about $ 10 million to bring such a drug to introduction in the United States.

The demanding drug regulatory requirements in the United States, the high development cost, the lack of a peer review group to arbitrate refusal of a New Drug Application, has led to cessation or reduction of contraceptive research in industry due to the unsatisfactory return on investment. Therefore, new chemical contraceptives will probably be developed and introduced first outside the United States.

In 1969 the Ford Foundation estimated the total funds required to achieve an optimum research effort in the contraceptive field at $ 150–200 million per year considering the extraordinary complexity of the scientific questions that need investigation, the relatively primitive state of scientific research in this field and the urgency of finding ways to slow down population growth. It is certain that such cost estimates are low today and very doubtful whether the required funding has been achieved for the goal set.

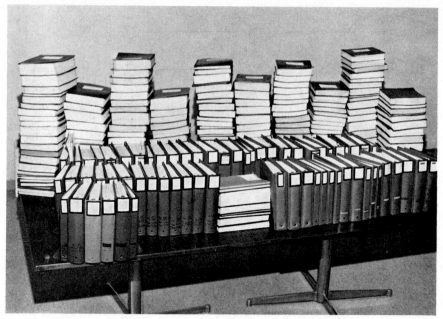

Fig. 5.
The information submitted to the U. S. Federal Drug Administration for a New
Drug Application of a Combination Oral Contraceptive.
From: Bennett (1974a).

For the above reasons and others listed in my recent paper outlining factors
limiting development of new contraceptives (Bennett 1974a) I feel our progress
in this area will be long delayed.

When the WHO Expanded Program was initiated I hoped that there was
a chance to introduce a new goal oriented approach to contraceptive development. However, it is apparent that WHO has tried to cover too wide an area
in its search for new contraceptives and is currently, in many cases, supporting
basic research in University departments more than contraceptive development.
In our program this week nearly all the papers are directed towards basic
studies of mechanisms of action without yet having a contraceptive product or
even a clear plan of how a contraceptive working on egg transport might be
used.

It is my contention that WHO should narrow its sights for the immediate
term to support directly goal oriented work likely to yield new contraceptives.

For whom is WHO developing new contraceptives, the developed or the
so-called developing or Third World?

If the answer is the developed world, I believe that we presently have effective contraceptives for these regions and will have the time available to pro-

duce novel contraceptive methods because of a lowering birth-rate in these countries.

If the answer is the developing countries, then I would ask do we need new contraceptives for these regions when agents exist such as the paper spermicide (e. g., C-Film) which can be used by male or female and can be identified with coitus or the paper oral hormonal contraceptives which are used in China? Although such contraceptive methods are not perfect, they would be easy to distribute and even at 50 % reduction in population growth would provide some relief and perhaps provide sufficient time for development of more suitable contraceptives for these regions.

Perhaps the funds of WHO may better be used at this time to assist introduction of available contraceptives by an intensive education and motivation program rather than to support research programs with funds insufficient to reach the goal of a new contraceptive before the serious consequences of population growth become evident.

In the context of our program I feel the question should be asked as to whether effects on egg transport can indeed produce a new, efficacious contraceptive in the human. Unless we first develop a method for ovulation prediction or detection, I believe the possibilities are poor. If, however, we do accept that a new contraceptive that affects egg transport is possible then it is evident we need a better model to screen likely groups of compounds. We have discussed some possibilities at this meeting.

Lastly, I would suggest that the funds supporting contraceptive research of both WHO and NICHD are out of phase with the rate of population growth in the Third World. We have little time left, indeed it may already be too late, to produce an effective program of fertility control before serious consequences occur in those countries.

I believe that funding agencies such as WHO must be realistic enough to place their funds where they do the most good in the shortest possible time and become more oriented to specific practical goals, if ever they are to succeed in arresting population growth. Possibly a 2 part funding system could be introduced with a drive developed to increase available funds. The major part should be used for the education and motivation of people in relevant countries to the use of simple, though imperfect contraceptives (not necessarily 100 % effective). The remainder should be divided between goal oriented contraceptive product-oriented research with some small funds going to very carefully selected basic research studies likely to yield the necessary knowledge to assist towards a new contraceptive product.

With the small funds available, and their present disbursement, the size of the problem, the constraints to development and the shortage of time available to achieve fertility control where it is needed, my prognosis for the future remains gloomy.

REFERENCES

Bencze W. L., Carney R. W. J., Barsky L. I., Renzi A. A., Dorfman L. and deStevens G. (1965) Synthetic estrogens and implantation inhibitors. *Experientia 21,* 261 (Abstr.).

Bennett J. P. (1967) Artificial insemination of the squirrel monkey. *J. Endocr. 37,* 473–474.

Bennett J. P. (1974a) Factors limiting the development of new contraceptives. *J. Reprod. Fertil. 37,* 487–498.

Bennett J. P. (1974b) In: *Chemical Contraception,* Ch. 6, pp. 99–132. Columbia University Press, New York.

Bennett J. P. and Kendle K. E. (1967) The effect of reserpine upon the rate of egg transport in the Fallopian tube of the mouse. *J. Reprod. Fertil. 13,* 345–348.

Bennett J. P., Kendle K. E., Vallance D. K. and Vickery B. H. (1966) A comparison of the antifertility and hormone activities of some new synthetic estrogens. *Acta endocr. (Kbh.) 53,* 443–454.

Bennett J. P., Vickery B. H. and Dorfman R. I. (1969) Some effects of progestins on pregnancy in the rabbit. Presented at *N. American Conf. Fertility and Sterility,* January 1969. Jamaica, West Indies.

Blye R. P. (1969) The effect of estrogens and related substances on embryonic viability. *Adv. Biosci. 4,* 323–343.

Bodkhe R. R. and Harper M. J. K. (1972) Changes in the amount of adrenergic neurotransmitter in the genital tract of untreated rabbits, and rabbits given reserpine or iproniazid during the time of egg transport. *Biol. Reprod. 6,* 288–299.

Boling J. L. (1969) Endocrinology of the oviductal musculature. In: Hafez E. S. E. and Blandau R. J., eds. *The Mammalian Oviduct,* Ch. 6, pp. 163–181. University of Chicago Press, Chicago.

Brundin J. (1969) Pharmacology of the oviduct. In: Hafez E. S. E. and Bdandau R. J., eds. *The Mammalian Oviduct,* Ch. 10, pp. 251–269. University of Chicago Press, Chicago.

Callantine M. R., Humphrey R. R., Lee S. L., Windsor B. L., Schottin N. H. and O'Brien O. P. (1966) Action of an estrogen antagonist on reproductive mechanisms in the rat. *Endocrinology 79,* 153–167.

Casas J. H. and Chang M. C. (1970) Effects of subcutaneous implantation or intrauterine insertion of silastic tube containing steroids on the fertility of rats. *Biol. Reprod. 2,* 315–325.

Chang M. C. (1964a) Effects of oral administration of medroxy progesterone acetate and ethinyl estradiol on the transportation and development of rabbit eggs. *Endocrinology 79,* 939–948.

Chang M. C. (1964b) Effects of certain antifertility agents on the development of rabbit ova. *Fertil. Steril. 15,* 97–106.

Chang M. C. (1967) Effect of progesterone and related compounds on fertilization, transportation and development of rabbit eggs. *Endocrinology 81,* 1251–1260.

Chang M. C. and Bedford J. (1961) Effects of various hormones on the transportation of gametes and fertilization in the rabbit. *Proceedings of the IVth International Congress on Animal Reproduction,* June 1961, 2, p. 367–370. The Hague.

Chang M. C., Casas J. H. and Hunt D. M. (1970) Prevention of pregnancy in the rabbit by subcutaneous implantation of silastic tube containing estrogen. *Nature (Lond.) 226,* 1262–1263.

461

Chang M. C. and Harper M. J. K. (1966) Effects of ethinyl estradiol on egg transport and development in the rabbit. *Endocrinology 78*, 860–872.

Chang M. C. and Hunt D. M. (1972) Effect of prostaglandin $F_{2\alpha}$ on the early pregnancy of rabbits. *Nature (Lond.) 236*, 120–121.

Chang M. C., Hunt D. M. and Polge C. (1973) Effects of prostaglandins (PG's) on sperm and egg transport in the rabbit. *Adv. Biosci. 9*, 805–810.

Chang M. C. and Yanagimachi R. (1965) Effect of estrogens and other compounds as oral antifertility agents on the development of rabbit ova and hamster embryos. *Fertil. Steril. 16*, 281–291.

Courrier R. and Raynaud R. (1934) Étude quantitative de l'avortement folliculinique chez la lapine par l'hormone cristallisée: réalisation d'un avortement partiel. *C. R. Séanc. Soc. Biol. 116*, 1073–1076.

Dafoe C. A., Thompson H. E., Moulding T. S. and Seitz L. E. (1972) Chemical occlusion at the uterotubal junction in monkeys. *Amer. J. Obstet. Gynec. 113*, 388–393.

Davis B. K. (1963) Termination of pregnancy in the rat with norethynodrel. *Nature (Lond.) 197*, 308–309.

Deanesly R. (1961) Effects of estrogen on tubal transport and ovo implantation in the guinea pig. *Proceedings of the IVth International Congress on Animal Reproduction 2*, 371–374. The Hague.

Duncan G. W., Lyster S. L., Clark J. J. and Lednicer D. (1963) Antifertility activity of two diphenyl-dihydronaphthalene derivatives. *Proc. Soc. exp. Biol. Med. 112*, 439–442.

Duncan G. W., Lyster S. C. and Wright J. B. (1965) Reproductive mechanisms influenced by a diazocine. *Proc. Soc. exp. Biol. Med. 120*, 725–728.

Duncan G. W., Stucki J. C., Lyster S. C. and Lednicer D. (1962) An orally effective mammalian antifertility agent. *Proc. Soc. exp. Biol. Med. 109*, 163–166.

Edwardson J. A. (1968) The effects of agroclavine, an ergot alkaloid, on pregnancy and lactation in the rat. *Brit. J. Pharmac. Chemother. 33*, 215P–216P.

Eliasson R. (1959) Studies on prostaglandin occurrence, formation and biological actions. *Acta physiol. scand. 46*, Suppl. 158, 71–73.

Ellinger J. V. and Kirton K. T. (1972) Ovum transport in rabbits injected with prostaglandins E_1 and $F_{2\alpha}$. *Biol. Reprod. 11*, 93–96.

Emmens C. W. (1965) Oestrogenic, anti-estrogenic and antifertility activities of various compounds. *J. Reprod. Fertil. 9*, 277–283.

Gardner J. N., Gnoj O., Watnick A. S. and Gibson J. (1964) New contraceptive agents with high activity in rats. *Steroids 4*, 801–813.

Greenwald G. S. (1959) The comparative effectiveness of estrogens in interrupting pregnancy in the rabbit. *Fertil. Steril. 10*, 155–161.

Greenwald G. S. (1961) A study of the transport of ova through the rabbit oviduct. *Fertil. Steril. 12*, 80–95.

Greenwald G. S. (1962) The role of the mucin layer in development of the rabbit blastocyst. *Anat. Rec. 142*, 407–415.

Greenwald G. S. (1963) *In vivo* recordings of intraluminal pressure changes in the rabbit oviduct. *Fertil. Steril. 14*, 666–674.

Greenwald G. S. (1965) Effects of a dihydronaphthalene derivative (U-11, 100A) on pregnancy in the rat. *Fertil. Steril. 16*, 185–194.

Greenwald G. S. (1967) Species differences in egg transport in response to exogenous estrogen. *Anat. Rec. 157*, 163–172.

462

Greenwald G. S. (1968) Hormonal regulation of egg transport through the mammalian oviduct. In: Behrman S. J. and Kistner R. W., eds. *Progress in Infertility*, pp. 157–179. Little Brown & Company, Boston.

Grover P. K., Chawla H. P. S., Anand N., Kamboj V. P. and Kar A. B. (1965) New antifertility agents. 2,2-diphenyl-benzofurans. *J. Med. Chem. 8*, 720–721.

Hafez E. S. E. and Aref L. (1974) Ova retention at the ampullary – isthmic junction and role of prostaglandin E_2 and prostaglandin $F_{2\alpha}$. *Fertil. Steril. 25*, 302 (Abstr.).

Harper M. J. K. and Walpole A. L. (1966) Contrasting endocrine activities of cis and trans isomers in a series of substituted triphenylethylenes. *Nature (Lond.) 212*, 81.

Harper M. J. K. and Walpole A. L. (1967) Mode of action of ICI 46,474 in preventing implantation in rats. *J. Endocr. 37*, 83–92.

Harrington E. F. (1965) Transportation of ova and zygotes through the genital tract of immature mice treated with gonadotrophins. *Endocrinology 77*, 635–640.

Haspels A. A. (1969) Morning-after pill – a preliminary report. *I. P. P. F. Med. Bull. 3*, 6.

Haspels A. A. (1970) The morning-after pill. *Int. J. Gynaec. Obstet. 8*, 113 (Abstr.).

Heckel G. P. and Allen M. M. (1939) Maintenance of the corpus luteum and inhibition of parturition in the rabbit by injection of estrogenic hormone. *Endocrinology 24*, 137–148.

Hodgson B. J., Fremming B. and Pauerstein C. J. (1974) Effects of oviductal denervation on ovum transport in the rabbit. *Gynecol. Invest. 5*, 15.

Horton E. W., Main I. H. M. and Thompson C. J. (1965) Effects of prostaglandins on the oviduct, studied in rabbits and ewes. *J. Physiol. (Lond.) 180*, 514–528.

Horton E. W. and Marley P. B. (1969) An investigation of the possible effects of prostaglandins E_1, $F_{2\alpha}$ and $F_{2\beta}$ on pregnancy in mice and rabbits. *Brit. J. Pharmacol. 36*, 188P–189P.

Jensen E. N. (1968) Antifertility properties of two diphenylethylenes. *Acta Pharmacol. Toxicol. 26*, Suppl. 1, p. 1–97.

Kamboj V. P., Chandra H., Setty B. S. and Kar A. B. (1970) Biological properties of 2-phenyl-3-p-(β-pyrrolidinoethoxy)-phenyl-(2:1,b)naphthofuran – a new oral antifertility agent. *Contraception 1*, 29–45.

Kamboj V. P. and Kar A. B. (1966) Anti-implantation effect of some aromatic sulphur derivatives. *Indian J. exp. Biol. 4*, 120–121.

Kar A. B., Setty B. S. and Kamboj V. P. (1968) Post-coital contraception by topical application of some steroidal and non-steroidal agents. *Amer. J. Obstet. Gynec. 102*, 306–307.

Kendle K. E. (1969) *Some pharmacological studies upon the factors controlling egg transport through the mouse oviduct*. Ph. D. Thesis. University of London.

Kendle K. E. and Bennett J. P. (1969a) Studies upon the mechanism of reserpine induced arrest of egg transport in the mouse oviduct. *J. Reprod. Fertil. 20*, 429–434.

Kendle K. E. and Bennett J. P. (1969b) Studies upon the mechanism of reserpine induced arrest in egg transport in the mouse oviduct. II. Comparative effects of some agents with actions on smooth muscle and tissue amines. *J. Reprod. Fertil. 20*, 435–441..

Ketchel M. M. and Pincus G. (1964) *In vivo* exposure of rabbit ova to estrogens. *Proc. Soc. exp. Biol. Med. 115*, 419–424.

Koester H. (1969) Tubal secretion and egg development. In: Raspé G., ed. *Advances in the Biosciences: Mechanisms Involved in Conception*, Vol. 4, pp. 181–187.

Koester H. (1970) Ovum transport. In: Gibian H. and Plotz E. J., eds. *Mammalian Reproduction*, pp. 189–228. Springer-Verlag, New York.

Kuchera L. K. (1971) Postcoital contraception with diethylstilbestrol. *J. Amer. med. Ass. 218*, 562–563.

Labhsetwar A. P. (1972) Effects of prostaglandin $F_{2\alpha}$ on some reproductive processes of hamsters and rats. *J. Endocr. 53*, 201–213.

Labhsetwar A. P. (1973) Effects of prostaglandins E_1, E_2 and $F_{2\alpha}$ on zygote transport in rats: Induction of delayed implantation. *Prostaglandins 4*, 115–125.

Lednicer D., Lyster S. C. and Duncan G. W. (1965) Mammalian antifertility agents II. Basic ethers of 3,4-diphenyl coumarins. *J. Med. Chem. 8*, 725–726.

Lerner L. J., Holthaus F. J. and Thompson C. R. (1958) A nonsteroidal estrogen antagonist 1-(p-2-diethylamino-ethoxyphenyl) 1-phenyl-2-p-methoxyphenol ethanol. *Endocrinology 63*, 295–318.

Liu T. C., Cho C., Chu L. C., Chen L. R., Cheng K. T., Sun I., Chiang K. T. and Ma T. N. (1970) Effect of prostaglandins $F_{2\alpha}$ and E_2 on fertilized ovum transport in the mice. *Acta Zool. Sin. 20*, 1–7.

Miyake R. and Takeda K. (1967) Epithioandrostanol, a new type of anti-estrogen. In: Martini L., Fraschini F. and Motta M., eds. *Proceedings of the Second International Congress on Hormonal Steroids, Milan*, pp. 616–627. Excerpta Medica, Amsterdam.

Morris J. M. and Dorfman R. I. (1971) The antifertility activity of *dl*-cis-bisdehydro-isynolic acid methyl ether. *Contraception 4*, 15–22.

Morris J. M. and Van Wagenen G. (1967a) Compounds interfering with ovum implantation and development. In: Westin B. and Wiqvist N., eds. *Proceedings of the Fifth World Congress on Fertility and Sterility*, Stockholm, June 1966, pp. 406–410. Excerpta Medica, Amsterdam, Series No. 133.

Morris J. M. and Van Wagenen G. (1967b) Postcoital oral contraception. In: Hankinson R. K. B., Kleinman R. L., Eckstein R. and Romero H., eds. *Proceedings of the 8th International Conference of the International Planned Parenthood Federation*, Santiago, Chile, April 9, 1967, pp. 256–259. International Planned Parenthood Federation, London.

Morris J. M., Van Wagenen G., Hurteau D. G., Johnston D. W. and Carlsen R. A. (1967a) Compounds interfering with ovum implantation and development. I. Alkaloids and antimetabolites. *Fertil. Steril. 18*, 7–17.

Morris J. M., Van Wagenen G., McCann T. and Jacob D. (1967b) Compounds interfering with ovum implantation and development. II. Synthetic estrogens and anti-estrogens. *Fertil. Steril. 18*, 18–34.

Nutting E. F. (1969) Antifertility activity of prostaglandin E_2 in hamsters, rabbits and rats. *Proc. Soc. Study Reprod.*, 2nd Meeting. Davis, Calif., p. 1.

Nutting E. F. and Cammarata P. S. (1969) Effects of prostaglandins on fertility in female rats. *Nature (Lond.) 222*, 287–288.

Parkes A. S. and Bellerby C. W. (1926) Studies on the internal secretions of the ovary. 2. The effects of injection of the estrus producing hormone during pregnancy. *J. Physiol. (Lond.) 62*, 145–155.

Pauerstein C. J. (1974) *The Fallopian Tube: A Reappraisal*, Ch. 3, pp. 29–68. Lea & Febiger, Philadelphia.

Pauerstein C. J., Fremming B. D. and Martin J. E. (1970) Estrogen induced tubal arrest of ovum: Antagonism by alpha adrenergic blockade. *Obstet. Gynec. 35*, 671–675.

Petrow V. (1966) Steroidal oral contraceptive agents. *Essays Biochem. 2*, 117–145.

464

Pincus G. (1965) *The Control of Fertility*. Academic Press, New York.

Pincus G., Banik U. K. and Jacques J. (1964) Further studies on implantation inhibitors. *Steroids 4,* 657–676.

Pincus G. and Kirsch R. E. (1936) The sterility in rabbits produced by injections of estrone and related compounds. *Amer. J. Physiol. 115,* 219–228.

Rezabek K., Semonsky M. and Kucharczyk N. (1959) Suppression of conception with D-6-methyl-8-cyanomethylergoline (1) in rats. *Nature (Lond.) 221,* 666–667.

Richart R. M., Neuwirth R. S. and Taylor H. C., Jr. (1972) Experimental studies on Fallopian tube occlusion. In: Richart R. M. and Prager R., eds. *Human Sterilization,* Ch. 31, pp. 360–361. C. C. Thomas, Springfield, Ill.

Robinson T. J. (1951) The control of fertility in Sheep II. *J. Agricult. Sci. (Cambridge) 41,* 6–63.

Rooks W. H., McCalla K. O., Kennedy C. and Dorfman R. I. (1971) The oral antifertility activity of dl-cis-bisdehydrodoisynolic acid methyl ether in rats. *Contraception 3,* 387–392.

Rowson L. E. (1951) Methods of inducing multiple ovulations in cattle. *J. Endocr. 7,* 260–270.

Segal S. J. and Nelson W. O. (1958) An orally active compound with antifertility effects in rats. *Proc. Soc. exp. Biol. Med. 98,* 431–436.

Segal S. J. and Nelson W. O. (1961) Antifertility action of chloramiphene. *Anat. Rec. 139,* 273. (Astr.).

Shelesnyak M. C. (1957) Some experimental studies on the mechanism of ova implantation in the rat. *Recent Progr. Hormone Res. 13,* 269–322.

Smith M. G. (1926) On the interruption of pregnancy in the rat by the injection of ovarian follicular extract. *Bull. Johns Hopkins Hosp. 39,* 203–214.

Spilman C. H. and Harper M. J. K. (1972) Effects of prostaglandins on oviduct motility in conscious rabbits. *Biol. Reprod. 7,* 106. (Abstr.).

Spona J., Matt K. and Schneider W. H. F. (1974) Study on the action of D-norgestrel as a postcoital contraceptive agent. *Contraception 11,* 31–43.

Vickery B. H. and Bennett J. P. (1969) Mechanisms of antifertility action of chlormadinone acetate in the rabbit. *Biol. Reprod. 1,* 372–377.

Wakeling A. (1965) Effect of norethynodrel on spontaneous ovulation and fertilization in adult female rats. *J. Reprod. Fertil. 10,* 1–7.

Watnick A. S., Talksdorf S., Kosierowski J. and Tabachnick I. (1966) Post-ovulatory contraceptive actions of 10β-hydroperoxy-17α-ethynyl-4-estren-17β-ol-3-one (SCH 10015) and norethynodrel. In: Martini L., Fraschini F. and Motta M., eds. *Proceedings of the Second International Congress on Hormonal Steroids,* Milan, p. 83 (Abstr.). Excerpta Medica, International Congress Series III, Amsterdam.

Wislocki G. and Snyder F. (1933) The experimental acceleration of the rate of transport of ova through the Fallopian tube. *Bull. Johns Hopkins Hosp. 52,* 379–386.

Zipper J. A., Medel M., Pastene L. and Rivera M. (1969) Intrauterine installation of chemical cytotoxic agents for tubal sterilization and treatment of functional metrorrhagias. *Int. J. Fertil. 14,* 280–288.

Zipper J. A., Stachetti E. and Medel M. (1970) Human fertility control by transvaginal application of Quinacrine on the Fallopian tube. *Fertil. Steril. 21,* 581–589.

465

SUMMARY OF DISCUSSIONS ON
CONTROL OF OVUM TRANSPORT IN THE OVIDUCT

Reporter: *C. E. Adams*

SUMMARY OF CURRENT KNOWLEDGE

Consideration of the morning's papers led to the conclusion that morphological studies, while having a place in confirming or negating a physiological hypothesis, are in themselves not helpful in defining mechanisms controlling oviductal function. Furthermore, scanning electron microscopic pictures are always subject to artefacts and must be interpreted with caution.

The reported studies on the pattern of ovum transport in various primates were felt to be most useful; however, it was recognized that much still remains to be done to define the best animal model for the human. It will not be necessary to perform comparative studies on pharmacological modification of ovum transport in both baboons and monkeys, since once the normal pattern of transport has been definitely identified, the species in which it most closely resembles the human can be chosen. It was felt that the results obtained to date in non-human primates, while suggestive, cannot be regarded as definitive owing to the poor recovery rate of ova. The fact that missing ova may be in different segments of the oviduct could invalidate the present results.

In the same context, the experiments on the normal rate of ovum transport in women using both surgical and non-surgical techniques are very promising and should be encouraged. It was emphasized that a better method of pinpointing the time of ovulation should be established. Recovery rates of ova from the human oviduct are already excellent (60 %) but may be further improved. It was noted that owing to the difficulty of pinpointing the time of ovulation there still appeared to be some discrepancy between the time taken for ovum transport in women when the data obtained by surgical techniques were compared to those obtained by non-surgical techniques.

The use of copper ovum surrogates in women was felt to be less justified than that of radiopaque plastic ones, owing to the possible toxic effects of the copper especially if some surrogates were expelled into the peritoneal cavity or remained lodged in the oviduct. It was also felt that placement of ovum surrogates in women should be done via laparoscopy wherever possible.

IDENTIFICATION OF NEEDED INFORMATION AND REQUIRED RESEARCH

There was general agreement that further studies are required to determine the normal time course of ovum transport in primates, including man. It was noted that if the rate of ovum recovery is low, interpretation of the results may be hazardous and the conclusions misleading, especially since in monotocous species a 50 % rate of ovum recovery means that in one-half of the cases no ovum is recovered. Undoubtedly, in some cases lack of knowledge of the precise time of ovulation is a serious handicap.

Establishing the normal time course of ovum transport in sub-human primates was considered essential in order to fulfill the following objectives:

1. to identify an animal model for man, if indeed one exists,

2. to establish a baseline against which to compare the effect of pharmacologic agents, and

3. to validate ovum surrogates.

It was considered that the criteria for validating animal models and ovum surrogates should include not only similarity of transport under basal conditions but also a similar response to pharmacologic doses of estrogen and progesterone.

The need for development of a better method of pinpointing the time of ovulation in order to provide the relevant reference point in ovum transport studies was stressed. Additionally, obtaining an endocrine profile was considered important, as it would permit the correlation of hormonal levels with ovulation and thus facilitate the location of ova.

The importance of synchronization of ovum and endometrial development for the successful establishment of pregnancy in experimental animals, including Lagomorphs, Rodents and Ungulates, is now well established. Whether such a strict relationship also applies in Primates is not yet known. Certainly, in women the relatively high incidence of oviductal ectopic pregnancy and reports of pregnancies following Estes' operation indicate that man occupies a unique position with regard to ovum survival under abnormal conditions.

Considerable interest was expressed in the observation on the differential retention of the unfertilized ovum in the oviduct of the mare. The suggestion

467

that the equine embryo may influence in part its own passage through the oviduct through the production of a humoral agent is a novel concept; if proved, it would provide another example of the contribution of the early embryo to the successful establishment of pregnancy. However, from a comparative standpoint, it is necessary to stress that in respect of the retention of unfertilized ova the mare appears to occupy a unique position. Clearly in species where the course of oviductal transport is similar, irrespective of whether or not the ovum (ova) is (are) fertilized, the possibility of the embryo playing an active role would appear remote.

Questions that could be answered experimentally which might resolve these various problems were formulated as follows:

(a) Can ectopic (oviductal) pregnancy be induced experimentally in non-human primates?

(b) Is the timing of the ovum's sojourn in the oviduct critical to fertility in the human?

(c) Do ovum surrogates really mimick normal rate of ovum transport in women? Further comparative studies in women should be performed.

(d) Does the fertilized primate ovum influence the rate of its own transport, or is this phenomenon confined solely to the horse?

ASSESSMENT OF FEASIBILITY AND COST OF SUCH APPROACHES

The major recommendations for future research were as follows:

Further studies on the normal pattern of ovum transport should be made in women, using surgical and non-surgical techniques, and in sub-human primates. The species in which ovum transport most closely resembles that in women should be chosen for further experiments.

High priority should be given to studies of the effects on ovum transport and fertility in sub-human primates of agents known to increase the motility of the oviduct, e. g. sympathomimetics, oxytocin and its analogues, estrogens and anti-estrogens, progestins, prostaglandins and gonadotrophins. The effects of drug combinations should also be determined since this may reduce the incidence of side effects.

Methodology should be developed to enable one to determine more easily the precise time of ovulation.

There is a need to gain an understanding of the mechanisms of oviductal pregnancy in women, and to determine whether oviductal pregnancy can be induced experimentally in sub-human primates.

Studies should be made in sub-human primates to determine whether the precocious entry of the fertilized ovum into the uterus is compatible with its further development and pregnancy.

The success rate of Estes' operation should be evaluated by reviewing available records, published or unpublished, and by keeping careful records of any such operations which may be performed now or in the future.

More funds should be provided for basic studies on oviductal physiology, including secretions.

It was recognized that while experiments involving humans and smaller laboratory animals were likely to be relatively inexpensive, studies using non-human primates could be costly. However, in view of the lack of suitability of the rabbit and in consideration of ethical limitations on human experimentation no other appropriate course of action was available. The various experiments to be undertaken to resolve the problem of oviductal pregnancies in non-human primates might cost at least $150,000/year for 2–3 years. However, such expenditure was regarded as justified in the light of the issues involved.

SECTION V

Effects of Estrogen and Progesterone on Contractility and Ovum Transport

MODERATORS

M. C. CHANG

and

G. S. GREENWALD

Worcester Foundation for Experimental Biology,
Shrewsbury, Massachusetts 01545, USA

ESTROGEN, PROGESTERONE
AND EGG TRANSPORT
– OVERVIEW AND IDENTIFICATION
OF PROBLEMS

By

M. C. Chang

ABSTRACT

This paper attempts to present a broad view, personal experience, and a few pertinent problems concerning the effects of estrogen and progesterone on egg transport for the development of fertility control. Administration of estrogen or other substances with estrogenic activity soon after ovulation can prevent pregnancy by the disturbance of egg transport and endometrial development. Such effects are dependent on compound, dosage, species, and time of administration. Estrogen however does not affect the course of human pregnancy once nidation has taken place. Administration of various progestins before ovulation also disturbs egg transport but the physiological mechanism is obscure. In many species, the uterotubal junction has an anatomical identity but the ampullary-isthmic junction is not distinctive. Although oviductal contractiliy is associated with estrogen and progesterone, its correlation with egg transport is not well demonstrated.

The oviduct is the site of fertilization, a critical phase of reproduction. Its function is to transport spermatozoa upwards and eggs downwards for their union.

It not only plays a role in the capacitation of spermatozoa, which involves many membrane and enzymic changes of spermatozoa, but also in the nourishment of the eggs during their cleavage, which involves again many biochemical reactions. The anatomy, physiology and pathology of the oviduct have been dealt with in several books to which many active research workers have contributed (Funck-Brentano 1955; Hafez and Blandau 1969; Woodruff and Pauerstein 1969; Johnson and Foley 1974). It is hard to give an unbiased review for any topic in connection with the physiology of the oviduct. Surely more findings and many controversies will be revealed during this timely conference. For the development of fertility control this paper attempts to present a broad overview, personal experience, and a few pertinent problems concerning the effects of estrogen and progesterone on egg transport.

I. EFFECT OF ESTROGEN ON EGG TRANSPORT AND IMPLANTATION

About 50 years ago it was reported that pregnancy could be interrupted by injection of "oestrin" in the mouse (Parkes and Bellerby 1926) and by injection of "follicular extract" in the rat (Smith 1926). This observation was confirmed in the guinea pig (Kelly 1931) and the rabbit (Courrier and Raynaud 1934). Since such treatment is more effective soon after ovulation when the eggs are in the oviduct, studies of the estrogenic effect on the development and transport of eggs in the mouse and rabbit (Burdick and Pincus 1935; Whitney and Burdick 1936) and on the fertility of rabbits (Pincus and Kirsch 1936) led to the discovery of so-called "tube-locking" by estrogen treatment. Since the estrogenic tolerance is higher in the rhesus monkey and man (van Wagenen and Morse 1944; Karnaky 1947) than other species and since the time of ovulation is difficult to determine in non-human primates and man, the administration of estrogen to interrupt pregnancy was not used in human medicine until recent years.

In the rabbit, egg transport through the oviduct (Greenwald 1961), interruption of pregnancy by administration of estrogen (Greenwald 1957), comparative effectiveness of various estrogens in interrupting pregnancy (Greenwald 1959) and species differences in egg transport in response to exogenous estrogen (Greenwald 1967) have been systematically investigated. However, a recent study of egg transport in the rabbit which used a freeze-clearing technique, produced data which differed from those obtained by oviductal flushings or autoradiography. This study indicated that the primary site for sphincteric activity was the uterotubal junction rather than the ampullary-isthmic junction (Howe 1970).

In my early experiments (Chang 1959, 1964) of the study of antifertility drugs (Segal and Nelson 1958; Duncan et al. 1962; Duncan and Lyster 1963), norethynodrel, clomiphene or a diphenylindene (U-11555A) were administered to rabbits for 3 days after insemination. The retention of eggs in the oviducts, rapid egg transport into the uterus and expulsion of eggs from the uterus were observed. These are very similar to what happened in the estrogen-treated rabbits. But when 6-day blastocysts from the untreated animals were transferred into the uterus of treated pseudopregnant rabbits, implantation and normal development was also disturbed in the animals treated with norethynodrel and diphenylindene but not with clomiphene (Chang 1964). This shows that these two compounds not only disturbed egg transport but also disturbed the physiological integrity of the endometrium required for proper implantation. Following treatments of an A-norsteroid (H241) which has estrogenic activity, estradiol cyclopentylpropionate (ECP), estrone, and diphenyl-dihydronaphthalene (U-11100A) for 3 days after mating in rabbits and hamsters, it was found that a higher dose level was required for the prevention of pregnancy in the hamster and that natural estrogen or other substances with estrogenic activity would be effective as antifertility compounds (Chang and Yanagimachi 1965). These observations are in agreement with those reported by Stone and Emmens (1964) and Emmens (1965) for the mouse and by Banik and Pincus (1964) for the rat.

The effectiveness of oral adminstration of ethinyl estradiol on egg transport and development in the rabbit was investigated by Chang and Harper (1966). We found that ethinyl estradiol is more effective than other estrogens and there is no difference in embryonic development whether the early blastocysts of treated animals were transferred to the uterus of normal rabbits or vice versa. Degeneration and disappearance of fertilized eggs and the failure of blastocyst formation were found in rabbits that had a Silastic tube containing estrogen implanted under the skin, but this did not occur with progestins (Chang et al. 1970). However, normal development occurred following transfer of early blastocysts from estrogen-implanted animals to untreated animals, but not following transfer of blastocysts from untreated animals to estrogen-implanted animals (Chang et al. 1971). This shows that prolonged estrogen treatment not only disturbs egg transport but also disturbs normal function of the endometrium for implantation and embryonic development. Although many contradictory facts have been reported concerning the effect of estrogen on egg transport I should like to repeat my previous statement once again; that "when administered before ovulation estrogen has no obvious effects on fertilization and development of eggs. When administered soon after ovulation and fertilization, it can interrupt pregnancy by different mechanisms, depending on the dosage of the particular compounds used, the species used for testing and, above all, on the time of administration" (Chang 1967a).

II. ESTROGENS AS POSTCOITAL CONTRACEPTIVES

Although estrogen affects the motility (Coutinho 1971), fluid flow (Mastroianni et al. 1961) and ciliary activity (Brenner 1969) of the oviduct in primates and women, "there is no evidence that estrogen alters egg transport in primates including man" (Blye 1973). This, however, still requires scientific investigation.

Morris and van Wagenen (1966) reported that 25 to 50 mg diethylstilbestrol or 2 to 5 mg ethinyl estradiol administered for the first few days following unprotected midcycle coital exposure was effective in preventing pregnancy. Haspels (1970) reported that following treatment with 5 mg ethinyl estradiol or 50 mg diethylstilbestrol daily administered within 48 h of coitus, no pregnancy was observed in a large number of women. Kuchera (1971) found that no pregnancy occurred after treatment with 50 mg diethylstilbestrol daily for 5 days starting within 72 h after coitus. Udry (1972) estimated that the over-all risk of pregnancy among those untreated women was about 1 in 10, and that therefore treatment with estrogen as a postcoital contraceptive was highly efficacious.

Based upon the reports that estrogen administered in the middle of the cycle reduced plasma progesterone (Board and Bhatnager 1971) and decreased the thermogenic effect of progesterone (Morris and van Wagenen 1967), Blye (1973) remarked that if estrogen is luteolytic in women as in other species, then its administration at the critical stage for the developing corpus luteum may prevent human pregnancy. Since proper implantation requires precisely timed developmental stages of both the embryo and the endometrium (Chang 1950), estrogen, provided that it does not disturb egg transport in women, could upset the process of implantation. Data concerning the estrogenic activity and the effectiveness of various estrogens as postcoital contraceptives have been compiled by Blye (1973). He concluded that "once nidation has taken place, exogenous estrogen does not affect the course of human pregnancy" and that "oral administration of estrogen should be instituted as soon as possible after coitus." To my mind the administration should be started soon after ovulation rather than soon after coitus. In this case, the determination of time of ovulation becomes of extreme importance for treatment with estrogen to provide effective contraception.

III. EFFECT OF PROGESTERONE ON EGG TRANSPORT

It takes about 3 to 4 days for the egg to reach the uterus in most mammals, regardless of the length of the oviduct (Hartman 1962). In the rabbit egg transport through the ampulla to the isthmus of the oviduct takes only a few minutes (Harper 1961, 1965) but 3 to 4 days are required for transport to the uterus

(Gregory 1930). Obviously, progesterone secreted from the developing corpus luteum must play an important role in the regulation of egg transport. The transport of eggs in cumulus through the ampulla of the rabbit oviduct was faster in estrus and at ovulation than during pseudopregnancy (Harper 1965). Ovariectomy decreased the rate of transport, and this was significantly further decreased by injection of progesterone; estrogen, however, restored the rate of transport (Harper 1966). Greenwald (1968) stated that "probably increasing levels of progesterone depress the muscular activity of the ampulla and so account for the retardation in the rate of egg transport." Recent systematic study of muscular contraction and egg transport in the rabbit led Boling and Blandau (1971) to conclude that "the acceleration of egg transport at the time of ovulation may be related to an increase in the secretion of progestins and fall in the level of estrogen."

As for the egg transport from the oviduct to the uterus, acceleration in pregnant and pseudopregnant rabbits was reported by Wislocki and Snyder (1933) showing that egg transport is affected by the corpus luteum. Black and Asdell (1959) reported acceleration of egg transport due to administration of progesterone to rabbits, but Adams (1958) described a delay of egg transport caused by injection of progesterone soon after ovariectomy.

A single injection of 5 mg progesterone given soon after mating accelerated egg transport through the oviduct of rabbits, but no eggs entered the uterus within 2 days after mating; a single injection of 25 mg progesterone caused an even more pronounced acceleration of egg transport within the tube but only one of 5 rabbits had her eggs in the uterus two days after mating; even with injection of 1 to 100 mg Delalutin®, a long-lasting progestin, only one of 12 rabbits had half the number of her eggs reaching the uterus (Greenwald 1961). It appears that following administration of progesterone after ovulation, egg transport from the oviduct to the uterus is not necessarily accelerated.

When 2 mg progesterone was given for 3 days before ovulation, however, 50 % of the eggs were found in the uterus of rabbits 12 h after ovulation (Chang and Bedford 1961). Further study revealed that disturbance of egg transport and degeneration of eggs were caused by administration of progestin before ovulation but not after ovulation, and that the effect of progestin administered before ovulation was very similar to that of estrogen administered after ovulation (Chang 1966a). From studies in which fertilized 1-day eggs were transferred into the ampullae of estrous non-ovulated rabbits treated with estrogen or progestin and the locations of the eggs examined at various times after transfer, it was concluded that endogenous or exogenous estrogen causes rapid egg transport from the oviduct to the uterus, while endogenous or exogenous progesterone counteracts the estrogenic effect and delays egg transport (Chang 1966b). The rapid egg transport after administration of progesterone before ovulation can be explained by a physiological "recovery" or "adaptation" of

477

the oviduct from the initial stimulation by progesterone. It may also be related to changes in the prostaglandin F level in the oviduct (Saksena and Harper 1975) but the physiological mechanism of such action is still obscure.

Further study of the effects of progesterone and related compounds administered before ovulation showed that their major effect is on egg transport, causing some disturbance of fertilization but mainly causing degeneration of the eggs in the uterus and their expulsion from the uterus (Chang 1967b). In the ferret the administration of medroxyprogesterone acetate before ovulation inhibited fertilization and hastened egg transport from the oviduct to the uterus; administration of estrogen after ovulation, however, had no effect on fertilization and egg transport but adversely affected embryonic survival (Chang 1967c). For this reason it has been suggested that accelerated transport of eggs from the oviduct to the uterus due to administration of progesterone before ovulation is not a universal phenomenon (Woodruff and Pauerstein 1969, page 99). In fact, following injection of pigs with progesterone 36 h before ovulation, 77 % of the eggs were recovered from the uterus 8 h after ovulation (Day and Polge 1968). How to use this knowledge for the development of a pre-ovulatory pill is a problem for consideration. Moreover, the effectiveness of the present pills given for 20 days during the menstrual cycle has been attributed not only to the inhibition of ovulation but also to the disturbance of gamete transport, fertilization and development of early embryos (Chang 1967a,b). In this respect, it would be the task of competent chemists and endocrinologists to find more effective drugs that can disturb gamete transport, fertilization, embryonic development, and implantation, without other side effects.

IV. AMPULLARY-ISTHMIC JUNCTION AND UTEROTUBAL JUNCTION

The uterotubal junction has an anatomical identity in many species (Hafez and Black 1969) but the ampullary-isthmic junction of the oviduct in the rabbit and other species is not so distinctive as in the mouse (Reinius 1969). If the ampullary-isthmic junction has the function to trap eggs in this portion of the oviduct, one can consider it as a physiological activity at this part of the oviduct rather than an anatomical obstruction. However, the critical time to interfere with egg transport is probably during the egg's passage from the oviduct to the uterus rather than during passage within the oviduct. Eggs can survive and develop in the oviduct for a long time, not only in the same species (Adams 1958) but also in the oviducts of different species (Hunter et al. 1962; Chang 1966c). Retention of eggs in the oviduct, however, is obviously not a good method for fertility control because of the hazard of oviductal pregnancy in women. The entry of eggs into the uterus, however, must be accurately timed for the subsequent development and implantation of the eggs.

The importance of egg transport in the oviduct for the regulation of fertility is based on the fact or assumption that the properly timed passage of the zygote, is of importance to normal implantation and pregnancy. If spermatozoa can fertilize eggs in the uterus and if fertilized eggs can develop and implant normally whenever they reach the uterus, then the study of egg transport through the oviduct is not as important as we may think. In the rabbit, fertilization can take place in the uterus but such fertilized eggs degenerate soon after fertilization (Chang 1955). In the hamster fertilization cannot take place in the uterus (Hunter 1968) and only a few eggs can be fertilized in the uterus with signs of early degeneration (Miyamoto and Chang 1973). In the human, the Estes' operation is well known (Estes 1924; Preston 1953) and an oviductal prosthesis which effectively places the ovary in contact with the uterine cavity for the restoration of fertility in women was again advocated recently (Taylor 1971). In this respect whether the importance of the oviduct and its function to transport eggs properly in women is as important as in other species should be determined.

V. STUDY OF OVIDUCTAL CONTRACTILITY AND FLUID FLOW

It is well known that the motility and contractions of the female tract are greater during the follicular phase than during the luteal phase and that estrogen increases and progesterone decreases such activities. A recent study has shown that alpha-receptors in the oviduct are stimulatory and beta-receptors are inhibitory and that estrogen potentiates alpha-receptors and progesterone potentiates the beta-receptors (Howe and Black 1973). However, it has been stated that "the changes in tubal motility are not necessarily associated with the rate of egg transport" (Greenwald 1968) and that "in addition to the disparate descriptions of the patterns of cyclic contractile activity and of the responses to administration of estrogen and progesterone, the relationship of contractile activity to ovum transport remained enigmatic" (Woodruff and Pauerstein 1969, page 92). Such statements lead us to question the importance of studying motility or contractility of the female tract without paying attention to gamete transport and egg development. If, as I have pointed out before, the critical point is the egg transport from the oviduct to the uterus, then we should pay more attention to the physiological activity of the oviduct 3 to 4 days after ovulation when the eggs pass to the uterus and try to devise measures to interfere at this time for contraceptive purposes.

From the observations of Hafez (1963), it seems that normal flow of fluid in the rabbit oviduct proceeds mainly in the direction of the peritoneal cavity except during the third or fourth day after mating. In the ewe (Bellve and

McDonald 1970) and cow (Carlson et al. 1970; Stanke et al. 1973) the maximal flow from the ovarian end and the maximal flow through the uterine end appears to be influenced by estrogen and progesterone. If the oviductal fluid, especially its direction, plays a role in egg transport from the oviduct to the uterus, investigation along this line should be undertaken, especially in non-human primates and man for the understanding of gamete transport and for the development of contraceptive measures. Moreover, considering the possibility that the unfertilized human egg reaches the uterus earlier than the fertilized egg (Croxatto et al. 1972) while unfertilized mare eggs are retained in the oviduct (Van Niekerk and Gerneke 1966; Betteridge and Mitchell 1974), one wonders whether or not the transport of eggs through the oviduct is also affected by the physiological condition of the eggs.

In conclusion I should like to refer to one of our pioneers in reproductive biology, Dr. Blandau (1973) who made the pertinent remark that although much information has been gathered in the study of gamete transport through the oviduct in different species, facts, assumptions and guesses are very mixed up. He particularly cautioned us about the danger of transfer of information from one species to another. I would like us all to bear his remarks in mind.

ACKNOWLEDGMENT

The writer is a recipient of a research career Award (HD 18,334) of National Institute of Child Health and Human Development.

REFERENCES

Adams C. E. (1958) Egg development in the rabbit: The influence of post-coital ligation of the uterine tube and ovariectomy. *J. Endocr. 16*, 283–293.

Banik U. K. and Pincus G. (1964) Estrogen and transport of ova in the rat. *Proc. Soc. exp. Biol. Med. 116*, 1032–1034.

Bellve A. R. and McDonald M. F. (1970) Directional flow of Fallopian tube secretion in the ewe at onset of the breeding season. *J. Reprod. Fertil. 22*, 147–149.

Betteridge K. J. and Mitchell D. (1974) Direct evidence of retention of unfertilized ova in the oviduct of the mare. *J. Reprod. Fertil. 39*, 145–148.

Black D. L. and Asdell S. A. (1959) Mechanism controlling entrance of ova into rabbit uterus. *Amer. J. Physiol. 197*, 1275–1278.

Blandau R. J. (1973) Gamete transport in the female mammal. In: Greep R. O. and Astwood E. B., eds. *Handbook of Physiology*, Chap. 38, pp. 153–163. The William & Wilkins Co., Baltimore.

Blye R. P. (1973) The use of estrogens as postcoital contraceptive agents. Clinical effectiveness and mode of action. *Amer. J. Obstet. Gynec. 116*, 1044–1050.

Board J. A. and Bhatnager A. S. (1971) Abstract. *7th Annual Meeting of the Southern Gynec. and Obstet. Society*, Miami Beach, Florida.

Boling J. L. and Blandau R. J. (1971) Egg transport through the ampulla of oviducts of rabbits under various experimental conditions. *Biol. Reprod. 4*, 174–184.

Brenner R. M. (1969) The biology of oviduct cilia. In: Hafez E. S. E. and Blandau R. J., eds. *The Mammalian Oviduct*, pp. 203–213. The University of Chicago Press, Chicago.

Burdick H. O. and Pincus G. (1935) The effect of oestrin injection upon the developing ova of mice and rabbits. *Amer. J. Physiol. 111*, 201–208.

Carlson D., Black D. L. and Howe G. R. (1970) Oviduct secretion in the cow. *J. Reprod. Fertil. 22*, 549–552.

Chang M. C. (1950) Development and fate of transferred rabbit ova or blastocyst in relation to the ovulation time of recipients. *J. exp. Zool. 114*, 197–216.

Chang M. C. (1955) Développement de la capacité fertilisatrice des spermatozoides du lapin a l'intérieur du tractus génital femelle et fécondabilité des oeufs de lapine. In: Funck-Brentano P., ed. *La Fonction Tubaire et Ses Troubles*, pp. 40–52. Masson & Cie, Paris.

Chang M. C. (1959) Degeneration of ova in the rat and rabbit following oral administration of (p-2 diethylaminoethoxyphenyl)-1-phenyl-2-p-anisylethanol. *Endocrinology 65*, 339–342.

Chang M. C. (1964) Effects of certain antifertility agents on the development of rabbit ova. *Fertil. Steril. 15*, 97–106.

Chang M. C. (1966a) Effects of oral administration of medroxyprogesterone acetate and ethinyl estradiol on the transportation and development of rabbit eggs. *Endocrinology 79*, 939–948.

Chang M. C. (1966b) Transport of eggs from the Fallopian tube to the uterus as a function of oestrogen. *Nature (Lond.) 212*, 1048–1049.

Chang M. C. (1966c) Reciprocal transplantation of eggs between rabbit and ferret. *J. exp. Zool. 161*, 297–306.

Chang M. C. (1967a) Physiological mechanisms responsible for the effectiveness of oral contraceptives. *Proc. 8th Int. Conf. Planned Parenthood Fed.*, Santagio, Chile, pp. 386–392.

Chang M. C. (1967b) Effects of progesterone and related compounds on fertilization, transportation and development of rabbit eggs. *Endocrinology 81*, 1251–1260.

Chang M. C. (1967c) Effects of medroxyprogesterone acetate and ethinyl oestradiol on the fertilization and transportation of ferret eggs. *J. Reprod. Fertil. 13*, 173–174.

Chang M. C. and Bedford J. M. (1961) Effects of various hormones on the transportation of gametes and fertilization in the rabbit. *Proc. IVth Int. Cong. Anim. Reprod.*, The Hague *1*, 367–370.

Chang M. C. and Harper M. J. K. (1966) Effects of ethinyl estradiol on egg transport and development in the rabbit. *Endocrinology 78*, 860–872.

Chang M. C. and Yanagimachi R. (1965) Effect of estrogens and other compounds as oral antifertility agents on the development of rabbit ova and hamster embryos. *Fertil. Steril. 16*, 281–291.

Chang M. C., Casas J. H. and Hunt D. M. (1970) Prevention of pregnancy in the rabbit by subcutaneous implantation of Silastic tube containing oestrogen. *Nature (Lond.) 226*, 1262–1265.

Chang M. C., Casas J. H. and Hunt D. M. (1971) Suppression of pregnancy in the rabbit by subcutaneous implantation of Silastic tubes containing various estrogenic compounds. *Fertil. Steril. 22*, 383–388.

481

Courrier R. and Raynaud R. (1934) Expériences d'antagonisme humoral ovarien réalises avec l'etalon internationale de folliculine cristallisée. *C. R. Soc. Biol. (Paris) 115*, 299–302.

Coutinho E. M. (1971) Tubal and uterine motility. In: Diczfalusy E. and Borell U., eds. *Control of Human Fertility. Proc. 15th Nobel Symposium*, pp. 97–115. Almqvist & Wiksell, Stockholm: John Wiley and Sons, New York.

Croxatto H. B., Diaz S., Fuentealba B., Croxatto H. D., Carrillo D. and Fabres C. (1972) Studies on the duration of egg transport in the human oviduct. I. The time interval between ovulation and egg recovery from the uterus in normal women. *Fertil. Steril. 23*, 447–458.

Day B. N. and Polge C. (1968) Effect of progesterone on fertilization and egg transport in pig. *J. Reprod. Fertil. 17*, 227–230.

Duncan G. W. and Lyster S. C. (1963) Effect of a diphenylindene derivative (U-11555A) on blastocyst survival *in utero. Fertil. Steril. 14*, 565–571.

Duncan G. W., Stucki J. C., Lyster S. C. and Lednicer D. (1962) An oral effective antifertility agent. *Proc. Soc. exp. Biol. Med. 109*, 163–166.

Emmens G. W. (1965) Oestrogenic, anti-oestrogenic and antifertility activities of various compounds. *J. Reprod. Fertil. 9*, 277–283.

Estes W. L. (1924) Ovarian implantation. *Surg. Gynec. Obstet. 38*, 394.

Funck-Brentano P. (1955) *La Fonction Tubaire et ses Troubles.* Masson & Cie, Paris.

Greenwald G. S. (1957) Interruption of pregnancy in the rabbit by administration of estrogen. *J. exp. Zool. 135*, 461–482.

Greenwald G. S. (1959) The comparative effectiveness of estrogens in interrupting pregnancy in the rabbit. *Fertil. Steril. 10*, 115–161.

Greenwald G. S. (1961) A study of the transport of ova through the oviduct. *Fertil. Steril. 12*, 80–95.

Greenwald G. S. (1967) Species differences in egg transport in response to exogenous estrogen. *Anat. Rec. 157*, 163–172.

Greenwald G. S. (1968) Hormonal regulation of egg transport through the mammalian oviduct. In: Behrman S. J. and Kistner R. W., eds. *Progress in Infertility*, pp. 157–179. Little Brown and Co., Boston.

Gregory P. W. (1930) The early embryology of the rabbit. *Contr. Embryol. Carneg. Instn 21*, 141–168.

Hafez E. S. E. (1963) The uterotubal junction and the luminal fluid of uterine tube in the rabbit. *Anat. Rec. 145*, 7–12.

Haftz E. S. E. and Black D. L. (1969) The mammalian uterotubal junction. In: Hafez E. S. E. and Blandau R. J., eds. *The Mammalian Oviduct*, pp. 85–120. The University of Chicago Press, Chicago.

Hafez E. S. E. and Blandau R. J. (1969) *The Mammalian Oviduct.* The University of Chicago Press, Chicaco.

Harper M. J. K. (1961) The mechanism involved in the movement of newly ovulated eggs through the ampulla of the rabbit Fallopian tube. *J. Reprod. Fertil. 2*, 522–524.

Harper M. J. K. (1965) Transport of eggs in cumulus through the ampulla of rabbit oviduct in relation to day of pseudopregnancy. *Endocrinology 77*, 114–123.

Harper M. J. K. (1966) Hormonal control of transport of eggs in cumulus through the ampulla of the rabbit oviduct. *Endocrinology 78*, 568–574.

Hartman C. G. (1962) *Science and the Safe Period.* The Williams & Wilkins Co., Baltimore.

Haspels A. A. (1970) *Proc. VIth World Congress of Gynec. Obstet.*, New York. Abstract no. 9.

Howe G. R. (1970) A study of egg transport in the rabbit using a freezing-clearing technique. *J. Reprod. Fertil. 21*, 339–341.

Howe G. R. and Black D. L. (1973) Autonomic nervous system and oviduct function in the rabbit. *J. Reprod. Fertil. 33*, 425–430.

Hunter R. H. F. (1968) Attempted fertilization of hamster eggs following transplantation into the uterus. *J. exp. Zool. 168*, 511–516.

Hunter G. L., Bishop G. P., Adams C. E. and Rowson L. E. A. (1962) Successful long-distance aerial transport of fertilized sheep ova. *J. Reprod. Fertil. 3*, 33–40.

Johnson A. D. and Foley C. W. (1974) *The Oviduct and its Functions.* Academic Press, New York and London.

Karnaky K. J. (1947) Estrogenic tolerance in pregnant women. *Amer. J. Obstet. Gynec. 53*, 312–316.

Kelly G. L. (1931) The effect of injections of female sex hormone (oestrin) on conception and pregnancy in the guinea pig. *Surg. Gynec. Obstet. 52*, 713–722.

Kuchera L. K. (1971) Postcoital contraception with diethylstilbestrol. *J. Amer. med. Ass. 218*, 562–563.

Mastroianni L., Shah U. and Abdul-Karim R. (1961) Prolonged volumetric collection of oviduct fluid in the Rhesus monkey. *Fertil. Steril. 12*, 417–424.

Miyamoto H. and Chang M. C. (1973) Fertilization of golden hamster eggs in the uterus. *J. Reprod. Fertil. 34*, 183–185.

Morris J. M. and van Wagenen G. (1966) Compounds interfering with ovum transplantation and development. *Amer. J. Obstet. Gynec. 96*, 804–813.

Morris J. M. and van Wagenen G. (1967) Post-coital oral contraception. *Proc. 8th Int. Conf. Planned Parenthood Fed.*, Santiago, Chile, pp. 256–259.

Parkes A. S. and Bellerby C. W. (1926) Studies of the internal secretions of the ovary. II. The effects of injection of the oestrus producing hormone during pregnancy. *J. Physiol. (Lond.) 62*, 145–155.

Pincus G. and Kirsch R. E. (1936) The sterility in rabbits produced by injections of oestrone and related compounds. *Amer. J. Physiol. 115*, 219–228.

Preston P. G. (1953) Transplantation of the ovary into the uterine cavity for the treatment of sterility in women. *J. Obset. Gynec. Brit. Cwlth 60*, 862.

Reinius S. (1969) *Morphology of Oviduct: Gametes and Zygotes as a Basis of Oviductal Function in the Mouse.* University of Uppsala. Almqvist & Wiksells Boktryckeri AB, Uppsala, Sweden.

Saksena S. K. and Harper M. J. K. (1975) Relationship between concentration of prostaglandin F in the oviduct and egg transport in rabbit. *Biol. Reprod. 13*, 68–76.

Segal S. J. and Nelson W. O. (1958) An orally active compound with anti-fertility effects in rats. *Proc. Soc. exp. Biol. Med. 98*, 431–436.

Smith Margaret G. (1926) On the interruption of pregnancy by injection of ovarian follicular extract. *Bull. Johns Hopk. Hosp. 39*, 204–214.

Stanke D. F., DeYoung D. W., Sikes J. D. and Mather E. C. (1973) Collection of bovine oviduct secretions. *J. Reprod. Fertil. 32*, 535–537.

Stone G. M. and Emmens C. W. (1964) The action of oestradiol and dimethylstilb-oestrol on early pregnancy and deciduoma formation in the mouse. *J. Endocr. 29*, 137–145.

Taylor R. (1971) The development of an artificial Fallopian tube. *J. Reprod. Fertil. 24*, 125 (abstract).

Udry J. R. (1972) 1,000 women use post-coital pills: No babies. *Family Planning Digest* *1*, 4.

Van Niekerk C. H. and Gerneke W. H. (1966) Persistence and parthenogenetic cleavage of tubal ova in the mare. *Onderstepoort J. vet. Res. 33*, 195–323.

van Wagenen G. and Morse A. H. (1944) Estrogen tolerance in pregnancy. *Yale J. Biol. Med. 17*, 301–309.

Whitney R. and Burdick H. O. (1936) Tube-locking of ova by oestrogenic substances. *Endocrinology 20*, 643–647.

Wislocki G. B. and Snyder F. F. (1933) The experimental acceleration of the rate of transport of ova through the Fallopian tube. *Bull. Johns Hopk. Hosp. 52*, 379–386.

Woodruff J. D. and Pauerstein C. J. (1969) *Fallopian Tube: Structure, Function, Pathology and Management*. Williams & Wilkins Co., Baltimore.

Dept. of Obstetrics & Gynecology
and Center for the Study of Reproductive Biology (CEBRE),
J. J. Aguirre Hospital, University of Chile, P. O. Box 6637, Santiago, Chile

IN VIVO HUMAN OVIDUCTAL MOTILITY:
EFFECTS OF ESTROGEN AND PROGESTERONE

By

Enrique Guiloff-Fische, Andrés Ibarra-Polo
and Carlos Gómez-Rogers

ABSTRACT

The effect of progesterone and estradiol valerate on oviductal motility
was investigated in 23 women by chronic recording of intraluminal
pressure with the microballoon technique. A total of 110 recording sessions comprising 164 hours were analyzed.

Treatment with 100 or 200 mg progesterone or with 10 or 20 mg estradiol
valerate increased the plasma levels of progesterone or estrogen respectively as determined by radioimmunoassay.

The number of outbursts per hour (Burst Hour Index) and the area under
the curve in ten min periods (Oviductal Activity), were used to quantitate
oviductal motility in the tracings.

In 12 patients treated with estrogen, no definite changes in oviductal
motility were seen; however, in 11 patients under progesterone treatment,
a consistent and significant increase in oviductal motility was observed.
It was concluded that pharmacological doses of estrogen and progesterone
have a different effect upon human oviductal motility *in vivo*.

It seems clear that oviductal responses to the female sex hormones are influenced to a great extent by the species under consideration, the dose given
and the time of treatment relative to ovulation (Pauerstein et al. 1974).

This study was supported by Research Grant H9/181/117(A) from The World Health
Organization.

Marked species differences in the oviductal response to estrogen and progesterone prevent one from extrapolating to the human species results obtained in other mammals.

Studies relating hormonal profiles to oviductal motility in women are scarce and controversial. Some of them report a predictable pattern of oviductal contractility responding to hormonal changes of the cycle (Rubin 1939, 1947; Coutinho and Maia 1970), whereas variability of oviductal contractions at different stages of the ovarian cycle has been observed by others (Sica Blanco et al. 1970, 1972; Ibarra-Polo, unpublished data). Megestrol acetate, a synthetic progestin, has been reported as having a relaxing and quiescent effect, when studied through chronic recordings of oviductal motility (Coutinho et al. 1975), but to our knowledge no other studies on the effect of exogenous steroids on human oviductal motility have been reported.

The purpose of the present work was to assess the effect of pharmacological doses of estrogen and progesterone upon the *in vivo* muscular activity of the oviduct in women.

MATERIALS AND METHODS

Twenty-three multiparous women who had requested surgical sterilization were selected for this study. Informed consent of the patients was obtained according to the guidelines given in the Helsinki Declaration. The sterilization procedure was approved by the Ethics Committee of our Department.

The methodology to record intratubal pressure was the same for all patients and has already been described (Maia and Coutinho 1968).

The quantification of oviductal contractility in the tracings was made by:

1.– *The Burst Hour Index:* (BHI). This is defined as the number of bursts of contractions in 60 min.

2.– *Oviductal Activity:* (OA). This is the area above the base line measured by planimetry. The results were expressed as square millimeters per 10 min.

Recordings were obtained at different stages of the cycle. The drug effects were evaluated comparing the recordings made 24 and/or 48 h before, and 24 and/or 48 h after treatment. Differences in the mean BHI and OA were analysed statistically, and P values less than 0.05 were considered significant.

Hormones and dosage used were:

A) Estradiol Valerate*, 10 mg. i. m. in a single dose in 3 patients, and 10 mg. i. m. every 12 h (total dose 20 mg.) in 9 patients,

---

* Primofol Depot®, Schering A. G., Berlin, Germany.

B) Progesterone, 100 mg. i. m. in a single dose in 3 patients, and 100 mg. i. m. every 12 h (total dose 200 mg.) in 8 patients. Both hormones were injected dissolved in vegetable oil.

In order to evaluate the hormonal changes induced by these compounds, blood samples were obtained before and 24 and/or 48 h after their administration.

Progesterone plasma levels were measured by the radioimmunoassay procedures described by Thorneycroft and Stone (1972). Estrogens were measured in plasma by the radioimmunoassay procedure described by Edqvist and Johansson (1972). The chromatographic step was omitted so that 17 β-estradiol and estrone were measured together.

RESULTS

Estrogen and progesterone plasma levels before and after treatment are shown in Tables 1 and 2 respectively. A definite increase in the plasma concentration of the corresponding hormone was observed in all cases and the more marked increases were seen in patients receiving the higher dose of each hormone.

The effect of estradiol upon BHI and OA is shown in Figs. 1 and 2. No

Table 1.
Changes induced in plasma estrogen levels after estradiol valerate treatment.

Subject	Cycle day	Before (pg/ml)	After (pg/ml)
BH*	A	200	450
OA**	A	125	1500
LF**	4	95	895
MF**	7	170	1995
ER**	16	250	1150
AO*	17	180	350
WN**	18	170	1770
IV**	19	245	1095
MU**	22	220	1220
AG*	23	175	525
MM**	24	125	2600
ACh**	26	500	4000

* Estradiol valerate 10 mg im single dose.
** Estradiol valerate 10 mg im every 12 h.
   Total dose 20 mg.
A Amenorrhea (lactation).

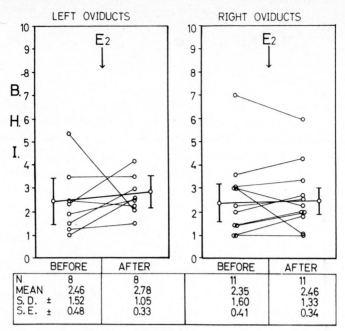

Fig. 1.

Burst Hour Index (BHI). Individual variations for each oviduct before and after estradiol (E₂) treatment are shown. Group averages ± 2 standard errors (SE) are also indicated.

Table 2.

Changes induced in plasma progesterone levels after progesterone treatment.

Subject	Cycle day	Before (ng/ml)	After (ng/ml)
JP**	A	2.60	15.00
IH**	A	5.20	11.50
MG**	4	1.00	92.00
TB**	6	0.33	37.00
GA**	13	2.20	113.00
LB*	15	1.85	4.50
AA*	21	0.60	16.00
MA*	21	1.40	8.00
HM**	21	6.50	10.30
AM**	22	3.40	65.00
CZ**	24	3.00	16.00

* Progesterone 100 mg im single dose.
** Progesterone 100 mg im every 12 h.
   Total dose 200 mg.
A Amenorrhea (lactation).

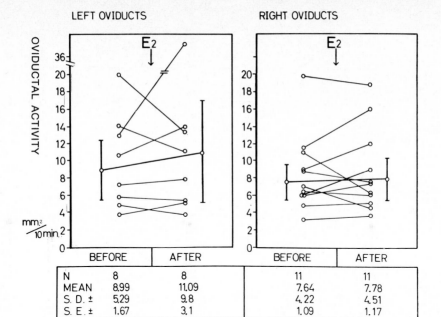

Fig. 2.

Oviductal activity. Individual values and group averages ± 2 SE before and after estradiol treatment (E_2).

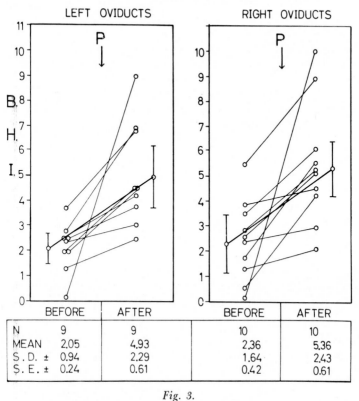

Fig. 3.

Burst Hour Index (BHI). Individual values and group averages ± 2 SE before and after progesterone treatment (P).

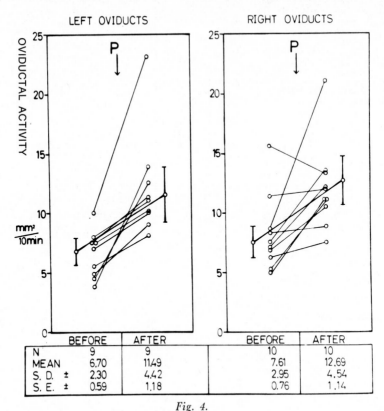

| | LEFT OVIDUCTS | | RIGHT OVIDUCTS | |
	BEFORE	AFTER	BEFORE	AFTER
N	9	9	10	10
MEAN	6.70	11.49	7.61	12.69
S. D. ±	2.30	4.42	2.95	4.54
S. E. ±	0.59	1.18	0.76	1.14

Fig. 4.

Oviductal activity. Individual values and group average ± 2 sᴇ before and after
progesterone treatment (P).

significant change in any of these parameters was observed. Actual recordings
are shown in Figs. 5 and 6.

The effect of progesterone upon BHI and OA is shown in Figs. 3 and 4. A
definite and significant increase in both parameters was observed in all subjects.
Representative examples of actual recordings are shown in Figs. 7, 8 and 9.
The intensity of this effect bore no relation to the stage of the menstrual cycle
and there was no apparent quantitative correlation between the response to
progesterone and plasma levels of this hormone attained after treatment.
Recordings obtained 24 h after treatment did not differ significantly from
those obtained at 48 h; therefore, in order to calculate the mean, the data were
pooled.

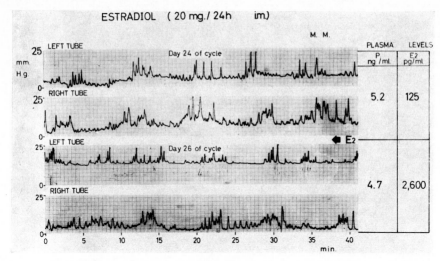

Fig. 5.

Effect of estradiol. *In vivo* recordings obtained on days 24 and 26 of the cycle. The plasma levels of progesterone (P) and estradiol (E₂) are shown before and after treatment. A slight decrease in oviductal motility can be seen after estradiol treatment.

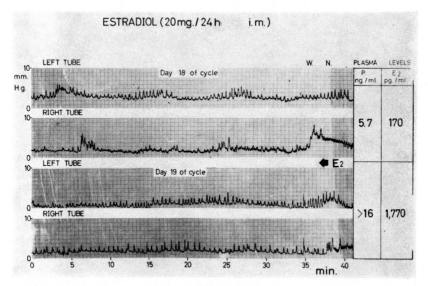

Fig. 6.

Effect of estradiol. *In vivo* recordings obtained on days 18 and 19 of the cycle. A decrease of oviductal motility can be observed after estradiol treatment. (Same conventions as Fig. 5).

491

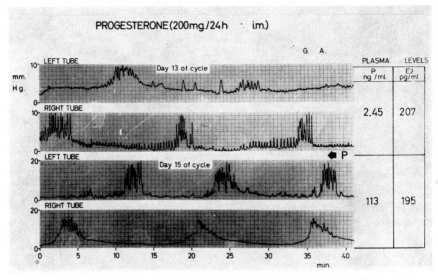

Fig. 7.

Effect of progesterone. *In vivo* recordings obtained on days 13 and 15 of the cycle. Increase in oviductal motility is found 48 h after treatment with progesterone. Notice the change in range (0–20 mmHg) in the record from day 15 of cycle. (Same conventions as Fig. 5).

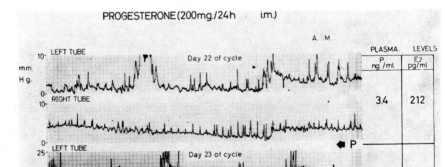

Fig. 8.

Effect of progesterone. *In vivo* recordings obtained on days 22 and 23 of the cycle. Same stimulatory response as the one described in Fig. 7. Notice the change of scale in the recording of day 23. (Same conventions as Fig. 5).

492

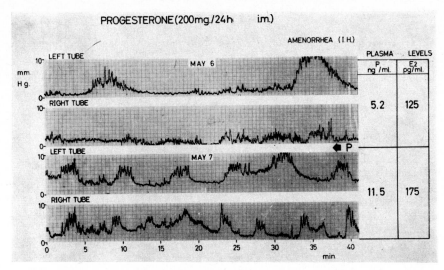

Fig. 9.
Effect of progesterone. *In vivo* recordings obtained on 2 consecutive days from an amenorrheic patient. A clear increase may be seen 24 h after progesterone treatment. (Same conventions as Fig. 5).

DISCUSSION

These results indicate that pharmacological doses of estrogen and progesterone have different effects upon human oviductal motility *in vivo* as evaluated by BHI and OA parameters. Stimulation of oviductal motility with progesterone was obtained in all cases regardless of pre-existing hormonal conditions. This response of the oviducts was observed consistently 24 or 48 h after the administration of this compound.

The response to estrogen treatment was variable and no predictable pattern was observed with doses used in this study.

The use of a microballoon to record changes of intraluminal pressure in the oviduct introduces an artifact which may disturb the physiologic activity of this organ or its responses to pharmacological stimulation. Keeping this in mind, the parameters used to quantitate oviductal motility in this study were sensitive enough to discriminate between the effects of estrogen and progesterone, but their meaning in terms of the role of the oviduct in the reproductive process in unclear. It would be of interest to investigate whether progesterone (or other compounds) which increase BHI and OA can change the rate of ovum transport in predictable manner.

Further work will be necessary to elucidate this question and to establish the time-course and dose-effect relationships of these compounds with regard to alteration of oviductal motility.

493

ACKNOWLEDGMENTS

We are indebted to Dr. Horacio Croxatto and the personnel of The Endocrine Laboratory of the Catholic University for carrying out the hormone assays in plasma.

REFERENCES

Coutinho E. M. and Maia H. (1970) The influence of the ovarian steroids on the response of the human Fallopian tubes to neurohypophysial hormones *in vivo. Amer. J. Obstet. Gynec. 108*, 194–202.

Coutinho E. M., Maia H. Jr. and Mattos C. E. R. (1975) Contractility of the Fallopian tube. *Gynec. Invest. 6*, 146–161.

Emment Y., Collins W. P. and Sommerville I. F. (1972) Radioimmunoassay of oestrone and oestradiol in human plasma. *Acta endocr. (Kbh.) 69*, 567–582.

Maia H. and Coutinho E. M. (1968) A new technique for recording human tube activity *in vivo. Amer. J. Obstet. Gynec. 102*, 1043–1047.

Pauerstein C. J., Hodgson B. J. and Kramen M. A. (1974) The anatomy and physiology of the oviduct. In: Wynn R. M., ed. *Obstet. Gynecol. Annual*, pp. 137–201. Appleton-Century-Crofts, New York.

Rubin I. C. (1939) The influences of the hormonal activity of the ovaries upon the character of the tubal contractions as determined by uterine insufflation. *Amer. J. Obstet. Gynec. 37*, 394–404.

Rubin I. C. (1947) *Intra-tubal Insufflation.* The C. V. Mosby Company, St. Louis.

Sica-Blanco Y., Cibils L., Remedio M. R., Rozada H. and Gil B. (1972) Isthmic and ampullar contractility of the human oviduct *in vivo. Amer. J. Obstet. Gynec. 111*, 91–97.

Sica-Blanco Y., Rozada H., Remedio M. R., Hendricks C. and Alvarez H. (1970) Human tubal motility *in vivo. Amer. J. Obstet. Gynec. 106*, 79–86.

Thorneycroft I. H. and Stone S. C. (1972) Radioimmunoassay of serum progesterone in women receiving oral contraceptive steroids. *Contraception 5*, 129–146.

18 Lennox Street, Gordon, Sydney, Australia

INFLUENCE OF ESTROGEN AND PROGESTERONE ON OVIDUCTAL FUNCTION

By

K. W. Humphrey

ABSTRACT

The disruption of oviductal function by antifertility compounds is dependent on the dosage and hormonal properties of the drug and most importantly on the time of administration. In laboratory rodents, estradiol administered when fertilised ova are present in the ampulla causes prolonged closure of the ampullary-isthmic junction and retention of ova – "ampulla-locking". Treatment later in pregnancy causes accelerated transport of ova from the isthmus to the uterus and vagina; loss through the infundibulum does not occur. The antiestrogenic compounds DMS, MER-25, MRL-37, U11100A and U11555A cause "ampulla-locking" only, without reducing the overall recovery of ova, whereas erythro-MEA and U10997 have similar effects to estradiol and produce both "ampulla-locking", accelerated transport and loss from the genital tract. These effects are not reversed by concurrent treatment with progesterone. None of the compounds were zygotoxic although "tube-locked" ova showed retarded development of the blastocele. "Tube-locked" ova implanted normally following transfer to pseudopregnant host mice. All compounds prevented decidualisation and implantation.

Since ectopic pregnancies can develop following "tube-locking", and since "tube-locked" ova may eventually enter the uterus and implant, it is desirable that antifertility drugs produce only accelerated transport of ova through the ampulla, isthmus, uterus and the associated sphincters and also prevent implantation of retained ova.

Many compounds, both estrogenic and anti-estrogenic, prevent implantation in rodents, although their precise mode and site of action is not always clear. A series of experiments was performed to analyse the antifertility actions of a number of anti-estrogens and of 17β-estradiol: the parameters examined were effects of these compounds on oviductal transport, ovum development, and decidualisation and implantation in intact and ovariectomized mice. An attempt was made to correlate the hormonal properties of the compounds with their effects on different aspects of early pregnancy in the mouse.

In this paper I will summarize my findings on the effects of 17β-estradiol and the anti-estrogens DMS (dimethylstilbestrol), MER-25 (1-P-2-diethyl-amino-ethoxyphenyl)-1-phenyl-2-anisylethane) and the corresponding ethane-MRL 37, U11100A (1-(2-(P-(3,4-dihydro-6-methoxy-2-phenyl-1-napthyl) phenoxy)ethyl-pyrrolidine hydrochloride), U11555A (2-(P-(6-methoxy-2 phenylinden-3-yl)-phenoxy)-triethylamine), U10997 (7,17-dimethyl-19-nortestosterone), erythro-MEA (erythro-a-ethyl-a-methyl-4,4'-dihydroxy-bibenzyl) on ovum transport and development.

MATERIALS AND METHODS

General procedures were as described by Humphrey, (1968a) and Humphrey and Martin (1968). The day of finding the vaginal copulatory plug was termed day 1 of pregnancy and coitus was assumed to have occurred at the preceding midnight.

The location and movement of ova in the tract was determined by microscopic *in vitro* examination of the straightened oviduct kept in buffer solution at 37°C or by examination of "squashed" specimens compressed under a cover slip. Histological preparations were also made.

RESULTS

In *in vitro* preparations progression of ova was due solely to contractions of the musculature of the ampulla and isthmus. Cilia were present only in the ampulla, and were apparently only necessary for the initial pick-up of ova from the distended bursa after ovulation; but otherwise cilia were not involved in ovum transport. Ova were suspended in fluid in a dilated loop of the isthmus, and were churned to and fro by peristaltic-antiperistaltic contractions of the distended oviductal loop. Only those sections of the oviduct containing fluid and ova showed peristaltic contractions, with the exception of loop 3, adjoining the ampullary-isthmic junction (AIJ). At all times from day 1 to day 4, peristaltic contractions were observed in this region, even though ova were not present. In the ampulla, and the isthmus, the presence of ova and fluid apparently was the stimulus to initiate and maintain peristaltic contractions, and ova were churned back and forth in a pendular fashion.

Table 1.

The effects of 17β-estradiol and antiestrogens on oviductal transport in the mouse. Results are mean numbers of ova flushed from the uterus or oviduct on day 4 of pregnancy following treatment with estradiol or an antiestrogen on days 1–3.

Treatment on days 1–3	Daily dose	Mean ovum count on day 4		
		Oviduct	Uterus	Total
Control vehicle only 76 mice		1.9	8.6	10.5
Estradiol-3,17β 20 mice/group	0.025 µg	1.4	7.1	8.5
	0.1	2.5	2.1	4.6
	0.4	3.0	0.4	3.4
	1.6	3.5	0.1**	3.6**
Erythro-MEA 8 mice/group	0.16 µg	0.3	11.0	11.3
	0.4	2.6	8.3	11.3
	1.0	2.6	1.0	3.6
	2.5	3.5	1.5	5.0
DMS 10 mice/group	0.025 µg	4.0	5.7	9.7
	0.1	7.2	2.1	9.3
	0.4	9.1	0.0	9.1
	1.6	8.0***	0.3***	8.3
U10997 8 mice/group	8 µg	5.3	8.0	13.3
	20	4.4	3.8	8.2
	50	2.5	2.6**	5.1
U11100A 8 mice/group	100 µg	10.3**	0.1*	10.4
U11555A 8 mice/group	178 µg	7.0	3.8	10.8
	267	13.3	1.1	14.4
	400	9.8	1.9	11.7
	600	11.3***	2.3***	13.6
MRL-37 8 mice/group	0.25 mg	5.2	7.3	12.5
	0.5	8.6	2.8	11.4
	1.0	10.9	0.0	10.9
	2.0	12.3	0.0	12.3
	4.0	8.1	1.6	9.7
	8.0	8.3***	0.4***	8.7
MER-25 20 mice/group	1.0 mg	1.8	7.3	9.1
	2.0	3.4	5.7	9.1
	4.0	3.3	6.2	9.5
	8.0	5.7**	4.2*	9.9

*** $P < 0.001$ ** $P < 0.01$ * $P < 0.05$.

Table 2.

Th effects on oviductal transport of a single injection of estradiol on day 1 *post coitum*. All results are mean ovum counts on day 4 for 8 mice/group.

Treatment on day 1	Dose	Ovum counts on day 4		
		Oviduct	Uterus	Total
Peanut oil	0.1 ml	0.0	8.2	8.2
Estradiol	0.1 µg	2.8	5.7	8.6
	1.6 µg	7.2	1.2	8.4

The AIJ and the uterotubal junction (UTJ) were very important blocks to the passage of ova which are retained at these points for 24 and 30–36 h respectively of the 72 h spent in the oviduct. Passage through the ampulla to the AIJ is very rapid – less than 1 h, and passage through the isthmus to the UTJ lasts only 12–18 h. Ova enter the uterus 72–75 h after coitus – the functional block previously present at the UTJ disappears at this time and ova and fluid can be forced through the final section of the oviduct either by a peristaltic rush in the last loop of the isthmus or by pressure on this section in compressed preparations.

The effects of 17β-estradiol, given on days 1–3, on ovum transport are summarized in Table 1. The mean ovum counts in the uterus and oviduct on day 4 are given. As the daily dose of estradiol was increased, the total recovery of ova was reduced by 60 %, very few ova were found in the uterus and many ova were found in the oviducts. Examination of oviducts *in vitro*, and of

Table 3.

The effects on oviductal transport of estradiol given on days 2 and 3 *post coitum*. Pregnant mice received estradiol (0.4 µg/day) or oil at 18.00 h on day 2 only or on day 2 (at 18.00 h) and day 3 (at 12.00 h). Results are mean ovum counts for 15 mice/group, killed on day 3 (09.00 h) or on day 4 (09.00 h) (expt. 8).

Treatment on day 2 or days 2 and 3	Daily dose	Day 3 (09.00 h)			Day 4 (09.00 h)		
		Oviduct	Uterus	Total	Oviduct	Uterus	Total
Peanut oil	0.1 ml	12.0	0.3	13.2	1.1	15.3	16.4
Estradiol	0.4 µg	1.5	5.6	7.1	1.5	4.2	5.7

Table 4.

The effects of unilateral ligation of the reproductive tract on the recovery of ova from control and estradiol-treated mice.
Pregnant mice received estradiol (0.4 μg/day) or oil on days 1, 2 and 3 after ligation of one side of the reproductive tract on day 1.
The results are mean numbers of ova flushed from each section of the tract on day 4.

Experiment #	Unilateral ligation on day 1	Treatment on days 1–3	Oviduct		Uterus		Totals		Grand total
			Ligatured	Not ligatured	Ligatured	Not ligatured	Ligatured	Not ligatured	
#9 (10 mice/group)	Sham-operation	Peanut oil	–	0.5	–	9.6	–	10.1	10.1
		Estradiol	–	1.5	–	0.2	–	1.7	1.7
#10 (20 mice/group)	Uterotubal junction	Peanut oil	6.2	0.5	–	4.7	6.2	5.2	11.4
		Estradiol	4.1*	1.9	–	0.0	4.1*	1.9	6.0
#11 (10 mice/group)	Uterine horn	Peanut oil	0.0	0.0	2.6*	5.5	2.6*	5.5	8.1
		Estradiol	1.3	1.1	0.4	0.2	1.7	1.3	3.0
#12 (10 mice/group)	Infundibulum	Estradiol	0.5	1.0	0.2	0.4	0.7	1.4	2.1

* These totals in ligatured sections are significantly different from those for non-ligatured side ($P < 0.01$).

histological specimens showed that most of the "tube-locked" ova in estradiol treated mice were in the ampulla, near the AIJ from day 1 to day 5.

When estradiol was given only on day 1 (Table 2) it was found that the total recovery of ova was not reduced, but that many ova were "tube-locked" (mainly in the ampulla).

When estradiol (0.4 μg/day) was given on days 2 and 3 (Table 3) it was found that within 15 h of the first injection, ova were prematurely in the uterus and that the overall recovery of ova was greatly reduced ($P < 0.001$).

In an attempt to determine why estradiol reduced the recovery of ova, different areas of the reproductive tract were unilaterally ligated on day 1. The infundibulum, UTJ, or the uterine horn close to the cervix were separately ligated on one side and the contralateral side served as a control. The mice were given estradiol or peanut oil on days 1–3 and the distribution of ova in the tract on day 4 was determined (Table 4).

In estradiol treated mice, ligation of the infundibulum or uterine horn did not increase the recovery of ova, but ligation of the UTJ did ($P < 0.001$). It was found that in control mice, ligation of the uterine horn significantly reduced the recovery of ova, perhaps because blood and tissue debris resulting from the ligation obscured ova in the flushings. It is likely that the recovery of ova from the ligated uteri of estradiol-treated mice was also underestimated and it appears that many ova prematurely enter the uterus in estradiol-treated mice.

The next experiment was to investigate the effects of estradiol on ovum transport in the uterus (Table 5). Pseudopregnant host mice were treated with estradiol or vehicle only on day 1, 2 and 3 of pseudo-pregnancy. On day 3, blastocysts were transferred to the uteri of these host mice, which were killed

Table 5.

The effects of estradiol on ovum transport in the uterus. Results are means for 5 mice/group, at various times after transfer of 5 ova to the uterus at noon on day 3.

Treatment on days 1–3	Daily dose	Hours after transfer	No. of mice with ova	Mean no. of ova	Location
Estradiol	0.4 μg	6	5	3.2	Uterus, cervices
		9	2	0.8	Uterus
		12	2	0.4	Uterus, cervices
		24	0	0.0	–
Peanut oil	0.1 ml	12	5	4.0	Uterus
		24	4	3.0	Uterus

at various times later, and the uteri flushed to recover the transferred ova. In control mice, most of the transferred ova were recovered 12 and 24 h later and appeared normal. However, in host mice, pretreated with estradiol the recovery of ova fell markedly 9 h after transfer.

The few ova recovered at 12 h had rough, partly dissolved zonae pellucidae and some naked morulae were found. A few ova were recovered from the cervices, showing that the rapid loss of ova in estradiol-treated mice is due to expulsion through the cervix to the vagina.

These experiments demonstrated that estradiol has multiple effects on ovum transport.

Treatment on day 1 when ova are still in the ampulla produce "ampulla-locking" of many ova, because of the prolonged retention at the AIJ.

Treatment on days 2 or 3 when ova are in the isthmus causes accelerated passage through the isthmus, UTJ, uterus and cervix apparently because of premature openening of the UTJ and increased motility of the uterus.

Treatment on days 1–3 causes both "tube-locking" and accelerated transport and loss, indicating that prolonged closure of the AIJ and premature opening of the UTJ can occur simultaneously.

Despite the findings that the AIJ and UTJ have a dominant role in controlling oviductal transport, I was unable to demonstrate any significant differences in the histological structure or the *in vitro* activity of these junctions, or in the pattern of oviductal contractions *in vitro* between control and estradiol-treated mice. A precise quantitative technique is obviously required.

Ovum transfer studies have shown that "tube-locked" ova implant normally following transfer to pseudo-pregnant host mice (Humphrey and Emmens, 1966).

It seems unlikely that ova which enter the uterus prematurely can remain, and eventually implant, but "tube-locked" ova can belatedly reach the uterus and implant.

In this and other experiments it was found that estradiol was luteolytic in the mouse, as well as the hamster (Greenwald 1965). However, concurrent administration of progesterone 2.0 mg/day and estradiol 0.4 μg/day on days 1–3 did not prevent "tube-locking" or increase the recovery of ova (not tabulated).

Table 1 summarizes the effects of various anti-estrogens on oviductal transport. All compounds produced "tube-locking" of ova, and decreased recovery of ova from the uterus. Only erythro-MEA, U10997 and to a lesser extent MRL 37 and DMS reduced the total recovery of ova. Examination of histological preparations and of oviducts *in vitro* showed that most of the "tube-locked" ova were in the ampulla near the AIJ from day 1 to day 6 or 7. At the dose levels used all compounds significantly reduced the numbers of mice with inplants on day 12, showing that even if "tube-locked" ova eventually reach the uterus then implantation is prevented. Ovum transfer studies, and experiments on delayed implantation and on decidualisation have shown that the "tube-locked" and uterine zygotes are viable, but that all these compounds prevent decidualisation (Humphrey 1967, 1968c, Humphrey and Emmens 1966, 1969).

Thus all compounds have actions similar to estradiol and produce "ampulla-locking" of many ova, but accelerated transport of ova in the isthmus through the UTJ and uterus does not occur. Simultaneous treatment with progesterone (2 mg/day) does not reverse the "tube-locking" effect of DMS, MRL 37 and MER 25 (Humphrey and Martin 1968). All of these compounds had some luteolytic actions.

In all of the preceding experiments it was found that the "tube-locked" ova had delayed development of the blastocele early on day 4. This delay in development was only temporary and large blastocysts with well developed blastocele were found in the ampulla on day 4 and zona-less blastocysts were flushed from the uterus on days 5 and 6.

DISCUSSION

In the mouse, the progression of ova through the oviduct is due to peristaltic-anti-peristaltic contractions of the musculature. Cilia are important in the pick-up of newly ovulated ova from the dilated bursa, but are otherwise not a major factor in ovum transport in the mouse or rabbit (Harper 1961, Humphrey 1968a).

In my observations ova were always suspended in a considerable quantity of fluid which distended that segment of the oviduct, and was the essential stimulus to contraction of the oviductal loop. Pendular or to and fro movement of ova and fluid is a constant feature of ovum transport in the mouse, rabbit guinea pig and ewe (Humphrey 1968a, Dukelow and Riegle 1974).

Passage through the isthmus is rapid in all species studied, but temporary blocks to the passage of ova occur in the isthmus *in vitro*. In observations in the straightened oviduct, small folds of mucosa were present at the end of each loop, but the presence or position of such folds in the coiled oviduct *in vivo* is not known. In the rabbit, local occlusion of the lumen of the isthmus occurs due to kinks in the oviduct (Stavorski and Hartman 1958).

However in most species control of the downward passage of ova is predominantly by the ampullary-isthmic and uterotubal junctions (Beck and Boots 1974). The anatomical structure of these junctions is well described by these authors.

The activity of the AIJ is controlled by hormonally induced shifts in the population of α- and β-adrenergic receptors (Brundin 1965, Brenner and West 1975).

502

In the mouse and also the rabbit and possibly other species the last section of the isthmus adjacent to the intramural segment acts functionally as part of the blocking mechanism (Black and Asdell 1959, Humphrey 1968a).

The functional activity of these junctions can be modified by neural or hormonal forces acting on the local vascular and lymphatic systems, or on the contractility of the musculature of the oviductal walls or mesenteries. Although the precise mechanism of regulation of these junctions is only slowly being elucidated, their functional significance is undoubted, and compounds which disrupt oviductal transport act largely on these segments.

Estrogens have been variously reported as causing "tube-locking" (in the ampulla) or accelerated transport, or a combination of both (Greenwald 1967, Humphrey 1968b). In the mouse the effects of estradiol depends largely on the time of treatment: estradiol causes delayed passage through the AIJ, accelerated passage through the UTJ and from the uterus. Thus, estradiol affects the AIJ, UTJ and the uterine musculature. Treatment with a wide variety of anti-estrogenic compounds produced only "ampulla-locking", and ovum transport through the isthmus, UTJ and in the uterus was not greatly affected.

The compounds MER 25 and MRL 37 caused retention of many ova in the ampulla until day 6 or 7.

This "ampulla-locking" action seems to be an estrogenic and not an anti-estrogenic effect. All of these substances, while not estrogenic in conventional vaginal smear assays in rodents, do exhibit some estrogenicity in other, more sensitive, assays, or in estrogen-dependent reactions (Humphrey 1967, 1968c; Humphrey and Martin 1965; Humphrey and Emmens 1969; Emmens et al. 1967; Emmens 1971; Emmens and Carr 1973).

Thus it is possible to produce hormonally active compounds that selectively affect limited aspects of oviductal physiology, in the case of the above compounds, they modify the function of the AIJ.

Estradiol at the doses used here does not completely prevent implantation, some "tube-locked" ova eventually pass through the UTJ and implant; further estradiol treatment on days 4–6 is needed to inhibit implantation.

The anti-estrogens tested inhibited decidualisation and estrogen-dependent aspects of implantation and exhibited both estrogenic and anti-estrogenic actions (Humphrey 1967, 1968c).

The compound U11100A and some triarylalkene derivatives have been shown to have prolonged anti-estrogenic effects after injection in rodents, apparently by prolonged prevention of replenishment of cytoplasmic estrogen receptors (Emmens 1971, Emmens and Carr 1973, Jordan 1975).

Compounds of this nature which have long term hormonal properties and which could selectively affect the transport of ova in the oviduct and uterus and also inhibit implantation would be most effective post-coital anti-fertility substances. Because of their prolonged activity, the time of administration in relation to ovulation is of reduced importance. Possibly it would be preferable for the compounds to accelerate selectively passage of ova to the uterus and vagina rather than to produce "tube-locking". However oviductal pregnancies are only common in the human, and the likelihood that anti-fertility compounds could inhibit implantation in both the uterus and the oviduct should not be overlooked.

ACKNOWLEDGMENTS

This work was performed while the author was at the Department of Veterinary Physiology, University of Sydney and was supported by grants from the Population Council and the Ford Foundation.

The help of Prof. C. W. Emmens is gratefully acknowledged.

REFERENCES

Beck L. R. and Boots L. R. (1974) The comparative anatomy, histology and morphology of the n ammalian oviduct. In: Johnson A. D. and Foley C. W., eds. *The Oviduct and its l'unctions*, pp. 1–52. Academic Press, New York.

Black D. L. and Asdell S. A. (1959) Mechanism controlling entry of ova into rabbit uterus. *Amer. J. Physiol. 197*, 1275–1278.

Brenner R. M. and West N. B. (1975) Hormonal regulation of the reproductive tract in female mammals. *Ann. Rev. Physiol. 37*, 273–302.

Brundin J. (1965) Pharmacology of the oviduct. In: Hafez E. S. E. and Blandau R. J., eds. *The Mammalian Oviduct*, pp. 251–270. Univ. Chicago Press, Chicago.

Dukelow W. R. and Riegle G. D. (1974) Transport of gametes and survival of the ovum as functions of the oviduct. In: Johnson A. D. and Foley C. W., eds. *The Oviduct and its Functions*, pp. 193–200. Academic Press, New York.

Emmens C. W. (1971) Compounds exhibiting prolonged antioestrogenic and anti-fertility activity in the mouse. *J. Reprod. Fertil. 34*, 29–40.

Emmens C. W. and Carr W. L. (1973) Further studies of compounds exhibiting prolonged antioestrogenic and antifertility activity in the mouse. *J. Reprod. Fertil. 34*, 29–40.

Emmens C. W., Humphrey K., Martin L. and Owen W. H. (1967) Antifertility properties of two nonoestrogenic steroids and MRL 37. *Steroids 9*, 235–243.

Greenwald (1965) Luteolytic effect of oestrogen on the corpora lutea of pregnancy in the hamster. *Endocrinology 76*, 1213–1219.

Greenwald G. S. (1967) Species differences in egg transport in response to exogenous estrogen. *Anat. Rec. 157*, 163–172.

Harper M. J. K. (1961) The mechanisms involved in the movement of newly ovulated eggs through the ampulla of the rabbit Fallopian tube. *J. Reprod. Fertil. 2*, 522–524.

Humphrey K. W. (1967) The antifertility actions of some antioestrogens in the mouse. *Proc. 3rd Asia Oceania Congr. Endocr.*, Manila. Pt. 2, pp. 784–789.

Humphrey K. W. (1968a) Observations on transport of ova in the oviduct of the mouse. *J. Endocr. 40*, 267–273.

Humphrey K. W. (1968b) The effects of oestradiol-3,17β on tubal transport in the laboratory mouse. *J. Endocr. 42*, 17–26.

Humphrey K. W. (1968c) The effects of some anti-oestrogens on the deciduoma reaction and delayed implantation in the mouse. *J. Reprod. Fertil. 16*, 201–209.

Humphrey K. W. (1969) Mechanisms concerned in ovum transport. In: Raspé G., ed. *Schering Symposium on Mechanisms Involved in Conception. Adv. Biosci. 4*, 133–148.

Humphrey K. W. and Emmens C. W. (1966) Site of action of oestradiol and some anti-oestrogens in preventing implantation in the mouse. *Proc. 2nd Int. Congr. Hormonal Steroids*, Milan, Italy, Abstr. 351.

Humphrey K. W. and Emmens C. W. (1969) Effects of a hexoestrol derivative, erythro-MEA, on early pregnancy in the mouse. *J. Reprod. Fertil. 20*, 247–253.

Humphrey K. W. and Martin L. (1968) The effects of oestrogen and anti-oestrogens on ovum transport in the laboratory mouse. *Aust. J. Biol. Sci. 21*, 1239–1248.

Jordan V. C. (1975) Prolonged antioestrogenic activity of ICI 46,474 in the ovariectomized mouse. *J. Reprod. Fertil. 42*, 251–258.

Stavorski J. and Hartman C. (1958) Uterotubal insufflation. A study to determine the origin of fluctuations in pressure. *Obstet. and Gynec. 11*, 622–639.

Central Drug Research Institute,
Lucknow, India

ESTROGEN, PROGESTERONE, OVIDUCTAL FUNCTION AND OVUM TRANSPORT

By

J. N. Karkun

ABSTRACT

Contraceptive approaches based on regulation of ovum transport are dependent on precise knowledge of oviductal function and its hormonal control. These are discussed with particular reference to functional changes in the ciliated cells and radioactive estradiol incorporation under altered hormonal conditions and during pregnancy. It is shown that (i) the ciliary function may also be involved during ovum transport through the isthmus, (ii) the threshold of the isthmus for estrogen may be higher for ciliary formation than that of the ampulla, and (iii) the isthmus may retain estrogen more tenaciously than the ampulla.

The idea that contraception could be achieved by interference with ovum transport originated from certain early experiments and their subsequent follow up (see Pincus 1965). It was shown that estrogen could interrupt pregnancy in laboratory rodents by either keeping the ovum within the oviduct beyond the normal period or transporting it from the oviduct to the uterus prematurely.

Acceleration and "tube-locking" of ova by natural and synthetic estrogens have since been confirmed and extended to several other animal species (see Greenwald 1967; Humphrey 1968a; Humphrey and Martin 1968). Greenwald (1967) observed that the first process requires lesser doses of the hormone and opined that acceleration of ovum transport under estrogen might offer a new approach to control of human fertility. However, estrogen could also induce contraception by its action on other vulnerable sites (see Blye 1973; Shearman 1973). Massive dosage of estrogen undoubtedly produced an antifertility effect in women (Morris and Van Wagenen 1973; Haspels and Andriesse 1973), but questions remained unanswered whether such effect was due to disturbance of ovum transport *solely* throught the oviduct.

Progesterone is also known to accelerate ovum transport in rabbits (Wislocki and Snyder 1933; Chang 1967; Chang and Hunt 1970 and others) and in gilts (Day and Polge 1968). However, it is a matter of common knowledge that the contraceptive action of progestins currently employed is exerted at other site(s), depending on dose and mode of treatment. Even in animals, progesterone might evoke antifertility effects by processes other than interference with ovum transport (Tinsley and Brennan 1972).

Thus, while the contraceptive effect of natural or synthetic estrogens and progestins, based on interference of ovum transport as demonstrated in animals, can not at present be put to immediate practical use in human contraception, it has become imperative for any future attack along these lines to know correctly the mode and mechanism(s) of ovum transport in different animals, including man, and how they are regulated under the influence of the ovarian hormones. The present article deals with certain aspects of these problems, along with other relevant work done by the author and his colleagues in this field.

MODE AND MECHANISM(S) OF OVUM TRANSPORT

According to the present consesus, the ovum immediately after pick-up from the ovary is quickly transported through the ampulla to be detained at the ampullary-isthmic junction (AIJ). Once released from the AIJ, it passes through the isthmus comparatively slowly but is detained for a second time at the uterotubal junction (UTJ), until a surge of fluid current pushes it rapidly into the uterus (see Karkun 1973). However, similar information for primates is still fragmentary. Only recently Jainudeen and Hafez (1973) showed that in the crab-eating monkey (*Macaca fasicularis*) the isthmus rather than the AIJ played an important role in such retention. The authors also questioned whether in humans the ovum is really blocked either at the AIJ or the UTJ, rather than in the isthmus.

Transport of the ovum within the oviduct is accomplished by the oviduct itself, by the ciliary action of its own epithelium, and the contractility of its musculature. This was shown in mice (Humphrey 1968a,b) and in rabbits (Harper 1961, 1965a, 1966) and is generally accepted to be true for all mammals.

The epithelium of the ampulla is heavily ciliated (Nilsson and Reinius 1969). However, despite this condition, the ciliary contribution to ovum transport within ampulla is suggested to be confined to only a small part of its distal end (Harper 1961, 1965a, 1966; Humphrey 1968b; Boling and Blandau 1971a). Koester (1970), however, opposed such a view and suggested that for normal ovum transport ciliary participation is essential along the entire oviduct. A correlative survey of ciliary changes with the presence or absence of ova in different oviductal segments of mated animals might resolve this pproblem. This was attempted by Gupta et al. (1970a), who by employing light microscopic techniques (LM) recorded the overall changes in ciliation in different parts of the oviductal epithelium of mated rabbits from 14 h *post coitum* (p. c.) to 70 h p. c. The planning of the experiment and the sacrifice of the animals were staggered in such a manner that specific ciliary changes could be evaluated in different parts, ampulla, AIJ and isthmus of the oviduct at several post-coital periods, viz., at 14, 24 and 70 h p. c., both in the presence and absence of the ovum. Estrous unmated rabbits served as the controls; it has previously been shown by the authors that in their rabbits the ovum is located at the aforesaid segments during the above-mentioned periods (Gupta et al. 1970b).

The results indicated that the ampullary cilia of estrous (control) rabbits increased in number when they were mated, but at 14 and 24 h p. c., i. e. at times when the ovum was at the distal and proximal ends of the ampulla respectively and had not passed into the isthmus, the ciliation in the last segment remained unchanged, but recorded a decrease at 70 h p. c.

The experiment was repeated later for electron microscopic observations (EM), and it was found that a large number of microvilli interspersed between the cilia made the above conclusion incorrect, since it was very difficult to distinguish the microvilli from the cilia using LM; using EM, a cilium could be recognized by the characteristic structure of its fibrils and also by the association of its prominent basal body. The results using EM (Shipstone et al. 1974) modified the findings by Gupta et al (1970a). The epithelium of the ampulla was found to exhibit greater ciliation at 24 and 70 h p. c. as compared to the corresponding values at estrus. Ciliation of the isthmus remained unaltered at 14 and 24 h but increased at 70 h p. c. An interesting change was found in the mitochondria; their position changed from random distribution in the supranuclear part of the ciliated cells at estrus to increased aggregation in the sub-apical region of the cells in both the ampulla and isthmus particularly at 70 h p. c. These findings are relevant to oviductal function, since mitochondria constitute the "power-pack" of a cell. Thus, their accumulation near the base of the cilia probably accounts for the increased ciliary activity by Borell et al. (1957) during days 2 and 3 p. c. The overall results of the ciliary change obtained in the above experiments also suggested that ciliary function in oviductal transport must be operative throughout the oviduct even later in the post-ovulatory period. Perhaps the increased activity of the cilia within the isthmus is necessary for rotating the ovum for uniform deposition of its mucin coat and/or for driving the ovum through the narrow isthmic lumen. Much more work on this problem using primates is necessary for exact definition of the role of the cilia in ovum transport in these species.

Observations concerning the influence of ovarian hormones on the growth and neogenesis of oviductal cilia are often contradictory. Part of such contradiction can probably be accounted for by the fact that the hormonal effect varies depending upon the species of animals examined, the time-lag between ovariectomy and hormonal treatment, and more importantly the difference in the response of different parts of the oviduct to the hormone under similar conditions. In a recent study, Brenner et al. (1974) have shown that while ovariectomy of rhesus monkeys for 6–12 months provokes atrophy of the entire oviductal epithelium, deciliation is less dramatic in the ampulla than in the isthmus. In the rabbit, however, long term ovariectomy reduces the number of cilia significantly below normal values in both the infundibulum (Odor 1969; Rumery and Eddy 1974) and the ampulla (Rumery and Eddy 1974). Estrogen treatment restores ciliary growth and provokes neogenesis of cilia (Odor 1969; Rumery and Eddy 1974 – rabbit; Nyak and Zimmerman 1971 – pig). In intact cyclic animals, ciliogenesis (with signs of new basal body formation etc.) is observed during the proliferative phase of the cycle (Brenner and Resko, 1972; Brenner et al. 1974 – monkey; Verhage et al. 1973 – dog). In women no cyclic shedding of the cilia occurs (Ludwig et al. 1972; Patek 1974). However, stilbestrol administered to women 5 days after delivery has been claimed to stimulate proliferation of the ciliary epithelium.

Thus while most of the results obtained by the above investigators suggest that estrogen has a favorable effect on ciliation, the electron microscopic study of Shipstone et al. (1974) revealed that ciliation in the rabbit was increased both in the oviductal ampulla and isthmus at 70 h p. c., i. e. at a time when the estrogen level should be at its nadir (Hilliard and Eaton 1971). A re-investigation of the effect of estrogen on the numbers of cilia in the epithelium of the ampulla and the isthmus of ovariectomized rabbits was, therefore, undertaken (Bajpai et al. 1975). Estrogen treatments were made at 2 dose levels (1 μg/kg and 5 μg/kg body wt per day) for 7 days, commencing 30 days after ovariectomy, and the animals were sacrificed 24 h after the last injection.

The results indicated that under the above conditions ovariectomy had no significant deterimental effect on the ampullary ciliated cells; they were present in good numbers. The number of cilia was comparatively low in the isthmus, but this was consistent with the normal relative pattern of ciliary distribution in the two segments of the oviduct of the intact adult rabbit. Some degenerative changes in the ciliary apparatus were noticed in the isthmic cells as indicated by the presence of ciliary debris within their cytoplasm. Similar findings were not apparent in the ampulla. With low doses of estrogen, the cilia increased in number and ciliogenesis was observed in both the segments of the oviduct. The pattern of distribution of mitochondria did not change, although their number increased in the isthmic region. With high doses of estrogen no further change in ampullary ciliation was observed; in the isthmic region, however, the number of cilia increased rather markedly. The numbers of mitochondria increased in both segments of the oviduct.

These results apart from confirming the favorable influence of estrogen on growth and neogenesis of cilia suggested also that under identical conditions the isthmus requires a higher dose of estrogen for ciliation than the ampulla. Whether this is the reason for the normal sparsity of cilia in the rabbit isthmus compared to the ampulla is not clear through the ciliary conditions observed in the two segments suggest such a possibility. The higher threshold of isthmus to estrogen for ciliary growth is also supported by the fact that degeneration after ovariectomy set in earlier in the ciliated cells of the isthmus then in the ampulla. A second important finding was that with low doses of estrogen, the mitochondria increased more in the isthmus than in the ampulla.

Since this experiment did not apparently furnish any clue concerning the increase of isthmic ciliation at 70 h p. c., a third experiment was performed in which the ovariectomized rabbits were treated with progesterone (5 mg/kg body wt day) from the day of ovariectomy for a period of 7 days. Appropriate controls were also done.

The results indicated that there was not much change either in the pattern of ciliary distribution or in the number of cilia between the two segments as compared to estrous or ovariectomized control animals. An interesting finding, however, was that mitochondriogenesis occurred, not only in the isthmus but also in the ampulla. The results failed again to account for the increased ciliation of the two segments of rabbit oviduct at 70 h p. c. The change may be due to high preovulatory estrogen (and/or progesterone), whose action becomes manifest only after 2 to 3 days p. c. However, simultaneous studies on the secretory cells provided us with some important and additional information. It was observed that with long term ovariectomy the secretory cells lost most of their secretory granules (S. Gs.) from both segments of the oviduct; these returned to normal only after estrogen administration. When progesterone was administered to rabbits immediately after ovariectomy (Bajpai et al. 1975), the S. Gs. were reduced but only in the ampulla; the isthmic cells remained completely filled with S. Gs. It appeared that progesterone might either antagonise (preovulatory) estrogen in the ampulla but not in the isthmus, or alternatively the isthmic region bound such (preovulatory) estrogen more tenaciously (and for a longer time) than the ampulla. Incorporation studies using estradiol-6,7-^{3}H suggest the latter possibility (vide infra).

The precise manner in which ovarian hormones regulate ovum transport has yet to be delineated. The most comprehensive study in this aspect was first undertaken by Harper (1961, 1964, 1965a,b, 1966), who used either artificial or natural ova and recorded their transport through the oviducts of ovariectomized rabbits treated with estrogen and/or progesterone. His view as explained in his later study (Harper 1966) is that estrogen accelerates, while progesterone retards ovum transport and that this is accomplished by the respective stimulation and depression of the activities of the oviductal muscles. Boling and Blandau (1971a,b), however, made just the opposite conclusion regarding the mode of working of the above hormones on the ampulla, and forcefully put forward the view that withdrawal rather than dominance of estrogen, increases the vigor and orderly programming of muscular contractions as well as the acceleration of ova. Progesterone administered to ovariectomized rabbits does not significantly change the rate of transport; however, given to intact or ovariectomized estrogen-treated animals (Boling and Blandau 1971a,b), it increases the amplitude and decreases the frequency of contractions: in this sense it may be considered facilitatory to ovum transport (de Mattos and Coutinho 1971). However, the contradictory views on the mechanism of hormonal regulation by the two groups still persist as just recently Spilman and Harper (1974) have reiterated the early views of Harper (1966). Part of the difference undoubtedly lies in the fact that in one case the studies were of chronic effects and in the other of acute effects of progesterone administration.

Interestingly, attempts to reproduce normal ovum transport failed using either (i) fixed doses of the ovarian hormones (Harper 1964) or (ii) daily changing dose schedules with gradually decreasing estrogen and increasing progesterone (Harper 1965b); the latter condition was thought to stimulate the normal hormonal environment of the post-ovulatory period. In the light of recent knowledge that in the mated rabbit, a rapid fall in estrogen and progestins (progesterone and 20α-hydroxyprogesterone) occurs after their immediate prevoulatory rise, this failure could be explained. In none of the above experiments (Harper 1964, 1965a,b, 1966) were such hormonal conditions created. However, a more pertinent question is whether the investigator would have obtained normal transport even if he had used optimal conditions. Brenner et al. (1974) have recently shown that in ovariectomized monkeys given sequential treatment with fixed doses of estrogen and progesterone, the estrogen receptors vary in different parts of the oviduct, with resultant manifestation of differential physiological responses. Earlier Roy et al. (1972) demonstrated that incorporation of estrogen *in vitro* by different parts of the oviduct was different in estrous rabbits; the incorporation by isthmus was significantly higher than that of the ampulla. The results run contrary to those of Kim et al. (1967) and Martin et al. (1970) but they were not done under identical conditions. However, what is significant are our recent findings that during ovum transport the incorporation capacity *in vitro* of the ampulla, AIJ, isthmus and the UTJ of the rabbit oviduct all change significantly but differently. The incorporation by the ampulla and AIJ gradually increase from a lowest values at 14 h p. c. to the highest at 70 h p. c., while those of the isthmus and UTJ remain unchanged at the highest level. The implication of these findings are not clear at present, but are sufficiently provocative to require further study under *in vivo* conditions. The findings also emphasize the need for assessment of estrogen and progesterone concentrations in the tissue before one can hope to reproduce normal ovum transport. Incidentally, the above data again indicate the higher retention capacity of isthmus (and UTJ) for estrogen (vide supra) and in addition furnish an answer why Black and Asdell (1959) failed to reduce estrogen-induced edema from the UTJ with Diamox®.

ACKNOWLEDGMENTS

The author is thankful to Dr. Nitya Anand, Director of the Institute for his interest in this work. Thanks are also due to his collaborators, Drs. D. N. Gupta, A. C. Shipstone, and V. K. Bajpai for the physiologic and electron microscopic work and to Drs. S. K. Roy (Sr. and Jr.) for the study on estrogen incorporation *in vitro*.

REFERENCES

Bajpai V. K., Shipstone A. C., Gupta D. N. and Karkun J. N. (1975) Studies on the ultrastructure of the Fallopian tube: Part III. Changes in the ciliated and secretory cells of the rabbit Fallopian tube after ovariectomy and estrogen treatment. *Indian J. exp. Biol.* (in press).

Black D. L. and Asdell S. A. (1959) Mechanism controlling entry of ova into rabbit uterus. *Amer. J. Physiol. 197*, 1275–1278.

Blye R. P. (1973) The use of estrogens as postcoital contraceptive agents. Clinical effectiveness and potential mode of action. *Amer. J. Obstet. Gynec. 116*, 1044–1050.

Boling J. L. and Blandau R. J. (1971a) The role of estrogens in egg transport through the ampulla of oviducts of castrated rabbits. *Fertil. Steril. 22*, 544–551.

Boling J. L. and Blandau R. J. (1971b) Egg transport through the ampulla of oviducts of rabbit under various experimental conditions. *Biol. Reprod. 4*, 174–184.

Borell U., Nilsson O. and Westman A. (1957) Ciliary activity in rabbit Fallopian tube during oestrus and after copulation. *Acta obstet. gynec. scand. 36*, 22–28.

Brenner R. M. and Resko J. A. (1972) Artificial oviductal cycles in the rhesus monkey. *Biol. Reprod. 7*, 121 (Abstr.).

Brenner R. M., Resko J. A. and West N. B. (1974) Cyclic changes in oviductal morphology and residual cytoplasmic estradiol-binding capacity induced by sequential estradiol-progesterone treatment of spayed Rhesus monkeys. *Endocrinology 95*, 1094–1104.

Chang M. C. (1967) Effects of progesterone and related compounds on fertilization, transportation and development of rabbits eggs. *Endocrinology 81*, 1251–1260.

Chang M. C. and Hunt D. M. (1970) Effect of various progestins and estrogen on the gamete transport and fertilization in rabbit. *Fertil. Steril. 21*, 683–686.

Day B. N. and Polge C. (1968) Effects of progesterone on fertilization and egg transport in the pig. *J. Reprod. Fertil. 17*, 227–230.

De Mattos C. E. R. and Coutinho E. M. (1971) Effects of the ovarian hormones on tubal motility of the rabbit. *Endocrinology 89*, 912–917.

Greenwald G. S. (1967) Species differences in egg transport in response to exogenous oestrogen. *Anat. Rec. 157*, 163–172.

Gupta D. N., Karkun J. N. and Kar A. B. (1970a) Studies on the physiology and biochemistry of the Fallopian tube: Histologic changes in different parts of the rabbit Fallopian tube during early pregnancy. *Indian J. exp. Biol. 8*, 162–166.

Gupta D. N., Karkun J. N. and Kar A. B. (1970b) Biochemical changes in different parts of the rabbit Fallopian tube during passage of ova. *Amer. J. Obstet. Gynec. 106*, 833–837.

Harper M. J. K. (1961) The mechanisms involved in the movement of newly ovulated eggs through the ampulla of the rabbit Fallopian tube. *J. Reprod. Fertil. 2*, 522–524.

Harper M. J. K. (1964) The effect of constant doses of oestrogen on the transport of artificial eggs through the reproductive tract of ovariectomized rabbits. *J. Endocr. 30*, 1–19.

Harper M. J. K. (1965a) Transport of eggs in cumulus through the ampulla of the rabbit oviduct in relation to day of pseudopregnancy. *Endocrinology 77*, 114–123.

Harper M. J. K. (1965b) The effects of decreasing doses of oestrogen and increasing doses of progesterone on the transport of artificial eggs through the reproductive tract of ovariectomized rabbits. *J. Endocr. 31*, 217–226.

Harper M. J. K. (1966) Hormonal control of transport of eggs in cumulus through the ampulla of the rabbit oviduct. *Endocrinology 78*, 568–574.

Haspels A. A. and Andriesse R. (1973) The effects of large doses of estrogens post-coitus in 2,000 women. *Euro. J. Obstet. Gynecol. Reprod. Biol. 3*, 113.

Hilliard J. and Eaton L. W., Jr. (1971) Estradiol-17β, progesterone and 20α-hydroxy-pregn-4-en-3-one in rabbit ovarian venous plasma. II. From mating through implantation. *Endocrinology 89*, 522–527.

Humphrey K. W. (1968a) The effect of oestradiol-3,17β on tubal transport in the laboratory mouse. *J. Endocr. 42*, 17–26.

Humphrey K. W. (1968b) Observations on transport of ova in the oviduct of the mouse. *J. Endocr. 40*, 267–273.

Humphrey K. W. (1969) Mechanisms concerned in ovum transport. In: Raspé G. ed. *Schering Symp. on Mechanisms involved in Conception. Adv. Biosci. 4*, 133–148.

Humphrey K. W. and Martin L. (1968) The effects of oestrogen and antioestrogens on ovum transport in the laboratory mouse. *Aust. J. Biol. Sci. 21*, 1239–1248.

Jainudeen M. R. and Hafez E. S. E. (1973) Egg transport in the Macaque (*Macaca fascicularis*). *Biol. Reprod. 9*, 305–308.

Karkun J. N. (1973) Physiology of the Fallopian tube. *Proc. Indian Nat. Sci. Acad. 39* (Part 3), 333–353.

Kim Y. J., Coates J. B. and Flickinger G. L. (1967) Incorporation and fate of estradiol 17β-6,7-^{3}H in rabbit oviduct. *Proc. Soc. exp. Biol. Med. 126*, 918–921.

Koester H. (1970) Ovum transport. In: Gibian H. and Plotz E. J., eds. *Mammalian Reproduction*, pp. 189–228. Springer-Verlag, Berlin.

Ludwig H., Wolf H. and Hildegard M. (1972) Scanning electron microscopy of the luminal surface in the human Fallopian tube. *Archiv. Gynaekologie 212*, 380–396.

Martin J. E., McGuire W. L. and Pauerstein C. J. (1970) Macromolecular binding of estradiol in the rabbit oviduct and uterus. *Gynec. Invest. 1*, 303–311.

Morris J. M. and Van Wagenen G. (1973) Interception: The use of postovulatory estrogens to prevent implantation. *Amer. J. Obstet. Gynec. 115*, 101–106.

513

Nilsson O. and Reinius S. (1969) Light and electron microscopic structure of the oviduct. In: Hafez E. S. E. and Blandau R. J., eds. *The Mammalian Oviduct*, pp. 57–83. The University of Chicago Press, Chicago.

Nyak R. K. and Zimmerman D. R. (1971) Effect of estrogen and progesterone on the ultrastructure of porcine oviductal epithelium. *J. Animal Sci. 33*, 1161 (Abstr.).

Odor D. L. (1969) Estrogen hormone and ciliogenesis in the infundibulum of the rabbit oviduct. *Anat. Rec. 163*, 236–237.

Patek E. (1974) The epithelium of the human Fallopian tube. (A surface ultrastructural and cytochemical study). *Acta obstet. gynec. scand. 53* (Suppl. 31), 1–28.

Pincus G. (1965) Free ovum development. In *The Control of Fertility*, pp. 103–110. Academic Press, New York.

Roy S. K., Jr., Roy S. K., Gupta D. N., Karkun J. N. and Kar A. B. (1972) Studies on the physiology and biochemistry of the Fallopian tube: *In vitro* uptake of estradiol 17β-6,7-^{3}H by different parts of the rabbit Fallopian tube, uterotubal junction, uterus, cervix and vagina. *Indian J. exp. Biol. 10*, 26–28.

Rumery R. E. and Eddy E. M. (1974) Scanning electron microscopy of the fimbriae and ampulla of rabbit oviduct. *Anat. Rec. 178*, 83–101.

Shipstone A. C., Bajpai V. K., Gupta D. N. and Karkun J. N. (1974) Studies on the ultrastructure of the Fallopian tube: Part I – Changes in the ciliated cells of the rabbit Fallopian tube during ovum transport. *Indian J. exp. Biol. 12*, 115–122.

Shearman R. P. (1973) Post-coital contraception: A review. *Contraception 7*, 459–476.

Spilman C. H. and Harper M. J. K. (1974) Comparison of the effects of adrenergic drugs and prostaglandins on rabbit oviduct motility. *Biol. Reprod. 10*, 549–554.

Tinsley F. C. and Brennan D. M. (1972) Antifertility effects of progestins in hamsters. *Fertil. Steril. 23*, 924–928.

Verhage H. G., Abel J. H., Jr., Tietz W. J., Jr. and Barrau M. D. (1973) Development and maintenance of the oviductal epithelium during the estrous cycle in the bitch. *Biol. Reprod. 9*, 460–474.

Wislocki G. B. and Snyder F. F. (1933) The experimental acceleration of the rate of transport of ova through the Fallopian tube. *Bull. Johns Hopk. Hosp. 52*, 379–386.

From the Center for Research and Training
in Reproductive Biology and Voluntary Regulation of Fertility
Department of Obstetrics and Gynecology,
The University of Texas Health Science Center at San Antonio,
7703 Floyd Curl Drive, San Antonio, Texas 78284

INFLUENCE OF TIMING AND DOSE OF PROGESTERONE ON OVUM TRANSPORT RATES

By

Maria Isabel Gonzalez de Vargas[1]
and Carl J. Pauerstein[2]

ABSTRACT

Previous investigators have demonstrated that 2.5 mg progesterone administered intramuscularly to rabbits on the day of ovulation and the 2 preceding days (days −2, −1, 0), significantly and consistently accelerates ovum transport. In contrast, when given on the day of ovulation and the 2 following days (days 0, +1, +2), progesterone does not accelerate ovum transport. The experiments reported here were designed to define more precisely the temporal relationships critical to progesterone-induced acceleration of ovum transport. Maximal acceleration, equal to that achieved by injection on days −2, −1 and 0 was attained by injection of 2.5 mg progesterone on days −2 and −1, significant acceleration was noted with treatment on either of these days alone. Although 2.5 mg progesterone given on day −2 only did not maximally accelerate transport, maximal acceleration was noted if 7.5 mg was given. The accelerating effect of progesterone was significantly antagonized if the injections were given on days −3, −2, −1 and 0. Injection of either 2.5 mg or 7.5 mg on day −3 only or on day 0 only did not affect transport rates.

[1] Rockefeller Foundation Post-Doctoral Fellow in Reproductive Biology.
[2] Recipient of NICHHD Research Career Development Award KO4 HD47279.

33*

Table 1.

Effects of progesterone and medroxyprogesterone acetate (MPA) on the development of rabbit ova*. Six animals in each group, examined on day 6.

Compounds, dosage (mg/rabbit) and route	Day of treatment**	No. of CL	Ova recovered							
			Total	%	From oviducts	From uteri			From vagina	% normal
					De-generate	De-generate	Small blasto-cysts	De-generate	Normal blasto-cysts	
Progesterone 2 mg oral	1, 2, 3	72	64	89	5	0	3	56	0	78
Progesterone 2 mg sc	1, 2, 3	58	52	90	6	1	1	44	0	76
Progesterone 2 mg oral	−2, −1, 0	67	50	75	0	2	0	48	0	72

Treatment									
Progesterone 2 mg sc	−2, −1, 0	66	14	21	1	13	0	0	0	0
MPA 2 mg oral	−2, −1, 0	87	36	41	3	21	0	0	12	0
MPA 1 mg oral	−2, −1, 0	78	40	51	1	23	6	10	0	13
MPA 0.5 mg oral	−2, −1, 0	79	52	66	0	27	3	22	0	28
MPA 0.1 mg oral	−2, −1, 0	67	60	90	0	21	9	36	0	54
Control 22 rabbits		238	216	21	3	10	9	192	2	81

* Reprinted with modifications from Chang (1966), Endocrinology 79 with permission from the J. B. Lippincott Co.

** Day of insemination was called day 0; −1, −2 1 and 2 days before day 0 respectively; and 1, 2, 3 the days after day 0.

CL = Corpora lutea.

Rabbit ova take a few minutes to reach the ampullary-isthmic junction of the oviduct, where they remain for several hours before entering the isthmus. They traverse the isthmus in about two days and arrive in the uterus 66 to 72 h after the ovulatory stimulus.

The rate of oviductal transport of rabbit ova is modified by progesterone. However, little unanimity exists in the experimental results concerning the influence exerted by progesterone on ovum transport.

Boling and Blandau (1971) demonstrated that administration of progesterone or 20 alpha dihydroprogesterone accelerated ovum transport through the ampullae of estrous rabbits. The average transport time from the ostium to the ampullary-isthmic junction in estrous rabbits was 9.4 ± 1.6 min, while it was 4.2 ± 0.5 min in rabbits treated 12–14 h prior to observations of ovum transport with 20 alpha dihydroprogesterone and 4.3 ± 1.0 min in rabbits treated with progesterone. These results are in direct contrast to those obtained by Harper (1965, 1966) who found that progesterone ((2 mg/day for 4 days) or pseudo-pregnancy roughly doubled ampullary transit time from 7.5 ± 0.7 min in estrous, to 15.4 ± 1.1 min in estrous animals treated with progesterone. It is difficult to reconcile such opposite results. However, the difference may be due to the

Table 2.

Effect of oral administration of medroxyprogesterone acetate (MPA) on fertilization and transportation of rabbit ova examined on day 2[*].

Compound, dosage (mg/rabbit) and day of treatment	No. of CL	No. of rabbits	Ova recovered				
			Total	Oviducts	Uteri	Vagina	Fertilized
Progesterone sc 2 mg on day −1, 0	6	55	31 56 %	17 55 %	11 36 %	3 10 %	23 74 %
MPA 2 mg on day −1, 0	6	56	37 66 %	31 84 %	5 14 %	1 3 %	30 81 %
MPA 2 mg on day −2	4	49	37 76 %	36 97 %	1 3 %	0	31 84 %
MPA 2 mg on day −1	6	74	56 76 %	53 95 %	3 5 %	0	54 96 %
MPA 2 mg on day 0	4	50	50 100 %	50 100 %	0	0	50 100 %
Control	6	58	55 95 %	55 100 %	0	0	50 91 %

[*] Reprinted with modifications from Chang (1966), Endocrinology *79* with permission from the J. B. Lippincott Co.

Table 3.

Ovum transport in non-ovulated estrous rabbits fed 2 mg medroxyprogesterone acetate (MPA)*.

Compounds and day of treatment	No. of recipients	No. of ova transferred	Time of examination (h after transfer)	Ova recovered			
				Total	Oviducts	Uteri	Vagina
MPA on day –2, –1, 0	4	41	40–42	33 80 %	1 3 %	31 94 %	1 3 %
MPA on day 0, 1	3	39	41	38 97 %	38 100 %	0	0
MPA on day 0, 1, 2	3	45	64–65	42 93 %	42 100 %	0	0
MPA on day 0, 1	3	51	65	31 61 %	1 3 %	29 94 %	1 3 %
Control	4	41	40–41	27 66 %	14 52 %	12 44 %	1 4 %

* Reprinted with modifications from Chang (1966), Endocrinology *79* with permission from the J. B. Lippincott Co.

fact the former experiments examined the effect of acute, and the latter of chronic, administration of progesterone. Further, one wonders whether the effect of any treatment on the rapid journey through the ampulla is a valid indicator of the effect on the longer, and more critical, travel through the isthmus.

Several other reports in the literature shed light on this question. In 1966, Chang studied the effect of oral and subcutaneous progesterone and oral medroxyprogesterone acetate (MPA) on the development, transport and fertilization of rabbit ova. He found that the oral administration of 2 mg/day of progesterone either before or after insemination was ineffective in preventing normal development of ova, but that the same dose given subcutaneously or oral administration of MPA (2 mg/rabbit/day) before insemination prevented development of ova. However, at dose levels below 2 mg/rabbit, MPA was progressively less effective (Table 1).

Chang (1966) demonstrated that injection of progesterone or feeding of MPA at a dosage of 2 mg/rabbit/day on day –1 and 0, hastened the transport of ova into the uterus. Injection of progesterone caused more rapid ovum transport than did feeding of MPA (Table 2).

In other experiments, one day old rabbit ova were transferred into the oviducts of estrous rabbits that had received MPA before, or at the time of, and after transfer. A high percentage of ova had reached the uterus in estrous recipients and also in those fed MPA before transfer. No ova were found in the uteri of recipients fed MPA after transfer, even when examined 41 or 65 h later (Table 3).

Pauerstein et al. (1974b) injected 2.5 mg progesterone intramuscularly (im) on the day of human chorionic gonadotropin (HCG) injection and on each of the two preceding days. The animals were sacrificed 20 h later to assess ovum transport. Only 31 percent of ova remained in the oviducts of the animals treated with progesterone. In contrast, 100 percent of ova were recovered from the oviducts of control animals, as long as 63 h after HCG injection (Table 4).

Pauerstein et al. (1970, 1973, 1974a), have demonstrated progesterone receptors in the rabbit oviduct, and bound progesterone-receptor complex to oviductal chromatin (1975).

Greenwald (1961) divided the oviducts into eight equal segments, each segment thus representing 12.5 percent of the total oviductal length. Morphologic studies revealed that the ampulla was contained in segments 1 through 4, or the distal 50 percent of the oviduct, the ampullary-isthmic junction was located in segment 5, 50 to 62.5 percent of the distance from the fimbriated end of the uterus. He investigated the effect of progesterone and of 17a-hydroxy-progesterone caproate (Delalutin®) administered 5 h after mating on ovum transport in the rabbit. Both 5 and 25 mg of progesterone produced some

Table 4.
Recovery rates of ova*.

Time after HCG (h)	No. of corpora lutea	Oviduct % recovery	Total % recovery
18	15	80	80
24	24	96	96
36	22	100	100
48	22	86	86
60	31	100	100
63	21	100	100
66	33	3	100
Progesterone			
20	41	37	76

* Reprinted with modifications from Pauerstein et al. (1974b), Amer. J. Obstet. Gynec. 120 with permission from the C. V. Mosby Company.

Table 5.
Effect of a single injection of progesterone (5 h after HCG) on oviductal transport*.

Treatment	Time of exa- mination (h)	No. of ani- mals	Distribution of ova in segment of oviduct								
			1	2	3	4	5	6	7	8	Uterus
Control	24	3				13	31	2			
Control	48	4				3	23	8	7		
Progesterone 5 mg	24	3				1	11	14	1		
Progesterone 5 mg	48	3					2	14	14		
Progesterone 25 mg	24	4				4	4	11		5	9
Progesterone 25 mg	48	1				1	6	1			

* Reprinted with modifications from Greenwald (1961), Fertil. Steril *12* with permission from the American Fertility Society.

acceleration of ovum transport (Table 5). A 1 mg dose of Delalutin yielded inconsistent results because few or no ova were recovered from the oviducts or cornua of some animals, whereas in others the ova were found in segments 4, 5 and 6. Increasing the dosage to as much as 100 mg caused some acceleration but the recovery rates were inconsistent, making interpretation difficult. In any case, no marked acceleration was noted, in the sense that ova were recovered from the uteri of only 1 of the 12 animals at autopsy performed 48 h after the injection of Delalutin.

Comparing these results with those of Chang and of Pauerstein et al. (1974a) leads naturally to the inference that the temporal relationship of progesterone administration to ovulation or ovum transfer strongly influences the effect of progesterone on ovum transport rates.

We then performed experiments designed to define more precisely this temporal relationship (Vargas et al. 1975). We tried to answer three questions: 1) Can a critical period during which progesterone exerts its effect on ovum transport be defined? 2) Can maximal acceleration of ovum transport be achieved with a single injection of progesterone, administered at the proper time? 3) Could we see any differences in the location of ova within the oviducts associated with variations in the timing of progesterone administration? To this

Table 6.
Design of experiment.

Group and dose	Day −3	Day −2	Day −1	Day 0	Day +1
Controls				HCG	
1 − 2.5 mg		PROG	PROG	HCG PROG	
2 − 2.5 mg	PROG	PROG	PROG	HCG PROG	
3 − 2.5 mg	PROG	PROG	PROG	HCG	
4 − 2.5 mg		PROG	PROG	HCG	
5 − 2.5 mg			PROG	HCG PROG	K
6 − 2.5 mg	PROG			HCG	I L L
7 − 2.5 mg		PROG		HCG	
8 − 2.5 mg			PROG	HCG	
9 − 2.5 mg				HCG PROG	
10 − 7.5 mg	PROG			HCG	
11 − 7.5 mg		PROG		HCG	
12 − 7.5 mg			PROG	HCG	
13 − 7.5 mg				HCG PROG	

PROG = progesterone.

end 70 New Zealand white does divided in 14 groups were used (Table 6). The groups differed in the amount and days of progesterone administration relative to HCG injection. Ovulation was induced by intravenous injection of 100 i. u. of HCG. All animals were killed 24 h after HCG injection. The ova were located and counted in the cleared oviducts by means of a dissecting microscope as previously described (Pauerstein et al. 1974b) and uterine ova were recovered by flushing the uterine horns (Pauerstein et al. 1973). Recovery rates were expressed by dividing the number of ova recovered (oviductal and total of oviductal plus uterine) by the number of ovulation points counted on the ovaries. The anatomic location was shown by dividing the oviduct into segments called distal ampulla (0–38 % of the total length of the oviduct), proximal ampulla (38–50 %), ampullary-isthmic junction (50–60 %), distal isthmus (60–75 %), and proximal isthmus (75–90 %). Thus, the distal ampulla corresponded to Greenwald's segments 1, 2 and 3, the proximal ampulla to segment 4, the ampullary-isthmic junction to segment 5, the distal isthmus approximated Greenwald's segment 6, and the proximal isthmus roughly to segment 7. The precentage of ova found in each segment was then mapped.

Maximal acceleration was observed in group 1 (2.5 mg progesterone on days –2, –1, and 0). All other treatments were therefore compared with both untreated controls, and with the maximal acceleration noted in group I (Table 7). A single injection of 2.5 mg progesterone on either day –3 or day 0 did not accelerate ovum transport. All other regimens induced some acceleration of transport, but maximal acceleration comparable to group 1 was only attained in group 4 (treatment on days –2 and –1) and in group 8 (treatment on day –1 only). Treatment for four days starting on day –3 (group 2) or moving the standard 3 day treatment ahead by one day (group 3) significantly diminished the acceleration.

In table 8 the effects of a dose of 7.5 mg (2.5 mg × 3 days = 7.5 mg) are compared with the effect of 2.5 mg in a single injection. Neither dose altered ovum transport when administered on either day –3 or day 0. The 7.5 mg dose induced maximal acceleration when given on either day –2 or –1, but the 2.5 mg dose failed to induce maximal acceleration if given on day –2. In contrast, 2.5 mg given on day –1 induced maximal acceleration.

Table 7.
Effect of injecting 2.5 mg progesterone on various days (in parentheses).

Group	No. of corpora lutea	% Recovery* of ova		Significantly different**	
		Oviductal	Total	From control	From group 1
Controls	50	100	100		
1 (–2, –1, 0)	52	34	75		
2 (–3, –2, –1, 0)	55	71	78	$P < 0.001$	$P < 0.001$
3 (–3, –2, –1)	55	85	87	$P < 0.01$	$P < 0.001$
4 (–2, –1)	55	28	75	$P < 0.001$	
5 (–1, 0)	42	62	77	$P < 0.001$	$P < 0.001$
6 (–3)	46	93	93		$P < 0.001$
7 (–2)	48	78	88	$P < 0.01$	$P < 0.001$
8 (–1)	41	54	83	$P < 0.001$	
9 (0)	55	97	97		$P < 0.001$

* Mean percentage recovery.
** By Chi^2.

Table 8.

Effect of injecting 2.5 mg vs. 7.5 mg progesterone on various days (in parentheses).

Group	No. of corpora lutea	% Recovery* of ova		Significantly different**	
		Oviductal	Total	From control	From group 1
Controls	50	100	100		
1 (−2, −1, 0)	52	34	75		
6 (2.5, day −3)	46	93	93		$P < 0.001$
10 (7.5, day −3)	50	97	97		$P < 0.001$
7 (2.5, day −2)	48	78	88	$P < 0.01$	$P < 0.001$
11 (7.5, day −2)	50	44	69	$P < 0.001$	
8 (2.5, day −1)	41	54	83	$P < 0.001$	
12 (7.5, day −1)	40	47	55	$P < 0.001$	
9 (2.5, day 0)	55	97	97		$P < 0.001$
13 (7.5, day 0)	43	89	89		$P < 0.001$

* Mean percentage recovery.
** By Chi^2.

Table 9 shows the anatomic location of the ova in the cleared oviducts in the different groups. Most of the control ova were found at the AIJ and in the distal isthmus. The same pattern is shown in all those groups in which all the ova remained in the oviduct. In those groups in which progesterone maximally accelerated ovum transport, fewer ova were found in the proximal isthmus than in the groups in which ovum transport was not maximally accelerated. These findings suggest that progesterone acts both at the ampullary-isthmic junction, and at the uterotubal junction, and that the latter is less sensitive to progesterone. Thus, treatments that induced significant, but less than maximal acceleration, decreased the number of ova retained at the ampullary-isthmic junction, but did not seem to decrease isthmic delay to the same degree. Similar trends can be discerned in Greenwald's data.

The effects of progesterone on ovum transport rates are related to both the timing of administration and the dose administered. In order to induce acceleration of ovum transport, treatment must begin earlier than 12 and not more than 60 h prior to ovulation. Further, although the oviduct becomes sensitive to progesterone about 60 h prior to ovulation and remains sensitive up to at least 36 h prior to ovulation, this sensitivity is greater at 36 h than at 60 h. These data also demonstrate that the mechanism, once "switched on", is dose

Table 9.
Per cent distribution of ova with various treatment schedules.

Group	Dose/mg	Days given	Distal ampulla	Proximal ampulla	AIJ	Distal isthmus	Proximal isthmus	Uterus
Control	0	Controls		12	32	50	6	
1	2.5	-2, -1, 0	10.8	16.2	8.1	8.1	2.7	54.0
2	2.5	-3, -2, -1, 0	9	27.2	29.5	15.9	9.0	9.0
3	2.5	-3, -2, -1		6.2	37.5	39.6	14.6	2.0
4	2.5	-2, -1			13.1	18.4		68.4
5	2.5	-1, 0	3.0			18.1	60.5	18.1
6	2.5	-3		18.6	37.2	41.9	2.3	
7	2.5	-2		9.5	28.5	26.1	21.4	14.3
8	2.5	-1		2.9	8.8	11.7	41.1	35.3
9	2.5	0		5.6	34.0	60.4		
10	7.5	-3		6.1	22.4	63.3	8.1	
11	7.5	-2		22	25	5	11	34
12	7.5	-1		0	16	33	33	16
13	7.5	0		9	40	46	3	

AIJ = ampullary isthmic junction.

dependent. Our results also suggest that the mechanism has a life of only about 3 days after the initial dose of progesterone.

These data provide some insight concerning the mechanism by which progesterone accelerates ovum transport. In addition, examinations of oviductal contractility, progesterone receptors and protein synthesis can now be more accurately defined temporally.

The reports summarized may also be relevant to the design of contraceptives. In order to develop contraceptives that act by accelerating ovum transport it is necessary to make at least two assumptions: 1) That it is possible pharmacologically to accelerate ovum transport in women and 2) that such acceleration would indeed be contraceptive. If the data summarized in this report hold true for the human, progesterone should be administered as a single dose within 30 to 60 h of ovulation. A change in ovum transport should not be expected from the administration of daily doses of progestin as in the oral contraceptives or maintainence of fairly constant blood levels of progestin as with medroxy-progesterone-loaded implants.

REFERENCES

Boling J. L. and Blandau R. J. (1971) Egg transport through the ampullae of the oviducts of rabbits under various experimental conditions. *Biol. Reprod. 4*, 174–184.

Chang M. C. (1966) Effects of oral administration of medroxyprogesterone acetate and ethinyl estradiol on the transportation and development of rabbit eggs. *Endocrinology 79*, 939–948.

Greenwald G. S. (1961) A study of the transport of ova through the rabbit oviduct. *Fertil. Steril. 12*, 80–95.

Harper M. J. K. (1965) Transport of eggs in cumulus through the ampulla of the rabbit oviduct in relation to day of pseudopregnancy. *Endocrinology 77*, 114–123.

Harper M. J. K. (1966) Hormonal control of transport of eggs in cumulus through the ampulla of the rabbit oviduct. *Endocrinology 78*, 568–574.

Pauerstein C. J., Anderson V., Chatkoff M. L. and Hodgson B. J. (1974b) Effect of estrogen and progesterone on the time-course of tubal ovum transport in rabbits. *Amer. J. Obstet. Gynec. 120*, 299–308.

Pauerstein C. J., Chatkoff M. L. and Fremming B. D. (1975) Unpublished data.

Pauerstein C. J., Fremming B. D., Hodgson B. J. and Martin J. E. (1973) The promise of pharmacologic modification of ovum transport in contraceptive development. *Amer. J. Obstet. Gynec. 116*, 161–166.

Pauerstein C. J., Fremming B. D. and Martin J. E. (1970) Influence of progesterone and alpha adrenergic blockade upon tubal transport of ova. *Gynec. Invest. 1,* 257–267.

Pauerstein C. J., Hodgson B. J., Fremming B. D. and Martin J. E. (1974a) Effects of sympathetic denervation of the rabbit oviduct on normal ovum transport and on transport modified by estrogen and progesterone. *Gynec. Invest. 5*, 121–132.

Vargas M. I., Hodgson B. J. and Pauerstein C. J. (1975) Temporal relationships critical to progesterone-induced acceleration of ovum transport. *Obstet. Gynec. 46*, 299–301.

Laboratorios de Endocrinología y Bioquímica,
Instituto de Ciencias Biológicas,
Universidad Católica de Chile, Santiago, Chile

PROGESTERONE BINDING PROTEIN
IN CYTOSOL FRACTION FROM HUMAN OVIDUCT

By

B. E. Fuentealba, G. Escudero and G. E. Swaneck

ABSTRACT

Progesterone binding components in cytosol obtained from oviducts of normal women have been detected by the dextran-charcoal technique. The specific binding components are proteins in nature, thermolabile, and different from plasma progesterone binding protein. Kd values estimated were in the range of 10^{-9} to 10^{-8} M.

This specific binding protein was found in mucosa, in the proximal and distal segments of the oviduct obtained from women in the late follicular or early luteal phase. The concentration of binding sites in these oviducts was determined.

In vitro uptake of ^{3}H-progesterone by human oviduct slices was studied. Uptake and retention of labelled progesterone was observed only in the ampullar segment, at midcycle.

The oviduct is involved in physiologic processes leading to fertilization and implantation and its functions are regulated by neuroendocrine mechanisms in which the ovarian steroids play a major role.

One of the first steps in the action of steroids upon target organs seems to be the interaction with specific macromolecule(s) found in the cytoplasm. Therefore, one can assume that the hormonal regulation of a target tissue depends,

527

not only on hormonal plasma levels, but also on the concentration of these specific macromolecules in or on the cell. These considerations imply the possibility of controlling some functions of the oviduct by changing the concentration of hormonal "receptors" in the tissue.

In vivo or *in vitro* uptake of estradiol or progesterone by the oviduct has been shown in a number of species (rabbit: Kim et al. 1967; rat: Rosner et al. 1970; human: Brush et al. 1967; Taylor et al. 1969; Mendizabal et al. 1971; Roy et al. 1972; and guinea pig: Sar and Stumpf 1974). Estradiol receptors in the oviduct have also been demonstrated (rabbit: Martin et al. 1970; Muechler et al. 1974; monkey: Brenner et al. 1974; human: Flickinger et al. 1974; Kumra et al. 1974).

Differences in estradiol binding capacity from different segments of the human oviduct were found. However, no significant differences were observed in the concentration of estrogen binding sites among oviducts obtained from proliferative and secretory phases (Flickinger et al. 1974).

Cyclic variations in the concentration of specific estradiol or progesterone receptors have been demonstrated in monkey oviduct (Brenner et al. 1974) and in guinea pig uterus (Milgrom et al. 1973).

Synthesis of progesterone receptors seems to be induced by estrogen (Milgrom et al. 1970) whereas progesterone is probably involved in their inactivation (Luu et al. 1973).

The present study was undertaken to explore the presence and regional distribution of specific receptors to progesterone in the human oviduct, and to investigate if they vary qualitatively or quantitatively throughout the menstrual cycle. Preliminary data on *in vitro* uptake by tissue slices and binding of ³H-progesterone to cytosol fractions are presented in this report.

MATERIALS AND METHODS

Oviducts were obtained by salpingectomy from normally menstruating women or in the *post partum* period. The intramural portion of the oviducts, and approximately one cm of the adjacent isthmic portion, were excluded from the sample due to the surgical techniques used. After salpingectomy, the ovaries were inspected to determine if ovulation had occurred and biopsies were taken from corpora lutea for histologic dating (Corner 1956). In some cases, a biopsy was also taken from the abdominal muscles, and endometrial tissue was obtained by dilatation and curettage on completion of surgery. All tissues obtained for incubation were placed in cold buffer immediately after removal. On the day of surgery, a blood sample was drawn to determine plasma levels of progesterone and estrogen by radioimmunoassay (RIA), as described below. The phase of the menstrual cycle, as indicated by the menstrual history, was confirmed by either estradiol and progesterone plasma levels, or endometrial or ovarian biopsy.

To determine *in vitro* uptake of ^{3}H-progesterone by tissue slices, oviducts and samples from endometrium and abdominal muscle were obtained from two women who were in their follicular and luteal phase, respectively. After excluding the fimbria, oviducts were divided in four segments of similar length, which were numbered from I to IV. Segments I and II corresponded to distal and proximal ampulla, respectively. Segment III corresponded to the ampullary-isthmic junction, and segment IV to the distal isthmus.

All other studies were carried out with cytosol fractions obtained from 27 oviducts removed from 14 women under various conditions. Usually, right and left oviducts or equivalent portions of them, obtained from each woman, were pooled in order to prepare the cytosol fraction.

The presence of specific progesterone binding protein in cytosol was determined in 6 oviducts from 3 women which were obtained during the follicular phase, luteal phase, and the 7th day after normal delivery respectively.

The regional concentration of progesterone binding proteins was studied in 10 oviducts which were obtained from 5 women on different days of the cycle. Each oviduct was divided into two segments. The distal segment corresponded to ampulla, and the proximal segment to the ampullary-isthmic junction and distal isthmus.

The concentration of specific progesterone binding protein in mucosal and muscle layers was determined in 4 oviducts obtained from 2 women in the luteal phase. Mucosa was separated from muscle by scraping with a glass slide, and cytosol was prepared from each layer separately.

Cytosol from 5 oviducts was used to investigate the nature and identity of the progesterone binding protein. For this purpose, these cytosols were either heated, treated with trypsin, or compared with corticosterone binding globulin (CBG) by ammonium sulfate precipitation, as described below.

Tissue incubations

In order to determine total uptake, tissue samples from endometrium, oviduct, and abdominal muscle were incubated in duplicate at 30°C in Hank's tissue culture medium (HTCM) with 6×10^{-9} M ^{3}H-progesterone (1,2-^{3}H-progesterone, 48 Ci/mM, New England Nuclear) for 15, 30, or 60 min. Simultaneously, other samples from the same tissues were incubated with ^{3}H-progesterone plus 100 fold non-radioactive progesterone under the same conditions. Radioactivity measured in these samples was considered to be due to non-specific uptake. Specific uptake was calculated from the difference between total and non-specific uptake.

Following incubation at 30°C, the samples were chilled on ice and washed twice with cold HTCM and weighed. After digestion with NCS (Amersham), and addition of 10 ml of toluene counting solution (PPO 4 g, dimethyl POPOP 50 mg and toluene to complete one liter), total tritium was determined.

Preparation of cytosol

Oviducts were washed with ice-cold buffer (0.01 M Tris, 1.5 mM EDTA, Glycerol 20 % pH 7.6) and weighed. After mincing, the tissue was homogenized in a blender (Waring Blendor), in 3 volumes (w/v) of cold buffer. Nuclei and cellular debris were removed by centrifugation at $800 \times g$ for 10 min at 4°C in a HB-4 Sorval rotor. The cytosol fraction was obtained by ultracentrifugation of the supernatant at $105,000 \times g$ for 60 min in a Beckman L-65 ultracentrifuge.

Assay procedure

In order to determine the presence of progesterone binding protein in cytosol, different concentrations of ^{3}H-progesterone (10^{-12} M to 10^{-10} M) were incubated for 2 h at 25°C with the same amount of cytosol (0.4 ml). After incubation, aliquots were mixed with 50 μl dextran-charcoal suspension (100 mg Norite A, 10 mg Dextran T70/ml buffer) for 5 sec and then they were centrifuged at 4°C for 5 min at 5,000 rpm. Radioactivity remaining in the supernatant was measured and the total binding was determined. Simultaneously, aliquots of cytosol were incubated with the same amount of ^{3}H-progesterone plus 1000 fold non-radioactive progesterone. After separation of the free hormone by the dextran-charcoal technique, the non-specific binding was measured. Specific binding was calculated by the difference between total and non-specific binding.

Cytosols obtained from distal segments and from mucosal layers were incubated for 15 min at 25°C. Cytosols prepared from proximal segments and from muscle layers were incubated at 25°C for 30 min. Preliminary experiments had shown that these periods of time were optimal for specific binding of ^{3}H-progesterone by the two segments of the oviduct. All aliquots were assayed at least twice.

The dissociation constant (Kd) and the concentration of binding sites were calculated by plotting the data according to the Lineweaver-Burk method.

Nature of steroid binding sites

To explore the nature of the progesterone binding components, cytosol was heated at 60°C for 20 min, or incubated with trypsin (Calbiochem) (25–50 μg per ml of cytosol) for 30 min at 25°C before the addition of the ^{3}H-progesterone (1×10^{-9} M). The binding was measured as described above.

In addition, cytosol and plasma supernatant fractions were treated with ammonium sulfate. Plasma obtained from a woman in 3rd trimester of pregnancy was centrifuged at $27,000 \times g$ for 15 min and the supernatant obtained was centrifuged for an additional 4 h at $27,000 \times g$. This supernatant, diluted 1:4 with buffer, and the cytosol were incubated separately with ^{3}H-progesterone (3×10^{-8} M) at 25°C for 2 h. After incubation at 25°C both fractions were chilled on ice and were kept at 0°C for 60 min after ammonium sulfate was added up to 30 % final concentration. After centrifugation at $27,000 \times g$ for 20 min, radioactivity was measured in the supernatant and in the resuspended pellet.

Protein assay

Protein was determined using the method of Lowry et al. (1951).

Measurement of radioactivity

Radioactivity from cytosols was measured in 10 ml of scintillation solution (naphthalene 60 g, PPO 4 g, dimethyl POPOP 200 mg, methanol 200 ml, ethyleneglycol 20 ml, and dioxane to complete one liter) in a liquid scintillation spectrometer (Mark I, Nuclear Chicago). The counting efficiency was determined in all the experiments for each vial by the external standard technique.

Hormone assays in plasma

Estrogen was measured by RIA, as described by Edqvist and Johansson (1972), except that the chromatographic step to separate estrone from estradiol was omitted. The antiserum to estradiol-17β-succinyl BSA used was a gift of Dr. E. Johansson (Uppsala).

Progesterone was measured by RIA as described by Thorneycroft and Stone (1972), using an antiserum to 4-pregnen-11 alpha-ol 3,20-dione hemisuccinyl BSA, prepared in rabbits.

Table 1.

In vitro uptake of ^{3}H-progesterone by oviducts, endometrium and muscle from a woman in the late follicular phase.

Tissue	Time of incubation					
	Total uptake	15 min non-specific uptake	Specific uptake	Total uptake	30 min non-specific uptake	Specific uptake
	$\times 10^{-15}$ moles/mg wet tissue			$\times 10^{-15}$ moles/mg wet tissue		
Endometrium	19.97	19.13	0.84	30.95	31.07	0.00
Muscle	26.55	12.35	14.20	21.00	33.52	0.00
Oviduct						
Segment I	10.13	7.90	2.22	20.19	16.85	3.34
Segment II	11.90	9.58	2.32	21.18	22.08	0.00
Segment III	11.40	3.26	8.15	26.23	27.01	0.00
Segment IV	11.50	4.32	7.18	–	–	–

Table 2.

In vitro uptake of ^{3}H-progesterone by oviducts, endometrium and muscle from a woman in the early luteal phase.

Tissue	Time of incubation					
	Total uptake	30 min non-specific uptake	Specific uptake	Total uptake	60 min non-specific uptake	Specific uptake
	$\times\ 10^{-15}$ moles/mg wet tissue			$\times\ 10^{-15}$ moles/mg wet tissue		
Endometrium	8.97	9.78	0.00	10.05	18.10	0.00
Muscle	8.01	10.80	0.00	8.12	9.91	0.00
Oviduct						
Segment I	7.35	5.29	1.16	9.38	8.06	1.33
Segment II	5.19	5.20	0.00	10.89	11.72	0.00
Segment III	5.70	5.70	0.00	9.20	9.35	0.00
Segment IV	4.72	5.09	0.00	–	–	–

RESULTS

In vitro uptake of ^{3}H-progesterone by oviduct, endometrium, and muscle

Uptake of progesterone was determined in two women. According to ovarian and endometrial biopsies, one donor was in the late follicular phase and the other in the early luteal phase (corpus luteum day 1). Results obtained in follicular phase specimens are shown in Table 1.

All segments of the oviduct, as well as endometrium and muscle, had specific uptake after incubation for 15 min. However, only segment I of the oviduct had specific uptake after incubation for 30 min.

Results obtained with the luteal phase specimens are shown in Table 2. Only segment I had specific uptake after incubation for 30 or 60 min. These results indicate that, in these conditions, only the distal ampulla shows specific uptake capacity for ^{3}H-progesterone at midcycle.

Determination of specific progesterone binding protein in cytosol fraction from human oviduct

A representative example of the determination of specific progesterone binding to cytosol is shown in Fig. 1. The Lineweaver-Burk plot of these specific progesterone binding data is shown in Fig. 2.

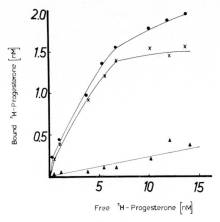

Fig. 1.

Binding of ³H-progesterone by cytosol fraction from the distal segment of human oviduct. Cytosol was incubated with ³H-progesterone (●) and with ³H-progesterone plus 1000 fold unlabelled progesterone (▲). Specific binding was calculated as the difference between the bound radioactivity of these two types of incubations (×). Oviducts were obtained from a women on day 19 of the cycle.

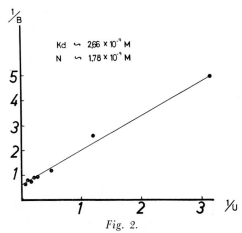

Fig. 2.

Lineweaver-Burk plot of specific binding progesterone from the data in Fig. 1. Kd was calculated as the reciprocal value of the intercept with the abscissa, and the concentration of binding sites (N) was estimated as the reciprocal value of the intercept with the y axis.

533

Table 3.
Kd values and concentration of progesterone binding sites in whole oviducts.

Phase	Kd at 25°C (M)	N (× 10^{-13} moles/mg protein)
Preovulatory	0.8×10^{-9}	5.7
Postovulatory	1.0×10^{-9}	2.5
Puerperal*	0.5×10^{-9}	0.9

* Oviducts were obtained 7 days after normal delivery.

The concentration of progesterone binding sites and Kd values determined in whole oviducts is shown in Table 2. In the post ovulatory case, the plasma progesterone level was still low, and corresponded to recent ovulation (corpus luteum day 1).

Concentration of progesterone binding sites determined on distal and proximal segments showed variations between segments and between women. The range of Kd values for four experiments in which distal segments obtained from luteal phase patients were used was $2.6–25 \times 10^{-9}$ M. For the corresponding proximal

Table 4.
Kd values and concentration of progesterone binding sites in distal and proximal segments of the oviducts on different days of the cycle.

Cycle phase	Distal segment		Proximal segment	
	N × 10^{-13} moles/mg protein	Kd at 25°C (M)	N × 10^{-13} moles/mg protein	Kd at 25°C (M)
Follicular	4.8	1.9×10^{-9}	4.0	1.5×10^{-9}
Luteal	1.9	25.0×10^{-9}	0.8	5.5×10^{-9}
	4.3	10.0×10^{-9}	6.2	4.5×10^{-9}
	3.7	4.0×10^{-9}	1.2	11.0×10^{-9}
	3.5	2.6×10^{-9}	0.5	4.0×10^{-9}

Table 5.

Effect of temperature on the progesterone binding capacity of the cytosol.

Cytosol	Total binding	Specific binding
25°C	2.88×10^{-10} M	2.22×10^{-10} M
60°C	0.12×10^{-10} M	0.01×10^{-10} M

segments, the range of Kd values was $4{-}11 \times 10^{-9}$ M (Table 4). Analysis of corpus luteum dating in these four cases indicated day 3 in two and day 4 and day 6 in the others. However, only one woman had high values of plasma progesterone (14 ng/ml); in the other cases, the levels were below 3.5 ng/ml.

The concentration of binding sites in the mucosa from each pair of oviducts analyzed was 0.72 and 0.17×10^{-13} M ³H-progesterone/mg of protein. Kd values determined in these samples were 0.25×10^{-9} M and 0.5×10^{-9} M. No binding sites were found in cytosol obtained from the muscle layer of the same two pairs of oviducts.

Nature of progesterone binding component

Total binding of ³H-progesterone to oviductal cytosol was partially inhibited after heating or after enzymatic digestion with trypsin. Both procedures inhibited completely the progesterone specific binding capacity of the control. The results are shown in Tables 5 and 6.

Results of ammonium sulfate precipitation are shown in Table 7. Essentially all plasma binding activity remained in the supernatant, while cytosol binding activity was distributed in the pellet and in the supernatant. ³H-progesterone bound per mg of protein in the pellet was two fold higher than in the supernatant.

Table 6.

Trypsin effect on the progesterone binding capacity of the cytosol.

Cytosol	Total binding	Specific binding
Control	5.18×10^{-10} M	2.48×10^{-10} M
Trypsin 25 μg	3.22×10^{-10} M	0.08×10^{-10} M
Trypsin 50 μg	2.88×10^{-10} M	0.00×10^{-10} M

535

Table 7.

Progesterone receptors distinguished from corticosterone binding globulin by
ammonium sulfate precipitation.

Fraction	^{3}H-progesterone bound in fraction*		Bound ^{3}H-progesterone recovered after precipitation**	Specific activity
				moles ^{3}H-progesterone/mg protein
	moles/ml	%	moles/ml	
Cytosol	1.7×10^{-12}	5.3		0.49×10^{-12}
Supernatant			0.30×10^{-12}	0.25×10^{-12}
Pellet			0.22×10^{-12}	0.55×10^{-12}
Plasma	11.3×10^{-12}	30.8		1.16×10^{-12}
Supernatant			3.10×10^{-12}	0.70×10^{-12}
Pellet			0.04×10^{-12}	0.01×10^{-12}

* $100 \times \dfrac{\text{bound } ^3\text{H-progesterone}}{\text{total } ^3\text{H-progesterone}}$ in the incubate.

** binding activity determined by dextran-charcoal technique.

DISCUSSION

These experiments confirm the progesterone binding capacity of the human
oviduct reported previously by Kumra et al. (1974). In addition, they demonstrate that progesterone binds to a thermolabile molecule of protein nature,
which seems to be different from CBG, as determined by ammonium sulfate
precipitation.

While essentially all plasma binding activity remained in the supernatant,
after ammonium sulfate precipitation, binding activity in the cytosol was separated into two populations of binding molecules, a pellet fraction that was pre-
cipitated by ammonium sulfate and was not present in plasma, and another
fraction that remained in the supernatant. This latter fraction could correspond
either to non-specific or other-specific binding molecules normally present in
the tissue. Contamination of cytosol with plasma components is unavoidable
but it is unlikely that one third of total binding activity of cytosol could derive
entirely from such contamination. In accordance with the observations of
Schrader and O'Malley (1972), who showed that specific progesterone binding
protein obtained from chick oviduct precipitates with ammonium sulfate, it is
likely that the binding activity present in the pellet corresponded to specific
progesterone binding protein. However, this needs confirmation.

Progesterone receptors were found in cytosol from ampullary and isthmic segments, and from the mucosal layer; but surprisingly, they were not detected in the muscular layer. This observation is in contrast with the presence of progesterone receptors in the human myometrium (Verma and Laumas 1973) and in the myosalpinx of guinea pig (Sar and Stumf 1974). On the other hand, it is in agreement with our finding, in most of the cases, of a larger concentration of binding sites in ampulla, where the mucosal layer is predominant, than in isthmus, where the muscle forms the thickest layer.

Variations in the concentration of binding sites between segments and between women were observed. The analysis of these preliminary data does not yet permit us to determine if these variations are significant and whether or not they correspond to cyclic variations.

In vitro uptake experiments showed that, at midcycle, only the distal ampulla can retain ^{3}H-progesterone. However, in experiments with cytosol, receptors were detected in both segments of the oviduct. The same difference was observed with endometrial tissue. In our experiments, uptake was not observed but binding of progesterone in the endometrial cytosol fraction has been reported by Haukkamaa and Luukkainen (1974) and Rao et al. (1974). This could indicate that cytosol binding capacity does not necessarily reflect the binding activity of intact cells.

ACKNOWLEDGMENTS

The authors are grateful to Dr. H. B. Croxatto for his constructive comments on the manuscript, and to Drs. G. Valenzuela, U. Pastore and J. Balmaceda for their help in providing the surgical material.

These investigations were supported in part by The Population Council, N. Y., Grant M71, 138/ICCR/RA-16 to Dr. H. B. Croxatto; by the Expanded Programme of Research, Development and Research Training in Human Reproduction of the World Health Organization; and Grant 113/74 del Fondo de Investigaciones de la Universidad Católica de Chile.

REFERENCES

Brenner R. M., Resko J. A. and West N. B. (1974) Cyclic changes in oviductal morphology and residual cytoplasmic estradiol binding capacity induced by sequential estradiol-progesterone treatment of spayed Rhesus monkey. *Endocrinology 95*, 1094–1104.

Brush M. G., Taylor R. W. and King R. J. B. (1967) The uptake of (6,7-^{3}H) oestradiol by the normal human female reproductive tract. *J. Endocr. 39*, 599–607.

Corner G. W. (1956) The histological dating of the human corpus luteum of menstruation. *Amer. J. Anat. 98*, 377–392.

Edqvist L.-E. and Johansson E. D. B. (1972) Radioimmunoassay of oestrone and oestradiol in human and bovine peripheral plasma. *Acta endocr. (Kbh.) 71,* 716–731.

Flickinger G. L., Muechler E. K. and Mikhail G. (1974) Estradiol receptor in the human Fallopian tube. *Fertil. Steril. 25,* 900–903.

Haukkamaa M. and Luukkainen T. (1974) The cytoplasmic progesterone receptor of human endometrium during the menstrual cycle. *J. Steroid Biochem. 5,* 447–452.

Kim Y. J., Coates J. B. and Flickinger G. L. (1967) Incorporation and fate of estradiol-17β-6,7-^{3}H in rabbit oviduct. *Proc. Soc. exp. Biol. Med. 126,* 918–921.

Kumra R., Sen K. K., Hingorani V. and Talwar G. P. (1974) Binding of progesterone in the human Fallopian tube. *Amer. J. Obstet. Gynec. 119,* 762–766.

Lowry O. H., Rosebrough N. J., Farr A. L. and Randall R. J. (1951) Protein measurement with the folin phenol reagent. *J. biol. Chem. 193,* 265–275.

Luu M., Baulieu E. E. and Milgrom E. (1973) Régulation par la progestérone de la concentration de ses récepteurs utérins. *C. R. Acad. Sci. (Paris) 276,* 2281–2284.

Martin J. E., McGuire W. L. and Pauerstein C. J. (1970) Macromolecular binding of estradiol in the rabbit oviduct and uterus. *Gynec. Invest. 1,* 303–311.

Mendizabal A. F., Rosner J., Martinez I. and Spaltro N. (1971) The uptake of (6,7-^{3}H) oestradiol by the normal Fallopian tube. *Excerpta medica International Congress Series No. 234b.*

Milgrom E., Atger M. and Baulieu E. E. (1970) Progesterone in uterus and plasma IV. Progesterone receptor(s) in guinea pig uterus cytosol. *Steroids 16,* 741–754.

Milgrom E., Luu Thi M. and Baulieu E. E. (1973) Control mechanisms of steroid hormone receptors in the reproductive tract. In *Karolinska Symposia on Research Methods in Reproductive Endocrinology.* 6th Symposium: Protein synthesis in reproductive tissue (Diczfalusy E., ed.), pp. 380–397.

Muechler E. K., Flickinger G. L. and Mikhail G. (1974) Estradiol receptors in the oviduct and uterus of the rabbit. *Fertil. Steril. 25,* 893–899.

Rao B. R., Wiest W. G. and Allen W. M. (1974) Progesterone "receptor" in human endometrium. *Endocrinology 95,* 1275–1281.

Rosner J. M., Macombe J. C., Castro-Vasquez A. and De Carli D. N. (1970) Rat oviductal uptake of estradiol. *Revista Argentina de Endocrinologia 16,* 45.

Roy S. K., Jr., Roy S. K., Dasgupta P. R, Engineer A. D. and Kar A. B. (1972) Biochemical composition and *in vitro* uptake of estradiol 6,7-^{3}H by the Fallopian tube: A preliminary study. *Amer. J. Obstet. Gynec. 112,* 299–300.

Sar M. and Stumpf W. E. (1974) Cellular and subcellular localization of [^{3}H]-progesterone or its metabolites in the oviduct, uterus, vagina and liver of the guinea pig. *Endocrinology 94,* 1116–1125.

Schrader W. T. and O'Malley B. W. (1972) Progesterone binding components of chick oviduct. *J. biol. Chem. 247,* 51–59.

Taylor R. W., Brush M. G. and King R. J. B. (1969) Intravenous and intraluminal administration of [6,7-^{3}H] oestradiol in *in vivo* uptake studies with human Fallopian tube. *J. Endocrinology 43,* lxii.

Thorneycroft I. H. and Stone S. C. (1972) Radioimmunoassay of serum progesterone in women receiving oral contraceptive steroids. *Contraception 5,* 129–146.

Verma U. and Laumas K. R. (1973) *In vitro* binding of progesterone to receptors in the human endometrium and the myometrium. *Biochim. biophys. Acta (Amst.) 317,* 403–419.

Departments of Obstetrics & Gynecology & Anatomy,
Ralph L. Smith Research Center,
University of Kansas Medical Center,
Kansas City, Kansas 66103

Discussion Paper

EFFECTS OF ESTROGEN AND PROGESTERONE ON EGG TRANSPORT: SUMMARY AND CONCLUSIONS

By

Gilbert S. Greenwald

The idea that exogenous estrogens could act as antifertility agents by affecting egg transport in the oviduct was first concretely expressed about 40 years ago. In 1936, Whitney and Burdick raised the questions: "Can a normally fertilized primate ovum be tube-locked by excess oestrin? Can pregnancy be prevented in primates by injections of oestrin soon after copulation?". Burdick's contributions in this field are especially noteworthy. He was the first to establish the dose-dependent acceleratory or retarding effects of estrogen on egg transport and introduced the concept of "tube-locking:" the retention of eggs in the oviducts beyond their normal period of oviductal sojourn.

Parkes et al. (1938) showed that orally administered ethinyl estradiol or stilbestrol interrupted early pregnancy in rabbits and rats. At the conclusion of their paper, they stated "The intensive work at present being carried out on the artificial production of oestrogenic substances may well result in the production of a compound also active by mouth, but more effective in suppressing the tubal and uterine changes necessary for implantation of the fertilized egg". It is always a humbling but salutary experience to review the work of our predecessors.

Since the pioneering studies of Burdick and others, the effects of steroids on egg transport have been extensively studied and the literature is too extensive to summarize on this occasion. Instead, the reader is referred to a series of recent review articles by Harper (1968, 1972), Kincl (1972) and Pauerstein (1974).

My own research on egg transport was initiated in 1954 while I was a post-doctoral fellow at the Department of Embryology of the Carnegie Institution of Washington. Over the next 13 years I published a series of studies which were summarized in a review article published in 1968 (Greenwald 1968). The research confirmed, and hopefully extended, some aspects of oviductal physiology and the salient findings were as follows:

1. The results stressed the importance of the ampullary-isthmic junction (AIJ) in regulating egg transport. In the rabbit, after a very rapid phase of ampullary transport, lasting a matter of minutes, eggs are retained for long periods at the AIJ. Therefore, isthmic transport of eggs is a relatively slow drawn-out process.

2. The anatomical organization of the oviduct is consistent with the rapid and slow phases of egg transport. Comparing the ampulla and isthmus, there are differences in the size of the lumen and its distensibility, development of the myometrium, number of cilia and the extent of sympathetic innervation. Hence, the oviduct is really a composite organ and one must specify what phase of egg transport is being analyzed and be aware that different hormonal levels and mechanisms may be involved depending on the level of the oviduct.

3. In the rabbit, small doses of estrogen accelerate egg transport and eggs are rapidly conveyed into the uterus and then lost *per vaginam*. The rapid egg transport induced by small doses of estrogen cannot be reversed by exogenous progesterone. The estrogen treatment does not interfere with normal progestational proliferation of the endometrium.

4. In the rabbit, large doses of estrogen lead to "tube-locking" at the AIJ for several days and also prevent the histologic transformation of the uterus normally attributable to progesterone. Estrogen levels are believed to be the controlling factor regulating the passage of eggs into the isthmus. In the normal rabbit, a decline in circulating levels of estrogen or an altered estrogen-progesterone ratio by days 2–3 *post-coitum* enables eggs to resume their migration through the oviduct.

5. Despite the accelerating or delaying action of low or high doses of estrogen on oviductal transport of eggs, the pattern of oviductal motility is the same following either treatment. This suggests that premature or delayed relaxation of a sphincter involving the AIJ or the isthmus as a whole accounts for the different rates of egg transport.

6. Profound species differences exist in the effects of exogenous estrogen on oviductal transport of eggs. At one extreme is the rat in which 1–500 μg of estradiol cyclopentylpropionate always accelerates egg transport; "tubal-locking" of eggs never occurs. This is most likely the reason why a number of anti-estrogens (which have weak inherent estrogenicity) are effective as anti-fertility agents in the rat. At the other end of the spectrum, the guinea pig and hamster are extremely resistant to large doses of estrogen, with luteal function affected before egg transport is disrupted.

For several reasons, I envisioned my 1968 review article as my last effort in oviductal physiology. For one thing, like most workers in the field, I had serious reservations about the recording systems then available and the obvious need for miniaturization and improved techniques in bioengineering. In other words, how much was artifact versus true physiologic changes in myosalpingeal activity. A second qualm was that I lacked the talent and temperament to master the electrophysiological techniques which were obviously essential to comprehend muscle physiology. Still a third reason for my uneasiness was Dr. Brundin's now classic contribution (1965) which revealed the rich adrenergic innervation of the oviduct, especially of the isthmus. This indicated that neuropharmacology would become increasingly important in the armamentarium of the oviductal physiologist. I therefore bowed out of the oviduct and therefore, in a sense, I am an interloper but still an interested bystander at this meeting.

Dr. Fuentealba's presentation this morning on progesterone receptors in the oviduct conjured up an analogy. At this stage of the meeting if cerebral memory receptor sites exist, they are all occupied and anything that I add will be of the nature of non-specific binding. Hence, I will limit my remarks to a few generalizations, a number of which have already been raised by previous participants.

(1) The correlation between oviductal contractility and egg transport is still very nebulous. Several examples have been cited at this meeting where diametrically different patterns of oviductal contractions were still associated with acceleration of egg transport. This is a problem which obviously still remains to be resolved.

(2) Several speakers pointed out the danger of interpretation of intraluminal pressure recording systems. This is an obvious caveat but science, like politics, is the art of the possible. As long as one recognizes the inherent artifacts in this technique, one must also recognize that in a number of situations these are the only procedures available and although their interpretation must be considered carefully, until more sophisticated techniques are available, the balloon recording system still has a definite place.

As a proponent of a sphincteric blocking mechanism operative at the level of the AIJ or of the isthmus as a whole, I was intrigued by Dr. Blair's technique for determining changes in the internal diameter of the isthmus. It will be interesting to compare this technique with oviductal contractility and egg transport.

(3) The problem of correlating animal models with the primate oviduct still exists. For several obvious reasons the rabbit has been the model par excellence, but one must take into consideration the very different anatomical organization and the presence of the mucin layer in extrapolating to primates. Another factor that must be taken into account is the different nature of luteotrophic support in the rabbit versus primates. Whereas in the rabbit estrogen is supportive to the corpus luteum, estrogen may be luteolytic in the case of the primates. One of the paradoxical situations in the rabbit is that low doses of estrogen accelerate egg transport whereas high doses delay transport. I wonder whether the accelerating effects of estrogen in the rabbit may not be due to a precocious increase in progesterone secretion and if the latter is not really responsible for the observed acceleration. The availability of radioimmunoassays for steroids may resolve this question.

(4) In numerous other instances assays for progesterone and estrogen in blood and tissue will facilitate the analysis of oviductal control. In other words, steroid profiles as an adjunct will greatly enhance the value of a number of studies of oviductal function.

(5) The discovery of the rich adrenergic supply of the oviductal isthmus by Brundin in 1965 and the further studies of Owman seemed to offer a logical explanation as to how hormones exert their effect on the isthmic region of the oviduct. It was, to say the least, disconcerting at this meeting to learn that a number of procedures which deplete the adrenergic nerves fail to affect egg transport. Whether there is still sufficient adrenergic reserve or hypersensitivity of the muscle which enable the animal to still display normal egg transport, are possibilities which cannot be excluded. Still, one's faith in the adrenergic regulation of the isthmus is somewhat shaken.

(6) A point raised by Dr. Moawad, however, deserves consideration, and that is that the oviduct represents a multifactorial system representing the interaction of ciliary and muscular activity, oviductal secretions, hormones, and the autonomic nervous system. It is possible that manipulation of one component can lead to compensatory changes in others so that "normal" transport may still occur.

(7) A point that was raised at the meeting that I have never considered before is the possible interaction between the mucosa and the myosalpinx. For example, the histochemical localization in the mucosa of prostaglandins and their known effects on oviductal contractions and egg transport. It would, therefore, be

interesting to try to dissociate these two factors. One possibility is that trans-luminal perfusion of the oviduct with various fixatives might destroy the mucosa and leave the muscle layers intact. Under these circumstances, recordings of oviductal contractility would be of interest. This may be a far fetched experiment, but it might be worth undertaking.

The 40 years that have elapsed between Burdick's questions and today have so far not resulted in the ultimate pay-off of a fertility control technique based on acceleration of egg transport. The fact that we have not gone from dream to reality in 40 years is no reason for discouragement. For too long the oviduct has been the orphan of the reproductive tract when one considers the enormous volume of work carried out, for example, on the ovary or the uterus. A much better perspective on the status of the oviduct, as Dr. Black mentioned yesterday, is the tremendous increase in knowledge represented at this meeting in comparison to the Pullman Conference of 1968. One cannot help being impressed by these new findings. Hopefully the next meeting will represent a further exponential increase in information and bring us that much closer to devising a new and revolutionary technique of fertility control.

REFERENCES

Brundin J. (1965) Distribution and function of adrenergic nerves in the rabbit Fallopian tube. *Acta physiol. scand. 66*, Suppl. 259, pp. 1–57.

Greenwald G. S. (1968) Hormonal regulation of egg transport through the mammalian oviduct. In: Behrman S. J. and Kistner R. W., eds. *Progress in Infertility*, pp. 157–179. Little, Brown and Company, Boston.

Harper M. J. K. (1968) Pharmacological control of reproduction in women. In: Jucker E., ed. *Progress in Drug Research 12*, 47–136. Birkhauser, Basel.

Harper M. J. K. (1973) Agents with antifertility effects during preimplantation stages of pregnancy. In: Moghissi K. S. and Hafez E. S. E., eds. *Biology of Mammalian Fertilization and Implantation*, pp. 431–492. C. C. Thomas, Springfield.

Kincl F. A. (1972) Estrogens as antifertility agents. In: *Pharmacology of the endocrine system and related drugs: Progesterone, Progestational Drugs and Antifertility Agents*, Vol. II, pp. 347–384. Pergamon Press, Oxford.

Parkes A. S., Dodds E. C. and Noble L. L. (1938) Interruption of early pregnancy by means of orally active oestrogens. *Brit. Med. J. 2*, 557–559.

Pauerstein C. J. (1974) *The Fallopian Tube: A Reappraisal.* Lea and Febiger, Philadelphia.

Whitney R. and Burdick H. O. (1936) Tube-locking of ova by oestrogenic substances. *Endocrinology 20*, 643–647.

Dept. of Maternal Health and Child Care,
Maternidade Climerio de Oliveira,
Federal University of Bahia School of Medicine,
Salvador – Bahia – Brazil

INTERFERENCE WITH OVUM TRANSPORT: IMPLICATIONS FOR FERTILITY CONTROL

By

Elsimar M. Coutinho

The evidence available in the human, as in many other species, suggests that following ovulation the ovum remains within the oviduct for a relatively long time (two to three days) before it is allowed to be transported into the uterus where it will implant (Blandau 1969; Betteridge and Mitchell 1972; Croxatto et al. 1972). It is assumed that this period of residence in the oviduct is necessary to synchronize ovum development with uterine receptivity to nidation. Receptivity to nidation includes supression of uterine motility and development of a secretory endometrium. The progestational changes which render the myometrium quiescent and the endometrium secretory are induced by estrogens and progesterone secreted by the corpus luteum, whose secretory activity increases rapidly fom days 2–3 to reach a peak 6 to 7 days after ovulation (Thorneycroft et al. 1971). The time needed by the corpus luteum to supress uterine motility and render the endometrium suitable for implantation should therefore be the lower limit of the time interval that the ovum must be retained within the oviduct. Because progesterone and its metabolites are responsible for the progestational changes which take place in the uterus after ovulation it is very appropriate that the same hormones acting on the musculature of the oviductal wall should regulate the passage of the ovum into the uterus. Indirect evidence suggests that indeed during the pre-ovulatory phase when the smooth musculature of the reproductive tract is under estrogen-domination, a block is established at the oviductal isthmus which prevents the passage of the oviductal contents into the uterus (Pauerstein et al. 1974; Croxatto 1974). This estrogen-induced isthmic block which may establish itself several days before ovulation and should last two to three days past ovulation, can be demonstrated in normally ovulating women by means of oviductal insufflation and serial hysterosalpingography (Coutinho 1974a). Retention of ova surrogates in the oviduct of women during the proliferative phase of the cycle has been reported recently, a finding which is undoubtedly the best available proof of an estrogen-induced oviductal block (Croxatto 1975). Paradoxically estrogen, a hormone which induces synthesis of contractile proteins and activates both the uterus and the oviduct, becomes through stimulation of oviductal musculature the first hormone to provide pregnancy protection. The estrogen block prevents the immature ovum from reaching an unprepared uterus, therefore reducing ovum wastage.

If in fact, the isthmic block induced by estrogen is the earliest mechanism of pregnancy protection, inhibition or reversal of the block should prevent implantation by allowing expulsion of the fertilized ovum from the oviduct as soon as it reaches the oviductal isthmus. Probably the best way to overcome an estrogen block is that used by nature, i. e., through progestational steroids. If progesterone secretion could be activated several days before ovulation, the block would probably be inhibited and as soon as the ovum reached the oviductal isthmus it would quickly pass into the uterus. Whether this may be achieved by appropriate gonadotrophin treatment is not known, but there is evidence that with proper doses and schedule, ovarian progesterone secretion may be increased without necessarily inducing ovulation (Jones and Nalbandov 1972; Nalbandov and Bahr 1974). The closest approach to this at present is through continuous progestin treatment. Here we certainly interfere with ovum transport as shown by the studies of Croxatto (1974b), who measured the duration of passage of ovum surrogates in women treated with the progestin, megestrol acetate*. Croxatto found, however, that in these women ovum transport was considerably delayed. That a delay rather than an acceleration of ovum transport occurred suggests that this progestin apparently inhibited the propulsive mechanism, an effect which is not shared by progesterone.

Studies of oviductal contractility in women show that even during pregnancy when uterine motility is almost completely inhibited by ovarian steroids secreted by the corpus luteum of pregnancy, the oviduct remains active (Coutinho 1974b) (Fig. 1). Continuous treatment with synthetic progestin on the other hand not only counteracts the action of estrogen, but also competes with progesterone itself, inducing partial atrophy of epithelial cells and reducing the activity and renewal of cilia. In view of the weak progestational effects of 19-norsteroids, it is possible that by using these compounds rather than the C21 progestins, the effects of estrogen on the isthmus may be inhibited without supression of oviductal motility. The ideal compound to be used in this approach should be

---

* 17-alpha-acetoxy-6α-methylpregna-4,6-diene-3,20-dione.

Ovum Transport

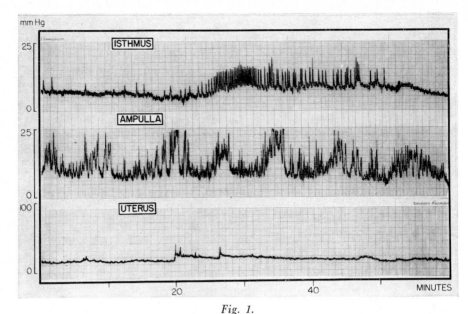

Fig. 1.

Oviductal activity during early pregnancy. *In vivo* recording. Note activity in both
the isthmus and the ampulla whereas the uterus is quiescent.
Reprinted from Coutinho (1974b) by permission of Butterworths.

an anti-estrogen with little anti-progesterone effect and no androgenicity, with
a minimum of intrinsic estrogenicity and high affinity for the oviduct. In fact
anti-estrogens may contribute to acceleration of ovum transport not only through
their potential effects in releasing the isthmic block, but also through activation
of oviductal motility by causing an acute estrogen deficiency. Estrogen withdrawal may stimulate rather than inhibit oviductal motility (Coutinho 1974b).
This effect of estrogen withdrawal may be seen following ovariectomy of
estrous rabbits, and in castrate and menopausal women following discontinuation
of estrogen treatment.

Some trieneoic steroids which are contraceptive at very low doses fulfill some
of above mentioned conditions for an ideal contraceptive acting on the oviduct.
Norgestrienone and ethylnorgestrienone (R-2323) have been used in subdermal
silastic capsules and found to be as effective as megestrol acetate in preventing
pregnancy for long periods of time (Coutinho and Silva 1974; Coutinho et al.
1975). R-2323 also prevented pregnancy when it was administered daily for
three days following ovulation (Sakiz et al. 1974). Although the anti-estrogenic
effect of R-2323 may interfere with other effects of estrogen which are required
for normal conception, one of the mechanisms of the contraceptive action of
R-2323 administered at mid cycle is probably the release of the isthmic block.

In an extensive evaluation of the effects of several steroids of the trienoic series on ovum transport and implantation Azadian-Boulanger (unpublished) found that in rats both R-2323 and 17-ethynyl-19-nortestosterone accelerate ovum transport whereas non-anti-estrogenic compounds such as R-5020 (17,21-dimethyl-19-norpregna-4,9-diene-3,20-dione) had no effect as compared to non-treated controls. The same mechanism probably applies to other norsteroids used post coitally. A significant anti-fertility effect is achieved for example with d-norgestrel given daily for a few days after coitus (Kesseru et al. 1973).

Other compounds which may cause the release of the isthmic block are beta-adrenergic receptor activators, and alpha-adrenergic receptor blockers (Pauerstein and Woodruff 1970; Polidoro et al. 1973). Adrenergic activation of oviductal musculature is probably the major mechanism through which the estrogen block occurs. Adrenergic agonists and antagonists however act on other smooth muscle structures such as vascular smooth muscle and in the heart, thus rendering their use problematic. Nevertheless, the potential use of these compounds as pre- or post coital contraceptives is being investigated. Some of the beta-adrenergic activators are well tolerated and their side effects predictable. Ritodrine® is one such compound. It is effective orally and inhibits oviductal contractility at relatively low doses (Coutinho et al. 1974). The standard dose of Ritodrine used to suppress uterine motility (10 mg) does not suppress oviductal motility but is probably sufficient to release the isthmic block. This is indicated by the partial inhibition of oviductal motility and the suppression of outbursts of activity which follow the administration of this drug to women during the ovulatory phase of the menstrual cycle (Fig. 2).

Another group of compounds which may interfere with ovum transport are prostaglandins. Prostaglandins (Pg) are apparently associated with oviductal function and may be responsible for the spontaneous contractility of the oviduct (Spilman and Harper 1975). PGF_2 alpha synthesis inhibitors such as aspirin and indomethacin reduce oviductal motility and should be able to suppress the isthmic block (Maia, Jr. and Coutinho 1974).

Inhibition of oviductal contractility and very likely of the isthmic block is also induced by PGE_2 (Coutinho and Maia 1971). PGE_2 occurs in human semen and may play an important role in faciliating sperm transport through the uterus and into the oviduct (Bygdeman and Eliasson 1973). Long acting prostaglandin analogs are now being tested which may through their prostaglandin-like effects or through competition with endogenous prostaglandins be used to interfere with ovum transport (Fig. 3).

Another possible way to interfere with ovum transport is through prolonged activation of oviductal motility. Although increased contractility of the oviduct without isthmic relaxation may be incapable of destroying the ovum, prolonged and intense activation of oviductal musculature, should be able to overcome the isthmic block.

547

35*

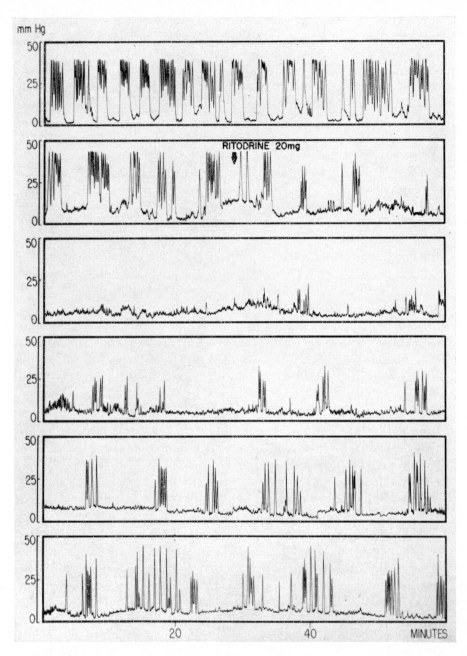

Fig. 2.
The effect of ritodrine on human oviductal activity. *In vivo* recording. Note that following the administration of 10 mg orally (arrow) oviductal activity is depressed for almost two hours. Reprinted from Coutinho et al. (1974) by permission of the American Fertility Society.

548

We have found that ergot compounds are powerful stimulants of oviductal motility inducing long lasting contractions with relatively small doses (Coutinho 1971; Coutinho 1971b). The response to ergot compounds may be induced at all stages of the menstrual cycle and is also recorded in women treated with progestational steroids (Fig. 4).

The oviduct responds to as little as 10 μg of ergonovine maleate given intravenously. A response lasting four h or longer is achieved with a standard dose of 0.20 mg which may be administered orally. Repeated administration at four or six h intervals will sustain an exaggerated oviductal activity continuously for 12 h or longer. Oviductal response to ergot compounds is depressed during the puerperium but returns fully when cyclic ovarian function is re-activated. (Coutinho et al., unpublished).

It is of interest to note that no activation by ergot derivatives has been recorded in the oviduct of other species, such as the rabbit (Coutinho et al. 1971) an animal whose oviductal function has been used frequently as a model for the human oviduct. The ergot compounds active on the oviduct do not have a comparable effect on the non-pregnant human uterus. The response of the non-pregnant uterus to ergonovine maleate is weak and short-lived.

Preliminary clinical trials with ergonovine maleate given at a daily dose of 0.20 mg orally indicated that the compound has a contraceptive effect (Coutinho and da Silva, unpublished). However the regimen did not provide full contraceptive protection, since several pregnancies occurred which were considered drug failures. In this study, 48 women took ergonovine maleate daily for 262 women months. It has been calculated that 30 to 40 pregnancies should occur

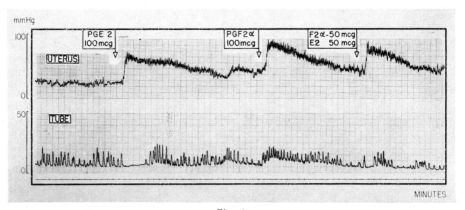

Fig. 3.

The effect of prostaglandins on human oviductal activity. *In vivo* recording. Note inhibition following the administration of PGE$_2$ and stimulation following PGF$_{2\alpha}$. Both compounds were injected intravenously. Reprinted from Coutinho and Maia (1971) by permission of the American Fertility Society.

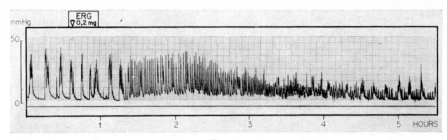

Fig. 4.

The response of the human oviduct to ergonovine maleate (ERG) *in vivo*. Recording
at slow paper speed. Note that following the administration of 0.20 mg of ergonovine
maleate orally oviductal motility is activated for several hours.

in this group if the women were unprotected. However only six pregnancies
occurred suggesting that the fertility of these women was reduced by the ergonovine maleate treatment.

Pilot studies in which ergonovine or methyl-ergonovine maleate are given
pre- or post coitally are also being conducted in our clinic, but in these studies
as in the daily regimen trial some contraceptive failures have been observed.

If implantation occurs following premature expulsion of the immature ovum
into the uterus in these ergonovine treated women, we have to assume that
complete pre-implantation development takes place in the uterus and that
shortening of the stay of the ovum in the oviduct is not always harmful. It
should be noted that transport does not end when the ovum leaves the oviduct.
To reach its implantation site the ovum must migrate further within the uterine
cavity. The slow and gentle motion of the progesterone-dominated uterus should
provide the propulsive mechanism. As the uterus remains almost undisturbed
when ergonovine maleate is administered to women during the luteal phase,
it is possible that the ovum ejected from the oviduct into the uterus develops
normally within the uterine cavity and implants. We propose therefore that
activation of uterine motility should be part of a treatment aiming for a contraceptive effect based on interference with ovum transport.

Most oxytocic drugs which have been screened for use as pre-implantation
uterine stimulants have serious limitations. The effect of oxytocin on the progesterone-dominated uterus is weak and short-lived (Coutinho 1968). Vasopressin
induces strong and long-lasting contractions on the non-pregnant uterus but
its repeated and chronic administration as required for a post coital contraceptive
is limited by its powerful vasopressor and anti-diuretic effects (Coutinho and
Vieira Lopes 1968). Prostaglandin $F_{2\alpha}$ which is a powerful stimulant of both
the oviduct and the uterus, has too many undesirable side effects resulting
mainly from its action on the gastro-intestinal tract and on the vascular bed for
repeated and frequent use (Anderson et al. 1971).

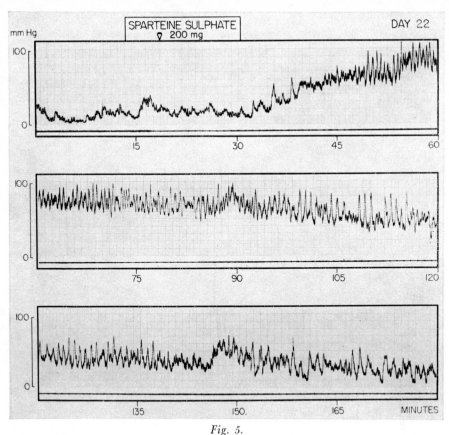

Fig. 5.

The response of the human non-pregnant uterus to sparteine sulfate. *In vivo* recording during the early luteal phase, the LH peak was recorded on day 15. Note marked and long lasting activation of uterine motility following the oral administration of sparteine sulfate.

Oxytocin or vasopressin analogs (Bengtsson 1974) devoid of anti-diuretic and vasopressor activity, but retaining the oxytocic action which vasopressin exerts on the non-pregnant uterus, would have potential use as pre-implantation uterine activators. None of the existing analogs however have as yet shown to possess these qualities. The same applies to prostaglandin and prostaglandin analogs. Attempts have been made to counteract the effects of $PGF_{2\alpha}$ on the gastro-intestinal tract by the simultaneous administration of drugs which specifically block the gastrointestinal response (Lauersen and Wilson 1974). This approach could be developed in connection with the use of prostaglandins for contraception. However, a proper formulation which would be effective and well tolerated by the majority of women may take many years to develop.

The only compound among the presently available oxytocics which qualifies as a potential pre-implantation uterine activator is sparteine sulfate. This alkaloid is effective on the progesterone-dominated uterus, inducing long lasting contractions in response to a single dose of 100 to 200 mg.

Sparteine sulfate is well tolerated and doses of up to 600 mg have been used to induce labor in women (Newton et al. 1966). It is of interest to note that the only side effect that obstetricians are seriously concerned with is related to its powerful and long lasting stimulation of uterine contractility which may be detrimental to the foetus (Brazeau 1970). The drug is administered usually by intramuscular injection or intravenous infusion, but we have recently used sparteine sulfate orally to activate the non-pregnant uterus with success. Approximately twenty min following the oral administration of 100-200 mg of sparteine sulfate uterine contractility is progressively increased reaching a peak of activity approximately 1 h later (Fig. 5). The time interval between ingestion of the drug and the onset of its effect on the myometrium varies considerably from patient to patient. It may be as short as 15 min or as long as two h. Usually one single dose of 200 mg is sufficient to maintain a high level of uterine activity for three h or longer. When sparteine sulfate is administered to women during the late luteal phase the uterus develops labor-like activity following a single dose of 200 mg.

Repeated administration (100–200 mg every 4 h for 3 days) produces sustained uterine contractions which may cause abortion. We have used this regimen for menstrual regulation instead of suction curettage. In most women bleeding starts on the first day of administration and no further treatment is necessary.

Although the administration of sparteine sulfate during early implantation should cause abortion its use as a contraceptive may require earlier administration. To be able to interfere with ovum transport and prevent implantation, the alkaloid should be given soon after the arrival of the ovum in the uterus. If a period of residence in the uterus longer than 24 h is required by the ovum before it is able to implant, the post-ovulatory daily administration of sparteine sulfate should suffice to prevent pregnancy in all cases. Another possible alternative is post coital administration from one to several days. In this case, consideration should be given to the fact that sparteine sulfate is a poor oviductal stimulant and as long as the ovum remains in the oviduct it is unaffected by the alkaloid's action on the uterus.

The latest approach that we now propose is the combined administration of ergonovine maleate and sparteine sulfate. The two alkaloids appear to have no pharmacological incompatibility and may be given simultaneously with no significant untoward reaction. When the two compounds are given simultaneoulsy by mouth, activation of oviductal motility by ergonovine occurs usually ten to thirty min before the onset of the effect of sparteine sulfate on the uterus (Fig. 6). The response to the combined administration of one capsule containing

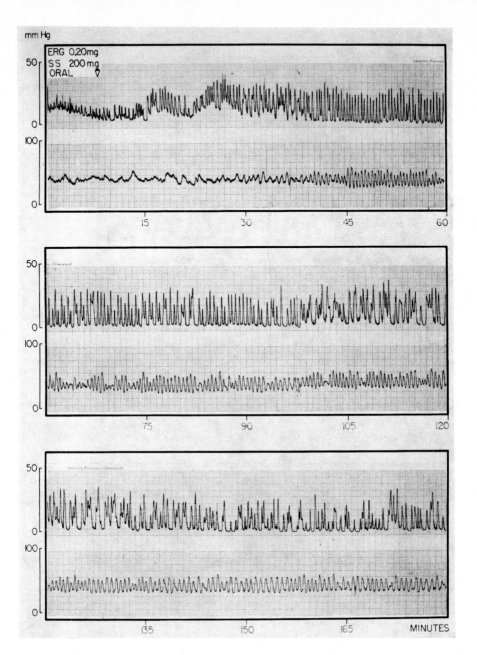

Fig. 6.

The response of human uterus and oviduct to ergonovine maleate and sparteine sulfate. Simultaneous recording *in vivo* (0–50 oviduct, 0–100 uterus). The subject received 0.20 mg or ergonovine maleate (ERG) and 200 mg of sparteine sulfate (SS) at the arrow. Note that activation of the oviduct in response to ergonovine maleate begins almost 30 min before the onset of the activation of the uterus by sparteine sulfate.

553

0.20 mg of ergonovine maleate and 200 mg of sparteine sulfate lasts in both the oviduct and the uterus longer than 3 h and may last as long as 6 h. Whether or not the ova will resist the combined action of these two compounds which should through their effects on the musculature quickly empty the genital tract, only expanded clinical trials will show.

Preliminary clinical trials suggests that the combined treatment may be effective and acceptable. Ergonovine maleate and sparteine sulfate are among the least toxic alkaloids and may be used repeatedly without apparent serious consequences. These compounds offer the first alternative for the development of a truly post coital contraceptive, whose anti-fertility action would derive exclusively from direct action on the lower circuit of the reproductive system leaving undisturbed the function of the endocrine glands.

ACKNOWLEDGMENTS

The studies reported here were supported by the International Committee for Contraceptive Research (ICCR), The Ford Foundation and The World Health Organization.

REFERENCES

Anderson G., Hobbins J., Cordero L. and Speroff L. (1971) Clinical use of prosta-glandins as oxytocin substances. *Ann. N. Y. Acad. Sci. 180,* 499–512.

Bengtsson L. Ph. (1974) Effect of a vasopressin analogue on myometrial activity in nonpregnant women. In: Coutinho E. M. and Fuchs F., eds. *Physiology and Genetics of Reproduction,* Part B, pp. 189–202. Plenum Press, New York.

Betteridge K. J. and Mitchell D. (1972) Retention of ova by the Fallopian tube in mares. *J. Reprod. Fertil. 31,* 515 (Abstr.).

Blandau R. J. (1969) Gamete transport – Comparative aspects. In: Hafez E. S. E. and Blandau R. J., eds. *The Mammalian Oviduct,* pp. 129–162. University of Chicago Press, Chicago.

Brazeau P. (1970) Drugs affecting uterine motility. Oxytocics, oxytocin and ergot alkaloids. In: Goodman L. S. and Gilman A., eds. *The Pharmacological Basis of Therapeutics,* 4th Ed., Chapt. 42, pp. 893–907. The Macmillan Co., New York.

Bygdeman M. and Eliasson R. (1963) The effect of prostaglandin from human seminal fluid on the motility of the human pregnant uterus *in vitro. Acta physiol. scand. 59,* 43–51.

Coutinho E. M. (1968) The effect of vasopressin and oxytocin on the genital tract of women.*Proc. VI World Cong. Fert. Steril,* The Israel Academy of Sciences and Humanities, Tel Aviv, pp. 182–188. Gordon and Breach, New York.

Coutinho E. M. (1971a) Tubal and uterine motility. In: Diczfalusy E. and Borell U., eds. Nobel Symposium 15: *Control of Human Fertility,* pp. 97–107. Almqvist and Wiksell, Stockholm; John Wiley & Sons, New York.

Coutinho E. M. (1971b) Physiologic and pharmacologic studies of the human oviduct. *Fertil. Steril. 22,* 807–815.

Coutinho E. M. (1974a) Motility of the Fallopian tube. In: Persianivov L. S., Cherva-
kova T. V. and Presl J., eds. *Recent Progress in Obstetrics and Gynecology*, pp. 576.
Excerpta Medica, Amsterdam.

Coutinho E. M. (1974b) Hormonal control of oviductal motility and secretory functions.
In: Greep R. O., ed. *Reproductive Physiology*, Physiology Series One, Vol. 8, MTP
International Review of Sciences, pp. 133–153. Butterworths, London.

Coutinho E. M. and da Silva A. R. (1974) One year contraception with norgestrienone
subdermal silastic implants. *Fertil. Steril. 25*, 170–176.

Coutinho E. M., da Silva A. R., Carreira M., Cacilda Chaves M. C. and Filho J. A.
(1975) Contraceptive effectiveness of silastic implants containing antiprogesterone
steroid (R-2323). *Contraception 11*, 625–635.

Coutinho E. M. and Maia H. (1971) The contractile response of the human uterus,
Fallopian tubes and the ovary to prostaglandins *in vivo*. *Fertil. Steril. 22*, 539–543.

Coutinho E. M., Maia H. and Filho J. A. (1974) The inhibitory effect of ritodrine on
human tubal activity *in vivo*. *Fertil. Steril. 25*, 596–601.

Coutinho E. M., Mattos C. E. R. and da Silva A. R. (1971) The effect of ovarian
hormones on the adrenergic stimulation of the rabbit Fallopian tube. *Fertil. Steril.
22*, 311–317.

Coutinho E. M. and Vieira Lopes A. C. (1968) Response of the nonpregnant uterus to
vasopressin as an index of ovarian function. *Amer. J. Obstet. Gynec. 102*, 479–489.

Croxatto H. B. (1974) The duration of egg transport and its regulation in mammals.
In: Coutinho E. M. and Fuchs F., eds. *Physiology and Genetics of Reproduction*,
Part B, pp. 159–166. Plenum Press, New York.

Croxatto H. B. (1975) Personal communication.

Croxatto H. B., Diaz S., Fuentealba B., Croxatto H. D., Carrillo D. and Fabres C.
(1972) Studies on the duration of egg transport in the human oviduct. I. The time
interval between ovulation and egg recovery from the uterus in normal women. *Fertil.
Steril. 23*, 447–458.

Jones E. E. and Nalbandov A. V. (1972) Effects of intrafollicular injection of gonadotrophins on ovulation or luteinization of ovarian follicle. *Biol. Reprod. 7*, 87–93.

Kesseru E., Larrañaga A. and Parada J. (1973) Post coital contraception with d-norgestrel. *Contraception 7*, 367–379.

Lauersen N. H. and Wilson K. H. (1974) Continuous extraovular administration of
prostaglandin $F_{2\alpha}$ for midtrimester abortion. *Amer. J. Obstet. Gynec. 120*, 273–280.

Maia H., Jr. and Coutinho E. M. (1974) Efeitos da indometacina a imidazol sobre a
contractilidade tubária *in vitro*. *Proc. VI Reunion Asoc. Latino Amer. Invest.*
Human Abstr. 311.

Nalbandov A. V. and Bahr J. M. (1974) Ovulation, corpus luteum formation and
steroidogenesis. In: Coutinho E. M. and Fuchs F., eds. *Physiology and Genetics of
Reproduction*, Part A, pp. 399–407. Plenum Press, New York.

Newton B. W., Benson R. C. and McCorriston C. C. (1966) Sparteine sulphate: A
potent capricious oxytocic. *Amer. J. Obstet. Gynec. 94*, 234–241.

Pauerstein C. J., Fremming B. D. and Martin J. E. (1970) Estrogen induced tubal
arrest of ovum: antagonism by alpha-adrenergic blockade. *Obstet. Gynec. 35*, 671–675.

Pauerstein C. J., Hodgson B. J. and Kramen M. A. (1974) The anatomy and physiology
of the oviduct. In: Wynn R., ed. *Obstetrics and Gynecology Annual*, pp. 137–201.
Appleton-Century-Crofts, New York.

Polidoro J. P., Howe G. R. and Black D. L. (1973) The effects of adrenergic drugs
on ovum transport through the rabbit oviduct. *J. Reprod. Fertil. 35*, 331–337.

Sakiz E., Azadian-Boulanger G., Laraque F. and Raynaud J. P. (1974) A new approach to estrogen-free contraception based on progesterone receptor blockade by mid cycle administration of ethyl-norgestrienone (R-2323). *Contraception 10,* 467–474.

Spilman C. H. and Harper M. J. K. (1975) Effects of prostaglandins on oviduct motility and egg transport. *Gynec. Invest. 6,* 186–205.

Thorneycroft I. H., Mishell D. R., Jr., Stone S. C., Kharma K. M. and Nakamura R. M. (1971) The relation of serum 17-hydroxyprogesterone and estradiol-17β levels during the human menstrual cycle. *Amer. J. Obstet. Gynec. 111,* 947–951.

SUMMARY OF DISCUSSIONS ON EFFECTS
OF ESTROGEN AND PROGESTERONE
ON CONTRACTILITY AND OVUM TRANSPORT

Reporter: *H. B. Croxatto*

SUMMARY OF CURRENT KNOWLEDGE

The preceding group of papers deals with the interactions between estrogens, progestins and some non-steroidal compounds with the oviduct and their effects upon ovum transport.

Of all the aspects reviewed by the speakers, the changes in the rate of ovum transport produced by treatment with estrogen stand as one of the earliest findings concerning the endocrine pharmacology of the oviduct. However, a comprehensive explanation to account for the remarkable variation in response obtained in different species or in a single species by changing the dose or time of administration of estrogen has not been offered. The involvement of ciliary, secretory, muscular or nervous components of the oviduct in the "tube-locking" effect or in the accelerating effect of estrogen treatment has not been clarified, and critical experiments to disclose whether these changes in the rate of ovum transport result from a direct action of estrogen upon the oviduct or from systemic effects of estrogen administration are yet to be done. In consequence, neither the site nor the mode of action have been elucidated, even though locking of ova in the oviducts of mice and rabbits treated with estrogenic substances was described by Burdick and Pincus 40 years ago (1935). Localized micro-injections of estrogen in selected regions such as the ampullary-isthmic junction, uterotubal junction or even the sympathetic ganglia located in the cervico-

557

vaginal region, where short neurons innervating the oviduct originate, should provide an experimental means to answer some of these questions. The mouse oviduct model described by Humphrey might be useful for *in vitro* studies concerning drug action on oviductal activity and ovum transport, and studies such as those presented by Karkun might shed more light on the participation of ciliated cells in hormonally-induced changes in the rate of transport.

In contrast to the abundant literature documenting effects of estrogen upon ovum transport in laboratory animals, a noticeable lack of information in primates was readily recognized and several discussants pointed out the need to characterize ovum transport in these species under the influence of exogenous estrogens.

The antifertility action of estrogen administered after coitus in animals has been reproduced in the human, but the degree to which altered oviductal function and ovum transport are involved in this effect has not been established. If anything, the reported high proportion of ectopic pregnancies with this treatment indicates that accelerated ovum transport may not be observed in primates.

The interaction of progesterone with the oviduct was analyzed from different angles by several speakers. Except for the action of progesterone given before ovulation, most of the data is controversial and, unfortunately, no generalizations can be offered at this point to make a coherent picture of the available information. The bulk of data reviewed by Chang indicates that, in contrast to the results with estrogen, progesterone administration after ovulation does not disturb significantly the passage of ova from the oviduct to the uterus, in rabbits. On the other hand, preovulatory treatment with progesterone or synthetic progestins is followed by pronounced acceleration of ovum transport. This was further stressed in the presentation of Vargas and Pauerstein, in which the optimal time of treatment for maximal acceleration in rabbits was carefully investigated and narrowed down to 36 h prior to ovulation.

Since we often see opposite effects on ovum transport with low and high pharmacological doses of estrogen, it is quite possible that these effects do not reflect the physiological role of the hormones in the regulation of transport. The use of antiestrogens in intact animals was expected to disclose the regulatory role of endogenous estrogens by counteracting their effects. However, the so called antiestrogens have, to a greater or lesser degree, some intrinsic estrogenic activity which complicates the interpretation of results.

Accelerated transport of transferred ova is observed in estrous rabbits under the physiologic influence of endogenous estrogens. However, among workers in this field, there seems to be greater awareness of the "tube-locking" effect of pharmacological doses. This accelerating effect of physiological estrogenic levels is counteracted by endogenous progesterone when ovulation is induced, or by exogenous progesterone given at the time of ovum transfer to estrous animals.

This retarding effect of progesterone in rabbits is, perhaps, the true physiological role of the hormone in the regulation of ovum transport.

Consideration of the physiological role of endogenous hormone, as opposed to the effects obtained with pharmacological doses, can lead to completely different approaches in the development of a contraceptive based on accelerating ovum transport. If the rabbit data were to be extrapolated to a spontaneous ovulator, we might expect fertility inhibition with two opposite treatments working in different ways: Administration of antiprogesterone around the time of ovulation would counteract the physiological or delaying effect of endogenous progesterone; whereas, administration of progesterone prior to ovulation would produce the known pharmacological or accelerating effect of premature progesterone action. Both treatments could, theoretically, produce untimely early arrival of ova in the uterus. Unfortunately, one of the obvious drawbacks is the need to time rather precisely drug administration in relation to ovulation. This consideration leads us to emphasize that such a requirement is not compatible with post-coital administration in humans, since intercourse in this species does not bear a constant relationship to ovulation.

Increased oviductal motility in women was reported by Guiloff et al. following pharmacological doses of progesterone, but not of estrogen, at all stages of the menstrual cycle. However, spontaneous oviductal motility studies throughout the menstrual cycle do not show a change from the follicular to the luteal phase corresponding with this observation. Instead, decreased motility has been described during the luteal phase at the time of progesterone dominance. Whether or not these pharmacologic effects, qualitatively different from the physiologic effects, are due to flooding of non-specific receptors in the tissue, is yet unresolved. Absence of specific progesterone receptors in the cytosol obtained from the muscular layer of human oviducts was reported by Fuentealba et al. If this observation is confirmed, an indirect pathway for the action of progesterone on oviductal motility should be sought. The finding of differential effects of progesterone and estrogen on oviductal activity provide the interesting possibility of studying ovum transport in women given these two treatments to assess the correlation between increased motility and rate of ovum transport. Such a study should also include a group treated with some of the ergot derivatives which increase oviductal motility. Activation of oviductal musculature by pharmacological means may result in rapid passage of ova into the uterus. This assumption gave the impetus for limited clinical trials to test the contraceptive effect of ergonovine maleate. The interesting proposition made by Coutinho to add another agent to stimulate myometrial activity and expel the ovum from the endometrial cavity could increase the modest antifertility effect obtained with ergonovine maleate alone. The concept that ovum transport can continue in the uterus and that this is also a vulnerable step of the reproductive process, offers a wider perspective to the efforts of the Task Force.

Much information exists on the effect of steroids and non-steroids on ovum transport but observations have been confined largely to laboratory animals, particularly the rabbit. Very little has been done in man or primates in general.

With reference to the action of progesterone – the dose level, time of treatment and species are particularly critical. Progesterone is rapidly metabolized and it might be questioned whether some of the effects attributed to this hormone are due to its withdrawal rather than its continued activity. Many studies on oviductal function should be confined to the period immediately preceding and following ovulation; they should also incorporate endocrine profiles and provide evidence of ovulation. Some treatments would even require ovulation prediction.

Throughout all the discussions the need for a method of detecting ovulation in women has been stressed. Also emphasized was the essential difference between "post-coital" and "post ovulatory" treatment since in man these two events often bear no relationship to each other unlike other animal species.

There appears to be a question as to the relationship between cellular events and circulating hormone levels. There is no correlation between hormone and drug studies and physiology. Steroids and other agents have been shown to modulate transport and/or contractility in women. The preovulatory state seems to be a critical period in control processes. Therefore studies of the mechanisms of drug action with particular emphasis on dose and timing should only be done during this period, and should only be performed in women after well controlled animal studies.

We suggest that an appropriate path to obtaining an effective antifertility agent acting on ovum transport would be: 1) obtain an appropriate animal model of human ovum transport: random studies on unproved animal models may confuse rather than help clarify the situation. 2) select drugs for in depth testing based on reasonable evidence from the animal model that ovum transport is accelerated and that fertility is suppressed. 3) if drugs pass this screen, then the question of whether mechanistic studies are useful must be considered, especially if the drug has many other effects (e. g. a prostaglandin might accelerate ovum transport and decrease fertility in appropriate animals, but could not be applied widely in clinical trials because of side effects. However, if the mechanism whereby it accelerates ovum transport could be elucidated then appropriate alternate drugs may be sought). 4) once a drug has passed to the point of being shown to accelerate ovum transport and inhibit fertility and can be expected not to cause serious side effects, then carefully designed trials containing appropriate controls (not exclusively retrospective controls) should be carried out.

Attempts should be made to correlate observations on oviductal activity with ovum transport. In all experimentation every effort should be made to reduce the influence of extraneous factors, i. e. in the external or internal environment – noise, temperature, nutrition, fertility of the animals before treatment and, in certain cases, also after treatment. Another recommendation was the need to standardize procedures in order to make possible comparison of results obtained by different laboratories.

There was considerable interest in the work on steroid receptors in the genital tract, and advances are likely to be made in this area. However, it was noted that at the present time such work only allows the estimation of binding capacities – it does not assist in the definition of mechanisms of action. With regard to steroid hormone action in general, it was noted that the response of a primed tissue continued long after the hormone was removed from the circulation – for example, uterine muscle may continue to behave as if under the influence of estrogen up to 20 days after ovariectomy. However, it must be recognized that the present results indicate that there are few specific receptors in the oviductal musculature, and that the majority are mainly located in the mucosa. Specificity of receptors also apparently varied throughout the oviduct. The half life of these receptors is not known at present, and further experiments are urgently needed to resolve some of these questions. It may be that the oviduct responds to progesterone only after a certain period of priming by estrogen, and following exposure to progesterone must again be re-primed by estrogen, before progesterone can again exert its effect. This seems well within the realm of probability since commencing progesterone injections on day –4 or –3 rather than day –2 reduces the effect of progesterone on ovum transport.

The effects of ergonovine maleate on the oviduct and sparteine sulfate on the uterus seem already well documented and it would appear that a combination of these drugs may provide an effective method of contraception. However, at present it is not possible to say with certainty that they are effective by virtue of propelling the ova through the oviduct and out of the uterus prematurely. Careful detailed studies on the time course of ovum transport in women and in sub-human primates following administration of these drugs should be performed as soon as possible. It is important to know whether they are acting on the oviduct, since they could be valuable tools in the assessment of methods of recording oviductal activity. Further trials of the clinical efficacy of the combination therapy combined with appropriate toxicological studies seem warranted.

ASSESSMENT OF FEASIBILITY
OF SUCH APPROACHES

Comments that have been made in previous sections again apply here. In general, the various groups concluded that there was more promise in pursuit of studies on the mechanism of action of hormones on the oviduct than of agents affecting the adrenergic system. Furthermore, although the combination treatment proposed by Coutinho appeared promising, confirmation awaits further trials. In general, empirical approaches, unless favoured by serendipity, are less likely to be successful than a carefully designed plan of action. In the absence of other obvious leads, studies on the action of hormones, prostaglandins, and ergot alkaloids may provide information permitting a more rational selection of compounds to be tested. Much of the success of the work of the Task Force clearly hangs on advances being made in other areas, e. g. prediction of ovulation, identification of suitable models for *in vitro* and *in vivo* testing, and even development of local delivery systems.

Thus much of what is proposed for future research in this area involves more basic studies than for the other sections. This is not the contradiction that it would at first sight appear to be since the drugs to be studied are known to be effective in lower animals at least, and may be effective in primates. In this context, the proposed experiments make good sense and will involve adequate but not excessively costly funding.

REFERENCE

Burdick H. O. and Pincus G. (1935) The effect of oestrin injections upon the developing ova of mice and rabbits. *Amer. J. Physiol. 111*, 201–207.

EPILOGUE

Implications for
the Development of a Clinically
Useful Contraceptive

BY

M. J. K. HARPER

and

C. J. PAUERSTEIN

IMPLICATIONS FOR THE DEVELOPMENT
OF A CLINICALLY USEFUL CONTRACEPTIVE

Our prejudices as organizers of this conference on behalf of the World Health Organization naturally lead us to the conclusion that this was a productive meeting. We hope that independent observers will concur. Many of the participants told us how much they enjoyed the meeting – not only because of the excellent Local Arrangements for which our thanks are due to Marie L. Pauerstein and Becca Price, the efficient and pleasant secretarial assistance provided by Ms. S. Harrison and Miss M. T. Rodriguez, but also because of the setting and the format of the meeting.

The mechanism of dividing the participants into separate discussion groups in the afternoon to review critically the morning's papers was felt by all to be most useful and productive. It was interesting that nearly all groups came to similar conclusions regarding each session. The division into smaller groups was felt to be more satisfactory than meeting in one large group since all participants had greater opportunity to express their opinions. Further, the author of a particular paper could sit in only one group, which thus permitted unbiased opinions on his findings from the five other groups.

The summaries of the discussions by the other editors show some overlap in views expressed, although they were written independently. Since most of the groups working on these various aspects of the physiology of the oviduct were represented at the meeting, these summations clearly represent a worldwide concensus of the present status of research in this field, and of the critical experiments that remain to be done. It is also clear that whereas all the experiments proposed need to be done, all do not have equal priority with regard to the goals of the World Health Organization Expanded Programme of Human Reproduction, and specifically of the Task Force on Methods for the Regulation of Ovum Transport: Section Control of Oviduct Function.

We do not intend here to reiterate all the experiments which the various groups thought should be done, but rather to draw attention to those areas which we consider most relevant to the objectives of the Task Force.

The idea of developing a contraceptive that acts by interfering with ovum transport stems from the observations that premature or delayed entry of fertilized ova into the uterus of infraprimates significantly interferes with fertility and fecundity. The transposition of these observations to human contraception is then based upon the following assumptions: 1) It should be possible to modify ovum transport rates in women by using pharmacologic agents. 2) Such drug-induced alterations of ovum transport would indeed be contraceptive in women.

Facts to convert these assumptions to truths were not available in 1973 when the Task Force first began. In order to seek the required information in the face of obstacles created by ethical and practical limitations upon the study of ovum transport in women, some preliminary or alternative approaches were suggested: 1) The overall duration and detailed time course of ovum transport in women and in infrahuman primates should be determined in an attempt to define a suitable animal model. These studies would answer questions such as: Is the ampulla rapidly traversed as in the rabbit? Is the ovum delayed at the ampullary-isthmic junction; or in the isthmus; or at the uterotubal junction? Such information is required before one can even speculate intelligently about control mechanisms that might be altered by contraceptive agents.

We now know that the mean duration of ovum transport in women is approximately 67 h. Although the data are incomplete, the pattern of ovum transport in women appears to consist of a relatively long sojourn in the ampulla (about 48 h), followed by relatively rapid passage through the isthmus into the uterus. This is in contrast to the rabbit, in which species ova rapidly traverse the ampulla, enter the isthmus at 24–36 h after coitus, and then spend a relatively long time in the isthmus. Thus, the rabbit may not be a good model for ovum transport in women. By contrast, the detailed time course of ovum transport in the rhesus monkey and in the baboon is quite similar to that in women.

In light of the difficulties of obtaining direct data on the pharmacologic alteration of ovum transport in women, various other groups have now been encouraged to commence studies similar to the pioneering ones of Dr. H. B. Croxatto. More rapid progress could be made with such experiments if the time of ovulation could be more easily pinpointed (or preferably predicted). In addition, the final delivery and effectiveness of a contraceptive interfering with ovum transport would be greatly facilitated by the ability to predict ovulation. The reliable detection of the time of ovulation has not been addressed in research undertaken by this Task Force, however a WHO Task Force on Methods for the Prediction and Detection of Ovulation is seriously studying this question.

Another approach encompasses the testing of the effects of pharmacologic agents on oviductal motility in women and in appropriate animal models. The rationale underlying this approach is as follows: If a consistent correlation between recording of motility and ovum transport rates can be identified, motility studies will be used to screen pharmacologic agents in the appropriate animal model for potential use in women. To this end, radioactive plastic ovum models which accurately mimick the detailed time-course of transport of natural ova in the rabbit have been developed. These models are accelerated and delayed by treatments that accelerate and delay the transport of natural ova, and the anatomic sites of delay and acceleration are identical to those where natural ova are delayed and accelerated. Current experiments with the ovum model are in the following directions: 1) Development of a telemetry system for chronic tracking of the surrogates. 2) Validation of the time course of transport of the surrogates in rhesus monkeys and baboons. 3) Validation of the time course of transport of surrogates in women. In the near future the surrogate-detection system should be sufficiently developed to begin screening drugs for their effects on transport rates. The plastic ovum models will then be used to correlate oviductal motility with transport rates. Several types of sensors (open-ended and balloon-tipped catheters, conductive silastic doughnut, and extraluminal strain gauges) will be tested. Recordings made with the various sensors under treatments known to accelerate and to retard ovum transport will be compared with each other, and with effects on the actual transport of the surrogates.

A number of drugs have been studied in humans and animals, for their effects on oviductal motility. They include steroids, catecholamine stimulating and blocking agents, prostaglandins, ergot derivatives, and oxytocics. From evidence to date, it does not appear that interference with catecholamines will interrupt pregnancy through effects on the oviduct. The role of prostaglandins is still obscure but long-acting prostaglandin analogues are now being tested. Ergonovine increased oviductal motility and reduced the incidence of pregnancy, but without the addition of sparteine sulphate was not wholly effective. The promising results described by Dr. E. Coutinho need to be urgently followed up on a larger scale.

Some data gathered by other members of the Task Force also suggest that drugs that increase oviductal motility in women also lower pregnancy rates. These data are inconclusive and the mechanism by which these treatments lower fertility remains undefined. Parallel experiments in rabbits failed to resolve this question. We hope that experiments to be undertaken this year in humans and infrahuman primates will define more precisely the role of the oviduct in the development of the primate ovum. If primate ova can develop normally despite premature entry into the uterus the basic assumption underlying the work of the Task Force is negated. Answers to this question should be provided by the ongoing experiments of the Task Force.

Little progress has been made in determining whether or not ovum transport rates can be altered in women. These studies will be continued during the coming year. More effort needs to be directed toward this question. The ability to alter pharmacologically ovum transport rates in the human is also central to the thesis of the Task Force.

Studies of the mechanisms controlling oviductal function should be continued. These studies are essential because they can provide new leads which may become important if the ones presently under investigation should fail to confirm their initial promise. For example, two laboratories are examining the mechanisms regulating oviductal contractility in *in vitro* studies utilizing human and animal tissue. Electrical and mechanical activity are recorded simultaneously and related to the ultrastructure of the tissue. Responses to various pharmacological agents are being characterized.

Comparing the work presented at this meeting with those of the Pullman Meeting, 1968, published in 1969 as "The Mammalian Oviduct", and of the Athens meeting, 1972, published in 1974 as "The Oviduct and its Functions" much progress has been made in the intervening periods. On the other hand we still lack some essential information. We hope that this symposium will focus attention on areas of research that merit renewed examination and will point out other areas where further study using current methodology may not be fruitful. If nothing else, we trust that the reader will have found this an enjoyable volume that will be a useful text for some time to come. We would like to thank the participants for making the conference and the book successful and WHO and the University of Texas Health Science Center at San Antonio for making it possible for scientists in ovum transport to come together to share their knowledge and ignorance.

Michael J. K. Harper, Ph.D.   Carl J. Pauerstein, M.D.

REFERENCES

Hafez E. S. E. and Blandau R. J. (1969) eds. *The Mammalian Oviduct*. The University of Chicago Press, Chicago.
Johnson A. D. and Foley C. W. (1974) eds. *The Oviduct and its Functions*. Academic Press, N. Y.